REHABILITATION
NUNSING

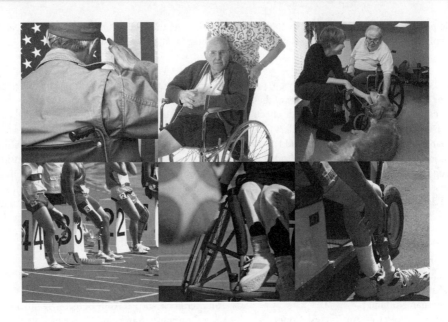

Edited by

KRISTEN L. MAUK, PhD, DNP, RN, CRRN, GNCS-BC, GNP-BC, FAAN

Professor of Nursing and Kreft Endowed Chair
Valparaiso University
Healthcare Consultant
Mauk Financial Solutions, LLC
Valparaiso, Indiana

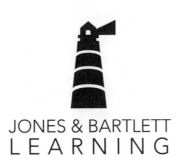

JONES & BARTLETT
LEARNING

World Headquarters

Jones & Bartlett Learning
40 Tall Pine Drive
Sudbury, MA 01776
978-443-5000
info@jblearning.com
www.jblearning.com

Jones & Bartlett Learning Canada
6339 Ormindale Way
Mississauga, Ontario L5V 1J2
Canada

Jones & Bartlett Learning International
Barb House, Barb Mews
London W6 7PA
United Kingdom

Jones & Bartlett Learning books and products are available through most bookstores and online booksellers. To contact Jones & Bartlett Learning directly, call 800-832-0034, fax 978-443-8000, or visit our website, www.jblearning.com.

Substantial discounts on bulk quantities of Jones & Bartlett Learning publications are available to corporations, professional associations, and other qualified organizations. For details and specific discount information, contact the special sales department at Jones & Bartlett Learning via the above contact information or send an email to specialsales@jblearning.com.

Production Credits

Publisher: Kevin Sullivan
Editorial Assistant: Rachel Shuster
Production Assistant: Sara Fowles
Marketing Manager: Meagan Norlund
V.P., Manufacturing and Inventory Control: Therese Connell
Composition: Publishers' Design and Production Services, Inc.
Cover Design: Kristin E. Parker

Printing and Binding: Malloy, Inc.
Cover Printing: Malloy, Inc.
Cover Images: (Clockwise from upper left) © Steve Cukrov/ ShutterStock, Inc.; © Andi Berger/Dreamstime.com; © iofoto/ShutterStock, Inc.; © Roger Dale Pleis/ShutterStock, Inc.; © Lucian Coman/Dreamstime.com; © Shariff Che'Lah/ Fotolia.com

To order this product, use ISBN: 978-1-4496-3447-6

Library of Congress Cataloging-in-Publication Data
Rehabilitation nursing: a contemporary approach to practice/edited by Kristen L. Mauk.
   p.;cm.
Includes bibliographical references and index.
ISBN 978-0-7637-8059-3
1.   Rehabilitation nursing.   I. Title.
[DNLM: 1.   Rehabilitation Nursing--methods.   WY 150.5]
RT120.R4M38 2011
610.73'6—dc22

2010043203

6048

Printed in the United States of America
15   14   13   12   11   10   9   8   7   6   5   4   3   2   1

CONTENTS

Preface   viii

Introduction   x

Contributors   xi

PART I   **General Concepts and Principles of Rehabilitation Nursing   1**

1   Overview of Rehabilitation   1
Kristen L. Mauk

2   Chronicity and Disability   14
Eileen T. French
Karen M. Allabastro

3   Settings for Care   22
Susan E. Maycock

4   Theories, Models, and Frameworks for Chronic Illness, Disability, Adaptation, and Coping   28
Penelope M. Kearney
Julie Pryor
Sandra Lever

5   Interdisciplinary Rehabilitation Team   51
Judi Behm
Nancy Brake Gray

6   Nursing Roles   63
Donna Williams
Stephanie Davis Burnett

PART II   **Promoting Self-Care in Rehabilitation Clients   84**

7   Improving Nutritional Status and Swallowing   84
Reatha Collingsworth

8   Maintaining Skin Integrity   100
Paula M. Anton

9   Bowel and Bladder Management   121
Jill Rye
Kristen L. Mauk

10   Promoting Mobility and Function   136
Sharleen Koenig
Joseph Teixeira
Elizabeth Yetzer

11   Enhancing Cognition, Communication, and Behavior   148
Jeffrey E. Evans
Dana Hanifan

12   Sexuality and Disability   161
Catherine Moore
Donald D. Kautz
Michelle Cournan

13   Educating Clients and Families   176
Pamela Farrell
Robin Raptosh

14   The Art of Caring: Addressing Psychosocial and Spiritual Issues:
Spirituality, Coping, Depression, Grieving, Adjustment,
and Adaptation   200
Gail L. Sims

PART III   **Clinical Rehabilitation Management for Persons with
Specific Health Alterations   215**

15   Stroke   215
Sylvia A. Duraski
Florence A. Denby
Linda V. Danzy
Susan Sullivan

16   Traumatic Brain Injury   255
Paula M. Anton

17   Spinal Cord Injury   268
Marsha Branche-Spelich
Ivy Ann Reyes
David Miller

18 Total Joint Replacement 283
Laura Horman
Ethan Roberts

19 Clinical Rehabilitation Management for Persons with Amputation 296
Elizabeth Yetzer
Edward Hansen
Yolanda Haskell
Sharleen Koenig
Judy Kapton
Edmond Ayyappa

20 Polytrauma 317
Lucille Raia
Lisa Perla

21 Cardiac and Pulmonary Disease 332
Catherine Biviano

22 Neurological Disorders 344
Matthew R. Sorenson

23 Other Chronic Illnesses 359
Ann Bonner

PART IV   Issues in Rehabilitation Nursing 373

24 Cultural Perspectives Within Rehabilitation Nursing 373
Margaret M. Andrews
Teresa L. Cervantez Thompson

25 Ethical and Legal Issues 386
Ryan Bratcher
James J. Farrell
Kathleen A. Stevens
Kevin W. Vanderground

26 Health Policy and Healthcare Financing 402
Anne F. Deutsch
James J. Farrell

PART V   **Unique Aspects of Rehabilitation Nursing   418**

27 Pediatric Rehabilitation   418
Cyndi Cortes

28 Gerontological Rehabilitation Nursing   437
Cheryl A. Lehman
Kristen L. Mauk
Kimberly Hickey

29 Animal-Assisted Therapy   459
Rachel M. Easton
Alan Beck

30 Life Care Planning: A Unique Practice Area for Nurses   471
Susan Wirt
Ava G. Porter

Glossary   487

Index   509

PREFACE

This book was designed to be a clinically focused rehabilitation nursing text that could be used for integrating rehabilitation into an academic curriculum for students, educating nurses new to the specialty, and serving as a reference for practicing nurses, including those preparing for certification.

In contrast to competing texts, this book has an interdisciplinary authorship that includes nearly 60 chapter authors from the disciplines of nursing, physical and occupational therapy, speech therapy, psychology, social work, orthotics, veterinary medicine, law, business, and others. For many chapters rehabilitation nurse experts collaborated with colleagues from other disciplines to bring a broader and valuable perspective to the book. Such an integrated text with various disciplines represented is true to the interdisciplinary nature of rehabilitation nursing.

This text contains some exciting chapters on such subjects as polytrauma, life care planning, and animal assisted therapy that were not included in prior competing texts. The age continuum is covered with special chapters on pediatric and geriatric rehabilitation authored by nurse experts. With the Baby Boomer generation entering the older age group in 2011, we have just a little time to adapt our nursing strategies to meet the needs of this unique cohort. The huge number of older adults in the population will mean more chronic illness and need for rehabilitation services. Rehabilitation of the future may need to take place in much different settings (more in the home environment), and future rehabilitation nurses will need to be expert educators of persons and families to help older adults age in place. Chapters on settings for care and educating patients and families provide practical guidance for rehabilitation practicing in many areas.

The strategic plan of the Association of Rehabilitation Nurses suggests that rehabilitation nursing needs to be incorporated into the nursing curriculum of all programs to prepare nurses who can provide quality rehabilitation care. Thus, each chapter has been written to assist students of rehabilitation nursing to acquire the essential knowledge and skills to provide excellent care. Competencies as set forth by the Association of Rehabilitation Nurses have been incorporated into the text to help direct students' learning. This is a text aimed at undergraduate level students and practicing rehabilitation nurses.

Chapter features include

- Learning objectives
- Key term list (with terms highlighted in chapter)
- Tables that summarize key points
- Boxes to highlight interesting information
- Evidence-based practice integrated
- Research and clinical practice guidelines
- Web exploration and links
- Notable quotes
- Pictures/diagrams/drawings
- Original photographs
- Critical thinking exercises
- Personal reflection exercises
- Case studies with questions

- Resource lists
- References (including websites)
- Recommended readings

Chapters reflect the competencies and specific areas identified as essentials by the Association of Rehabilitation Nurses. Common threads in each chapter are medications, ethics, research/evidence-based practice, related web links, and client–family teaching.

An online instructor's manual is available to assist educators, both in clinical settings and in academe, to teach the content from the text. The instructor's manual includes PowerPoint slides for each chapter, suggested activities in the classroom and clinical settings, a glossary of key terms, Web links, and a TestBank with relevant questions.

INTRODUCTION

Rehabilitation nursing is a growing specialty area. This is recognized at the national level by the Association of Rehabilitation Nurses (ARN), who has set forth a strategic plan whose core purpose is to advance rehabilitation nursing practice. The ARN's envisioned future goal is "to reshape healthcare by integrating rehabilitation nursing concepts into care for all people" (ARN, 2007, paragraph 7). To accomplish this goal, there must be more available resources to educate nurses in rehabilitation. This book is a contribution to the literature in rehabilitation. The editor hopes that students of this specialty in all settings, from academe to practice, will find this a useful resource.

Reference

Association of Rehabilitation Nurses. (2010). Strategic plan. Retrieved from http://www.rehabnurse.org/about/content/vision.html

CONTRIBUTORS

Karen M. Allabastro, BSN, RN, CRRN
Interim Nurse Manager
Center for Stroke Rehabilitation
Rehabilitation Institute of Chicago
Chicago, Illinois

Margaret M. Andrews, PhD, RN, CTN, FAAN
Director and Professor of Nursing
University of Michigan, Flint
Flint, Michigan

Edmond Ayyappa, CPO, FAAOP
V.A. Clinical Manager, Prosthetics
Veteran Affairs Medical Center
Long Beach, California

Paula M. Anton, RN, MS, CRRN, ACNS-BC
Clinical Nurse Specialist
Adjunct Clinical Faculty
University of Michigan Health System
Ann Arbor, Michigan

Alan Beck, MA, ScD
Director, Center of the Human Animal Bond
Dorothy N. McAllister Professor of Animal
    Ecology
School of Veterinary Medicine, Purdue University
Lafayette, Indiana

Judi Behm, RN, MSN, CRRN
Clinical Nurse Specialist–Rehab/Clinical Educator
The Drake Center
Cincinnati, Ohio

Catherine Biviano, MA, ONC, RN-BC
Hospital for Special Surgery
Nurse Manager-Private Ambulatory Practices
New York, New York

Ann Bonner, RN, PhD
Associate Professor
School of Nursing, Midwifery & Indigenous Health
Wagga Wagga Campus
Charles Sturt University
Wagga Wagga, New South Wales, Australia

Marsha Branche-Spelich, BSN, RN, CRRN
Barrow's Neurological Institute
Phoenix, Arizona
Former Nurse Manager SCI Unit
Rehabilitation Institute of Chicago
Chicago, Illinois

Ryan Bratcher, JD
Attorney
Bratcher & Vanderground, P.C.
Valparaiso, Indiana

Stephanie Davis Burnett, DNP, RN, ACNS-BC,
    CRRN
Advanced Nursing Coordinator
Rehabilitation Nursing and Safe Touch Program
UAB Hospital
Birmingham, Alabama
Adjunct Faculty
Tennessee State University
School of Nursing
Nashville, Tennessee

Reatha Collingsworth, MS, RN, CNS, CRRN
Rehabilitation Clinical Nurse Specialist
Department of Veterans Affairs Medical Center
    (VAMC)
Dayton, Ohio

Cyndi Cortes, DrPH, MSN, CRNP-PC
Associate Professor, IVMSON
Samford University
Birmingham, Alabama

Michelle Cournan, DNP, RN, CRRN, ANP-BC
Director of Education and Resources
Sunnyview Rehabilitation Hospital
Schenectady, NY

Linda V. Danzy, RN, BSN, CRRN
Clinical Instructor III
Rehabilitation Institute of Chicago
Chicago, Illinois

Florence A. Denby, RN, MS, ANP-BC, CRRN
Nurse Practitioner
Center for Stroke Rehabilitation
Rehabilitation Institute of Chicago
Chicago, Illinois

Anne F. Deutsch, PhD, RN, CRRN
Clinical Research Scientist
Rehabilitation Institute of Chicago
Chicago, Illinois
Research Assistant Professor
Department of Physical Medicine and
    Rehabilitation
Feinberg School of Medicine
Northwestern University
Evanston, Illinois

Sylvia A. Duraski, RN, MS, ANP-BC, CRRN
Nurse Practitioner
Brain Injury Medicine and Rehabilitation Program
Rehabilitation Institute of Chicago
Chicago, Illinois

Rachel M. Easton, DVM
Veterinarian
Montrose Veterinary Clinic
Montrose, Colorado

Jeffrey E. Evans, PhD
Clinical Associate Professor
Department of Physical Medicine and
    Rehabilitation
Rehabilitation Psychology and Neuropsychology
Head, First Year Seminar Program
Residential College
University of Michigan
Ann Arbor, Michigan

James J. Farrell, RN, MBA, CRRN
Chief Nursing Officer
Healthsouth Lakeview Rehabilitation Hospital
Elizabethtown, Kentucky

Pamela Farrell, MSN, RN, CRRN
Clinical Educator/Owner/Consultant
Rehab Classworks, LLC
Riverton, Utah
Clinical Educator
Intermountain Healthcare
Salt Lake City, Utah

Eileen T. French, MSN, RN, CRRN
Nurse Manager, 4th Floor
Rehabilitation Institute of Chicago
Chicago, Illinois

Nancy Brake Gray, BSN, RN, CCM, MSN(c)
University of Cincinnati
Former Manager, Case Management
The Drake Center
Cincinnati, Ohio

Dana Hanifan, MA, CCC
Speech-Language Pathologist II
University of Michigan Health System
Ann Arbor, Michigan

Edward Hansen, MSN RN
Rehabilitation Nursing Educator, PACT Program
Veterans Affairs Medical Center
Long Beach, California

Yolanda Haskell, PT, DPT
Amputee/Back PT Program Manager
Veterans Affairs Medical Center
Long Beach, California

Kimberly Hickey, MSN, APRN, BC
Clinical Nurse Specialist, Geriatrics
Nurse Practitioner
University of Michigan Hospitals and Health Centers
Ann Arbor, Michigan

Laura Horman, MSN, RN-BC, CRRN
Total Rehab Care
Washington County Health System
Hagerstown, Maryland

Judy Kapton, RN
Former Case Manager for Rehabilitation
Veterans Affairs Medical Center
Long Beach, California

Donald D. Kautz, PhD, RN, CRRN, CNE
Director, Hickory Outreach Program
Associate Professor of Nursing
UNC Greensboro School of Nursing
Greensboro, North Carolina

Penelope M. Kearney, RN, DipAppSci(Nursing),
    BHlthSci(Nursing), MN(Hons), PhD, MCN
Associate Director
Rehabilitation Nursing Research & Development Unit
Ryde, New South Wales, Australia

Sharleen Koenig, PT, DPT
Inpatient and Outpatient Amputee Care
Veteran Affairs Medical Center
Long Beach, California

Cheryl A. Lehman, PhD, RN, CNS-BC, RN-BC, CRRN
CNS Program Coordinator
Associate Professor
Clinical School of Nursing
University of Texas Health Science Center
Nurse Educator/Researcher
Polytrauma Rehabilitation Center
Audie L. Murphy VA Hospital
San Antonio, Texas

Sandra Lever, RN, BHM, MN(Rehabilitation), GradDipHlthSci(Sexual Health), MRCNA
Clinical Nurse Consultant–Rehabilitation
Royal Rehabilitation Centre Sydney
Sydney, Australia

Kristen L. Mauk, PhD, DNP, RN, CRRN, GNCS-BC, GNP-BC, FAAN
Professor of Nursing and Kreft Endowed Chair
Valparaiso University
Healthcare Consultant
Mauk Financial Solutions, LLC
Valparaiso, Indiana

Susan E. Maycock, MSN, RN
Clinical Nurse Specialist
Unit 6B Acute Care Medicine
University of Michigan Health System
Ann Arbor, Michigan

David Miller, BSN, RN, CRRN
Rehabilitation Institute of Chicago
Chicago, Illinois

Catherine Moore, RN, MSN
Director of Nursing Practice and Education
North Carolina Nurses Association
Raleigh, North Carolina

Lisa Perla, MSN, ARNP, CNRN
Polytrauma/TBI Rehabilitation Planning Specialist
U.S. Department of Veterans Affairs
Rehabilitation Services
Washington, DC

Ava G. Porter, DNP, RN, CNE
Nursing Department Chair
Associate Professor
Jefferson College of Health Sciences
Roanoke, Virginia

Julie Pryor, RN, RM, BA, GradCertRemoteHlth, MN, PhD
Director, Rehabilitation Nursing Research & Development Unit
Royal Rehabilitation Centre Sydney
Sydney, Australia

Lucille Raia, MS, RN, NEA-BC, ARNP, CBIST
Associate Chief of Nursing Education
Director of James A. Haley VA Nursing Academy (VANA)
James A. Haley VA Hospital
Tampa FL

Robin Raptosh, RN, MS(C), BSN, CRRN
Staff Nurse/Orthopedic Team Leader
St. Alphonsus Regional Medical Center
Boise, Idaho

Ivy Ann Reyes, BSN, RN, CRRN, CMSRN
Assistant Nurse Manage, SCI
Rehabilitation Institute of Chicago
Chicago, Illinois

Ethan Roberts, PT, OCS
Orthopedic Program Team Leader
Total Rehab Care at Robinwood
Hagerstown, Maryland

Jill Rye, MA, RN, CRRN, CNL
Unit Supervisor
Rehabilitation Nursing
Avera McKennan Hospital
Sioux Falls, South Dakota

Gail L. Sims, RN, MSN, CRRN
Nurse Manager
Kaiser Foundation Rehabilitation Center
Vallejo, California

Matthew R. Sorenson, PhD, RN
Department of Nursing
DePaul University
Chicago, Illinois
Clinical Scholar, Department of Physical Medicine and Rehabilitation
Northwestern University, Feinberg School of Medicine

Kathleen A. Stevens, PhD, RN, CRRN, NE-BC
Director of Nursing Education
Rehabilitation Institute of Chicago
Assistant Professor, Department of Physical Medicine
    and Rehabilitation
Feinberg School of Medicine
Northwestern University
Chicago, Illinois

Susan Sullivan, RN, BSN, CRRN
Staff Nurse
Rehabilitation Institute of Chicago
Chicago, Illinois

Joseph Teixeira, OTR/L
Acute Inpatient Rehabilitation Therapy for SCI,
    Orthopedics, and Neurologic Conditions
Veterans Affairs Medical Center
Long Beach, California

Teresa L. Cervantez Thompson, PhD, RN, CRRN
Dean and Professor
Madonna College of Nursing and Health
Detroit, Michigan

Kevin W. Vanderground, JD
Attorney, Bratcher & Vanderground, P.C.
Valparaiso, Indiana
Adjunct Professor of Business
Grace College
Winona Lake, Indiana

Donna Williams, RN, MSN, CRRN
RNS Health Care Consultants, Inc.
Santa Barbara, California

Susan Wirt, BSN, RN, CRRN, CCM, CLCP, CRP
Wirt & Associates, LLC
Catawba, Virginia

Elizabeth Yetzer, MA, MSN, RN, CRRN
Former Preservation, Amputation Care and Treatment
    (PACT) Coordinator
Veterans Affairs Medical Center
Long Beach, California

SECTION EDITORS

Section I: Stephanie Burnett, MSN, DNP(c), RN,
    CRRN, ACNS-BC

Section II: Paula Anton, MS, RN, CRRN, ACNS-BC

Section III: Cheryl Lehman, PhD, RN, CNS-BC,
    RN-BC, CRRN

Sections IV and V: Kathleen Stevens, PhD, RN, CRRN,
    NE-BC

SPECIAL ASSISTANTS TO THE EDITOR

Kenneth G. Easton, Jr., BS(c)
Personal Assistant, Mauk Financial Solutions, LLC

Daniel P. Easton
Personal Assistant, Mauk Financial Solutions, LLC

REVIEWERS

Paula M. Anton, RN, MS, CRRN, ACNS-BC
Clinical Nurse Specialist
Physical Medicine & Rehabilitation
University of Michigan Health System
Ann Arbor, Michigan

Dorothy Baker
Wilmington University
Georgetown, Delaware

Stephanie Davis Burnett, RN, MSN, DNP(c), CRRN,
    ACNS-BC
Advanced Nursing Coordinator
Program Coordinator, Safe Touch
UAB University Hospital-Spain Rehabilitation Center
Birmingham, Alabama

Theresa Cowan
Director, Nursing Education
Salem International University
Salem, West Virginia

Daniel P. Easton
Consultant and Personal Assistant
Mauk Financial Solutions, LLC
Valparaiso, Indiana

Kenneth G. Easton, Jr., BS(c)
Consultant and Personal Assistant
Mauk Financial Solutions, LLC
Valparaiso, Indiana

Debra J. Hain
Christine E. Lynn College of Nursing
Florida Atlantic University
Boca Raton, Florida

Cheryl A. Lehman, PhD, RN, CNS-BC, RN-BC, CRRN
CNS Program Coordinator
Associate Professor, Clinical
School of Nursing
University of Texas Health Science Center
San Antonio, Texas

Kristen L. Mauk, PhD, DNP, RN, CRRN, GNCS-BC, GNP-BC, FAAN
Professor of Nursing and Kreft Endowed Chair
Valparaiso University
Healthcare consultant
Mauk Financial Solutions, LLC
Valparaiso, Indiana

Kathleen A. Stevens, PhD, RN, CRRN, NE-BC
Director of Nursing Education
Rehabilitation Institute of Chicago
Assistant Professor, Department of Physical Medicine and Rehabilitation
Feinberg School of Medicine
Northwestern University
Chicago, Illinois

Jessica Vera
Hollywood, Florida

ACKNOWLEDGMENTS

I extend a special thank you to my exceptional section editors who worked tirelessly to ensure the completion of this work: Stephanie, Cheryl, Kathy, and Paula. Thank you so much. Your combined expertise is a shining testimony to rehabilitation nurses everywhere.

Thanks to my children who each helped with the completion of this book in their own special way: Rachel, Kenny, Daniel, Elizabeth, Jordan, Vika, and little Daniel. Thank you for believing Mom can do anything.

And finally, thanks to my husband, Jim, who reluctantly seems to understand and accept my need to leave a legacy for the nurses who will carry this profession into the future.

CHAPTER 1

Overview of Rehabilitation

Kristen L. Mauk

LEARNING OBJECTIVES

At the end of this chapter, the reader will be able to

- Define rehabilitation.
- State three common goals of rehabilitation across disciplines.
- Describe significant historical events in the development of rehabilitation as a specialty in nursing and medicine.
- Discuss major concepts of rehabilitation.
- Recognize the scope of practice of the rehabilitation nurse.
- Identify 16 basic competencies of rehabilitation nursing.

KEY CONCEPTS AND TERMS

Adaptation	Chronicity	Quality of life
Association of Rehabilitation Nurses (ARN)	Competencies	Rehabilitation
	Holistic care	Self-care
Certification	Interdisciplinary team	
Certified registered rehabilitation nurse (CRRN)		

This is an exciting time to be in the specialty of **rehabilitation** and rehabilitation nursing. Many new developments within the discipline make this a challenging and desirable field in which to work. When one considers the present conflicts continuing in Iraq and Afghanistan coupled with the existing number of aging veterans, the area of rehabilitation should be booming, and indeed there are never-before-seen injuries and effects of war to challenge the **interdisciplinary team**. Polytrauma has emerged as a significant specialty area within rehabilitation, and the benefits of these services extend to the civilian population as well. Technological advances in prosthetics for those with multiple limb amputations continue to push the limits of current knowledge in biomedical engineering. The devastating effects of catastrophic world events such as the 2010 earthquake in Haiti, the tsunami in Indonesia, or Hurricane Katrina in New Orleans suggest that there is a worldwide need for rehabilitation to help those with life-changing injuries to learn to live again. There are also the individuals seen daily in healthcare facilities with stroke, brain injury,

spinal cord injury, neurological disorders, and chronic illnesses from a variety of causes who need rehabilitative care. The purpose of this text is to provide the reader with a solid foundational background about rehabilitation and to set forth the necessary knowledge to meet basic **competencies** in rehabilitation nursing.

PHILOSOPHY

Rehabilitation is founded on the premise that all individuals have inherent worth and have the right to be experts in their own health care (Gender, 1998). Each person is viewed as a unique, comprehensive, holistic being. Rehabilitation nurses, and the rest of the team, are responsible for providing the education and training to equip the person with the needed knowledge and skills to maximize **self-care**.

The philosophy of rehabilitation is distinctly different from acute care. In acute care the patient's survival is a primary focus. Nurses provide care provision that involves performing activities of daily living *for* persons, whereas rehabilitation focuses on educating persons to be able to perform activities of daily living for themselves. Promoting self-care is key to rehabilitation.

The process of rehabilitation is best undertaken with the coordinated and deliberate assistance of an interdisciplinary team of experts who each bring specific knowledge and skills to the rehabilitation program for each patient or client. Such a healthcare team may consist of a variety of team members including physicians, nurses, therapists, social workers, case managers, nutritionists, orthotists, prosthetists, and vocational counselors, to name a few. The client functions as the center of the interdisciplinary team (see Chapter 5), which is composed of knowledgeable specialists who work together, share common goals, and collaborate to help clients reach their personal goals.

DEFINITIONS OF REHABILITATION

Rehabilitation is a process of **adaptation** or recovery through which an individual suffering from a disabling or functionally limiting condition, whether temporary or irreversible, participates to regain maximal function, independence, and restoration. Rehabilitation "refers to services and programs designed to assist individuals who have experienced a trauma or illness that results in impairment that creates a loss of function (physical, psychological, social, or vocational)" (Remsburg & Carson, 2006, p. 579). The National Cancer Institute (2007) defined rehabilitation as "a process to restore mental and/or physical abilities lost to injury or disease, in order to function in a normal or near-normal way" (p. 1). For some, this may be a lifelong process. For others, rehabilitation is of short duration. For example, a gymnast may injure her arm and need 3 months of rehabilitation to resume her former activity with full range of motion. But for an individual diagnosed with a severe stroke or a war veteran with head trauma, the rehabilitation may be continuous, even lifelong. Table 1.1 provides examples of conditions that may be improved with rehabilitation.

GOALS

Although goals are mutually established for each individual who participates in rehabilitation, there are underlying principles that guide the development of the plan of care. Habel stated that "rehabilitation goals are the desired outcomes for each rehabilitation client" (1993, p.3). All members of the rehabilitation team, although concentrating on a particular area, share similar goals for

TABLE 1.1   Examples of Conditions That May Benefit from Rehabilitation
Spinal cord injury
Stroke
Traumatic brain injury
Multiple sclerosis
Guillain-Barré syndrome
Polytrauma
Amputation
Disfiguring burns
Parkinson's disease
Functional debility
Joint replacement
Rheumatoid arthritis
Cerebral palsy
Muscular dystrophy
Chronic obstructive pulmonary diseases
Polio
Certain types of cancer
Alzheimer's disease and other dementias

the client. These include promoting self-care, maximizing independence, maintaining and restoring function, preventing complications, and encouraging adaptation. Table 1.2 lists the common goals of the rehabilitation team. The client's achievement of these is measured by considering outcomes based on the care planning of the interdisciplinary team, as discussed in Chapter 5.

TABLE 1.2   Common Goals of the Rehabilitation Team
Foster self-care, self-sufficiency
Encourage maximal independence level
Maintain function
Prevent complications
Restore optimum function
Promote maximum potential
Emphasize abilities
Promote adaptation
Restore acceptable quality of life
Maintain dignity
Reeducate
Assist with community reintegration/reentry
Promote optimal wellness

In addition to helping the client set goals in each needed discipline, interdisciplinary team members also meet regularly and establish realistic goals and objectives that team members can address together. A team goal is one in which two or more disciplines participate, is mutually established with the patient, and is time limited, realistic, and measurable. An example of a team goal related to patient safety might be the following: *Mr. Smith will lock his wheelchair brakes 100% of the time with cues from staff by discharge.* From this goal, one can see that it is patient oriented (Mr. Smith and his actions are the focus), has a definite time limit (by discharge), is measurable (100% of the time), and includes interventions or reminders from a variety of team members working with the client throughout the day. This is the type of goal the team can evaluate during weekly team conferences in which individual staff members provide updates about progress toward desired outcomes for each patient.

HISTORY

The development of rehabilitation principles occurred over a number of years in history, but rehabilitation was not recognized as a specialty until much later. As early as thousands of years ago, an Egyptian physician recorded his observations of a patient with a spinal cord injury, describing a dislocated vertebra in the neck, paralysis, and urinary incontinence (Martin, Holt, & Hicks, 1981). The earliest record of crutches appeared on an Egyptian tomb in 2380 B.C. (Mumma, 1987). During 300 to 400 B.C., Hippocrates, known as the Father of Medicine, stated that "exercise strengthens and inactivity wastes," recording the use of artificial limbs in a patient with amputation (Mumma, 1987).

Several nurses are credited with playing a significant role in the promotion of rehabilitation concepts. Florence Nightingale organized professional nursing in England in 1854. By using rehabilitation principles, Nightingale was able to significantly decrease the mortality rate during the Crimean War. Isabel Adams Hampton (1860–1910) was one of the leaders in the development of the nursing profession in North America. In a book on nursing principles and practice, Hampton pointed out to her pupils the importance of cleanliness and asepsis at all times to prevent secondary infections, saying "no department of a nurse's work should appeal more forcibly to her than the attention to the hygiene of the sick-room. She should thoroughly grasp the general principles which underlie the subject, and endeavor to apply them in the minutest detail" (Hampton, 1893, p. 93).

> Nightingale saved "more lives in the Crimean War than the entire British medical department, using hygiene and rehabilitation principles practiced by the ancient Romans."
>
> Christine Mumma, early ARN leader and author (1987, p. 5)

Although early records of the use of such exist, it was not until the world wars ensued that significant gains were made in the field of rehabilitation. This first occurred through the armed forces, with rehabilitation services not generally being available to civilians. In fact, the increased number of disabled veterans returning from battle provided the impetus for medical advancement and federal legislation. Before this time, the need for rehabilitation was not nearly as great. One can see that a major influence on the development of rehabilitation was war.

World War I presented the United States with many causalities but little hope of rehabilitation for injured soldiers. However, in 1917 the American Red Cross Institute for Crippled and Disabled men was created in the United States to provide vocational training for wounded military personnel. Several federal as well as individual state laws were passed in an attempt to help the disabled, but nothing was done on a wide scale.

After World War I, the life expectancy of a spinal cord–injured patient was less than 1 year. Mortality rates from these types of condition were high, and rehabilitation was generally minimized. Howard Rusk, a pioneer in rehabilitation medicine, recounted that the care for those with spinal cord injuries was poor. The founder of the Rehabilitation Institute of Chicago recounted that in these days a person with spinal cord injury or stroke might be laid in a box of sawdust in the basement of the hospital, given little therapy, and waiting to die.

> "They got terrible bed-sores, developed kidney and bladder problems, and simply lay in bed, waiting for death. It was almost the same with strokes."
>
> Dr. Howard Rusk, pioneer in rehabilitation medicine (1977, p. 43)

The Veterans Administration was created after World War I to care for those with service-related disabilities, but the initial care provided in the early 1940s was custodial, not rehabilitative. However, significant legislative decisions, such as the Vocational Rehabilitation Act of 1943, provided funding for training and research with the disabled. In addition, the United Nations Rehabilitation Administration drew the involvement of 44 countries in the planning of care for wounded and disabled veterans.

As a result of the development of sulfa drugs and better medical treatment, more wounded had survived World War II and the world now had to decide what to do with its disabled. According to Rusk (1977), although there had been many people concerned with the fate of the disabled, there was no organized movement to promote their rehabilitation. Fortunately, he persevered in his belief that there was **quality of life** beyond disability. Rusk's philosophy, which he developed and practiced during World War II, was to treat the whole man—that it was not enough just to heal the body. He pleaded his cause to anyone who would listen, pioneering a field that other doctors refused to accept as legitimate, until rehabilitation services were available to civilians as well as military patients. His experiences touched an entire nation, and his expertise influenced care of the disabled around the world.

The American Academy of Physical Medicine and Rehabilitation was established in 1938 and the American Board of Physical Medicine and Rehabilitation in 1947. However, if was not until well into the 1950s that rehabilitation began to be widely accepted as a viable medical specialty. During this time books were published by physicians on the subject, and over the next two decades several pieces of legislation were enacted, including many amendments to the Vocational Rehabilitation Act of 1943, the Architectural Barriers Act of 1968, and the Rehabilitation Act of 1973. The most significant piece of legislation passed in the 1990s was the Americans with Disabilities Act. This statute mandated employers to make reasonable accommodation for disabled workers, preventing discrimination on the basis of physical impairment. Table 1.3 summarizes major historical and legislative highlights.

TABLE 1.3	Selected Major Historical and Legislative Highlights Related to Health Care and Disability
Year	**Highlight**
1601	Poor Relief Act (England): provided assistance for the poor and disabled.
1854	Florence Nightingale organized professional nursing in England; used hygiene and rehabilitation principles practiced by the ancient Romans.
1873	First school of nursing at Bellevue Hospital in New York.
1883–1902	A wave of hospitals, homes, and institutes established for "crippled children."
1910	Nurse Susan Tracy published "Studies of Invalid Occupation"; the beginning of occupational therapy.
1911	Workers' Compensation Laws enacted.
1914–1918	World War I American Red Cross Institute for Disabled Men provided vocational training for injury soldiers.
1918–1938	Post–World War I: mortality rate of those wounded, particularly with spinal cord injuries, was high. Rehabilitation was minimized. Veterans Administration was created to care for those with service-related disabilities.
1919	First issue of *Archives of Physical Medicine and Rehabilitation*.
1920	First Civilian Rehabilitation Act passed by Congress (Smith-Fess Act): provided vocational rehabilitation services. First civilian rehabilitation program formed.
1935	Social Security Act enacted.
1938	American Academy of Physical Medicine and Rehabilitation formed.
1939–1945	World War II
1941	Dr. Frank Krusen wrote the first comprehensive book on physical medicine and rehabilitation.
1942	Sister Kenny Institute established: Sister Kenny's research led to the development of the profession of physical therapy and boosted support for physiatry as a specialty.
1943	Vocational Rehabilitation Act: provided funding for training and research with the disabled (amendments follow through the 1960s). UN Rehabilitation Administration was formed. Representatives from 44 countries met to plan care for disabled WWII veterans. The number of disabled veterans increased as a result of the development of sulfa drugs and better medical treatment.

TABLE 1.3   Selected Major Historical and Legislative Highlights Related to Health Care and Disability *(Continued)*

Year	Highlight
1945–present	Post–World War II : greater number of disabled civilians because of increased industrialization and transportation accidents.
1946	Hill-Burton Act (Hospital Survey and Construction Act)
1947	Dr. Howard Rusk brought the first medical rehabilitation services to a U.S. Hospital (Bellevue). The American Board of Physical Medicine and Rehabilitation was formed. Rehabilitation became a board-certified specialty.
1951	Alice Morrissey, RN, wrote the first textbook for rehabilitation nursing.
1958	Dr. Rusk and collaborators first published *Rehabilitation Medicine*.
1966	Medicaid enacted. The Commission on Accreditation and Rehabilitation Facilities was established.
1968	Architectural Barriers Act: set accessibility standards for federal buildings.
1973	Federal Rehabilitation Act: increased awareness of the needs of those with disabilities; influenced accessibility and employability.
1974	Association of Rehabilitation Nurses (ARN) formed; rehabilitation nursing emerges as a specialty.
1975	*ARN Journal* was first published.
1981	ARN publishes *Rehabilitation Nursing: Concepts and Practice—A Core Curriculum*. Another comprehensive rehabilitation nursing text published. The *ARN Journal* was renamed to *Rehabilitation Nursing*.
1984	The first certification exam for rehabilitation nurses (CRRN) was given
1990	Americans with Disabilities Act: mandated "reasonable accommodation" by employers for those with disabilities.
1993	Family Leave Act enacted to assist those with caregiver and family responsibilities.
1995	ARN publishes a core curriculum for advanced practice in rehabilitation nursing; the first advanced practice nurse certification examination in rehabilitation is offered to obtain the credentials CRRN-A
2009–present	The CRRN-A credential is terminated. All nurses who wish to certify in rehabilitation nursing obtain the basic CRRN. In response to the growing number of injured veterans from continuing wars in Iraq and Afghanistan, the VA established four Polytrauma Rehabilitation Centers and 21 Polytrauma Network Sites as well as many other Polytrauma Support Clinic Teams to provide support and rehabilitation to returning soldiers.
2010	Final rule for IRF prospective payment system implemented that affects payment for rehabilitation services through Medicare

The **Association of Rehabilitation Nurses (ARN)** was established in 1974 by Susan Novak to address the need for nurses in this specialty area. In 1976 the ARN was recognized as a specialty nursing organization by the American Nurses Association (ARN, 2010a). The first rehabilitation nursing journal was published in 1975 and then a core curriculum in 1981. The first **certification** exam for rehabilitation nurses was given in 1984. As of 2010 there were about 10,000 certified rehabilitation nurses in the United States. See Box 1.1.

BOX 1.1   Web Exploration

Visit the ARN website at www.rehabnurse.org. Explore the resources available through the ARN and examine the ARN-CAT.

Although the roots of rehabilitation may have been slow to take hold, growth continues to be evident. By the early 1990s rehabilitation was one of the top specialty choices of medical students. Certifications now exist for many types of specialists related to rehabilitation, including physiatrists, nurses, counselors, case managers, life care planners, and insurance representatives. Interestingly, the current wars in Iraq and Afghanistan have again propelled rehabilitation services into the forefront with the development of polytrauma centers that address the complex medical and rehabilitation needs of war veterans experiencing the after-effects of new explosives and tactics of war.

In addition to the influence of war on the development of rehabilitation, payment systems also play a role. The impact of reimbursement and prospective payment systems has become a driving factor in the availability and accessibility of rehabilitation services in the United States.

"Section 4421 of the Balanced Budget Act of 1997 (Public Law 105-33), as amended by section 125 of the Medicare, Medicaid, and SCHIP (State Children's Health Insurance Program) Balanced Budget Refinement Act of 1999 (Public Law 106-113), and by section 305 of the Medicare, Medicaid, and SCHIP Benefits Improvement and Protection Act of 2000 (Public Law 106-554), authorizes the implementation of a per discharge prospective payment system (PPS), through section 1886(j) of the Social Security Act, for inpatient rehabilitation hospitals and rehabilitation units—referred to as inpatient rehabilitation facilities (IRFs). The IRF PPS will utilize information from a patient assessment instrument (IRF PAI) to classify patients into distinct groups based on clinical characteristics and expected resource needs. Separate payments are calculated for each group, including the application of case and facility level adjustments." (Centers for Medicare & Medicaid Services, 2009, paragraph 1)

With changes in reimbursement that have occurred at many different points during the past few decades as rehabilitation became a specialty, there have also been wide variations in length of stay. During the late 1980s and early 1990s, persons with spinal cord injury and stroke were able to stay in acute rehabilitation for months until they were ready to be discharged. Home passes allowed them to leave the hospital and spend overnights with family and still return for therapy. Changes in payment resulted in decreased length of stay and more pressure on the interdisciplinary team to discharge patients "quicker and sicker." Less time was available for nurses and therapists to teach patients and family members what they needed to successfully adapt to life after a disability. Outpatient therapy became more popular, and the number of clinics increased, putting new pressure on

inpatient facilities to maintain their census. (These issues are discussed further in Chapter 26.)

New rules from the Centers for Medicare & Medicaid Services that were effective in January 2010 may again impact the affordability of rehabilitation services. The ARN is active in the development of health policy and advocacy at the national level and has made this a priority for the future. A number of white papers state ARN's position on important issues. These are accessible through the ARN website (http://www.rehabnurse.org/advocacy/position.html). See Box 1.2.

BOX 1.2   Web Exploration

Visit http://www.rehabnurse.org/advocacy/activities.html and browse the various activities of the ARN with regard to health policy and advocacy. Choose a link and read an issue brief or correspondence to Congress.

CONCEPTS AND PRINCIPLES

Concepts provide a way of categorizing or considering some major factors that may influence rehabilitation. In Part I of this text, many concepts are discussed that lay the framework for the rest of the book. Clinical reference books, texts, and healthcare research provide a fine body of literature on concepts related to rehabilitation such as adaptation, **holistic care**, **chronicity**, quality of life, coping, and self-care. The literature is filled with many helpful rehabilitation quotes from a variety of sources. Most of these "sayings" can be placed into one of several categories. Examples of general guiding principles used by rehabilitation professionals, with supporting concepts, follow.

"I think nurses should encourage all clients and patients to practice self-care. Orem's Self-Care Deficit Nursing Theory is an excellent theoretical model for rehabilitation nurses. As one progresses from a state of dependence to independence, self-care becomes a cardinal attribute of independence."

Paul Nathenson, ARN leader (ARN Network, 2008, p. 9)

Promote Adaptation, Not Just Recovery

The physical and emotional challenges that come with a disabling condition make a patient's experience intensely personal. Rehabilitation professionals understand that their role, no matter how great the contribution to the client's success, can only support and encourage strength and resourcefulness within the person.

All too often in healthcare terminology one hears the word *recovery* applied to the process that occurs after an accident or illness. This term purports the notion that a person can be completely restored to a former state of health and that this is the goal of treatment, but such is not often the case with long-term illnesses or injuries. Indeed, when considering the concept of recovery, one must wonder whether a patient ever truly returns to the exact premorbid state, because a change has occurred necessitating rehabilitative care.

The process of rehabilitation helps individuals adjust or adapt to life-altering situations without giving false hope of total recovery. In addition, patients may use the word *recovery* with a different meaning from that assigned to it by health professionals (Easton, 1999). Words such as *adaptation* suggest that clients may not return to the way they were before the illness or accident but that they can learn to make adjustments in their lifestyle to cope with changes that have occurred.

Those who experience chronic illnesses or disability come to the hospital with quite different needs from those who arrive for acute problems. Having a leg amputated is not akin to having an appendix removed. One condition may require a brief period of convalescence with complete recovery, whereas the other requires an extended period of rehabilitation with lifelong changes. In the case of an amputation, the client does not "get fixed," go home, and then resume life as before. Adjustments must be made. From a long-term health deviation, often there is no complete "recovery" but rather adaptation.

Persons recently diagnosed with multiple sclerosis or suffering a spinal cord injury are facing a life-altering situation. What has happened will change the way they live, think, and interact with others. For these individuals, the road of life will never be traveled the same again. They soon realize they will not return to their former state. Their life has been forever altered, and they may experience feelings of hopelessness, powerlessness, and sorrow.

Rehabilitation often makes the difference between positive adjustment and negative outcomes. As patients participate in therapeutic activities, the likelihood of successful reintegration into the community increases. Although this process may be long and arduous, patients and families who participate in it acknowledge feeling better about themselves and often express a greater ability to cope and improved acceptance of their new roles and self-image (Easton, Rawl, Zemen, Kwiatkowski, & Burczyk, 1995). The rehabilitation team assists clients back toward independence and the achievement of personal goals. When an individual's condition is acute, the services of the interdisciplinary team may be minimal. But if the state is chronic, a significant amount of therapy may be indicated.

Also of note is that persons with long-term health deviations may deal with chronicity throughout their lives, but they also experience acute problems too. Chapter 2 provides more detailed information on chronicity and disability and how individuals cope with long-term health concerns. Chapter 4 provides additional theories and frameworks for chronic illness, disability, adaptation, and coping.

Many persons living with functional deficits do not consider themselves disabled. There are things they cannot do, but other things they can do. Rehabilitation assists these persons in making the most of abilities and strengths that remain and working with what they have. Thus, the process of adaptation and recovery engaged in by those with physical limitation must be optimistic in nature and center on developing and maximizing the functions that remain.

Emphasize Abilities

People who have experienced a major health crisis have reason enough to think negatively. If rehabilitation focused on what patients had lost, then there would indeed be cause for despair. An amputated limb may not be restored, but an artificial one can return the function of ambulation. A hemiplegic arm may no longer be able to write, but it can help provide balance and stability. A traumatic brain injury may have robbed a person of speech, but with speech therapy, effective communication may be restored. Likewise, individuals with several physical impairments may choose to capitalize on their intellectual capabilities, exploring areas that were perhaps previously neglected.

Rehabilitation professionals offer hope and an optimistic outlook for the future to those whose lives have been devastated by a life-altering condition. Goal attainment is one way to measure a patient's progress. Setting mutually agreed on, realistic, achievable goals, both short term and long term, allows clients to participate in the rehabilitation process. Clients feel a sense of accomplishment when they overcome obstacles to meet their objectives. For some patients, being able to walk or talk again is a major step toward regaining independence. For others, meaningful progress is measured in smaller gains, such as being able to talk on the telephone, play cards, or resume a prior hobby.

Treat the Whole Person

The concept of the person as a holistic being is inherent to the rehabilitation process. Every person is a unique individual, worthy of the same respect and consideration as any other, regardless of age, race, gender, creed, or functional capacity. When a life-changing event occurs, it is essential for healthcare professionals to remember that the person being treated brings with them all past experiences, problems, values, and beliefs. The rehabilitation process strives to utilize these prior experiences to the individuals' benefit, not to remake the person.

Professionals treat the person, not the disease. Although this should be true in all of health care, it is one of the founding principles of rehabilitation. A disability affects not only the individuals' health, but everything about his or her body, relationships, environment, and community. Patients requiring a long period of treatment experience multiple changes in their lives. Financial considerations may be a great burden to some. Others may worry about role adjustments and the effect of their illness on family. Still others struggle with anger and depression. Denial and nonacceptance of one's limitations are barriers to successful adaptation. Therefore, a patient's preferences, culture, religious beliefs, values, developmental stage, social support, cognitive and physical abilities, and stress and coping patterns are all assessed by the interdisciplinary team when formulating a plan of care.

Rehabilitation is one specialty in which knowledge of the principles of adult learning is essential. Assessing the patient's prior knowledge and experience provides insight into his or her life philosophy and goals. Using this information, the team can get a better idea of the whole person and develop appropriate plans of care. Because team members engage in a large amount of educative activities with patients, drawing on an individual's background as a basis for teaching and learning can be helpful.

Disability Affects the Entire Family

Grieving is a normal part of the rehabilitation process for those who have suffered loss. This includes both the patient and those close to him or her. The client's family will also grieve. Research has demonstrated that the wives of stroke patients often remain in the depression phase of grieving longer than the patient (Rosenthal, Pituch, Greninger, & Metress, 1993) and that caregivers of stroke survivors have unique needs themselves (King & Semik, 2006; Pierce, Steiner, Hicks, & Holzaepfel, 2006). Coping with a chronic health problem requires many changes to the patient's entire support system. Thus, a long-term illness or disability affects the entire family.

The interdisciplinary team assists the patient and family to attain a quality of life that is acceptable to them. Family members often have unrealistic expectations of the client, making comments such as "when he gets over this and things return to normal, then I'll be all right." The grieving process may take time and continue long after the patient has been discharged. The team works together to identify appropriate resources, whether financial, emotional, or spiritual, to assist the family. Times of respite for the caregiver may be indicated, and the nurse should be able to identify community resources for the family before discharge, anticipating future needs. Follow-up programs can also have a positive impact on long-term coping skills (Easton et al., 1995).

Rehabilitation Begins "Day One" With Preventing Complications

Today's healthcare professionals are more aware of the need for preventive care. The move toward primary health care, health maintenance organizations, preventive medicine, and expanded roles for nurse practitioners indicates this. Yet the push toward primary prevention has not always resulted in the prevention of secondary complication so often seen in rehabilitation patients.

Take, for example, the situation of Mrs. Smith, who was admitted with the diagnosis of acute cerebral vascular accident to the intensive care unit (ICU) of a large, reputable hospital. As a result of the severity of her condition, Mrs. Smith twice experienced cardiac arrest and was successfully resuscitated. For three days Mrs. Smith was essentially unresponsive and had to rely on others for all her basic care needs. During this crucial time, however, Mrs. Smith developed black spots on her heels, indicating pressure ulcers. The nurses caring for her did not remember that "rehabilitation begins day one" and had been short-sighted in their thinking, not paying close enough attention to complications that could have been prevented. Once medically stable, Mrs. Smith was transferred to inpatient rehabilitation for concentrated therapy. After one week in rehabilitation she told her rehab nurse, "In ICU, I died and they revived me twice, but I didn't feel alive after my stroke. The people in rehabilitation have brought me back to life in a different way. They helped me to live again!" Mrs. Smith's determination propelled her through the rehabilitation program, and she began gait training. However, the black areas on her heels broke open once she became ambulatory. She told the rehabilitation nurses that she had not been turned for days while in the ICU. The stage IV wounds now on both heels required whirlpool therapy twice daily to control the copious amounts of drainage. The pain and bulky dressings greatly inhibited Mrs. Smith's ability to walk, setting her rehabilitation progress back. In addition, her wounds continued to require extensive outpatient treatment months after discharge, and Mrs. Smith and her family brought suit against the hospital to cover the cost of her ICU-acquired pressure sores. Aside from the obvious legal implications of this case, Mrs. Smith experienced unnecessary pain, suffering, and interference with her rehabilitation as a result of events occurring in the acute care unit. Rehabilitation must begin as soon as the patient is hospitalized to prevent secondary complications that could have devastating consequences later.

Other examples that demonstrate how postacute rehabilitation can be impeded if not practiced from the first day include the development of contractures. The nurse in the acute care setting who does not educate the patient with a new below-the-knee amputation about the contraindication of using a pillow under the knee joint may well promote a contracture that prohibits the complete range of motion necessary for wearing a prosthesis later to ambulate. Likewise, a person with a complete spinal cord injury and paraplegia may be dependent on the acute care staff to maintain skin integrity. If a sacral pressure ulcer forms, that client would be unable to develop needed wheelchair skills and perhaps be confined to a prone position until the wound heals. In addition, stroke patients who have been in acute care even one week or less if not given proper range of motion exercises and those who are allowed to stay in the "stroke position" will have to undo the ill effects of immobilization while embarking on intensive therapy. Such a patient may permanently have a contracted hemiplegic arm and hand. All these conditions are likely preventable when the healthcare professional applies the concepts and principles of rehabilitation.

REHABILITATION NURSING

> Evidence-based practice is the cornerstone of practice excellence, used for the development of standards of practice and to influence policy and legislation impacting those with chronic illness and disability.
>
> Stephanie Burnett (2012, p. 29)

Rehabilitation nursing is a nationally recognized specialty with a core body of knowledge and its own curriculum and research base, specialty organization, and certifica-

TABLE 1.4   Role Description Brochures Available From the ARN at www.rehabnurse.org

- The Gerontological Rehabilitation Nurse
- The Home Care Rehabilitation Nurse
- The Pain Management Rehabilitation Nurse
- Pediatric Rehabilitation Nursing
- Rehabilitation Nurse Manager
- The Rehabilitation Admissions Liaison Nurse
- The Advanced Practice Rehabilitation Nurse
- The Rehabilitation Nurse Case Manager
- The Rehabilitation Nurse Educator
- The Rehabilitation Staff Nurse
- The Rehabilitation Nurse Researcher

tion (ARN, 1996, 2000, 2007). Rehabilitation nursing was first recognized as a specialty by the American Nurses Association in 1976 (ARN, 2010a). The ARN was established in 1974 due to the emerging need for a network and support for those practicing rehabilitation in a growing number of areas. Presently, the ARN has developed 11 role description brochures (Table 1.4) to address the practice of rehabilitation nurses across a variety of settings and populations. This attests to the growth of this specialty area.

The ARN discusses rehabilitation nursing broadly by stating that "rehabilitation nurses help individuals affected by chronic illness or physical disability to adapt to their disabilities, achieve their greatest potential, and work toward productive, independent lives. They take a holistic approach to meeting patients' medical, vocational, educational, environmental, and spiritual needs" (ARN, 2010a, paragraph 1). The roles of the rehabilitation nurse are discussed more explicitly in Chapter 6, so this chapter only briefly introduces rehabilitation nursing.

Rehabilitation nurses practice in a wide variety of settings, including acute care hospitals, long-term care facilities, retirement communities, the community at large, hospice, the military, and academe. Similarly, rehabilitation nurses may specialize in working with various populations such as adults, pediatrics, or geriatrics, or they may focus on a particular aspect of rehabilitation care, such as pain, case management, legal nurse consulting, or life-care planning. Others may specialize in care of persons with stroke, brain injury, polytrauma, or burns. Therefore, rehabilitation nurses can be found everywhere, but what sets them apart is their holistic, long-term perspective and unique set of skills they bring to each setting and group with whom they interact.

Most members of the interdisciplinary team have expertise in given areas of rehabilitation. For example, physical therapists are particularly knowledgeable about muscles, movement, and gait. Occupational therapists focus on activities of daily living and home maintenance functions. Speech-language pathologists are experts in dysphagia, cognition, and speech disorders. Physiatrists are medical doctors with physical medicine and rehabilitation as their specialty. Likewise, rehabilitation nurses have several domains that fall under their scope of practice.

Some of the common areas addressed by the rehabilitation nurse include pain management, behavior, skin, bowel and bladder, medications, patient and family education, and nutrition. As an essential member of the rehab team, and the only professional who provides 24-hour-per-day care in acute rehabilitation, the rehab nurse brings a skill set to the team that makes her or him uniquely qualified to provide holistic care that should be highly valued by the patient, family, and fellow team members.

Rehabilitation nursing is a specialty just like perioperative nursing, oncology, or orthopedics. Rehabilitation requires special knowledge, skill sets, and expertise to achieve positive patient outcomes. Rehabilitation nurses use the roles of caregiver, teacher, case manager, counselor, and advocate (ARN, 2000). This type of care cannot be provided without education and a solid knowledge about rehabilitation (Lin & Armour, 2004; Pryor, 2002; Remsburg & Carson, 2006). Sadly, most nursing programs today do not include adequate content in rehabilitation, and few, if any, graduate programs in rehabilitation nursing currently exist. However, "far from being categorized as 'enthusiastic amateurs,' nurses aspire to be 'rehabilitators par excellence,' but there is little evidence in the literature that the necessary educational preparation is available or undertaken to achieve this, despite a number of studies supporting the overall view that specific educational preparation is required" (Booth, Hillier, Waters, & Davidson, 2004, p. 466).

Nurses validate their knowledge and skills in rehabilitation in several ways. Two of the most common are meeting basic competencies and obtaining certification in the specialty.

COMPETENCIES AND CERTIFICATION

In 1994 the ARN published a document entitled *Basic Competencies for Rehabilitation Nursing Practice*. This manual was designed to help preceptors or staff educators teach and orient new nurses to the specialty practice of rehabilitation. It was divided into three phases to be covered over 12 months. Months 1 to 3 were orientation, months 4 through 6 were midyear development, and months 7 through 12 included first-year competencies. Under each phase was listed a number of specific competencies that for the entire program totaled 89. Although this publication is no longer available to the general public, it presented a significant marker in the development of the specialty and a logical step in delineating rehabilitation nursing. In 2006 ARN moved to an evidence-based practice focus with its new publication *Evidence-based Rehabilitation: Common Challenges and Interventions* (Edwards, 2007).

Today, the ARN has listed 16 basic competencies (Table 1.5) recently updated from the 14 previous competencies set forth in the ARN-Competencies Assessment Tool (CAT). The ARN-CAT is a Web-based tool available at no cost from the ARN website to assist managers and educators in evaluating the rehabilitation knowledge of their staff in basic areas. Each competency area is tested with 10+ multiple-choice questions. The person taking the test must log in before taking the exam. The computer

TABLE 1.5   Sixteen Basic Competency Areas Included in the ARN-CAT
Autonomic dysreflexia
Bladder function
Bowel function
Communication
Disability
Dysphasia
Gerontology
Musculoskeletal/body mechanics/functional transfer techniques
Neuropathophysiology (CVA, SCI, TBI) and functional assessment
Pain
Patient and family education
Pediatrics
Rehabilitation
Safe patient handling
Sexuality
Skin and wound care

CVA, cerebrovascular accident; SCI, spinal cord injury; TBI, traumatic brain injury.

then provides a printout of the person's score along with rationale for the correct answer to each question and citation of one reference that supports the correct response. The questions were updated in late 2009 to reflect more current practice. However, no reliability or validity statistics are available for the ARN-CAT.

Certification in one's specialty area has been associated with increased knowledge and more positive patient outcomes (Carey, 2001; Kendall-Gallagher & Blegen, 2009; Nieburh & Biel, 2007). In a landmark study by Nelson and colleagues (2007), the researchers used a prospective observational design to examine nursing staffing patterns and the impact on patient outcomes in rehabilitation. The team of researchers studied 54 rehabilitation facilities stratified by geography and randomly selected to participate. This was the first study to report on relationships between nursing staffing and patient outcomes. A significant finding was that certification in rehabilitation was inversely related to length of stay in rehabilitation patients. More specifically, a 6% increase of nurses certified in rehabilitation on the unit was associated with an approximate one day decrease in length of stay. Additionally, nurses certified in rehabilitation report valuing their certification and expressed that it added knowledge, confidence, and professional recognition to their practice (Leclerc, Holdway, Kettyle, Ball, & Keither, 2004).

The credential for certified rehabilitation nurses is **certified registered rehabilitation nurse (CRRN)**. About 10,000 nurses in the United States hold the CRRN certification. To obtain the CRRN designation, nurses must pass an examination. Requirements to sit for the CRRN examination include having an unrestricted registered nurse license and either 2 years of experience in rehabilitation or 1 year of experience and a year of graduate study in nursing beyond the bachelor's level (ARN, 2010b). Certification tells employers and patients that the nurse has expertise in this specialty area. To maintain certification, nurses must meet additional criteria and renew every 5 years either by examination or portfolio that documents continued education and activity in rehabilitation nursing. Certification is a way of validating one's expertise, gaining additional knowledge in the specialty area, and promoting credibility within the community.

SUMMARY

This introductory chapter provides a brief overview of the history, philosophy, and major concepts in rehabilitation. In the chapters that follow in Part I, the foundations of the specialty are discussed. In Part II, rehabilitation nursing competencies mentioned in this chapter are expounded upon using a variety of evidence-based content and teaching-learning strategies to help the reader ef-

TABLE 1.6 Selected Books Written by Those Experiencing Significant Health Alterations			
Title	**Author**	**Date**	**Topic**
Tuesdays with Morrie	Albom	1997	Retired teacher dying from ALS
Bed Number Ten	Baier	1985	Mom with Guillain-Barré syndrome
The Diving Bell and the Butterfly	Bauby	1998	Editor-in-chief with brain-stem stroke/locked-in syndrome
Flying without Wings	Beisser	1989	Physician with polio
My Stroke of Insight: A Brain Scientist's Personal Journey	Bolte Taylor		Neuroanatomist with stroke
My Stroke of Luck	Douglas	2003	Actor with stroke
Always Looking Up: The Adventures of An Incurable Optimist	Fox	2009	Actor with Parkinson's disease
Change in the Weather: Life After Stroke	McEwen	2008	TV weatherman with stroke
Still Me	Reeve	1999	Actor with spinal cord injury
Speechless: God and Brain Injury	Williamson	2005	Man with traumatic brain injury and aphasia
In an Instant	Woodruff	2007	TV journalist with brain injury acquired while covering war story

ALS, amyotrophic lateral sclerosis.

fectively retain and apply the information provided. Part III provides clinical guidance in caring for persons with various specific rehabilitative problems. Part IV presents contemporary and relevant issues related to practice, and Part V offers unique aspects of the discipline such as geriatrics, pediatrics, animal assisted therapy and life care planning. Rehabilitation nurses are encouraged to continue the pursuit of knowledge in this specialty area and read additional materials such as those books suggested in Table 1.6 and listed as additional resources throughout the other chapters in this text.

CRITICAL THINKING

1. Go to the ARN website at www.rehabnurse.org and log on to take the ARN-CAT. Choose the competency of "rehabilitation" and take the multiple-choice assessment. See how you scored and review any incorrect answers.
2. Visit a local public building in your town. Evaluate how accessible the building is to persons with the following adaptive devices: a wheelchair, a walker, a prosthetic leg.
3. Consider visiting a local veterans group and talking to some war veterans. Find out from them first hand what it was like to be soldiers, what common injuries they or their friends sustained, what long-lasting effects they experienced, and what part rehabilitation has played since their return from war. Ask them about the importance of maintaining independence and performing self-care after being wounded.

PERSONAL REFLECTION

- Do you have any friends or relatives with physical challenges that make mobility difficult? If so, how does this make you feel when you are doing activities with them? Are you more or less sensitive to others who may need to use adaptive equipment?
- How do you feel when you hear these terms applied to persons with physical limitations: crippled, invalid, wheelchair bound? What other terms might be preferable to use when discussing persons with altered physical capabilities?
- Imagine that tonight when you go home from school or work you are in a serious car accident that was not your fault. As a result, you have a complete C-2 spinal cord injury with tetraplegia and will be dependent on others for most of your care for the rest of your life.

How would your life change? What kinds of feelings would you be dealing with? How would you cope with this loss of function? What resources do you have that could help you in adapting to a new life?

REFERENCES

Association of Rehabilitation Nurses (ARN). (1996). *Scope and standards of advanced clinical practice in rehabilitation nursing.* Glenview, IL: Association of Rehabilitation Nurses.

Association of Rehabilitation Nurses (ARN). (2000). *Standards and scope of rehabilitation nursing practice.* Glenview, IL: Association of Rehabilitation Nurses.

Association of Rehabilitation Nurses (ARN). (2007). *Role description brochures.* Retrieved from http://www.rehabnurse.org/db/members/fs

Association of Rehabilitation Nurses (ARN). (2010a). About ARN. Retrieved from http://www.rehabnurse.org/about/definition.html

Association of Rehabilitation Nurses (ARN). (2010b). CRRN certification. Retrieved from http://www.rehabnurse.org/certification/index.html

Booth, J., Hillier, V. F., Waters, K. R., & Davidson, I. (2004). Effects of a stroke rehabilitation education programme for nurses. *Journal of Advanced Nursing, 49*(5), 465–473.

Carey, A. (2001). Certified registered nurses: Results of the study of the certified workforce. *American Journal of Nursing, 101*(1), 44–52.

Centers for Medicare & Medicaid Services. (2009). *Overview of inpatient rehabilitation facility PPS.* Retrieved from http://www.cms.hhs.gov/inpatientrehabfacpps

Easton, K. L. (1999). The post-stroke journey: From agonizing to owning. *Geriatric Nursing, 20*(2), 70–75.

Easton, K., Rawl, S., Zemen, D., Kwiatkowski, S., & Burczyk, B. (1995). The effects of nursing follow-up on the coping strategies used by rehabilitation patients after discharge. *Rehabilitation Nursing Research, 4*(4), 119–127.

Edwards, P. (2007). Rehabilitation nursing: Past, present, and future. In K. L. Mauk (Ed.), *The specialty practice of rehabilitation nursing: A core curriculum.* Glenview, IL: ARN.

Gender, A. (1998). Scope of rehabilitation and rehabilitation nursing. In P. A. Chin, D. Finocchiaro, & A. Rosebrough (Eds.), *Rehabilitation nursing practice* (pp. 3–20). New York: McGraw-Hill.

Habel, M. (1993). Rehabilitation: Philosophy, goals, and process. In A. E. McCourt (Ed.), *The specialty practice of rehabilitation nursing: A core curriculum* (pp. 2–5). Skokie, IL: Rehabilitation Nursing Foundation.

Hampton, I. A. (1893). *Nursing: Its principles and practice.* Philadelphia: W. B. Saunders.

Kendall-Gallagher, D., & Blegen, M. A. (2009). Competence and certification of registered nurses and safety of patients in intensive care units. *American Journal of Critical Care, 19*, 106–114.

King, R. B., & Semik, P. E. (2006). Stroke caregiving: Difficult times, resource use, and needs during the first 2 years. *Journal of Gerontological Nursing, April*, 37–44.

Leclerc, A., Holdway, K., Kettyle, D., Ball, A., & Keither, L. (2004). Nurses perceptions of rehabilitation certification. *Canadian Nurse, 100*(2), 22. Retrieved from http://proquest.umi.com/pqdlink?did=548152401&Fmt=3&clientid=5302&RQTVVName=PQD

Lin, J. L., & Armour, D. (2004). Selected medical management of the older adult rehabilitative patient. *Archives of Physical Medicine and Rehabilitation, 85*(Suppl. 3), S76–S82.

Martin, N., Holt, N., & Hicks, D. (Eds.) (1981). *Comprehensive rehabilitation nursing*. New York: McGraw-Hill.

Mumma, C. M. (1987). *Rehabilitation nursing: Concepts and practice* (2nd ed.). Evanston, IL: Rehabilitation Nursing Foundation.

Nathenson, P. (2008). The role of complimentary alternative medicine in treating patients: A conversation with Paul and Nancy Nathenson. *ARN Network, 25*(1), 9–10.

Nelson, A., Powell-Cope, G., Palacios, P., Luther, S. L., Black, T., Hillman, T., Christiansen, P., Nathenson, P., & Coleman Gross, J. (2007). Nurse staffing and patient outcomes on rehabilitation settings. *Rehabilitation Nursing, 32*(5), 179–202.

Nieburh, B., & Biel, M. (2007). The value of specialty nursing certification. *Nursing Outlook, 55*, 176–181.

Pierce, L. L., Steiner, V., Hicks, B., & Holzaepfel, A. L. (2006). Problems of new caregivers of persons with stroke. *Rehabilitation Nursing, 31*(4), 166–172.

Pryor, J. (2002). Rehabilitative nursing: A core nursing function across all settings. *Collegian, 9*(2), 11–15.

National Cancer Institute. (2007). Rehabilitation. Retrieved from http://www.cancer.gov/Templates/db_alpha.aspx?CdrID=441257e

Remsburg, R., & Carson, B. (2006). Rehabilitation. In I. Lubkin & P. Larsen (Eds.), *Chronic illness: Impact and interventions* (pp. 579–616). Sudbury, MA: Jones and Bartlett Publishers.

Rosenthal, S., Pituch, M., Greninger, L., & Metress, E. (1993). Perceived needs of wivesof stroke patients. *Rehabilitation Nursing, 19*(3), 148–153.

Rusk, H. A. (1977). *A world to care for*. New York: Random House.

CHAPTER 2

Chronicity and Disability

Eileen T. French
Karen M. Allabastro

LEARNING OBJECTIVES

At the end of this chapter, the reader will be able to

- Define disability and chronic illness.
- Discuss the criteria for chronic illness.
- State the major chronic problems experienced by Americans today.
- Describe ways in which Healthy People 2010 aims to promote health among older adults and those with long-term health problems.
- Identify the purpose of organizations such as CARF and ARN.
- Recognize the impact of the aging population on the need for rehabilitation services.

KEY CONCEPTS AND TERMS

Activity limitations	Commission on Accreditation	Mental
Americans with Disabilities Act	of Rehabilitation Facilities	People with disabilities
(ADA)	(CARF)	Physical
Association of Rehabilitation	Communication	Self-efficacy
Nurses (ARN)	Disability	Union of Physically Impaired
Chronic disease	Environmental factors	Against Segregation
Chronicity	Individual with a disability	

People with disabilities have been described since Biblical times, in terms ranging from objects of pity and scorn to heroes to be admired for overcoming challenges. They currently comprise a significant portion of the U.S. population. According to the U.S. Census Bureau, in 2005 of the 291 million people in the United States, 54.4 million, or 18.7%, had some level of disability and 35 million (12%) had what was described as a severe disability. In addition, 11 million people (4.1%) 6 years of age and older were found to need assistance with one or more activities of daily living (Brault, 2008).

DEFINING DISABILITY

Healthy People 2010 defined **disability** as "the general term used to represent the interactions between indi-

viduals with a health condition and barriers in their environment" (U.S. Department of Health and Human Services, 2000, p. 6–25). They further define **people with disabilities** as "people identified as having an activity limitation or who use assistance or who perceive themselves as having a disability"(p. 6–26); **activity limitations** as "problems in a person's performance of everyday functions such as communication, self care, mobility, learning, and behavior"(p. 6–25); and **environmental factors** as "the policies, systems, social contexts, and physical barriers or facilitators that affect a person's participation in activities, including work, school, leisure, and community events" (p. 6–25).

As described by the Americans with Disabilities Act (ADA) of 1990, people with disabilities in part are those who have "a physical or mental impairment that substantially limits one or more major life activities" (U.S. Department of Justice, 1990, Title 42, ch. 126, sec. 12111). Individuals with disabilities were asked questions by the U.S. Census Bureau about their ability to perform functional and participatory activities. Based on the individuals' responses related to the difficulty of performing these activities, further questioning indicated severe or nonsevere disability. The U.S. Census Bureau provides definitions of the severity of disability and activities of daily living (Table 2.1). Disability was further categorized by the Bureau into three domains: **physical**, such as spinal cord injury, arthritis, or stroke; **mental**, such as a learning disability or Alzheimer's Disease; or **communication**, such as blindness, deafness, or a speech disorder (Brault,

TABLE 2.1 Definition of Disability, Functional Limitations, Activities of Daily Living (ADLs), and Instrumental Activities of Daily Living

Types of Disabilities	Age < 3 yr	Age 3–5	Age 6–14	Age ≥ 15 yr
Used a wheelchair, a cane, crutches, or a walker			SD	SD
Had difficulty performing one or more functional activities (seeing, hearing, speaking, lifting/carrying, using stairs, walking, or grasping small objects)				NSD
Unable to perform or needed help to perform one or more of the functional activities				SD
Had difficulty with one or more ADLs, which includes getting around inside the home, getting in or out of bed or a chair, bathing, dressing, eating, and toileting			NSD	NSD
Unable to perform or needed help to perform one or more ADLs			SD	SD
Had difficulty with one or more instrumental activities of daily living (IADLs), which includes going outside the home, keeping track of money and bills, preparing meals, doing light housework, taking prescription medicines in the right amount at the right time, and using the telephone				NSD
Unable to perform or needed help to perform one or more IADLs				SD
Had one or more specified conditions: a learning disability or some other type of mental or emotional condition			NSD	NSD
Had one or more specified conditions: mental retardation or another developmental disability, or Alzheimer's disease				SD
Had any other mental or emotional condition that seriously interfered with everyday activities				SD
Had a condition that limited the ability to work around the house or made it difficult to remain employed				SD
Had one or more specified conditions: autism, cerebral palsy, mental retardation, or another developmental disability			SD	
Had difficulty performing one or more functional activities (seeing, hearing, speaking, walking, running, or taking part in sports)			NSD	
Developmental delay	NSD	NSD		
Difficulty walking, running, or playing		NSD		
Difficulty moving arms or legs	NSD			

Note: The concepts and methods used to define "disability," ADLs, or IADLs are not unique to this report. The definitions for ADLs and IADLs are consistent with those used by other agencies, including the Medicare Current Beneficiary Survey and the National Health Interview Survey. See Related Materials and Appendix A, Background on the Concept of Disability in Four National Household Surveys for more details about the questionnaire or definitions of disability.

NSD, nonsevere disability; SD, severe disability.

Source: Adapted from Brault (2008).

TABLE 2.2   Definitions of a Disability in a Communication, Mental, or Physical Domain

For people 15 years and older, types of disability were categorized into domains (communication, mental, or physical) according to the following criteria:

People with disabilities in the communication domain reported one or more of the following:

1. Difficulty seeing, hearing, or having their speech understood.

2. Being blind or deaf.

3. Blindness or a vision problem, deafness or a hearing problem, or a speech disorder as a condition contributing to a reported activity limitation.

People with disabilities in the mental domain reported one or more of the following:

1. A learning disability, mental retardation or another developmental disability, Alzheimer's disease, or some other type of mental or emotional condition.

2. Some other mental or emotional condition that seriously interfered with everyday activities.

3. Difficulty managing money/bills.

4. Attention deficit hyperactivity disorder, autism, a learning disability, mental retardation, mental or emotional problems, senility, dementia, or Alzheimer's disease as a condition contributing to a reported activity limitation.

People with disabilities in the physical domain reported one or more of the following:

1. Use of a wheelchair, cane, crutches, or walker.

2. Difficulty walking a quarter of a mile, climbing a flight of stairs, lifting something as heavy as a 10-pound bag of groceries, grasping objects, or getting in or out of bed.

3. Arthritis or rheumatism, back or spine problems, broken bones or fractures, cancer, cerebral palsy, diabetes, epilepsy, head or spinal cord injury, heart trouble or atherosclerosis, hernia or rupture, high blood pressure, kidney problems, lung or respiratory problems, missing limbs, paralysis, stiffness or deformity of limbs, stomach/digestive problems, stroke, thyroid problems, or tumor/cyst/growth as a condition contributing to a reported activity limitation.

Source: Adapted from Brault (2008).

2008) (Table 2.2). Some of the underlying contributing factors to the increased number of persons noted to have disabilities are related to advances in medicine, especially neonatal, emergency, and trauma care, and increases in longevity for both individuals with disability and the population in general (Smart, 2001).

HEALTH PROMOTION OF INDIVIDUALS WITH DISABILITY

> *The commitment in rehabilitation nursing is to assist the person with a disability to maintain independence beyond hospitalization, with the goals of preventing complications, restoring and maximizing function, reintegrating into the community, and promoting self-esteem and life satisfaction (ARN, 2006).*

In 2000 the U.S. Department of Health and Human Services introduced the initiative *Healthy People 2010: Objectives for Improving Health* as "a statement of national health objectives designed to identify the most significant preventable threats to health and to establish national goals to reduce these threats" (U.S. Department of Health and Human Services, 2000, p. 6-2).

One important objective in Healthy People 2010 is to "promote the health of people with disabilities, prevent secondary conditions, and eliminate disparities between people with and without disabilities" (U.S. Department of Health and Human Services, 2000, p. 6-3). The health of persons with disabilities has often been addressed as an issue of medical care and rehabilitation or the cost of long-term care. Healthy People 2010 described several misconceptions resulting from this. If disability is thought of as a medical condition, then a standard definition of disability is not needed and all persons with disabilities are assumed to have poor health. In this scenario public health efforts should focus solely on preventing disabilities and not on the role the environment plays in defining disabilities.

The early frameworks of disability followed either the individual model or the social model and had a goal to improve the health and quality of life for individuals with physical disabilities. The individual model of disability was first introduced by Nagi (1966). The focus of this model is the disease process and the individual problems that arise as a result of the disabling illness or injury. The goal within this model for persons with disability is to return the individual to normal functioning and their ability to function in their former or expected roles in society. Further, the goal is the prevention or cure of the disabling condition or, if that is not possible, then caring for the disabled individual (Marks, 1997). Chapter 4 provides more detailed discussion of models and theories related to disability.

Like the individual model, the goal of the social model was to improve the quality of life for persons with disabilities. Social models identify the locus of the problem of disability as barriers in the physical/social environments due to societal/environmental discrimination, prejudice, and stigmatization (Hahn, 1993). The social model has its roots in part in the disability movement that has focused attention on the environmental barriers and social oppression of the individuals with disability. One key group in this movement was the **Union of Physically Impaired Against Segregation**, whose aim was to replace segregated facilities with opportunities for people with impairments to participate fully in society, to live independently, to undertake productive work, and to have full control over their lives (Shakespeare, 2006).

The environment affects people with disabilities in a myriad of ways. The weather can affect wheelchair mobility or the ability to use a walker safely. However, basic healthcare services, work, school, opportunities to promote fitness, or participate in leisure activities and community events may not be available due to buildings, offices, and equipment that are physically inaccessible. In addition, social policy, social norms, or caregiver issues may inhibit people with disabilities from participating fully in society.

The shift in focus on the concept of disability as it relates to barriers lead in part to changes in the legislation. The most significant change was the formation of the **Americans with Disabilities Act (ADA)**. The ADA of 1990 was enacted to mandate that people with disabilities are afforded legal protection and are provided with essential public services. The ADA defines an **individual with a disability** as a person who "has a physical or mental impairment that substantially limits one or more major life activities" (U.S. Department of Justice, 1990, Americans with Disabilities Act, Title 42, ch. 126, sec. 12102). The Act covers discrimination in three areas: employment, public services, and public accommodations.

Despite changes in the legislation, people with disabilities often do not receive the healthcare services they require to achieve optimal health. Beatty et al. (2003) surveyed 800 adults with arthritis, spinal cord injury, multiple sclerosis, and cerebral palsy to assess patterns of access to healthcare services among people with chronic or disabling conditions. They found that only half of those surveyed believed they received the rehabilitation services they needed, and those in the poorest health and with the lowest incomes were the least likely to receive needed services. Those with fee-for-service plans were more likely to see specialists than those with managed care plans, despite the complexities in their conditions. Rehabilitation services were received by only half of those who reported needing them. More responsive healthcare delivery models are needed to care for people with complex disabling conditions.

The **Commission on Accreditation of Rehabilitation Facilities (CARF)** was implemented in 1966 as an independent, nonprofit accreditor of rehabilitation services. Their stated mission is to promote the quality, value and optimal outcomes of rehabilitation services (CARF International, 2010). This group has helped develop evidence-based standards for several disabilities, including spinal cord injury, stroke, and brain injury. These standards help to ensure quality specialized care for patients in need of rehabilitative services. The **Association of Rehabilitation Nurses (ARN)** is another organization that seeks to promote quality rehabilitation. Its stated mission is to "promote and advance professional rehabilitation nursing practice through education, advocacy, collaboration, and research to enhance the quality of life for those affected by disability and chronic illness" (ARN, 2010, p. 1). After World War II acute inpatient rehabilitation settings were developed to provide specialized care for patients with disabling conditions. These units were often part of a larger territory hospital setting or they were free-standing facilities. Patients admitted to these units were required to participate in therapy several hours each day. The care team consisted of physiatrists; rehabilitation nurses; physical, occupational, and speech therapists; social workers; care managers; rehabilitation counselors; recreational therapists; and the patients and families.

> *CARF's mission is to promote the quality, value and optimal outcomes of rehabilitation services (CARF International, 2010).*

INDIVIDUALS WITH CHRONIC ILLNESS AND DISEASE

According to the Centers for Disease Control and Prevention (CDC), **chronic diseases**, including diabetes, cancer, arthritis, heart disease, and stroke, are the most common and costly as well as the most preventable health problems in the United States. In 2005 nearly one of every two adults in the United States (133 million people) had one or more chronic illness. Approximately one in four of those with a chronic condition described it as limiting their daily activities. The CDC attributes much of the illness and early death related to these chronic conditions to four health behaviors: lack of physical activity, poor nutrition, tobacco use, and excessive consumption of alcohol, all of which are modifiable (CDC, 2009). Despite this, a significant portion of the population engages in these behaviors.

Chronic illness was originally defined by the Commission on Chronic Illness as "all impairments or deviations from normal which have one or more of the following characteristics: are permanent, leave residual disability, are caused by a nonreversible pathological condition, require special training of the patient for rehabilitation, may be expected to require a long period of supervision, observation or care" (Strauss, 1975, p. 1).

Gloria Donnelly (1993) described the development of the concept of **chronicity** over the years. The Commission of Chronic Diseases in 1949 defined chronic illness as an impairment or deviation from the norm with the features of permanence, residual disability due to nonreversible pathology, need for rehabilitation, and for a long period of supervision, observation, or care (Roberts, 1955). In the 1980s definitions were broadened to include mental illness, such as the one set forth by Cluff (1981) as a condition that is not cured by medical intervention and that requires monitoring and supportive care to manage the illness and to maximize the person's function and self-care (Table 2.3). Adaptation to chronic illness was

TABLE 2.3   Examples of Common Chronic Illnesses and Conditions Resulting in Chronic Health Alterations
HIV/AIDS
Diabetes
Multiple sclerosis
Spinal cord injury
Traumatic brain injury
Amyotrophic lateral sclerosis
Cerebral palsy
Muscular dystrophy
Other neuromuscular disorders
Polio
Disfiguring burns
Amputation
Parkinson's disease
Rheumatoid arthritis
Many, but not all, types of cancer
Schizophrenia
Fibromyalgia
Alzheimer's disease and other forms of dementia
Chronic obstructive pulmonary disease
Some types of stroke (which leave residual functional limitations)

also studied during that time. Pollock, Christian, and Sands (1990) stated that "adaptation to chronic illness is a complex process and implies a balance between the demands of the situation and the ability of an individual to respond to the demands" (p. 300). This gave way to more complex models in the 1990s that emphasized the impact of chronic illness on families and society.

Current models may focus on maximizing adaptation to and successful management of chronic illness. Weinert, Cudney, and Spring (2008) developed the "women to women conceptual model for adaptation to chronic illness" (p. 364), which used computers to provide health information and teach self-management skills. These skills include problem-solving, resource utilization, collaboration with a healthcare professional, and promotion of **self-efficacy**, or the confidence that one can perform the behaviors needed to reach one's goals (Weinert et al., 2008).

OUR AGING POPULATION

As of 2007 approximately one in every eight Americans is aged 65 or older, and those reaching 65 have a life expectancy of 20 additional years for women and 17 years for men. It is projected, however, that by the year 2030, 20% of the U.S. population will be over 65 (CDC & the Merck Institute of Aging and Health, 2007). Older women outnumber older men, 58% to 42%. About 30% of noninstitutionalized older persons live alone, although half of women aged 75 or older do so (U.S. Department of Health and Human Services, Administration on Aging, 2007).

Aging has an impact on both disability and chronic disease. The prevalence of disability increases steadily with age, affecting 8.8% of people under age 15 and 71% of people aged 80 and over. Elderly persons with disabilities comprise 97.3% of the population in long-term care facilities (Brault, 2008). The health of our aging population is a high public health priority, with the CDC working to assist older adults to live "longer, high quality, productive and independent lives" (CDC & the Merck Institute of Aging and Health, 2007, p.3). The World Health Organization supports the concept of active aging, which is affected by gender, culture, economic status, personal and social support systems, and social and physical environments (Hardin, 2006).

Aging is universal but is highly individual and occurs to all humans. "Society provides many myths and cruel humor about aging that unfortunately mold older adults' beliefs about themselves and their worth, however inaccurate" (Radwanski, 2008, p. 655). One myth is that confusion is a normal part of aging, when in fact changes in cognitive status in older adults could often be the result of medication, dehydration, infection, and other treatable causes (Amella, 2004). Another myth is that falling is normal in older persons, when it could indicate an acute illness or underlying medical conditions. Urinary incontinence is another condition often considered expected in older adults, but in fact it could be related to treatable conditions like urinary tract infections, functional limitations, or side effects of medications (Mauk, 2008b).

The older adult in an acute rehabilitation setting typically is more debilitated, is more likely to have experienced problems during his or her hospitalization, and is more likely to be undernourished and fatigue more easily than a younger person with a disability. Conversely, older adults often have strategies that have served them well throughout their life, and the rehabilitation team can assist them in applying these behaviors to new situations (Jacelon, 2007). Healthcare professionals can also assist people with disability or chronic illness to maintain health by promoting education and behavior modification programs aimed at modifiable behaviors such as nutrition, exercise, smoking cessation, and moderate intake of alcohol (Mauk, 2008a). Maintaining health in older adults with disabilities or chronic conditions may be challenging because of limitations in activities from these conditions, along with issues of accessibility, social support, and economic hardship.

The state of aging and health in America was assessed by the Merck Institute of Aging and Health (MIAH), the CDC, and the Gerontological Society of America (GSA) in 2004. Their call to action for improving the health of older Americans included the following strategies (MIAH, CDC, & GSA, 2004):

- Monitoring recent physical health. Self-reports of physical health can be a marker for a new illness or point to areas the need improved management.
- Increasing physical activity among older adults. Physical activity should be made more accessible to older adults for them to reap the benefits of activity in improving overall health. Several program for exercise in older adults exist, such as from the National Institute on Aging (see Box 2.1)

BOX 2.1   Web Exploration

Browse the website for the National Institute on Aging at www.nia.nih.gov/exercisebook/index.htm and explore the various exercise programs available to older adults.

- Increasing the use of clinical preventative services. Use of screening for early detection of illnesses coupled with preventative vaccines can be effective in prevention and early treatment of diseases.
- Promoting healthy behaviors in older adults. Simple measures such as physical activity, improved diet, and combating obesity and smoking can improve the health of older adults, but these measures require improved communication between patient and provider and increased access to community resources.
- Implementing a national falls prevention program. Prevention of serious fall-related fractures, such as hip fractures, helps prevent death, disability, and decrease in quality of life in older adults but requires a coordinated program at a national level to significantly improve this problem.
- Addressing frequent mental distress, which may be associated with risky and/or unhealthy behaviors that can affect the recovery from illness or lead to new physical or mental issues.
- Improving oral health, which is important in avoiding tooth loss and infection.
- Preparing our healthcare workforce for an aging society. Recommendations include increased geriatric education in all levels of health care, incorporating new research, and increased recruitment into the field of geriatrics.

ROLE OF HEALTHCARE PRACTITIONERS

Rehabilitation nurses have a long tradition and experience in helping patients with traumatic illnesses but are now increasingly dealing with patients experiencing the ramifications of aging and chronic illness. Because modern health care is allowing persons with chronic illnesses to survive much longer than in the past, older adults today are dealing with the challenges of chronic disease as well as access to and funding for healthcare services to a degree not seen in the past. The leading causes of death in the United States today are chronic diseases and degenerative illnesses, whereas a century ago they were infectious diseases and acute illnesses. Persons reaching 75 years old today, on average, have three chronic illnesses and take five prescription medications (MIAH, CDC, & GSA, 2004). Thus, the costs of health care and medications today are a major concern for seniors and often take up a significant portion of their finances.

It is important that healthcare practitioners understand the needs and goals of the individual and the barriers to achieving them in persons with a disability, chronic condition, or advanced age. By listening to the needs and goals of the individual, healthcare practitioners can assist in that individual in achieving optimal quality of life. Adults with chronic and/or degenerative diseases have often been coping with their illnesses for a number of years and may be less receptive to new strategies. Healthcare practitioners may be more successful in introducing new strategies if they are integrated with the client's existing knowledge and those strategies already found to be successful.

CRITICAL THINKING

1. Explore some of the websites listed in Box 2.2. How could you use some of these resources in your practice as a rehabilitation nurse? What services are provided by these websites? Which ones would be more useful in your particular practice?
2. Discuss with a fellow student or colleague the difference between a chronic illness and a disease. What differences do you find?
3. How would you classify a stroke with no residual limitations? Is stroke a chronic illness in this case? Or would you define it differently? Is stroke progressive?

BOX 2.2 Rehabilitation Resources
Association of Rehabilitation Nurses www.rehabnurse.org
CARF International www.carf.org
Centers for Disease Control and Prevention www.cdc.gov
U.S. Department of Health and Human Services, Administration on Aging: A Profile of Older Americans: 2007 http://www.agingcarefl.org/aging/AOA-2007profile.pdf
Healthy People 2010 www.healthypeople.gov
Merck Institute of Aging and Health (MIAH), Centers for Disease Control and Prevention (CDC), & Gerontological Society of America (GSA). The state of aging and health in America 2004. http://www.cdc.gov/aging/pdf/State_of_Aging_and_Health_in_America_2004.pdf

PERSONAL REFLECTION

- Have you cared for persons with chronic illness and/or disabilities? If so, how did you feel about these experiences? What was most memorable about caring for a person with a long-term health problem?

What challenges did you note were most difficult for that client?
- Think about how you would feel if you were just diagnosed with a chronic illness such as multiple sclerosis or diabetes. How would it change your life? What adaptations would you have to make to continue your present lifestyle? What would you change?
- If you were responsible for caring for a loved one with a disability, what resources would you access? Where would you go for help or advice?

CASE STUDY 2.1

Joan Giovanazzo is a divorced, 51-year-old woman who was diagnosed 3 years ago with multiple sclerosis (MS). As yet, she is still able to live independently, although she has noticed some problems with her gait and feels more unsteady than she used to. She has three grown children and lives alone in a rural farmhouse and has limited financial resources. Joan gives herself injections to manage her MS and states that her biggest problem is fatigue.

Questions
1. Is Joan's problem classified as a chronic illness?
2. What resources might be most helpful for Joan at this point?
3. What rehabilitation nursing interventions can be done for those such as Joan who are living in the community and do not yet require inpatient rehabilitation interventions on a regular basis?

Answers
1. Yes. Although there are several recognized clinical patterns of MS, most are generally progressive with accumulated disability over time.
2. Joan could access information online through national organizations, check out area support groups for networking, or become involved in a local community group or church to strengthen her social supports.
3. Refer Joan to any community resources, support groups, or services available. Be sure she has current information about her disease and that she has discussed the clinical patterns and expectations for the future with her physician or nurse practitioner. Joan should also be kept informed about new treatments that are on the horizon, such as oral medications to treat MS. She should also be aware of the facility where she could receive the best inpatient rehabilitation management if she requires this in the future.

REFERENCES

Amella, E. J. (2004). Presentation of illness in older adults. *American Journal of Nursing, 104*(10), 40–51.

Association of Rehabilitation Nurses (ARN). (2006). Inclusion of rehabilitation concepts as a component of generic content in BSN programs: an ARN position statement (pp. 1–2). Retrieved from www.rehabnurse.org

Association of Rehabilitation Nurses (ARN). (2010). About ARN. Retrieved from www.rehabnurse.org

Beatty, P. W., Hagglund, K. J., Neri, M. T., Dhont, K. R., Clark, M. J., & Hilton, S. A. (2003). Access to health care services among people with chronic or disabling conditions: Patterns and predictors. *Archives of Physical Medicine and Rehabilitation, 84*(10), 1417–1425.

Brault, M. (2008). Americans with Disabilities: 2005. Current population reports. U.S. Census Bureau, 70–117. Retrieved from www.census.gov/prod/2008pubs/p70-117.pdf

CARF International. (2010). CARF's mission, vision, core values, and purposes. Retrieved from www.carf.org

Centers for Disease Control and Prevention (CDC). (2009). Chronic diseases and health promotion. Retrieved from www.cdc.gov/chronicdisease/stats/index.htm

Centers for Disease Control and Prevention (CDC) & the Merck Institute of Aging and Health. (2007). The state of aging and health in America. Whitehouse Station, NJ: The Merck Company Foundation.

Cluff, L. (1981). Chronic disease, function and the quality of care. *Journal of Chronic Diseases, 34*, 299–304.

Donnelly, G. F. (1993). Chronicity: Concept and reality. *Holistic Nurse Practitioner, 8*(1), 1–7.

Hahn, H. (1993). The political implications of disability definitions and data. *Journal of Disability Policy Studies, 4*(2), 45–51

Hardin, S. R. (2006). Promoting quality of life. In K. L. Mauk (Ed.), *Gerontological nursing: Competencies for care* (pp. 703–734). Sudbury, MA: Jones and Bartlett.

Jacelon, C. S. (2007). Older adults in rehabilitation. *ARN Network*, February/March 2007. Glenview, IL: Association of Rehabilitation Nurses.

Marks, D. (1997). Models of disability. *Disability and Rehabilitation, 19*, 85–91.

Mauk, K. L. (2008a). *Our aging society*. ARN Network. Glenview, IL: Association of Rehabilitation Nurses.

Mauk, K. L. (2008b). *Myths of aging*. ARN Network. Glenview, IL: Association of Rehabilitation Nurses.

Merck Institute of Aging and Health (MIAH), Centers for Disease Control and Prevention (CDC), & Gerontological Society of America (GSA). (2004). The state of aging and health in America 2004. Retrieved from http://www.cdc.gov/aging/pdf/State_of_Aging_and_Health_in_America_2004.pdf

Pollock, S. E., Christian, B. J., & Sands, D. (1990). Responses to chronic illness: analysis of psychological and physiological adaptation. *Nursing Research, 39*(5), 300–304.

Nagi, S. Z. (1966). Some conceptual issues in disability and rehabilitation. In M. B. Sussman (Ed.), *Sociology and rehabilitation* (pp. 100–113). Washington, DC: American Sociological Association.

Radwanski, M. L. (2008). Gerontological rehabilitation nursing. In S. P. Hoeman (Ed.), *Rehabilitations nursing: Prevention, intervention and outcomes* (pp. 655–673). St. Louis, MO: Mosby Elsevier.

Roberts, D. (1955). The concept and the reality. *Journal of Chronic Diseases, 1*, 149–155.

Shakespeare, T. (2006). The social model of disability. In L. J. Davis (Ed.) *The disability studies reader* (pp. 197–204). New York: Routledge.

Smart, J. (2001). *Disability, society and the individual*. Gaithersburg, MD: Aspen.

Strauss, A. L. (1975). *Chronic illness and the quality of life*. St. Louis, MO: C.V. Mosby.

U.S. Department of Health and Human Services. (2000). Healthy People 2010: Objectives for Improving Health. Retrieved April 2010 from www.healthypeople.gov

U.S. Department of Health and Human Services, Administration on Aging. (2007). A profile of older Americans: 2007. Retrieved from http://www.agingcarefl.org/aging/AOA-2007profile.pdf

U.S. Department of Justice, (1990). Americans with Disabilities Act of July 26, 1990. Retrieved from www.ada.gov/pubs/ada.htm

Weinert, C., Cudney, S., & Spring, A. (2008). Evolution of a conceptual model for adaptation to chronic illness. *Journal of Nursing Scholarship, 40*(4), 364–372.

CHAPTER 3

Settings for Care

Susan E. Maycock

LEARNING OBJECTIVES

At the end of this chapter, the reader will be able to

- Describe the various settings in which rehabilitation may take place.
- Compare the similarities and differences between acute rehabilitation settings, long-term settings, and community-based settings.
- Consider various ethical dilemmas that may occur in the rehabilitation setting.
- Appreciate the value of evidence-based research to guide nursing practice in rehabilitation settings.
- Recognize implications for nurses related to rehabilitation for geriatric clients.

KEY CONCEPTS AND TERMS

Acute rehabilitation	Impact analysis	Outcomes research
Autonomy	Informed decision	Stakeholder
Benchmarking	Justice	Skilled nursing facility (SNF)
Beneficence	Nurse-sensitive indicators	Subacute rehabilitation
Community settings	Outcomes management	
Home health rehabilitation	Outcomes measurement	

A variety of patient situations may necessitate the need for rehabilitation services after acute care hospitalization. These situations include but are not limited to complicated orthopedic problems resulting from trauma or amputations; neurological deficits resulting from brain injury, stroke, or spinal dysfunction; burns; cardiac events; or complex medical conditions resulting in debilitation. The goal of rehabilitation, regardless of the setting, is to help patients achieve optimal physical function. Multiple criteria influence the decision of which type of rehabilitation setting is most appropriate for a patient: the patient's diagnosis, the patient's payer source, the patient's ability to participate in rehabilitation activities, and the patient's postrehabilitation discharge plan. Table 3.1 lists settings for rehabilitation nursing practice discussed further in this chapter.

> The goal of rehabilitation, regardless of the setting, is to help patients achieve optimal function.

TABLE 3.1 Settings for Practice as Set Forth by the Association of Rehabilitation Nurses

- Freestanding rehabilitation facilities
- Hospitals (inpatient rehabilitation units)
- Long-term subacute care facilities/skilled nursing facilities
- Long-term acute care facilities
- Comprehensive outpatient rehabilitation facilities
- Private practice
- Home healthcare agencies
- Clinics and day rehabilitation programs
- Community and government agencies
- Insurance companies and health maintenance organizations
- Schools and universities

Source: From Association of Rehabilitation Nurses. (n.d.). *Rehabilitation nurses make a difference* (p. 2). Glenview, IL: Author.

ACUTE REHABILITATION SETTINGS

Acute rehabilitation takes place in a hospital setting. The setting can be a freestanding rehabilitation hospital or a separate rehab unit in an acute care hospital. Acute rehabilitation is a comprehensive program of coordinated, integrated, interdisciplinary services provided under the direction of physicians qualified in rehabilitation. Other members of the interdisciplinary team include registered nurses, social workers, physical therapists, occupational therapists, dieticians, and neuropsychologists.

If a patient has sustained a significant loss of function in mobility, activities of daily living, swallowing, emotional functioning, communication, or bowel/bladder control but has demonstrated rehabilitation potential with expectation for improvement through identifiable rehabilitation goals, he or she may qualify for acute rehabilitation. Patients may be admitted from acute care hospitals, nursing homes, or home. The admission process begins with a comprehensive physical assessment by the physician. The patient must require comprehensive, post–acute medical rehabilitation, be able to participate in at least 3 hours of therapy a day, require therapy from two or more disciplines, with an expected discharge within a few weeks. Although another stipulation is that patients require 24 hour specialty nursing availability, the patient must be clinically stable with low risk for medical instability. Once the patient is admitted for acute rehabilitation, a physician provides medical rehabilitation services, program coordination, and general oversight at least three times per week (Centers for Medicare & Medicaid Services [CMS], 2010).

Payment for acute rehabilitation may be provided by third-party payers such as commercial insurance, Medicare, or Medicaid. If a patient does not have insurance to cover fees, out-of-pocket payment may be an option. Continued third-party payment requires periodic documentation that provides evidence of regular progress toward treatment goals (CMS, 2010).

LONG-TERM AND/OR SUBACUTE REHABILITATION SETTINGS

Subacute rehabilitation takes place in **skilled nursing facilities (SNFs)** or nursing home settings that can be freestanding or hospital based. Subacute rehabilitation settings satisfy the need for a significant group of patients who do not meet criteria for acute rehabilitation but nevertheless need a 24-hour care rehabilitation environ-

ment. Patient placement into subacute rehabilitation is determined by a variety of factors. Admission criteria includes an acute functional disability, a recent 3-day acute care hospitalization, a qualifying diagnosis, medical or surgical condition that limits the stamina required for participation in more intensive rehabilitation, and the ability to participate in at least 1 hour of therapy per day. Patients admitted to subacute rehabilitation generally have a slower rate of recovery, with length of stays generally ranging several days to several months. Many programs encourage patient socialization through dining and recreation experiences in a homelike setting as a total care approach to recovery. In addition to physician services, programs in this setting provide 24-hour nursing supervision, physical therapy, occupational therapy, case management services, and speech therapy as members of the interdisciplinary team (CMS, 2008).

COMMUNITY SETTINGS FOR REHABILITATION

Community settings for rehabilitation include therapy gymnasiums housed in free-standing facilities or located in acute care or rehabilitation hospitals. Rehabilitation occurring in these settings may be referred to as outpatient rehabilitation therapy. A patient who has had an inpatient hospitalization may qualify for community-based rehabilitation if he or she has a medical or surgical condition deemed stable enough for discharge to home but has a residual acute physical disability. In addition, patients that have not have had a recent inpatient hospitalization may qualify for rehabilitation in community settings as well. These patients must have an acute medical or surgical condition and can be referred for rehabilitation in community settings by healthcare providers practicing in various outpatient clinic venues. Eligibility for rehabilitation in a community setting includes the ability to participate in moderate-intensity rehabilitation therapies for at least ½ to 2 hours per session, the ability to demonstrate progress in the therapy, and commitment to fiscal responsibility by the patient and/or third-party insurer (CMS, 2009).

Home Health Rehabilitation

A patient that is in need of professional rehabilitation services but is unable to leave home (except for medical care) may be eligible to receive rehabilitation therapies within his or her home. The most common in-home therapies are physical therapy, occupational therapy, and speech therapy. Criteria for in-home therapy include an acute disability, the ability to participate and show progress in low-intensity rehabilitation therapy for at least ½ to 1 hour per session, and agreement to fiscal responsibility by the patient and/or third-party payers. Most third-party payers place limits on the number of sessions that a patient may receive in his or her home (CMS, 2005).

ETHICAL CONSIDERATIONS

The issues of resource allocation, patient selection, and goal setting may occasionally create ethical dilemmas during the rehabilitation setting selection process. If only one type of setting for rehabilitation existed, there would be no conflict. Ethical dilemmas arise when there is conflict between principles or alternatives. When one considers the ethical dilemma, the question of perspective arises. To whom are the solutions acceptable? How is the superiority of one set of principles over another determined (Bruckner, 1987)? Ultimately, it is imperative that decision making is based on the major ethical principles of **autonomy**, **beneficence**, and **justice** (Hamric & Delgado, 2009).

The issues of access to rehabilitation, criteria for rehabilitation, length of stay, or a patient's noncompliance with treatment and rehabilitation are but a few of the ethical dilemmas that may evolve (Association of Rehabilitation Nurses, 2009). After considering the influencing factors and the possible alternatives, a setting is chosen. Given that an ethical dilemma is a conflict of principles or alternatives, it is conceivable that no solution is ever totally satisfactory.

EVALUATION OF OUTCOMES

Ongoing outcome analysis is vital in evaluating which rehabilitation settings return patients most effectively to the desired level of function (Weinrich, Stuart, & Hoyer, 2005). It seems fairly reasonable to pose the question of whether rehabilitation really works in all settings. Patients, insurers, employers, decision makers, government, and society in general all have a stake in patient outcomes (Zuzelo, 2007). There are measurement principles and concepts that assist in outcome evaluation of the various rehabilitation settings. In all settings, standard metrics are used to identify patient progress toward goals. Additional principles and concepts include **benchmarking** with like facilities, **impact analysis**, **outcomes measurement**, **outcomes research**, **outcomes management**, program evaluation, quality of care, and patient satisfaction

TABLE 3.2   Key Definitions Related to Outcome Measurement in Rehabilitation

Benchmarking: Standard of best practices by which healthcare settings and processes can be measured or judged.

Impact analysis: Process of assessing the merits or magnitude of a proposed alternative when comparing outcome versus cost.

Nurse-sensitive indicators: Indicators of patient outcomes that are sensitive to interventions that may be independently initiated and performed by nurses.

Outcomes management: Assessment of data and identification of preferred interventions that lead to the desired clinical outcome.

Outcomes measurement: Evaluation of the results of programs, processes, or interventions and their comparison with the intended results.

Outcomes research: Seeks to understand the end results of specific healthcare practices and interventions.

(Table 3.2) Of further interest in inpatient rehabilitation settings, SNFs, and long-term care facilities are **nursing-sensitive indicators**, influenced by nursing care practice, which are used interdependently with multidisciplines to influence general patient outcomes.

Diverse diagnoses for patients that require rehabilitation make it difficult to generalize regarding the efficacy of rehabilitation in various settings. A comparison of data related to the major diagnoses (i.e., major joint replacements, hip fractures, and stroke) provide the most valuable evaluation of outcomes (Weinrich et al., 2005).

A review of data for patients who undergo elective major joint replacements reveals that there is no significant difference in outcomes between patients who discharge directly home versus those who undergo inpatient rehabilitation. Furthermore, extensive reviews suggest that patients with hip fractures showed equivalent outcomes whether treated in rehabilitation hospitals or SNFs. A comparison of home rehabilitation versus outpatient rehabilitation noted substantially better outcomes with intensive outpatient rehabilitation regimens. Evaluations of outcomes for patients who have suffered strokes conclude that, generally, better functional outcomes are gained with acute, inpatient rehabilitation rather than in SNFs. However, the studies also indicate that outpatient rehabilitation is effective in maintaining the functions gained once they are discharged back to the community.

EVIDENCE-BASED PRACTICE

Evidence-based practice for nurses in various rehabilitation settings is guided by the same principles used in other areas of health care. The best theory-based systematic research evidence is integrated with clinical expertise and respect for the patient's values and expectations to guide decisions about delivery of care to patients (Depalma, 2009). Making the transition from long-standing rehabilitation traditions to evidence-based practice, especially with regard to settings of care, may be challenging for some. There is, however, increasing demand from **stakeholders** for decisions to be made based on critically appraised evidence as to their effectiveness (Valdes, 2010).

CLIENT–FAMILY TEACHING

Patient teaching is a vital component to the selection of an appropriate setting for rehabilitation. Each patient and his or her family has the right to receive health information and teaching that is pertinent to his or her rehabilitation needs. The nurse must first assess patient/family baseline knowledge of the various settings of care. Next, to initiate teaching the nurse should choose the most logical approach, using available resources individualized to patient/family needs so that an **informed decision** and subsequent plan may be determined. The nurse should be specific regarding any restrictions (i.e., length of stay, number of visits that may be received, or anticipated out-of-pocket expenses the patient may incur). In addition, the patient/family should understand that multiple levels of rehabilitation care may be needed while progressing toward the patient's goals. Chapter 13 provides additional discussion about patient and family education across rehabilitation settings.

GERIATRIC CONSIDERATIONS

The steady growth of the elderly population increases the need for rehabilitation nurses in all settings to enhance understanding of complex issues that may have a profound impact on patient goals and outcomes. Elderly patients may face many physical and emotional changes that can affect the return of function and well-being during rehabilitation. Studies show the average length of stay is longer for older adults than for younger adults. Therefore, the older adult may arrive in rehabilitation more debilitated from a hospitalization than a younger adult with a similar diagnosis. In addition, adjusting to changes from an acute care setting to a rehabilitation setting may take additional time for older adults that in turn may affect the length of time spent in the rehabilitation setting (Jacelon, 2007). In addition to normal age-related changes, other issues common to this patient population may include depression, sensory impairment, cognitive impairment, or chronic medical illness burdens. Whatever the setting, rehabilitation may be essential to promote functional independence in the geriatric patient population.

SUMMARY

As advances in medical technology have expanded, survival of patients involved in accidents and survival of patients afflicted with chronic illnesses have extended exponentially. Consequently, the need for rehabilitation is climbing. All settings of rehabilitation care are comprised of multidisciplinary team members who can meet the challenges of disability in this surging population of patients.

CRITICAL THINKING

1. Critical thinking is more than a set of skills. Nurses that think critically have the ability to think through, project, and anticipate the results of interventions or actions. This allows critical thinkers to provide justification for probable outcomes in the various rehabilitation settings. How could a rehab nurse use critical thinking in the care of patients in the various settings discussed in this chapter?

2. Rehabilitation nurses who integrate critical thinking into their daily practice provide safe and competent quality care that can result in positive patient outcomes and improved rehabilitation care environments (Simpson & Courtney, 2008). Given, this, how do you use critical thinking in your daily practice? How is this application of critical thinking skills different in the particular setting in which you work? Do you believe you would practice these skills differently if you were in a SNF versus acute rehabilitation within a hospital setting? If so, why?

3. What resources are available in your local community for each of the levels of care discussed in this chapter? Do you have SNFs available? Are rehabilitation services in acute care hospitals, freestanding rehabilitation facilities, or both?

PERSONAL REFLECTION

Think of a clinical situation that involved you and then reflect on the following questions:

- Do you believe the type of rehabilitation setting played a role in the situation?
- Why? What was your role in the situation? Did your role make you feel comfortable or uncomfortable?
- What actions did you take? How did others act? Did it seem appropriate at the time? How could you have improved the situation for the patient, yourself, or others involved?
- What would you change in the future? Did you learn anything new about yourself?
- Did you expect anything different to occur? What? Why? Has it changed your way of thinking in any way?

CASE STUDY 3.1

M. J., a 78-year-old woman, has been admitted to an acute care hospital for a right hip arthroplasty and right tibial traction pin. She was in her usual state of health until she tripped on a throw rug in her bathroom, sustaining a right hip fracture. Her past medical history includes diabetes mellitus Type 2 diagnosed at age 66. She has been on oral hypoglycemic agents since that time. In addition, M.J. has taken hydrochlorothiazide 25 mg daily for hypertension during the same time. Other than a history of osteoarthritis, she denies other medical issues. Her immediate postoperative course has been complicated by an infection at the surgical site, resulting in prolonged hospitalization. She will need to discharge with a continuation of intravenous antibiotic therapy twice daily for 10 days.

Before the acute care admission, M.J. was living independently with her husband of 50 years in the rural ranch-style farmhouse in which they had raised their four children. Her children, who are very attentive, still live close by on adjacent farmlands.

Post-acute discharge rehabilitation has been recommended for M.J. You are the rehabilitation nurse that is part of the multidisciplinary team that has come to evaluate M.J. for placement in the appropriate level of rehabilitation setting. Initially, M. J. appears very motivated to regain her prehospitalization functional status. She speaks enthusiastically about an inpatient acute rehabilitation admission. However, upon learning that her insurance would pay for a skilled nursing facility but not for an acute rehabilitation admission, she adamantly refuses further participation in development of a discharge plan for rehabilitation. She states, "Those places are horrible! I will not be put away in a nursing home."

Questions

1. What is your priority with this patient?
2. What are some of the possible explanations for M.J.'s change of attitude toward rehabilitation?
3. What interventions would you consider implementing at this time?
4. What other alternatives might work?
5. How will you create a plan with which this patient will comply?

REFERENCES

Association of Rehabilitation Nurses. (2009). Health policy & advocacy position statement. Retrieved from http://www.rehabnurse.org/advocacy/pethical.html

Bowden, S. (2003). Enhancing your professional nursing practice through critical reflection. *Abu Dhabi Nurse*, 28–31.

Bruckner, J. (1987). Physical therapists as double agents: Ethical dilemmas of divided loyalties. *Physical Therapy, 67*(3), 383–387.

Centers for Medicare & Medicaid Services (CMS). (2005). Medicare benefit policy manual. Retrieved from http://www.cms.gov/manuals/Downloads/bp102c07.pdf

Centers for Medicare & Medicaid Services (CMS). (2008). Medicare benefit policy manual. Retrieved from http://www.cms.gov/manuals/Downloads/bp102c08.pdf

Centers for Medicare & Medicaid Services (CMS). (2009). Medicare benefit policy manual. Retrieved from http://www.cms.gov/manuals/Downloads/bp102c12.pdf

Centers for Medicare & Medicaid Services (CMS). (2010). Medicare benefit policy manual. Retrieved from http://www.cms.gov/manuals/Downloads/bp102c01.pdf

Depalma, J. A. (2009). Research. In A. B. Hamric, J. A. Spross, & C. M. Hanson (Eds.), *Advanced practice nursing* (4th ed., pp. 217–248). Philadelphia: Saunders Elsevier.

Hamric, A. B., & Delgado, S. A. (2009). Ethical decision making. In A. B. Hamric, J. A. Spross, & C. M. Hanson (Eds.), *Advanced practice nursing* (4th ed., pp. 315–346). Philadelphia: Saunders Elsevier.

Jacelon, C. S. (2007, February). ARN Network. Retrieved from http://www.rehabnurse.org

Simpson, E., & Courtney, M. (2008). Implementation and evaluation of critical thinking skills in Middle Eastern nurses. *International Journal of Nursing Practice, 14*, 449–454.

Valdes, K. (2010). Overcoming the challenges to incorporate evidence-based medicine into clinical practice. *Journal of Hand Therapy, 23*(3), 239–240.

Weinrich, M., Stuart, M., & Hoyer, T. (2005). Rules for rehabilitation: An agenda for research. *Neurorehabilitation and Neural Repair, 19*(2), 72–83.

Zuzelo, P. (2007). Evidence based nursing and qualitative research: A partnership imperative for real-world practice. In P. Munhall (Ed.), *Nursing research: A qualitative perspective* (4th ed). (pp 48–57). Sudbury, MA: Jones & Bartlett Publishers.

CHAPTER 4

Theories, Models, and Frameworks for Chronic Illness, Disability, Adaptation, and Coping

Penelope M. Kearney
Julie Pryor
Sandra Lever

LEARNING OBJECTIVES

At the end of this chapter, the reader will be able to

- Discuss frameworks for thinking about chronic illness and disability.
- Recognize the multiple influences related to defining chronic illness and disability within rehabilitation practice.
- Debate the relevance of the International Classification of Functioning, Disability and Health to rehabilitation practice.
- Explain why people respond and adapt to chronic illness and disability in different ways.
- Recognize the impact of chronic illness and disability as a life event.
- Discuss the strengths and limitations of applying specific models to practice situations.

KEY CONCEPTS AND TERMS

Adaptation	Life changes and losses	Primary appraisal
Appraisal	Life thread model	Quality of life
Biographical disruption	Loss of the assumptive world	Reconfiguring the future
Chronic illness	Mauk model of poststroke recovery	Secondary appraisal
Chronic illness trajectories		Shifting perspectives model
Chronic sorrow	Meaning reconstruction	Social construction model
Coping	Medical model	Social model
Dimensions of adaptability	Narrative repair	Stage models
Disability	Narrative representation	Transition in chronic illness
Grief	Phenomenological approaches	Transition theory
International Classification of Functioning, Disability and Health (ICF)	Personal tragedy model	Well-being

CHRONIC ILLNESS AND DISABILITY

The distinction between illness and **disability** used to be reasonably clear-cut. Even though causally related—illness can cause disability and disability can lead to illness—there is a conceptual difference between them.

Illness has carried a commonsense meaning of a temporary disease or condition that can be either cured or controlled by treatment, whereas disability is thought of as permanent and moderated only by rehabilitation (Couser, 1997). However, today these distinctions are blurred because increasing numbers of people in the

Western world are living with diseases and conditions that continue indefinitely, such as asthma, diabetes, and renal disease, that once would have been fatal. These people live with **chronic illness** and often experience disability. Many others now survive devastating disease or trauma, such as cancer, stroke, and burns, and even though recovered from illness subsequently live with significant disability.

Chronic illness (which is sometimes referred to as chronic disease) and disability have been typically thought of as physical conditions, but along with their increasing prevalence has come greater recognition of them as existential entities—they are about people's lives. Concepts of illness and disability have come to embody the human experience of symptoms and suffering and refer to how these are perceived, responded to, and lived with by individuals and families. For these reasons chronic illness and disability are intertwined and are here considered jointly.

Advances in the management of chronic illness and disability have also caused an expansion of the traditional view of them as only a series of losses. Such conceptualizations are relevant and still powerful, but in recent decades there has been a shift in focus from loss and burden toward concepts of **well-being** within illness, such as transformation and normality (Thorne & Paterson, 1998).

The many ways of thinking about chronic illness and disability have an impact on how we interpret the experiences of people we work with and also how rehabilitative nursing care and rehabilitation services are delivered. In the following sections, various interpretations, models, and theories are presented. Although no single model or theory is able to capture or explain the complex processes involved in living with illness and disability, each may contribute unique components to our understanding. There are relationships between some of these ways of thinking and often the boundaries are blurred, but it is useful for us to consider them separately so that we can examine how our interpretations are influenced.

The terms, interpretation, model, and theory are related and often used interchangeably; however, there are differences in meanings between them:

- Interpretation: making sense of the *meaning* of a complex situation or process
- Model: a *representation* of a complex situation or process that enables insight
- Theory: an analytic structure developed for the *explanation* of a complex situation or process

In this chapter the terms "interpretations," "models," and "theories" are grouped together as "frameworks for thinking" about chronic illness and disability.

FRAMEWORKS FOR THINKING ABOUT CHRONIC ILLNESS AND DISABILITY: INTERPRETATIONS, MODELS, AND THEORIES

This section introduces the major frameworks for thinking about chronic illness and disability: biomedical, social, psychosocial, and biopsychosocial. It shows the development of thinking over many decades and highlights the contributions of different ways of thinking to the experience of chronic illness and disability and the multiple influences on practice. By tracking this movement, we can see how a rehabilitative focus on the body has expanded to consider the impact of physiological impairment on individuals' lives that includes the environment and society. The section illustrates different ways of thinking by using Archie's story (see Case Study 4.1).

CASE STUDY 4.1

Archie was 56, tall, strong and fit, and loved his long-held job as a tug boat driver in a large and busy port. He was happily married with two grown children and spent his weekends involved in sporting activities for the children in his community, camping out in the bush with his mates, and going canyoning in wild places. He took his kayak out onto rivers and the harbor whenever possible because he loved the challenges and the peace of being on the water on his own. He was attending his regular session at the gym when he found his legs would not respond. He slowly stopped and fell off the exercise bike. He knows this because his stroke was captured on video.

Gym staff administered oxygen and called the ambulance. Archie reached the emergency department of the large hospital within 45 minutes of his episode where a CT revealed a clot in his left middle cerebral artery. His wife, Sally, arrived from work and was shaken by his appearance and lack of response. She saw that his right side was paralyzed, his face drooped severely on the right, and he was drooling and unable to speak. He responded to her only with moans and appeared restless, confused, and frightened. The doctor explained Archie's condition, making clear to Sally that if her husband survived, he would be severely disabled if the clot was not dissolved as soon as possible. Permission was given for thrombolysis with (tPA) tissue plasminogen activator, which was commenced intravenously 2½ hours after his stroke.

Sally was astounded as she watched Archie "come back to life" as she later described the effect of the tPA. He enjoyed his evening meal and chatted with his family, who were all very grateful for the prompt treatment. However, shortly the family noticed Archie's speech slowing and slurring. He was transferred to the ICU where a basal cerebral hemorrhage was diagnosed. Sally was bluntly told by the neurologist that Archie would "never drive a tug again, never work, never drive, never figure out written instructions, never kayak. . .." She was devastated. After 3 weeks in ICU and the stroke unit, Archie was admitted to a rehabilitation facility.

Note: Archie's story is used in the chapter (Boxes 4.1 through 4.4) to illustrate issues that are highlighted using different frameworks for thinking about chronic illness and disability.

Biomedical Frameworks

Biomedical frameworks conceptualize chronic illness and disability as disease and physiological impairment that manifest in individuals as dysfunctions in the body's organs and systems and as disruptions in physical and mental function. Attention is directed toward etiology, symptoms, pathophysiology, epidemiology, the course of disease, prognosis, and treatments, which may be summarized as "cause and remediation." Acute management and rehabilitation focus on cure and recovery (Craig & Perry, 2008; Wade & Halligan, 2004; Williams, 2001).

Biomedical ways of thinking are captured in the **medical model**, which drives health and illness practice in the Western world. The medical model views disability and chronic illness solely as the consequence of impairment of an individual's body or mind structures and functions (Mitra, 2006; Swain, Finkelstein, French, & Oliver, 1993). Figure 4.1 illustrates this linear relationship.

A central concern is to medically diagnose disablement, with treatments, services, policy, and government benefits often dictated by diagnosis. External factors are not significant, and management is directed at curing or

---

BOX 4.1   Thinking About Archie Within a Biomedical Framework

Admission to Rehabilitation

- Fit 56-year-old man, well nourished and previously active
- Stroke 3 weeks ago. Clot in right middle cerebral artery → successful clot thrombolysis with tissue plasminogen activator (tPA) → hemorrhage in right basal ganglia (putamen).
- Hypertension and atrial fibrillation identified after acute admission.
- Family history of early deaths due to cardiovascular disease.
- Nonsmoker. Occasional social drinker. Denies history of hypertension or atrial fibrillation but states that "heart sometimes races" and that he was experiencing bouts of unexplained fatigue. Patient has not seen a medical practitioner in "years."
- Right hemiparesis. Right sensory deficits. Mild dysphagia. Moderate expressive dysphasia and some receptive dysphasia. Dyspraxia. Right homonymous hemianopia.

Interventions

- Physiotherapy, speech therapy, occupational therapy, nursing directed toward safety, improving function, and enhancing activities of daily living (ADLs). Screen for depression.

Outcomes

- Archie worked at all activities with persistence and determination and made good progress. There were no indications of depression.
- After 4 weeks he was discharged home and attended rehabilitation as an outpatient for a further 6 weeks.

Discharge

- At completion of rehabilitation, Archie used a walking stick and walked with a limp, managed normal food and fluids, spoke slowly, was compensating for hemianopia, and had some difficulties with planning. Reading and interpretation of complex materials and instructions remained impaired, with expressive language improved significantly. Some mild right sensory impairment remained but did not significantly affect function. He experienced considerable fatigue and was advised to rest.
- Professional opinion agreed that although he was now disabled and would not be able to return to work or drive a car, Archie's function had improved significantly. They told Archie he had made an excellent recovery and although he might make some small gains in the ensuing months, further recovery was unlikely. Archie was discharged from services.

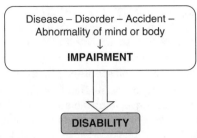

FIGURE 4.1   The medical model—Disability as a consequence of individual impairment.

changing patients' physiological and functional states. Patients are passive recipients of treatment, although they are expected to cooperate and might be held responsible for failing to achieve change (Forhan, 2009; Wade & Halligan, 2004). The medical model has dominated modern professional practice, policy, and societal arrangements for people with disabilities (Longmore & Umansky, 2001.

The medical model assumes disadvantage and reduced quality of life to the point where disability is understood as an individual and family tragedy and is known as the **personal tragedy model**. Through this lens, chronic illness and disability are viewed as medical issues and as personal problems. People are "victims" of their impairments and are "confined by" and "suffering from" their conditions. Such perceptions are maintained by medical dialogue and reinforced in popular culture, which is permeated with representations and the language of tragedy and suffering (Kearney & Pryor, 2004). As an example, we see such "tragedy" in the everyday media where people with disabilities are presented as suffering victims of their conditions and where the perceptions are exploited in charitable fundraising enterprises. People with disabilities claim this thinking defines them and contributes to their segregation from society and to the invalidation of their lives (French & Swain, 2004; Hughes, 2000).

With its emphasis on the management of physiological factors that has reduced mortality and morbidity, the medical model has made powerful contributions to rehabilitation. However, its dominance has resulted in the neglect of psychosocial aspects of rehabilitation, along with the view that disability is "abnormal."

Social Frameworks

Social frameworks move understandings of disability and chronic illness from impairments of individuals' bodies and minds to an emphasis on social environments. Social frameworks argue that disability cannot be understood outside cultural and social contexts. There has been

increasing recognition that social factors are essential in influencing an individual's experience of disability because they determine beliefs, expectations, and roles. Although consideration of social and cultural contexts is now generally included in thinking about disability, it was the development of the social model of disability that challenged the dominance of the medical model. Social frameworks have been expressed in a number of models, such as the social model of the United Kingdom, the social construction model of the United States, the oppressed minority model, the independent living model, and the discrimination model (Pfeiffer, 2001).

In general, social models see disability as a social construct rather than as an attribute of individual people. The most well-known of these, the **social model**, refers to an influential body of work that originated in the experiences of disabled activists in the United Kingdom. The social model emphasizes the collective, structural, and social origins of disability, such as discrimination, oppression, and barriers to participation, rather than the individual, personal, and medical origins (Oliver, 1990) (Figure 4.2).

Oliver (1996, p. 22) summarized the core definition of disability derived from the U.K. activists' more detailed descriptions as follows:

> In our view, it is society which disables physically impaired people. Disability is something imposed on top of our impairments by the way we are unnecessarily isolated and excluded from full participation in society.

We can see from this perspective that disability exists only insofar as it is imposed on people with impairments who are marginalized by societal views of normality. The social model asserts that society disables by creating barriers to independence and that the management of disability requires social action. The social model aligns with others, such as minority group and discrimination models. Whereas the medical model assumes individuals with disabilities must adapt to society, the social model

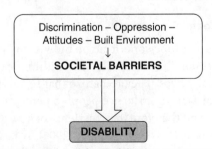

FIGURE 4.2   The social model—Disability as a consequence of societal barriers.

demands adaptations in social structures to accommodate the needs of all people.

The **social construction model** emphasizes the central roles played by language, social interaction, values and beliefs, power relationships, and culture in the construction of meaning in human contexts. It holds that things we believe to be real or factual are actually *constructed* in our thoughts, words, and actions (Danforth, 2001). For example, the notion of *disability* is socially and historically constructed as negative and conjures up a multitude of meanings because of the ways in which people with disabilities have been ridiculed, segregated, oppressed, and excluded from society. To demonstrate such treatment, Bogdan (1986) traced the exhibition of disabled people between 1850 and 1940 in circuses and fairs for the amusement of others and sometimes for the profit of their masters. Less than 50 years ago (and still sometimes today) people with disabilities were frequently hidden away in large institutions, and Blatt and Kaplan's (1966) classic photographic essay is a harrowing catalogue of state-sanctioned abuse in five such facilities. Bogdan and Taylor (1994) argue that the social meanings of intellectual disability are embedded in these past practices, whereas Ferguson, Ferguson, and Taylor (1992) show how such meanings affect life and relationships for disabled people along with their impact on services and professional practice. These examples, and many more besides, demonstrate the powerful force of culture, history, and language on the social construction of disability and the remnants to be found in current thinking and attitudes (Charlton, 1998).

There is a tendency for theoretical discussions about disability and chronic illness to be split and separated according to medical *or* social perspectives. However, binary (medical vs. social) and reductionist (*the* medical model) ways of thinking about chronic illness and disability do not account for the human experience of disability as involving body, the mind and its emotions, and society. Therefore, frameworks that consider the interactions between people and the sociocultural environment are crucial.

Psychosocial Frameworks

Psychosocial frameworks focus on individuals' personal experiences of illness and disability within the contexts of their daily lives. They recognize that social and psychological factors influence people's perceptions and responses and therefore the experience of how it is to be ill or disabled (Wade & Halligan, 2004). A large body of literature theorizes these experiences from different perspectives, and this section outlines some models

---

BOX 4.2   Thinking About Archie Within a Social Framework

- Archie faced major hurdles in returning to life because of societal attitudes and social and physical barriers.
- Although his functional status made return to his former job as a tug boat driver impossible, it is unlikely that he would gain other employment because of his disability and age.
- Although supported by sick leave because of the many years in his job, the family income was compromised and they are now forced to sell their home and move to a smaller property.
- Archie is now perceived as "disabled."
- Because Archie can no longer drive, he is dependent on others for getting out in the world. The suburb he lives in has poor public transport. Even though moving to another house, Archie and Sally want to live in the same area because their community and the gym with Archie's friends are located there.
- His general physical, cognitive, and language "slowness" is perceived negatively by others, and this will be a barrier to social participation.
- The local children who once thought of him as a hero will now make fun of him.

---

and theories that have influenced current thinking and practice, along with some newer approaches and interpretations.

Strauss and Glaser's (1975) groundbreaking work introduced the concept of **chronic illness trajectories** to explain the course of chronic illness. Chronic illness trajectories are more than the medical course of illness. They are linked with people's individual expectations, so that each person defines his or her illness course differently. Individuals' views of their trajectories, along with shifting social relations, affect personal identity, and efforts to maintain social relationships and build new ones contribute to a changed sense of identity. Essential to this interpretation of trajectory is that people play an active role in shaping the illness course over time. This course is affected by the nature of the illness and individual responses, along with input from others such as family, friends, and health professionals. The concept was expanded to a theoretical framework that identified various trajectory phases, along with associated problems and management strategies (Corbin & Strauss, 1988). The framework was translated into a nursing model for chronic illness management (Corbin & Strauss, 1992) and continues to have influence in some approaches to rehabilitation nursing, particularly when considering stroke recovery as a trajectory (Burman, 2001; Burton, 2000; Kirkevold, 2002)

Bury's (1982) classic conceptualization of chronic illness as **biographical disruption** is a continuing theme in much literature related to the experience of illness and disability that interprets the life course as an individual's life plot or *biography* (Becker, 1997; Gisquet, 2008; Kaufman, 1988; Rimmon-Kenan, 2002; Williams, 2000; Yaskowich & Stam, 2003). Bury described three aspects of disruption during chronic illness:

- Disruption of taken-for-granted assumptions and behaviors. People may ask, "What is going on here?"
- Disruptions in explanatory systems that lead to rethinking of individual biography and self-concept. Questions here are of a "Why me?" or "Why now?" nature.
- Practical responses to disruption that include the mobilization of resources. Here context becomes important as resources available to individuals affect consequences and signify meaning.

McAdams (2006) theorizes such disruption as the loss of thematic *coherence* of a person's self-narrative caused by the traumatic nature of an illness event that is difficult to integrate into the plot of the life as it was lived (the past life story). The value of biographical disruption theory lies in its recognition of the meaning of illness and disability as grounded in individuals' own biographies. This is in contrast to models of illness that see illness and disability as diagnostic entities that have predictable responses and courses. According to Bury (1988), illness meanings are unpredictable and emerge as products of change that interact with the structures of everyday life.

In recent times **narrative representations** of chronic illness and disability are receiving increasing attention as ways of understanding and acknowledging experience (Bury, 2001; Mattingly & Garro, 2000; Steffen, 1997). Personal illness narratives *tell* not simply the course of illness but rather of lives altered by illness. They *show* individuals' psychoemotional responses and changes, and also how social contexts and cultural knowledge shape those responses and people's stories (Couser, 1997; Garro, 1994). Frank (2001) notes people's responses to illness as a loss of control and presents storytelling as a process of regaining a new sense of control in that it "confines the catastrophe" (p. 229). Narrative representations provide explanation and meaning to people, with illness and disability narratives differing according to individuals' context and cultural knowledge. For example, a doctor's explanatory narrative of her patient's stroke includes its etiology as an infarct in the left middle cerebral artery caused by a clot associated with atrial fibrillation; her patient's story explains the stroke as caused by a rod falling on her head when she was replacing curtains after their monthly washing. Such differences in story transformed the famous neurologist Oliver Sacks (1984), who wrote an intense experiential account of terror, isolation, alienation, and strange emotional reactions when recovering from a traumatic leg injury. He was astounded by the medical description of "uneventful recovery" exclaiming "Recovery uneventful? It *consists* of events" (p. 124).

Although models and theories are useful as neat summaries of *how things are for people* (populations), they do not tell us *how things are for persons* (individuals). Practice expertise and imagination are enhanced by multiple stories of experience so that difference and particulars for individuals are recognized and valued—an accumulation of such stories contributes to "communities of meaning" (Frank, 2001, p. 243). Classic texts that make significant and continuing contributions to the narrative understanding of illness and disability include Frank (1995, 2002), Kleinman (1988), Moore (1991), Murphy (1990), Sacks (1984), and Zola (1982a, 1982b). Newer works are also making an impression, and they contribute to the growing literature on how things are for persons. Examples include Bauby's (1997) extraordinary *The Diving Bell and the Butterfly* in which he dictates with eye blinks his autobiography although locked-in following a stroke, along with noteworthy accounts by Carel (2008), Hale (2003), Mairs, (1996), McCrum (1998), Oakley (2007), and Seymour (1998).

These experiential frameworks are sometimes referred to as **phenomenological approaches** because they distinguish between the biological body and the lived body. Such frameworks argue that illness and disability are experienced primarily as disruptions to the lived body rather than as bodily impairments and that chronic illness and disability redefine individuals' relationships to their worlds (Carel, 2007, 2008; Toombs, 2001).

Biopsychosocial Frameworks

Recent years have seen changes in the way individuals with chronic illnesses and disability are viewed in society. It is evident that disability is not a consequence of either individual pathology or societal barriers alone but rather is a multidimensional concept experienced by people in multiple ways. Disability and chronic illness are life experiences composed of a complex interplay between the body, the person, and the wider physical, social, and political environment (Imrie, 2004). Biopsychosocial frameworks integrate these biological, psychological, and social dimensions of illness and disability experiences.

Apart from Nagi (1965), few models have addressed the multidimensional nature of disability. However, the World Health Organization's (2001) **International**

BOX 4.3   Thinking About Archie Within a Psychosocial Framework

- Archie and Sally were confused by the information regarding *recovery* and predictions about "little further improvement."
- After being at home for a while, it is evident to them that he is not *recovered*. However, they believe if he continues with rehab he will get better.
- Archie experiences his stroke as a life event—he is shocked and his world is irrevocably changed.
- His hopes and expectations for the future are shattered.
- His sense of self is shattered—he is a different person.
- His identity, grounded in strength, fitness, and control, is lost. He now feels useless.
- Knowing his family's cardiac history, he worked hard at being fit to avoid a similar fate. Now he wonders if excessive exercise might have caused his stroke.
- His doctors have identified hypertension and atrial fibrillation as the likely cause, but he doesn't understand how this would have developed, given his healthy lifestyle.
- He becomes overwhelmed by his losses and, at times when home alone, thinks about suicide.
- Sally increases her work hours.
- Sally takes on responsibility for family life and decisions.
- Sally sees great potential and consults with a language therapist and neuropsychologist for further assessment for Archie and activities to improve his cognitive-perceptual functions.
- Sally insists on Archie working at cognitive exercises (puzzles, workbooks, etc.) when she is at work.
- Sally encourages Archie to return to the gym where he is supported and encouraged by his friends to get moving and fit again. They take an active part in his return to life.
- Sally contacts the local stroke support group and arranges for him to participate.
- Sally mobilizes family and friends to assist with Archie's transportation to gym, stroke group, and household shopping.
- Archie's outlook improves, and he becomes more hopeful.
- Archie decides to undertake driver assessment and training. Over time, he learns to compensate for his hemianopia.

Classification of Functioning, Disability and Health (ICF) was developed after years of international consultation and now has wide recognition and application. It underpins much rehabilitation research and practice across disciplines, undergoes constant debate, revision, and development; and is achieving increasing levels of sophistication (Allan, Campbell, Guptill, Stephenson, & Campbell, 2006; Barbier, Penta, & Thonnard, 2003; Bilbao et al., 2003; Boldt et al., 2005; Dahl, 2002; Duggan, Albright, & Lequerica, 2008; Simeonsson, 2003; Stucki, Ewart, & Cieza, 2003).

The ICF provides a model that represents individual function as a relationship between health conditions and contextual factors. It focuses on components of health and provides a framework for understanding chronic illness and disability as complex products of dynamic interactions between several health domains and personal and environmental contextual factors.

Health domains consist of the following:

- Body functions and structures—and impairments of them (e.g., traumatic spondylolisthesis of L5–S1 causing sciatic pain when walking and standing)
- Activities—and limitations in their performance, (e.g., needs to use walking stick, and very limited tolerance for standing and walking interferes with daily activities such as showering, dressing, cooking, cleaning, work that involves walking around site)
- Participation—and restrictions to it (e.g., unable to use public transportation to go to work due to walking distances to access, and lack of adequate seating on buses and trains; unable to participate in outings that involve walking)

Contextual factors are as follows:

- Physical and social environment—which may hinder or facilitate (e.g., is the physical environment readily accessible? Does a person have family support? Is social and attitudinal environment supportive of people with disabilities?)
- Personal factors—moderate an individual's response to disability (e.g., a person with a resilient personality will adapt more readily; age may have an impact; roles and identity will contribute to the impact of impairment).

Figure 4.3 illustrates these interactions and presents disability as a consequence of breakdowns in health domains and individual contextual factors. Inclusion of the environment and personal factors show how these aspects interact to influence the impact of impairment, illness, or disease on individuals. Simplistically, this means a person with good coping skills, a supportive family, and a flexible and supportive job will likely adapt to a disabling condition more readily than a person with low resilience and little family or social support. In the above example of spondylolisthesis, a person aged 65 who is a teacher and not physically fit may adapt to the situation more easily than a 37-year-old policeman whose identity is grounded in fitness and athleticism. Such interactions help us understand why people with similar impairments and functional losses respond and adapt very differently. Some people do well in the face of significant impairment, whereas others make poor progress and are overwhelmed by their situations.

The ICF provides not only a model for understanding the concept of disability, but also serves as a basis for rehabilitation practice that is both restorative and adaptive (Gladman, Radford, & Walker, 2006). It allows identification of interventions that may target any or all of the domains of health, such as those that reduce impairment, improve activity performance, and promote participation, for example, by treating disease, using exercise therapy, supporting families, and modifying environments.

As previously discussed, beliefs about disability and chronic illness have moved away from an emphasis on biomedical causes to an expanded view that incorporates biomedical, social, and psychosocial frameworks. It is now recognized that the differences between impair-

ments arising from disease and trauma are less important than the shared psychological, social, and economic consequences. This is because the biological courses of different diseases and impairments are of lesser concern than the *impact* of living with symptoms on domains of lives: identity, self-esteem, sexuality, family, education, work, and leisure (Williams, 2001). It is this human experience of illness and disability that matters to individuals and their families, and professional practice is now incorporating concepts that synthesize the impact of pathology and contextual factors on a person's functioning capacity and participation in the world. It is crucial to understand that chronic illness and disability can affect all dimensions of personhood (Johnson & Chang, 2008).

LIVING WITH CHRONIC ILLNESS AND DISABILITY: APPRAISAL AND ADAPTATION

The analytic frameworks for studying chronic illness and disability have shifted away from those that emphasize loss, disruption, and suffering toward more optimistic orientations of health and well-being (Thorne & Paterson, 1998). However, it is important to understand that, particularly in the earlier phases of illness and disability, people's lives are often thrown into chaos and turmoil, multiple losses may be experienced, and emotional distress and grief are frequently experienced. Although specific impairments, illnesses, and their associated disabilities have their own dynamics and components

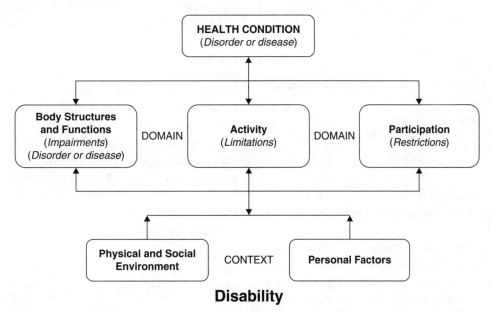

Disability

FIGURE 4.3   Disability as a consequence of dynamic interaction between breakdowns in health domains and individual contextual factors.
(*Source:* after WHO, 2001)

BOX 4.4   Thinking About Archie Within a Biopsychosocial Framework

- All information outlined in Boxes 4.1, 4.2, and 4.3 is now brought together to think about Archie.
- He had a cerebral event (health condition) that was treated with medicine and therapy. However, many functional limitations (impairments) of the stroke remain with him and interfere with his daily activities and participation in the world.
- For Archie and his family he has not recovered, because he is unable to return to his former life. They are experiencing a catastrophic life event.
- Archie has worked hard to support his family, to participate in his community, and to avoid the family history of cardiovascular disease.
- Archie's life roles have been turned upside down, and his identity is threatened. His identity is closely linked with his job, his fitness, being the head of his family, being in control, and being a strong man in his circle of friends.
- However, his strength and fitness can now be harnessed to improve physical function.
- His wife, Sally, is developing an inner strength she didn't realize she had. She is now taking charge and encouraging and organizing her husband to keep working at recovery and to develop hope.
- Sally realizes that Archie will not regain his tug boat license so is organizing the sale of their house and making other arrangements so they will survive financially.
- Even though only 56 years old, Archie will be able to access his superannuation funds.
- Archie really wants to regain his car driving license because he will then be able to get about, not be so dependent, and will get some control over his life.
- Over time, Archie becomes increasingly determined, works hard at fitness, cognitive-perceptual training, and driver training. After 18 months Archie is driving.
- Archie takes over the household activities because Sally increased her work hours.
- He is able to return to many activities and begins kayaking again, although now always in the company of another kayaker.

---

of physical, psychological, and social losses, common threads of response and **adaptation** have been identified (Harvey, 2000).

Chronic illness and disability are commonly associated with multiple **life changes and losses**. Despite certainty about life being only an illusion, people generally take for granted they are following a predictable path over which they have control. The onset of illness and disability may throw lives into chaos where uncertainty

and loss of control prevail. People may have little idea of what is happening or what their futures might now hold. Familiar physical, cognitive, and language functions may be lost; family relationships and roles may change; working capacity may be changed or lost; friends may be lost; autonomy and self-agency may be lost; and identities and selves are changing. Lives are changed—sometimes slowly and in small ways and sometimes suddenly in ways that overwhelm.

For some, these changes and losses are of such significance they are theorized as *shattered assumptions* or as **loss of the assumptive world** (Janoff-Bulman, 1992; Kauffman, 2002a). This theory is grounded in Parkes' (1971, p. 103) classic work on psychosocial transitions where he defined the assumptive world as follows:

> . . . the only world we know and it includes everything we know or think we know. It includes our interpretation of the past and our expectation of the future, our plans and our prejudices. Any or all of these may need to change as a result of changes in the life space.

This theory also resonates with Bury's (1982) descriptions of disruptions of taken-for-granted assumptions, behaviors, and explanatory systems. Life events that involve change or loss may invalidate our assumptions, and when traumatic loss is involved such as may be associated with major illness and injury, assumptive worlds are shattered, along with the ability to believe or assume. The self is violated, the world is no longer secure, and feelings of connection and belonging are severed (Kauffman, 2002b). Such *shattering* is likely to result in distress, grief, and possibly depression. This theoretical construct has been applied in studies related to stroke (Glass & Maddox, 1992; Kearney, 2009), and implicitly underpins much work related to the expanding field of transition theory, which is presented in the section on Adapting to Chronic Illness and Disability.

The following sections first consider how people appraise and cope with changes brought about by illness and disability. Coping theory is presented as a moderator of response and adaptation, and then frameworks for thinking about adaptation to chronic illness and disability are presented.

APPRAISAL OF AND COPING WITH CHRONIC ILLNESS AND DISABILITY

Some illnesses, such as multiple sclerosis and motor neuron disease, creep up slowly and may take time to manifest and be diagnosed. Others, such as arthritis, are manageable for a time but often progress to be severely disabling. And others, such as stroke and traumatic injuries, have a sudden onset. Nevertheless, at some point the personal meaning or relevance of the chronic illness or disability is considered by an individual (Lazarus, 1999).

This initial personal judgment about the meaning or relevance of the situation is known as **primary appraisal** (Lazarus & Folkman, 1984). According to Lazarus (1999), appraising is an active process. Through primary appraisal, Kennedy (2008) notes that the person makes an "initial conceptualization" (p. 60) or representation of their chronic illness or disability and the accompanying emotions (Reynolds & Alonzo, 2000).

According to Reynolds and Alonzo (2000), construction of the representation involves considerations of identity, timeline, and cause of illness or disability and its controllability and consequences. The outcome of primary appraisal is a determination, by individuals, of their situation as positive, neutral, or negative. Situations are deemed negative or stressful when they relate to loss or harm (already sustained or anticipated) and are challenges to be mastered (Lazarus & Folkman, 1984; Taylor, 1999).

Primary appraisal of a situation as negative or stressful triggers **secondary appraisal**, which is an evaluation of the adequacy of available abilities and resources to manage the situation (Taylor, 1999). Chronic illness and disability are commonly appraised as stressful. Recognition that a chronic illness or disability requires additional effort to manage leads to consideration of what might or can be done, another aspect of secondary appraisal. In relation to chronic illness and disability, Moos and Holahan (2007) explain that personal resources, health-related factors, and the social and physical context influence **appraisal**. Consequently, individuals have singular and different appraisals shaped by factors such as culture, social context, biography, family circumstances, age, personality, support systems, nature of the diagnosis and prognosis, and limitations, among others. Song and Nam's (2010) research illustrates how culture seems to account for differences between the coping strategies used by a sample of Asian people with spinal cord injuries and previous studies of Westerners.

Situations may be appraised as taxing or exceeding available resources and endangering well-being, and so stress is the consequence of individual appraisal processes (Lazarus & Folkman, 1984; Taylor, 1999). Livneh and Martz (2007, p. 8) describe the experience of stress as follows:

[A] subjective dynamic, unfolding, and only partially controllable, often unpredictable, and a typically negatively-valenced experience that is triggered by an intricate interaction of internal and external conditions and that disrupt the existing equilibrium.

Consideration of how one might cope with stress associated with chronic illness and disability and undertake adaptive tasks is part of secondary appraisal.

Coping is a powerful mediator and stabilizing factor in psychosocial adaptation to stress. It is classically defined as "constantly changing cognitive and behavioral efforts to manage specific external and/or internal demands that are appraised as taxing or exceeding the resources of the person" (Lazarus & Folkman, 1984, p. 141). Coping, therefore, is work done by an individual "to solve challenges and difficulties" (Middleton & Craig, 2009, p. 24). The specific strategies used by people to cope have been studied both qualitatively and quantitatively. For example, in one qualitative study, 28 older African American adults reported using the following coping strategies to deal with their chronic health conditions: dealing with it, engaging in life, exercising, seeking information, relying on God, changing dietary patterns, medicating, self-monitoring, and self-advocacy (Loeb, 2006). Quantitative studies use a range of coping inventories to investigate specific domains of coping strategies. Two representations of these domains seem to have been particularly influential:

- The domains of problem-focused and emotion-focused coping (Folkman & Lazarus, 1988; Lazarus & Folkman, 1984)
- The domains of approach and avoidance strategies (Holahan, Moos, & Schaefer, 1996; Moos & Holahan, 2007)

Problem-focused coping strategies are directed at the problem or stressor, whereas emotion-focused strategies generally seek to reduce emotional distress (Lazarus & Folkman, 1984). The Ways of Coping Questionnaire (Folkman & Lazarus, 1988), which was informed by the understanding of either problem- or emotion-focused coping strategies, lists eight coping strategies: accepting responsibility, planful problem solving, positive reappraisal, seeking social support, confrontive coping, self-controlling, distancing, and escape-avoidance.

The second representation, approach and avoidance, indicates that a person will try to either tackle a problem or avoid it by focusing on managing the emotional response (Moos & Holahan, 2007). When considering approach and avoidance, both can include behavioral and cognitive strategies (Holahan et al., 1996; Moos & Holahan, 2007). This expands the original two domains into four, with each comprising two coping strategies (Moos & Holahan, 2007):

- Cognitive approach coping (logical analysis and the search for meaning and positive reappraisal)
- Behavioral approach coping (seeking guidance and support and taking problem-solving action)
- Cognitive avoidance coping (cognitive avoidance or denial and acceptance and resignation)
- Behavioral avoidance coping (seeking alternative rewards and emotional discharge)

The choice of coping strategies and functional outcomes seems to be linked to primary appraisal (Moos & Holahan, 2007; Middleton & Craig, 2008). For example, in a study of 122 subjects by Ramirez-Maestre, Esteve, and Lopez (2008), the appraisal of chronic musculoskeletal pain as a challenge was associated with high levels of active (i.e., approach) coping and daily functioning, whereas appraisal of harm, loss, or threat was associated with high levels of passive (i.e., avoidance) coping and low levels of daily functioning, plus more pain and impairment.

This makes reappraisal, a time when new information can be taken into account (Lazarus, 1999; Lazarus & Folkman, 1984), a powerful opportunity for transforming or modifying the appraised meaning and decreasing the threat of chronic illness or disability (Park & Folkman, 1997). This involves comparison of the initial appraised meaning with one's own personal values and beliefs (Park & Folkman, 1997) and evaluation of the effectiveness of the coping strategies being used (Reynolds & Alonzo, 2000).

Although several studies have concluded that some coping strategies are more effective than others, in particular that problem-focused and approach coping strategies are better than emotion-focused and avoidance strategies, Livneh and Martz (2007, p. 20) provide a caution: "effective, or successful, coping requires a flexible and versatile repertoire of coping strategies. . . . Problem-focused coping may be more adaptive under changeable and controllable conditions, while emotion-focused coping may be more adaptive under unchangeable and uncontrollable situations."

Although, generally speaking, coping strategies are used to reestablish "a psychological homeostasis" (Livneh & Martz, 2007, p. 10), the specific functions of coping can be many and varied. Box 4.5 provides Livneh and Martz's summary of these.

BOX 4.5   Functions of Coping

1. Securing accurate information about the demands imposed by the external (i.e., social and physical) environment.
2. Maintaining adequate internal mechanisms to process incoming information and initiating action.
3. Creating stable psychological (emotional) equilibrium that successfully directs energy and skilled behaviors to meet external demands.
4. Making decisions after a search and evaluation of the obtained information.
5. Reducing and, if possible, eliminating harmful environmental conditions.
6. Maintaining a positive self-image and psychological well-being.
7. Increasing tolerance of negative events and situations or changing those situations that trigger stressful experiences.
8. Controlling the meaning of the stressful experiences to thwart their deleterious nature.
9. Reducing existing psychological stress or conflict while it is being experienced.
10. Maximizing the probability of returning to prestress activities.

Source: From Livneh and Martz (2007, p. 13).

In addition to these specific functions, effective or successful coping may also be a moderator of physiological health outcomes. Diamond (2009/2010) warns that chronic health conditions, such as elevated serum glucose, increased blood pressure, and suppression of immune responses, can result from chronic activation of the stress reaction. This makes adapting to chronic illness and disability vital for physiological as well as psychological well-being.

ADAPTING TO CHRONIC ILLNESS AND DISABILITY

Although rehabilitation aims to restore function, this is not always possible, and compensatory function is promoted and taught. Whatever the outcomes, the ultimate goal of rehabilitative practice is to assist individuals to live well and achieve well-being even when living with chronic illness and disability. Therefore, it is important for practitioners to understand adaptation to enable clients and families to move forward toward well-being.

Carel (2007, p. 96) asks, "Can I be ill and happy?", and proposes that a concept of *health within illness* captures the experience of well-being reported by many who live with chronic illness and disability. This concept of health within illness reflects biopsychosocial models of illness because it extends illness and disability from a focus on bodily impairment to include a person's being. This being lives in relationship with the physical and social environment. Studies that analyze such well-being use inductive phenomenological approaches to enable exploration of a diversity of illness experiences that often identify factors such as personal growth, adaptability, self-awareness, meaningfulness, and health (Lindsey, 1996; Moch, 1998). It is now understood that impairment levels do not correlate with subjective health and well-being (Clarke & Black, 2005; deRoon-Cassini, de St. Aubin, Valvano, Hastings, & Horn, 2009; Dunn & Brody, 2008; Wyller & Kirkevold, 1999). We see many people living well despite seemingly overwhelming impairment and disability, whereas others struggle and are miserable in the face of relatively minor conditions.

Albrecht and Devlieger (1999) interviewed 153 people with disabilities of whom 54% with moderate to severe disabilities reported having an excellent or good **quality of life**. They proposed a "balance framework" (p. 986) for understanding quality of life, which depends on finding a balance between body, mind, and spirit in the self and maintaining harmonious relationships with social contexts and external environments. A shift in thinking is required to see health and illness as a continuum or a blend rather than as mutually exclusive opposites, along with a revisioning of possibilities for living a good life within illness and disability (Adame & Knudson, 2008; Carel, 2007; Jarrett, 2000; Sunderland, Catalano, & Kendall, 2009). It is important for rehabilitation practitioners to assist clients to find ways of living well and developing well-being within illness and disability. Understanding adaptation enables us to help clients map their paths.

In the past it was postulated that people needed to pass through a series of stages to cope and adjust adequately to the changes and losses associated with chronic illness and disability. Collectively known as **stage models**, these approaches are based largely on responses to bereavement, most famously Elizabeth Kubler-Ross' (1969) classic work, which holds that people pass through designated psychological stages of shock, denial, anger, bargaining, and depression before coming to *acceptance*. These models had a profound impact on both professional and public thinking, and we see variations and remnants of them in some texts and also applied in practice. Although responses such as shock, anxiety, anger, hostility, denial, and depression are well documented (Livneh & Antonak, 2005), there is now recognition that linear models of adjustment do not account for the complexity

and unpredictability of adapting to illness and disability that is associated with multiple and ongoing stresses and fluctuations (Middleton & Craig, 2009)

Newer theories and models of living with the **grief** engendered by loss stress the complex, nonlinear, dynamic, and self-organizing nature of adaptation that defies clear prediction (Livneh & Parker, 2005). These theories and models also emphasize the normality of a range of individual responses that do not necessarily result in *acceptance* but rather recognize that people may function and live well while grieving for their past lives. Grieving while reconstructing a new life are dual processes that occur in tandem and move recursively and discontinuously (Stroebe & Schut, 2001). When people focus on losses and past lives, grief predominates, but over time as energies shift new lives are forged and reconstruction (adaptation) occurs (even though still grieving). Neimeyer (2001), a leading thinker in current grief practice and theory, holds that **meaning reconstruction** in response to loss is the central process in grieving. These newer models have application for rehabilitation practice as recognized by Roman (2006, 2008) and Kearney (2009), who, in a narrative study of poststroke transition, developed a model that draws on these notions of dual processes of loss and meaning reconstruction. This is expanded on and presented later in this section.

Chronic sorrow was initially described in the 1960s by Olshansky (1962, 1966), a leading rehabilitation counselor, writer, and thinker who developed the concept in his clinical practice with parents of mentally retarded children. He described a persistent and pervasive phenomenon of sorrow which intensified episodically as parents were reminded of their relentless loss. His thinking represented a major and compassionate paradigm shift, because in contrast to prevalent theories that saw extended grief as pathological, Olshansky considered its chronic and recurrent nature as a natural response to a tragic event. Unlike the grief associated with some losses, chronic sorrow cannot be resolved and closure is impossible because the source of the loss continues—it is a "living loss" (Roos, 2002).

In recent decades research has theoretically strengthened the concept (Eakes, Burke, & Hainsworth, 1998), and it now has broad application. It is particularly relevant when working with individuals and families experiencing the enduring losses of "what was" and "what might have been" associated with illness and disability (Ahlström, 2007; Bowes, Lowes, Warner, & Gregory, 2009; Eakes, 1993, 1995; Hainsworth, 1994; Hobdell et al., 2007; Isaksson, Gunnarsson, & Ahlström, 2007; Kearney & Griffin, 2001; Lichtenstein, Laska, & Clair, 2002; Lindgren, Burke, Hainsworth, & Eakes, 1992; Lowes & Lyne, 2000; Stricklin, 2005). Work in the area of chronic sorrow as it relates to people who "are living in the presence of unending losses sustained by the self or a significant other" (Neimeyer, 2002, p. ix) is gathering momentum, and its utility for therapeutic practice is recognized (Gordon, 2009; Roos & Neimeyer, 2007). This is believed to be related to the increasing prevalence of chronic sorrow associated with advancing technology in medicine that increases survival rates and life spans of people with serious illness and disability (Roos & Neimeyer, 2007).

Roos (2002) published a significant book that integrates extant theory and research with experiential accounts and also provides practice guidance for clinicians. Her definition of chronic sorrow, synthesized from the variations in use, captures the elements of chronic sorrow theory (Roos, 2002, p. 26):

> A set of pervasive, profound, continuing, and recurring grief responses resulting from a significant loss or absence of crucial aspects of oneself (self loss) or another living person (other loss) to whom there is a deep attachment. The way in which the loss is perceived determines the existence of chronic sorrow. The essence of chronic sorrow is a painful discrepancy between what is perceived as reality and what continues to be dreamed of. The loss is ongoing since the source of the loss continues to be present. The loss is a living loss.

Roos proposes a dimensional model of chronic sorrow built from this definition that provides a structure for organizing key aspects of loss and its effects. The broad dimensions are

- Characteristics of the loss
- Continuity of the loss
- Initial, continual, and recurring grief responses
- Discrepancy between perceived reality and the continuing fantasy or dream
- Continuing presence of the source or object of the loss

The model can function as a framework for assessment that distinguishes the extent to which personal and environmental factors affect individuals' responses and thus is congruent with ICF.

Adjusting to the *living losses* associated with chronic illness and disability is complex, unpredictable, fluctuating, and individual. In the following sections some ways of thinking about this are presented.

Concepts of **narrative repair** are grounded in models of chronic illness and disability as biographical disruption and are a logical consequence of theories of identity as narrative construction. People have individual biographies, composed of fluid interactions between the many stories surrounding things of value from both self and other perspectives; these constitute selves and identities over time and reflect the culture in which the life is lived and the stories told (McAdams, 2006; Nelson, 2001). When these biographies are disrupted or shattered, efforts are directed toward restoration: living the same stories, living those same lives, being those same people, being in control. However, because illness and disability sometimes have such an overwhelming impact, lives and biographies lose continuity, necessitating their repair and reconstruction.

Western culture places high value on physical attractiveness and ability, as well as cognitive capacity, independence, and self-determination or agency. Societies have particular role expectations related to age, gender, families, work, and communities. Illness and disability hurl people into unimagined lives that challenge self-definitions and identity, for example, when a young football-playing trainee surgeon finds himself with paraplegia after spinal cord injury, or a mother of young children confronts the limitations and progressive prognosis associated with a diagnosis of rheumatoid arthritis. Immediate responses of shock and anger to such situations reflect the internal turmoil and distress caused by the implications and meanings of impairment. However, over time new stories that redefine selves are constructed. The young surgeon, with enormous determination, will eventually switch his studies and specialize in rehabilitation where his experience enhances empathy, insight, and hope. The mother with pain, skeletal deformity, and limited function will take great pride in her children who, of necessity, have become capable, caring, supportive, and interdependent young people. These life stories are rewritten because unanticipated traumatic events resulted in the inability to make sense of the known life stories (Neimeyer, 2006). Such narrative repair, which is also referred to as *reauthoring the self* or *restorying a life*, involves reconstructing self and identity, regaining agency, and creating a new coherent life narrative (Roe & Davidson, 2005; Smith & Sparkes, 2008; Sparkes & Smith, 2005, 2008). Such narrative repair often symbolizes a quest for triumph over time, but within an enduring context of chronic sorrow (Roos & Neimeyer, 2007).

Adapting to chronic illness and disability is a time of change. **Transition theory**, with its emphasis on movement in terms of passing from one state or stage to another or changing into something different, is gathering strength as a framework for thinking about adaptation to chronic illness and disability. Parkes (1971) introduced the concept of psychosocial transitions as a way of thinking about peoples' perceptions of changes in their life worlds. Unexpected major life changes may affect the assumptive world, require the restructuring of ways of looking at the world and plans for living in it, and trigger enduring changes. It is a useful concept in terms of its breadth and inclusiveness and provides conceptual links between phenomena: It does not anticipate stress and crisis, includes notions of the self in interaction with the world, integrates restructuring of the life world, is associated with loss of confidence in the world as secure and reliable, involves processes of realization, and takes account of grief as a consequence of discrepancies between the world as it is and the world as it should be, leading to transitions that involve giving up one set of assumptions for another.

According to Parkes (1971), for satisfactory transition to occur an individual must give up long-held views of the self and the assumptive world and acquire others that are more realistic in the circumstances. He recognized that such transitions do not apply only to individuals but also to families and wider social settings. Parkes' concept of psychosocial transition has contributed to studies related to health/illness transitions. These include living with chronic illness (Jarrett, 2000), adjustment to cancer (Brennan, 2001), transitions for parents after diagnosis of diabetes in their children (Lowes, Gregory, & Lyne, 2005), and life after stroke (Glass & Maddox, 1992; Kearney, 2009; Rittman et al., 2004).

The theoretical development of transition in nursing has been largely driven by Schumacher and Meleis (1994), who conceptualized transitions as occurring during periods of instability precipitated by developmental, situational, health/illness, or organizational change. Such changes are deemed important for nursing because they may generate profound life alterations for individuals and significant others that have implications for health and well-being (Chick & Meleis, 1986). Universal properties of such transitions have been identified as

- Processes that occur over time involving development, flow, or movement
- Processes in which change occurs, the nature of which relates to identities, roles, relationships, abilities, and patterns of behavior in individuals and families, or the structure, function, and dynamics of organizations

These properties differentiate transitions from nontransitional changes and so mark the difference between the changes in chronic illness and the adjustments of self-limiting, acute illness (Schumacher & Meleis, 1994).

In research that focused on the chronic illness experiences of mid-life women, Kralik (2000, 2002) conceptualized the transition experience as a *quest for ordinariness*. Subsequent work has described the process as one of *moving on* in which the reconstruction of a valued self-identity is essential (Kralik et al., 2005). These notions are encapsulated in the definition of transition as "a process of convoluted passage during which people redefine their sense of self and redevelop self agency in response to disruptive life events" (Kralik, Visentin, & van Loon, 2006, p. 321). The concept of transition brings together a range of theoretical frameworks—disruption, illness trajectories, loss of self, and identity reconstruction in biographical work—and is thus significant when thinking about adaptation to chronic illness and disability.

In an effort to derive core theoretical understandings of what it is like to live with chronic illness, Thorne et al. (2002) conducted a metastudy that analyzed and synthesized 292 qualitative inquiries that explored the illness experience of adults. The researchers concluded that there is no single conceptualization to facilitate understanding, practice, or policy but rather a complex tapestry of perspectives influenced by numerous contradictory factors. Their findings are articulated in the **shifting perspectives model** (Paterson, 2001, 2003) which reflects the tensions and fluctuations of daily living with chronic illness. The perspective of chronic illness incorporates elements of illness and wellness that shift in relationship to the degree they are in the foreground or background of individuals' "worlds." Perspectives are representative of values, beliefs, perceptions, expectations, and experiences that dictate the meaning of chronic illness within a certain context. Such perspectives determine response and adaptation to situations affected by illness. As the illness experience progresses and contexts change, individuals' perspectives shift (Paterson, 2001). The model is illustrated in Figure 4.4.

The shifting perspectives model concisely captures and describes the paradox of living with chronic illness and enables an explanation of changes seen in individuals. For example, it is common for people who are newly diagnosed and in the earlier stages of illness to be over-

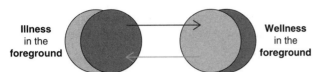

FIGURE 4.4   **The shifting perspectives model of chronic illness.**
(*Source:* after Paterson, 2001)

whelmed by their illness experience. This "illness in the foreground perspective" is characterized by suffering, loss, burden, a focus on the body, and absorption in the illness. By contrast, the "wellness in the foreground perspective" integrates illness into everyday life and focuses on the self as the source of identity, rather than the impaired body. Appraisals of living with chronic illness change over time and are related to many factors, with perceptions of threats to control having the greatest influence (Paterson, 2001). However, perspectives are not static and may shift rapidly according to need and circumstances. For example, poorly controlled pain might necessitate an illness focus, whereas the need to earn a living might promote a wellness perspective. The model succinctly incorporates many of the previously presented concepts and provides an effective interpretive framework for working with clients. Rather than applying a negative label of "denial" to a spinal-injured patient's optimism for the future, we can interpret this as a wellness in the foreground perspective and see it as a healthy shift in perspective.

Dimensions of Adaptability

Most frameworks for thinking about adaptation to chronic illness and disability focus on psychological adjustment; however, Carel (2007) draws attention to the diversity of adaptation at different levels. She highlights the physical, psychological, social, and temporal dimensions of individual adaptability that may occur simultaneously and blend into each other because we are embodied, thinking, relational creatures (de la Mare, 2005). The importance of Carel's thinking lies in its recognition of the need for adaptability arising as responses to changes in the body, not because of a new environment. If the body did not experience negative disruptive change, there would be no need for response and adaptation. However, it is the creative **dimensions of adaptability** that enable people to achieve health within illness, rather than focusing on the negative aspects of the bodily changes. Her thinking draws together much of the preceding frameworks and, with its attention to the body and individual contexts, sits well alongside the ICF. The following examination

of these dimensions of adaptability enables us to see the links.

Diminished bodily capacity (links with ICF domains of impairment and activity limitations) necessitates physical solutions that often happen without thinking. People usually automatically and subconsciously respond and adapt to their changed bodies—slowing down, allowing extra time, taking alternative routes to avoid hills or stairs—and the taken-for-granted nature of the body is replaced with sensitivity to its demands. Most rehabilitative practice is directed at either restoration of or compensation for lost function, and the conscious development of strategies to compensate for lost and altered capacities—learning to walk with a cane, learning to use an electric wheelchair, learning to self-catheterize, learning to communicate using an electronic device—are innovative and creative acts that can promote personal satisfaction and improve quality of life.

Psychological adaptability is usually of a conscious nature and associated with individual resilience, emotional responses, and coping strategies (links with ICF context of personal factors). In this chapter we have considered a number of frameworks that address themes of biographical disruption, meaning, loss, loss of the assumptive world, changes to self and identity, grief and reconstruction, chronic sorrow, narrative repair, and transitions. Such responses to disruption are affected by the availability of resources, such as medical, cultural, social, and financial, and accompanied by their mobilization (links with ICF context of physical and social environment).

Social adaptability (links with ICF domain of participation) takes many forms and is influenced by personality and the environment (links with ICF contexts of physical and social environment and personal factors). The maintenance of social identity or the development of new ones can be difficult in the presence of chronic illness or disability, particularly when impairments of cognition or communication are involved or when role disruption is significant (Rochette, Desrosiers, Bravo, St. Cyr-Tribble, & Bourget, 2007). Social participation is recognized as a major factor in adapting to illness and disability and attaining well-being (Isaksson, Josephsson, Lexell, & Skär, 2007). For some, this may mean continuing with valued activities, whereas for others it means finding new ones to be shared with others when the previous activities are no longer possible. A person with worsening vision might abandon tennis in favor of Tai Chi, or a stroke survivor with hemiplegia and aphasia might sadly leave the patchwork group to participate in a support group where identity can be renegotiated in safety and strength may be gained from a group identity (Barker & Brauer, 2005; Shadden & Agan, 2004; Steffen, 1997).

The temporal dimension of adaptation is ill defined with frequent disparities between objective biomedical concepts of functional "recovery" and the lived experience of illness and disability. Professionals tend to see recovery after injury as time-limited and related to physical outcomes, task achievement, and measured function, whereas for survivors it is an ongoing process that is about identity before the illness; related to being, social existence, and lifestyle; and about meaning (Bendz, 2003; Kearney, 2009). Usually, it takes people considerable time to realize they will not return to those past lives (losses) and adapt to their changed lives and selves. Concepts of transition accommodate temporal dimensions of adaptation.

The preceding sections presented some frameworks for thinking about chronic illness and disability and considered interpretations of living with chronic illness and disability in terms of how people respond and adapt to changed lives. It is evident from the examination of interpretations, models, and theories that living with illness and disability cannot be reduced to a set of coping strategies used by individuals or families and health professionals cannot take a formula approach to clients and families. Rather, a person's full biography and family context, along with the movement backward and forward through illness or injury, rehabilitation, and recovery or adaptation to a changed life must be considered.

In the following section some models that have incorporated aspects of the preceding interpretive frameworks and theories of appraisal and adaptation are presented. It will be useful to consider and identify these aspects as you read.

REFLECTIONS OF INTERPRETIVE FRAMEWORKS: SOME SPECIFIC MODELS

Models that represent the complexity of living with and adapting to chronic illness and disability enable insight that can enhance our professional practice. Following are some models in which we see many reflections of the concepts and interpretive frameworks presented in the previous sections of this chapter.

Researchers in Australia (Koch, Kralik, & Eastwood, 2002; Kralik, Koch, & Eastwood, 2003) have undertaken a series of interrelated inquiries over some years to explicate **transition in chronic illness**. They say that transition is an internal reorientation that occurs over time

when adapting to change (Kralik & Telford, 2005). Kralik and colleagues' model of transition describes movement through phases of "familiar life," "ending," "limbo," and "becoming ordinary." Central to the model is the process of "moving on" when living with chronic illness, and seven interrelated concepts are seen to constitute the process (Kralik et al., 2005):

- Knowing one's response to illness
- Developing inner conviction
- Refraining from making comparisons
- Prioritizing what is important
- Sharing stories with others
- Awareness of shifting one's self-identity
- Being in tune with the process of learning.

This body of work is making significant contributions to self-management programs and the facilitation by health professionals of enabling clients to move on to live well with chronic illness (Koch & Kralik, 2001; Koch, Jenkin, & Kralik, 2004; Kralik, Koch, Price, & Howard, 2004; Kralik & van Loon, 2008; Kralik, van Loon, & Visentin, 2006).

The **Mauk model of poststroke recovery** (Easton, 1999; Mauk, 2006) outlines a six-phase model focusing on the process of stroke recovery. It suggests a framework to guide rehabilitation practice by enabling nursing interventions to be targeted at appropriate times. Mauk emphasizes the nonlinear, multidimensional nature of adaptation to stroke and says that phases may be experienced simultaneously, in different proportions, and over long periods of time. A core concept is that progress to positive adjustment is evident, even though this temporal dimension may be extended. Mauk's six phases, along with their characteristics and survivor tasks, are summarized in Table 4.1.

The **life thread model**, which uses the metaphor of "threads" as stories that represent past lives and future plans, was initially articulated by Ellis-Hill (1998) and has since been developed through research and practice (Ellis-Hill & Horn, 2000; Ellis-Hill, Payne, & Ward, 2000, 2008). The model is grounded in a life narrative approach in which identity change and interpersonal relationships are fundamental. It recognizes stroke recovery as a combination of complex physical, psychological, and social processes taking place over a long time span. After stroke, predictability is lost and threads unravel and fray in a process frequently identified as "biographical disruption." To move on with life and find a new identity, people need to be able to manage the life threads, find a "new me," and learn new rules in an unfamiliar

TABLE 4.1	Mauk Model of Poststroke Recovery	
Phase	**Characteristics**	**Survivor Task**
Agonizing	Fear, shock/surprise, loss questioning, denial	Survival
Fantasizing	Mirage of recovery, unreality	Ego protection
Realizing	Reality, depression, anger, fatigue	Facing reality
Blending	Hope, learning, frustration, dealing with changes	Adaptation
Framing	Answering why, reflection	Reflection
Owning	Control, acceptance, determination, self-help	Moving on

Source: From Mauk (2006).

world. The life thread model supports a view of stroke as a time of transition rather than simply of loss, and its importance lies in the recognition of rehabilitation as not merely a physical process but as important psychological and social processes as well.

Kearney (2009) has extended Ellis-Hill and colleagues' life narrative approach and incorporated concepts of traumatic loss and changes to the assumptive world to represent poststroke transition as a dynamic process that oscillates between grief and reconstruction.

In this model (Figure 4.5), stroke means a loss of expected life and of the future because the assumptive world, with its hopes and expectations, is shattered. Stroke survivors and their families grieve for their losses and their narratives are embedded in the past. However, over time many engage in rebuilding their lives and constructing new meanings and stories. These are concurrent and recursive processes where, as time moves on and energies shift, we see future vision expanding and forward movement escalating. Transition to well-being, interpreted as **reconfiguring the future**, is depicted as a function of meaning reconstruction and the reconfiguration of new life plots. Although this model is derived from an inquiry with only 26 stroke survivors and family members, it holds promise for further development and application in situations where people's lives are unexpectedly shattered by catastrophic illness or injury that has long-term consequences.

SUMMARY

Theories of chronic illness, disability, coping, and adaptation have shifted from relatively simplistic, linear, and predictable models where people are expected to adapt and accept. In the past, failure to adapt and accept has been negatively interpreted by professionals, whereas today we recognize response and adaptation as individual, complex, dynamic, and ambiguous. These conceptual changes have implications for rehabilitation practice in

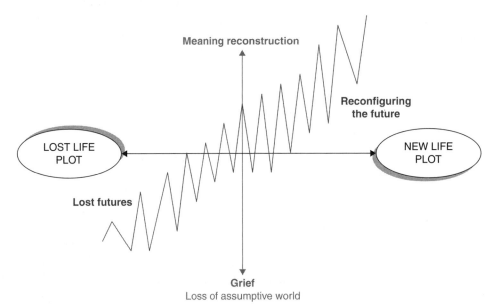

FIGURE 4.5   **Reconfiguring the future: A model of post-stroke transition.**
(*Source:* Kearney, 2009, p.175)

terms of shifts from thinking of clients as "our patients" to working with them as partners (Thorne & Patterson, 1998), along with an emphasis on their capacities rather than their deficits. Today it is vital that we work with clients in terms of their functionality, that is, what people can do within the limitations imposed by their changed bodies (Carel, 2008). We must emphasize capacities and, by competent rehabilitative practice that harnesses individuals' strengths and modifies and makes the most of the environment, enhance and maximize those capacities and develop capabilities using practical opportunities (Mitra, 2006). To do this, practitioners must develop narrative competence that enables effective comprehensive assessment and "tuning in" to critical aspects of people's lives. Narrative competence does not replace scientific competence and a sound knowledge base, rather it allows all that a professional knows to be placed at the service of clients (Charon, 2006).

CRITICAL THINKING

1. Identify aspects of theories, concepts, and frameworks presented in the sections "Frameworks for Thinking About Chronic Illness and Disability" and "Living With Chronic Illness and Disability: Appraisal and Adaptation" that are reflected in the specific models at the end of the chapter.
2. Do you agree or disagree with the comment on p. 38 that relates to Kearney's model: "Although this model is derived from an inquiry with only 26 stroke survivors and family members, it holds promise for further development and application in situations where people's lives are unexpectedly shattered by catastrophic illness or injury that has long-term consequences"? Think about your reasons for agreement or disagreement.

PERSONAL REFLECTION

Imagine you have sustained a catastrophic injury and are undergoing rehabilitation. Think about the things that would be important to you. Try to order these into priority. In your experience of rehabilitation practice, do you believe your priorities would match those of health professionals?

RECOMMENDED READINGS

Blatt, B., & Kaplan, F. (1966). *Christmas in Purgatory: A photographic essay on mental retardation*. Boston: Allyn and Ba-

con. [Photos available at the Disability History Museum at http://www.disabilitymuseum.org/lib/docs/1782card.htm. The site is worth viewing to develop some understanding of the roots of the social meanings of disability.]

Bruyere, S. M., Van Looy, S. A., & Peterson, D. B. (2005). The International Classification of Functioning, Disability and Health: Contemporary literature overview. *Rehabilitation Psychology, 50*(2), 113–121. [Excellent overview of ICF.]

Ellis-Hill, C., Payne, S., & Ward, C. (2008). Using stroke to explore the life thread model: An alternative approach to understanding rehabilitation following an acquired disability. *Disability & Rehabilitation, 30*(2), 150–159. [Brings together life concepts addressed in this chapter for rehabilitation practice.]

Ferguson, P. M., Ferguson, D. L., & Taylor, S. J. (1992). *Interpreting disability: A qualitative reader*. New York: Teachers College Press. [Collection of papers that demonstrates where we derive many of our understandings, interpretations and attitudes to disability.]

Roos, S. (2002). *Chronic sorrow: A living loss*. New York: Brunner-Routledge. [Provides greater detail on chronic sorrow model.]

Royal District Nursing Service of South Australia website: http://www.rdns.org.au/research/projects.php [Many resources, including a series of 11 booklets, related to a large body of work on transition, chronic illness, and self-management.]

REFERENCES

Adame, A. L., & Knudson, R. M. (2008). Recovery and the good life: How psychiatric survivors are revisioning the healing process. *Journal of Humanistic Psychology, 48*(2), 142–164.

Ahlström, G. (2007). Experiences of loss and chronic sorrow in persons with severe chronic illness. *Journal of Clinical Nursing, 16*(3A), 76–83.

Albrecht, G. L., & Devlieger, P. J. (1999). The disability paradox: High quality of life against all odds. *Social Science & Medicine, 48*, 977–988.

Allan, C. M., Campbell, W. N., Guptill, C. A., Stephenson, F. F., & Campbell, K. E. (2006). A conceptual model for interprofessional education: The international classification of functioning, disability and health (ICF). *Journal of Interprofessional Care, 20*(3), 235–245.

Barbier, O., Penta, M., & Thonnard, J. L. (2003). Outcome evaluation of the hand and wrist according to the International Classification of Functioning, Disability, and Health. *Hand Clinics, 19*(3), 371–378.

Barker, R. N., & Brauer, S. G. (2005). Upper limb recovery after stroke: The stroke survivors' perspective. *Disability & Rehabilitation, 27*(20), 1213–1224.

Bauby, J. D. (1997). *The diving-bell and the butterfly*. London: Fourth Estate.

Becker, G. (1997). *Disrupted lives: How people create meaning in a chaotic world*. Berkeley: University of California Press.

Bendz, M. (2003). The first year of rehabilitation after a stroke—from two perspectives. *Scandinavian Journal of Caring Sciences, 17*(3), 215–222.

Bilbao, A., Kennedy, C., Chatterji, S., Ustun, B., Barquero, J. L. V., & Barth, J. T. (2003). The ICF: Applications of the WHO model of functioning, disability and health to brain injury rehabilitation. *NeuroRehabilitation, 18*(3), 239–250.

Blatt, B., & Kaplan, F. (1966). *Christmas in Purgatory: A photographic essay on mental retardation.* Boston: Allyn and Bacon.

Bogdan, R. (1986). Exhibiting mentally retarded people for amusement and profit, 1850–1940. *American Journal of Mental Deficiency, 91*(2), 120–126.

Bogdan, R., & Taylor, S. J. (1994). *The social meaning of mental retardation.* New York: Teachers College Press.

Boldt, C., Brach, M., Grill, E., Berthou, A., Meister, K., Scheuringer, M., & Stucki, G. (2005). The ICF categories identified in nursing interventions administered to neurological patients with post-acute rehabilitation needs. *Disability and Rehabilitation, 27*(7/8), 431–436.

Bowes, S., Lowes, L., Warner, J., & Gregory, J. W. (2009). Chronic sorrow in parents of children with type 1 diabetes. *Journal of Advanced Nursing, 65*(5), 992–1000.

Brennan, J. (2001). Adjustment to cancer—coping or personal transition? *Psycho-Oncology, 10*(1), 1–18.

Burman, M. E. (2001). Family caregiver expectations and management of the stroke trajectory. *Rehabilitation Nursing, 26*(3), 94–99.

Burton, C. R. (2000). Re-thinking stroke rehabilitation: The Corbin and Strauss chronic illness trajectory framework. *Journal of Advanced Nursing, 32*(3), 595–602.

Bury, M. (1982). Chronic illness as biographical disruption. *Sociology of Health and Illness, 4*(2), 167–182.

Bury, M. (1988). Meanings at risk: The experience of arthritis. In R. Anderson & M. Bury (Eds.), *Living with chronic illness: The experience of patients and their families* (pp. 90–116). London: Unwin Hyman.

Bury, M. (2001). Illness narratives: Fact or fiction? *Sociology of Health and Illness, 23*(3), 263–285.

Carel, H. (2007). Can I be ill and happy? *Philosophia, 35*(2), 95–110.

Carel, H. (2008). *Illness: The cry of the flesh.* Stocksfield, UK: Acumen Publishing Limited.

Charlton, J. I. (1998). *Nothing about us without us: Disability, oppression and empowerment.* Berkeley: University of California Press.

Charon, R. (2006). *Narrative medicine: Honoring the stories of illness.* Oxford, UK: Oxford University Press.

Chick, N., & Meleis, A. I. (1986). Transitions: A nursing concern. In P. L. Chinn (Ed.), *Nursing research methodology* (pp. 237–257). Rockville, MD: Aspen.

Clarke, P., & Black, S. E. (2005). Quality of life following stroke: Negotiating disability, identity, and resources. *Journal of Applied Gerontology, 24*(4), 319–336.

Corbin, J. M., & Strauss, A. (1988). *Unending work and care: Managing chronic illness at home.* San Francisco: Jossey-Bass.

Corbin, J. M., & Strauss, A. (1992). A nursing model for chronic illness management based upon the trajectory framework. In P. Woog (Ed.), *The chronic illness trajectory framework: The Corbin and Strauss nursing model* (pp. 9–28). New York: Springer.

Couser, G. T. (1997). *Recovering bodies. Illness, disability and life writing.* Madison, Wisconsin: University Press.

Craig, A., & Perry, K. N. (2008). *New South Wales State Spinal Cord Injury Service: Guide for health professionals on the psychosocial care of people with a spinal cord injury.* Sydney, Australia: NSW Health.

Dahl, T. H. (2002). International Classification of Functioning, Disability and Health: An introduction and discussion of its potential impact on rehabilitation services and research. *Journal of Rehabilitation Medicine, 34*(5), 201–204.

Danforth, S. (2001). A pragmatic evaluation of three models of disability in special education. *Journal of Developmental and Physical Disabilities, 13*(4), 343–359.

de la Mare, B. (2005). The experience of stroke and the life of the Spirit. *Medical Humanities, 31*(2), 105–108.

deRoon-Cassini, T. A., de St. Aubin, E., Valvano, A., Hastings, J., & Horn, P. (2009). Psychological well-being after spinal cord injury: Perception of loss and meaning making. *Rehabilitation Psychology, 54*(3), 306–314.

Diamond, W. J. (2009/2010). Allostatic medicine: Bringing stress, coping, and chronic disease into focus. Part 1. *Integrative Medicine, 8*(6), 40–44.

Duggan, C. H., Albright, K. J., & Lequerica, A. (2008). Using the ICF to code and analyse women's disability narratives. *Disability & Rehabilitation, 30*(12), 978–990.

Dunn, D. S., & Brody, C. (2008). Defining the good life following acquired physical disability. *Rehabilitation Psychology, 53*(4), 413–425.

Eakes, G. G. (1993). Chronic sorrow: a response to living with cancer. *Oncology Nursing Forum, 20*(9), 1327–1324.

Eakes, G. G. (1995). Chronic sorrow: The lived experience of parents of chronically mentally ill individuals. *Archives of Psychiatric Nursing, 9*(2), 77–84.

Eakes, G. G., Burke, M. L., & Hainsworth, M. A. (1998). Middle-range theory of chronic sorrow. *Image: Journal of Nursing Scholarship, 30*(2), 179–184.

Easton, K. L. (1999). The poststroke journey: From agonizing to owning. *Geriatric Nursing, 20*(2), 70–76.

Ellis-Hill, C., Payne, S., & Ward, C. (2008). Using stroke to explore the life thread model: An alternative approach to understanding rehabilitation following an acquired disability. *Disability & Rehabilitation, 30*(2), 150–159.

Ellis-Hill, C. S. (1998). New world, new rules: Life narratives and changes in self-concept in the first year after stroke. Unpublished doctoral dissertation, University of Southampton, Southampton, UK.

Ellis-Hill, C. S., & Horn, S. (2000). Change in identity and self-concept: a new theoretical approach to recovery following a stroke. *Clinical Rehabilitation, 14*(3), 279–287.

Ellis-Hill, C. S., Payne, S., & Ward, C. (2000). Self-body split: issues of identity in physical recovery following a stroke. *Disability & Rehabilitation, 22*(16), 725–733.

Ferguson, P. M., Ferguson, D. L., & Taylor, S. J. (1992). *Interpreting disability: A qualitative reader*. New York: Teachers College Press.

Folkman, S., & Lazarus, R.S. (1988). *Ways of coping questionnaire sampler set manual*. Test booklet, scoring key. Palo Alto, CA: Mind Garden.

Forhan, M. (2009). An analysis of disability models and the application of the ICF to obesity. *Disability & Rehabilitation, 31*(16), 1382–1388.

Frank, A. (2001). Experiencing illness through storytelling. In S. K. Toombs (Ed.), *Handbook of phenomenology and medicine* (pp. 229–245). The Netherlands: Kluwer Academic.

Frank, A. W. (1995). *The wounded storyteller: Body, illness, and ethics*. Chicago: University of Chicago Press.

Frank, A. W. (2002). *At the will of the body: Reflections on illness*. Boston: Mariner Books.

French, S., & Swain, J. (2004). Whose tragedy? Towards a personal non-tragedy view of disability. J. Swain, S. French, C. Barnes, & C. Thomas (Eds.), *Disabling barriers: enabling environments* (2nd ed., pp. 34–40). London: Sage.

Garro, L. C. (1994). Narrative representations of chronic illness experience: Cultural models of illness, mind, and body in stories concerning the temporomandibular joint (TMJ). *Social Science & Medicine, 38*(6), 775–788.

Gisquet, E. (2008). Cerebral implants and Parkinson's disease: A unique form of biographical disruption? *Social Science & Medicine, 67*(11), 1847–1851.

Gladman, J., Radford, K., & Walker, M. (2006). Letter to the editor. *Clinical Rehabilitation, 20*(7), 635–636.

Glass, T. A., & Maddox, G. L. (1992). The quality and quantity of social support: Stroke recovery as psycho-social transition. *Social Science & Medicine, 34*(11), 1249–1261.

Gordon, J. (2009). An evidence-based approach for supporting parents experiencing chronic sorrow. *Pediatric Nursing, 35*(2), 115–119.

Hainsworth, M. A. (1994). Living with multiple sclerosis: the experience of chronic sorrow. *Journal of Neuroscience Nursing, 26*(4), 237–240.

Hale, S. (2003). *The man who lost his language*. London: Penguin.

Harvey, J. H. (2000). *Give sorrow words: Perspectives on loss and trauma*. Philadelphia: Brunner/Mazel.

Hobdell, E. F., Grant, M. L., Valencia, I., Mare, J., Kothare, S. V., Legido, A., & Khurana, D. S. (2007). Chronic sorrow and coping in families of children with epilepsy. *Journal of Neuroscience Nursing, 39*(2), 76–82.

Holahan, C. J., Moos, R. H., & Schaefer, J. A. (1996). Coping, stress resistance, and growth: Conceptualizing adaptive functioning. In M. Zeidner & N. S. Endler (Eds.) *Handbook of coping: Theory, research, applications* (pp. 24–43). New York: John Wiley & Sons.

Hughes, B. (2000). Medicine and the aesthetic invalidation of disabled people. *Disability & Society, 15*(4), 555–568.

Imrie, R. (2004). Demystifying disability: a review of the International Classification of Functioning, Disability and Health. *Sociology of Health and Illness, 26*(3), 287–305.

Isaksson, A. K., Gunnarsson, L. G., & Ahlstrom, G. (2007). The presence and meaning of chronic sorrow in patients with multiple sclerosis. *Journal of Clinical Nursing, 16*(11c), 315–324.

Isaksson, G., Josephsson, S., Lexell, J., & Skär, L. (2007). To regain participation in occupations through human encounters—Narratives from women with spinal cord injury. *Disability & Rehabilitation, 29*(22), 1679–1688.

Janoff-Bulman, R. (1992). *Shattered assumptions: Towards a new psychology of trauma*. New York: The Free Press.

Jarrett, L. (2000). Living with chronic illness: a transitional model of coping. *British Journal of Therapy and Rehabilitation, 7*(1), 40–44.

Johnson, A., & Chang, E. (2008). Chronic illness and disability: An overview. In E. Chang & A. Johnson (Eds.), *Chronic illness and disability: Principles for nursing practice* (pp. 1–13). Sydney, Australia: Elsevier.

Kauffman, J. (2002a). *Loss of the assumptive world: A theory of traumatic loss*. New York: Brunner-Routledge.

Kauffman, J. (2002b). Safety and the assumptive world: A theory of traumatic loss. In J. Kauffman (Ed.), *Loss of the assumptive world: A theory of traumatic loss* (pp. 205–211). New York: Brunner-Routledge.

Kaufman, S. (1988). Illness, biography, and the interpretation of self following a stroke. *Journal of Aging Studies, 2*(3), 217–227.

Kearney, P. M. (2009). *Reconfiguring the future: Stories of post-stroke transition*. PhD thesis. Adelaide: University of South Australia.

Kearney, P. M., & Griffin, T. (2001). Between joy and sorrow: Being a parent of a child with developmental disability. *Journal of Advanced Nursing, 34*(5), 582–592.

Kearney, P. M., & Pryor, J. (2004). The International Classification of Functioning, Disability and Health (ICF) and nursing. *Journal of Advanced Nursing, 46*(2), 162–170.

Kennedy. P. (2008). Coping effectively with spinal cord injuries. In A. Craig & Y. Tran (Eds.), *Psychological aspects associated with spinal cord injury rehabilitation* (pp. 55–70). New York: Nova Biomedical Books.

Kirkevold, M. (2002). The unfolding illness trajectory of stroke. *Disability & Rehabilitation, 24*(17), 887–898.

Kleinman, A. (1988). *The illness narratives: Suffering, healing and the human condition*. New York: Basic Books.

Koch, T., Jenkin, P., & Kralik, D. (2004). Chronic illness self-management: Locating the "self." *Journal of Advanced Nursing, 48*(5), 484–492.

Koch, T., & Kralik, D. (2001). Chronic illness: Reflections on a community-based action research programme. *Journal of Advanced Nursing, 36*(1), 23–31.

Koch, T., Kralik, D., & Eastwood, S. (2002). Constructions of sexuality for women living with multiple sclerosis. *Journal of Advanced Nursing, 39*(2), 137–145.

Kralik, D. (2000). *The quest for ordinariness: Midlife women living through chronic illness.* Doctoral dissertation. Adelaide, South Australia: Flinders University.

Kralik, D. (2002). The quest for ordinariness: Transition experienced by midlife women living with chronic illness. *Journal of Advanced Nursing, 39*(2), 146–154.

Kralik, D., Koch, T., & Eastwood, S. (2003). The salience of the body: Transition in sexual self-identity for women living with multiple sclerosis. *Journal of Advanced Nursing, 42*(1), 11–20.

Kralik, D., Koch, T., Price, K., & Howard, N. (2004). Chronic illness self-management: Taking action to create order. *Journal of Clinical Nursing, 13*(2), 259–267.

Kralik, D., & Telford, K. (2005). *Transition in chronic illness. Booklet 1. Constant change: The shifting experience of illness.* Adelaide, South Australia: Royal District Nursing Service Research Unit.

Kralik, D., Telford, K., Campling, F., Koch, T., Price, K., & Crouch, P. (2005). "Moving on": The transition to living well with chronic illness. *Australian Journal of Holistic Nursing, 12*(2), 13–22.

Kralik, D., & van Loon, A. (2008). Community nurses facilitating transition. In D. Kralik & A. van Loon (Eds.), *Community nursing in Australia.* Oxford, UK: Wiley Blackwell.

Kralik, D., van Loon, A., & Visentin, K. (2006). Resilience in the chronic illness experience. *Educational Action Research, 14*(2), 187–201.

Kralik, D., Visentin, K., & van Loon, A. (2006). Transition: A literature review. *Journal of Advanced Nursing, 55*(3), 320–329.

Kubler-Ross, E. (1969). *On death and dying.* New York: MacMillan.

Lazarus, R. (1999). *Stress and emotion: A new synthesis.* New York: Springer.

Lazarus, R. S., & Folkman, S. (1984). *Stress, appraisal, and coping.* New York: Springer.

Lichtenstein, B., Laska, M. K., & Clair, J. M. (2002). Chronic sorrow in the HIV-positive patient: Issues of race, gender, and social support. *AIDS Patient Care and STDs, 16*(1), 27–38.

Lindgren, C. L., Burke, M. L., Hainsworth, M. A., & Eakes, G. G. (1992). Chronic sorrow: A lifespan concept. *Scholarly Inquiry for Nursing Practice: An International Journal, 6*(1), 27–40.

Lindsey, E. (1996). Health within illness: Experiences of chronically ill/disabled people. *Journal of Advanced Nursing, 24*(3), 465–472.

Livneh, H., & Antonak, R. F. (2005). Psychosocial adaptation to chronic illness and disability: A primer for counselors. *Journal of Counseling & Development, 83*(1), 12–20.

Livneh, H., & Mattz, E. (2007). An introduction to coping theory and research. In E. Martz & H. Livneh (Eds.), *Coping with chronic illness and disability: Theoretical, empirical and clinical aspects* (pp. 3–27). New York: Springer.

Livneh, H., & Parker, R. M. (2005). Psychological adaptation to disability: Perspectives from chaos and complexity theory. *Rehabilitation Counseling Bulletin, 49*(1), 17–28.

Loeb, S. J. (2006). African American older adults coping with chronic health conditions. *Journal of Transcultural Nursing, 17*(2), 139–147.

Longmore, P. K., & Umansky, L. (2001). *The new disability history: American perspectives.* New York: New York University Press.

Lowes, L., Gregory, J. W., & Lyne, P. (2005). Newly diagnosed childhood diabetes: A psychosocial transition for parents? *Journal of Advanced Nursing, 50*(3), 253–261.

Lowes, L., & Lyne, P. (2000). Chronic sorrow in parents of children with newly diagnosed diabetes: A review of the literature and discussion of the implications for nursing practice. *Journal of Advanced Nursing, 32*(1), 41–48.

Mairs, N. (1996). *Waist-high in the world: A life among the nondisabled.* Boston: Beacon Press.

Mattingly, C., & Garro, L. C. (Eds.). (2000). *Narrative and the cultural construction of illness and healing.* Berkeley: University of California Press.

Mauk, K. L. (2006). Nursing interventions within the Mauk model of poststroke recovery. *Rehabilitation Nursing, 31*(6), 257–264.

McAdams, D. P. (2006). The problem of narrative coherence. *Journal of Constructivist Psychology, 19*(2), 109–125.

McCrum, R. (1998). *My year off: Recovering life after a stroke.* New York: W. W. Norton.

Middleton, J., & Craig, A. (2009). Psychological challenges in treating persons with spinal cord injury. In A. Craig & Y. Tran (Eds.), *Psychological aspects associated with spinal cord injury rehabilitation: New directions and best evidence* (pp.3–53). New York: Nova Science.

Mitra, S. (2006). The capability approach and disability. *Journal of Disability Policy Studies, 16*(4), 236–247.

Moch S.D. (1998). Health-within-illness: Concept development through research and practice. *Journal of Advanced Nursing, 28*(2), 305–310.

Moore, T. (1991). *Cry of the damaged man.* Sydney: Picador.

Moos, R. H. & Holahan, C. J. (2007). An introduction to coping theory and research. In E. Martz & H. Livneh (Eds.), *Coping with chronic illness and disability: Theoretical, empirical and clinical aspects* (pp. 107–126). New York: Springer.

Murphy, R. F. (1990). *The body silent.* New York: W. W. Norton.

Nagi, S. Z. (1965). Some conceptual issues in disability and rehabilitation. In M. B. Sussman (Ed.), *Sociology and rehabilitation* (pp. 100–113). Washington, DC: National Academy Press.

Neimeyer, R. A. (2001). *Meaning reconstruction and the experience of loss.* Washington, DC: American Psychological Association.

Neimeyer, R. A. (2002). Series editor's foreword. In S. Roos (Ed.), *Chronic sorrow: A living loss* (pp. ix–xi). New York: Brunner-Routledge.

Neimeyer, R. A. (2006). Restorying loss: Fostering growth in the posttraumatic narrative. In L. G. Calhoun & R. G. Tedeschi (Eds.), *Handbook of posttraumatic growth: Research and practice* (pp. 68–80). Mahwah, NJ: Lawrence Erlbaum.

Nelson, H. L. (2001). *Damaged identities, narrative repair*. Ithaca, NY: Cornell University Press.

Oakley, A. (2007). *Fracture: Adventures of a broken body*. Bristol, UK: The Policy Press.

Oliver, M. (1990). *The politics of disablement*. London: Macmillan.

Oliver, M. (1996). *Understanding disability. From theory to practice*. Basingstoke, England: Macmillan Press Ltd.

Olshansky, S. (1962). Chronic sorrow: A response to having a mentally defective child. *Social Casework, 43*, 190–193.

Olshansky, S. (1966). Parent responses to a mentally defective child. *Mental Retardation, 5*(4), 21–23.

Park, C. L., & Folkman, S. (1997). Meaning in the context of stress and coping. *Review of General Psychology, 1*(2), 115–144.

Parkes, C. M. (1971). Psychosocial transitions: A field for study. *Social Science & Medicine, 5*, 101–115.

Paterson, B. L. (2001). The shifting perspectives model of chronic illness. *Journal of Nursing Scholarship, 33*(1), 21–26.

Paterson, B. L. (2003). The koala has claws: Applications of the shifting perspectives model in research of chronic illness. *Qualitative Health Research, 13*(7), 987–994.

Pfeiffer, D. (2001). The conceptualization of disability. In B. M. Altman & S. Barnartt (Eds.), *Exploring theories and expanding methodologies* (Vol. 2). *Research in social science and disability*. Oxford: Elsevier.

Ramirez-Maestre, C., Esteve, R. & Lopez, A. E. (2008). Cognitive appraisal and coping in chronic pain patients. *European Journal of Pain, 12*, 749–756.

Reynolds, N. R., & Alonzo, A. A. (2000). Self-regulation: The commonsense model of illness representation. In V. H. Rice (Ed.) *Handbook of stress, coping and health: Implications for nursing research, theory, and practice* (pp. 483–494). Thousand Oaks, CA: Sage.

Rimmon-Kenan, S. (2002). The story of "I": Illness and narrative identity. *Narrative, 10*(1), 9–27.

Rittman, M., Faircloth, C., Boylstein, C., Gubrium, J. F., Williams, C., Van Puymbroeck, M., & Ellis, C. (2004). The experience of time in the transition from hospital to home following stroke. *Journal of Rehabilitation Research & Development, 41*(3A), 259–268.

Rochette, A., Desrosiers, J., Bravo, G., St. Cyr-Tribble, D., & Bourget, A. (2007). Changes in participation after a mild stroke: quantitative and qualitative perspectives. *Topics in Stroke Rehabilitation, 14*(3), 59–68.

Roe, D., & Davidson, L. (2005). Self and narrative in schizophrenia: Time to author a new story. *Medical Humanities, 31*(2), 89–94.

Roman, M. W. (2006). The process of recovery: a tale of two men. *Issues in Mental Health Nursing, 27*(5), 537–557.

Roman, M. W. (2008). Lessons learned from a school for stroke recovery. *Topics in Stroke Rehabilitation, 15*(1), 59–71.

Roos, S. (2002). *Chronic sorrow: A living loss*. New York: Brunner-Routledge.

Roos, S., & Neimeyer, R. A. (2007). Reauthoring the self: Chronic sorrow and posttraumatic stress following the onset of CID. In E. Martz & H. Livneh (Eds.), *Coping with chronic illness and disability: Theoretical, empirical and clinical aspects* (pp. 89–106). New York: Springer.

Sacks, O. (1984). *A leg to stand on*. London: Picador.

Schumacher, K. L., & Meleis, A. l. (1994). Transitions: a central concept in nursing. *Journal of Nursing Scholarship, 26*(2), 119–127.

Seymour, W. (1998). *Remaking the body: Rehabilitation and change*. Sydney, Australia: Allen & Unwin.

Shadden, B. B., & Agan, J. P. (2004). Renegotiation of identity: the social context of aphasia support groups. *Topics in Language Disorders, 24*(3), 174–186.

Simeonsson, R. J. (2003). Classification of communication disabilities in children: Contribution of the International Classification on Functioning, Disability and Health. *International Journal of Audiology, 42*(1), S2–S8.

Smith, B., & Sparkes, A. C. (2008). Changing bodies, changing narratives and the consequences of tellability: A case study of becoming disabled through sport. *Sociology of Health & Illness, 30*(2), 217–236.

Song, H. Y., & Nam, K. A. (2010). Coping strategies, physical function, and social adjustment in people with spinal cord injury. *Rehabilitation Nursing, 35*(1), 8–15.

Sparkes, A. C., & Smith, B. (2005). When narratives matter: Men, sport, and spinal cord injury. *Medical Humanities, 31*(2), 81–88.

Sparkes, A. C., & Smith, B. (2008). Men, spinal cord injury, memories and the narrative performance of pain. *Disability & Society, 23*(7), 679–690.

Steffen, V. (1997). Life stories and shared experience. *Social Science & Medicine, 45*(1), 99–111.

Strauss, A. L., & Glaser, B. G. (1975). *Chronic illness and the quality of life*. St. Louis, MO: Mosby.

Stricklin, S. M. (2005). Nursing diagnosis: Chronic sorrow. *Journal of Christian Nursing, 22*(3), 37–38.

Stroebe, M. S., & Schut, H. (2001). Meaning making in the dual process model of coping with bereavement. In R. A. Neimeyer (Ed.), *Meaning reconstruction and the experience of loss* (pp. 55–73). Washington, DC: American Psychological Association.

Stucki, G., Ewert, T., & Cieza, A. (2003). Value and application of the ICF in rehabilitation medicine. *Disability & Rehabilitation, 25*(11–12), 628–634.

Sunderland, N., Catalano, T., & Kendall, E. (2009). Missing discourses: Concepts of joy and happiness in disability. *Disability & Society, 24*(6), 703–714.

Swain, J., Finkelstein, V., French, S., & Oliver, M. (1993). *Disabling barriers—Enabling environments*. London: Sage.

Taylor, S. E. (1999). *Health psychology* (4th ed.). Boston: McGraw-Hill.

Thorne, S., & Paterson, B. (1998). Shifting images of chronic illness. *Image: Journal of Nursing Scholarship, 30*(2), 173–178.

Thorne, S., Paterson, B., Acorn, S., Canam, C., Joachim, G., & Jillings, C. (2002). Chronic illness experience: Insights from a metastudy. *Qualitative Health Research, 12*(4), 437–452.

Toombs, S. K. (2001). *Handbook of phenomenology and medicine.* The Netherlands: Kluwer Academic.

Wade, D. T., & Halligan, P. W. (2004). Do biomedical models of illness make for good healthcare systems? *BMJ, 329*(7479), 1398–1401.

Williams, G. (2001). Theorizing disability. In G. L. Albrecht, K. D. Seelman, & M. Bury (Eds.), *Handbook of disability studies* (pp. 123–144). Thousand Oaks, CA: Sage.

Williams, S. J. (2000). Chronic illness as biographical disruption or biographical disruption as chronic illness? Reflections on a core concept. *Sociology of Health & Illness, 22*(1), 40–67.

World Health Organization. (2001). *International Classification of Functioning, Disability and Health.* Geneva: World Health Organization.

Wyller, T. B., & Kirkevold, M. (1999). How does a cerebral stroke affect quality of life? Towards an adequate theoretical account. *Disability & Rehabilitation, 21*(4), 152–161.

Yaskowich, K. M., & Stam, H. J. (2003). Cancer narratives and the cancer support group. *Journal of Health Psychology, 8*(6), 720–737.

Zola, I. K. (1982a). *Ordinary lives: Voices of disability and disease.* Cambridge, MA: Applewood Books.

Zola, I. K. (1982b). *Missing pieces. A chronicle of living with a disability.* Philadelphia: Temple University Press.

CHAPTER 5

Interdisciplinary Rehabilitation Team

Judi Behm
Nancy Gray

LEARNING OBJECTIVES

At the end of this chapter, the reader will be able to

- Define the term *interdisciplinary team*.
- Recognize the benefits of team collaboration.
- Discuss the roles of each member of the interdisciplinary team.
- Contrast various team models used in rehabilitation.
- Describe characteristics of an effective interdisciplinary team.
- Recognize benefits and challenges of working within interdisciplinary teams.

KEY CONCEPTS AND TERMS

Advanced practice nurses	Interdisciplinary model	Physical Medicine and
Case manager	Interdisciplinary teams (IDTs)	Rehabilitation
Collaboration	Medical model	Physical therapists
Collaborative discussion	Multidisciplinary model	Psychologists
Dieticians	Nurses	Speech-language pathologist
Emotional intelligence	Occupational therapists	Social workers
Group dynamics	Physiatrists	Team competence

BACKGROUND AND HISTORY

Rehabilitation involves the successful and productive interaction of many stakeholders. The patient and family, physician, nurses, psychologists, therapists, social workers and case managers, dieticians, chaplains, payers, and, at times, even lawyers and employers are all collaborators in a process of joint decision making with a goal of achieving a sustainable outcome: return to the highest level of productivity possible for the patient. Central to contemporary rehabilitation philosophy, well-functioning **interdisciplinary teams (IDTs)** are critical for service integration and successful outcomes (Strasser, Uomoto, & Smits, 2008). The ever-increasing complexity of healthcare interventions and the myriad challenges that impede patients in their quest to return to productivity demand an interface between all healthcare professionals.

> *The interdisciplinary team continues to provide more combined knowledge and skill, clinical expertise, sensitivity, compassion, and understanding for individuals with disabilities than can be found in any other area of health care. . . .The individual team members each bring a unique perspective and expertise to the collective planning of the group. But the team shares similar goals for the patient.*
>
> *Easton, 1999, p. 31*

Ample evidence in multiprofessional, peer-reviewed literature supports collaborative practice as a strategy to produce optimal patient outcomes, and the IDT is one vehicle to implement that strategy. As early as 1900, interdisciplinary healthcare teams were active in the mission hospitals of India. In the United States the concept of teamwork was advanced by nursing theorist, Dorothy

Rogers (1932), as a means of achieving professional acceptance for nursing and allied health professionals. The IDT, as it is known today, emerged after World War II in response to the complex needs of wounded soldiers who survived injuries due to advances in medical care, such as antibiotics. The mandate to provide comprehensive treatment for service men and women with severe injuries and disabilities that could not be managed by a single-discipline medical model gave rise to the notion that multiple healthcare professionals could effectively and efficiently meet the needs of this population. From that point, the IDT (composed of all members of the treatment team as well as the patient and family) became the gold standard for the care coordination process. Eventually, the IDT became the cornerstone of a new field of medicine, **Physical Medicine and Rehabilitation** (Strasser et al., 2008), which focused on the restoration of patient capabilities.

Concurrently, in the 1950s social and behavioral scientists made substantial contributions to the structure, function, and process of small groups. Social psychologist, Kurt Lewin (1951), led the field of pioneers in **group dynamics** by proposing that a group is more than the sum of individuals in it. Lewin offered a context whereby well-functioning groups could be evaluated and proposed that effective group process could be taught and developed. This heralded the recognition that team leaders must possess particular skills. Today, it is accepted that interpersonal skills, including communication and negotiation skills, a willingness to compromise, and an ability to value and accept individual differences, are vital to the IDT process. Also understood is that effective team membership requires an awareness of one's own talents, limitations, and biases as well as an appreciation of the talents, limitations, and biases of other team members (Rossen, Bartlett, & Herrick, 2008).

Interest in interdisciplinary **collaboration** has exploded in the past two decades due to the increasing complexity of patient care and efforts to manage escalating healthcare costs. Research studies indicate that IDT collaboration enhances patient compliance, improves patient satisfaction, reduces costs, lowers mortality, reduces length of stay, and increases team member job satisfaction (Rubenfeld and Scheffer, 2010). That kind of efficiency is necessary in today's healthcare climate because consumers expect healthcare teams that are not only technically and emotionally competent, but that also are capable of blending professional boundaries when it is in the patient's best interest. Regulatory and accredi-

tation bodies, such as the Joint Commission, Commission on Accreditation of Rehabilitation Facilities, state departments of health, and the Centers for Medicare & Medicaid (Box 5.1) have identified IDTs as necessary for patient safety and quality care, and each organization has specific criteria to demonstrate compliance related to IDT function.

BOX 5.1   Web Resources
The Joint Commission: http://www.jointcommission.org
The Commission for Accreditation of Rehabilitation Facilities (CARF): http://www.carf.org
Institute of Medicine (IOM): http://www.iom.edu

The IDT is widely accepted in healthcare today, particularly in the areas of mental health and rehabilitation. The goal of the IDT is to provide well-coordinated care by marshaling the talents of multiple professionals in concert with the patient (Bokhour, 2006). Healthcare consumers expect high-quality, transparent care with optimal outcomes. Because of a variety of available World Wide Web databases, consumers are able to "shop" for care that meets the necessary criteria. All payers, whether managed care organizations or government entities, challenge healthcare organizations to demonstrate efficacy and value. Maintenance of provider–payer contracts hinges on providing metrics that support the "value-added" benefit of IDT-based treatment programs. Ultimately, in an unpredictable economy it is imperative that multisystem interventions by an IDT use combined skills to meet the rehabilitative needs of patients with complex injuries to ensure optimal outcomes at the lowest cost in the shortest possible lengths of stay.

In the final analysis, the value of the IDT can be attributed to one basic fact: Decisions made synergistically produce higher quality solutions than those made independently (Gage, 1998). To become an effective member of an IDT, it is important to understand not only the origins of the concept, but the variety of team models, members, and their roles and how to achieve IDT competence and success.

BOX 5.2   Web Exploration
Visit this interesting website that offers articles, games, activities, and books about team building at http://teambuildingportal.com

TEAM MODELS

The healthcare field, like the corporate world, has identified that working together toward a common goal or project is cost effective and more productive than working individually. Looking for ways to improve quality and decrease the cost of health care has been an ongoing goal, and in pursuit of that goal four main models of professional teams have been developed and practiced over the years: medical, multidisciplinary, interdisciplinary, and transdisciplinary models.

Medical Model

In the **medical model** the physician directs all care (Figure 5.1). This model can be effective in physician offices and sometimes in acute care settings when few professionals outside of medicine and nursing are involved in the patient's care. It is not an effective model in rehabilitation settings because the philosophy and goals are not consistent with rehabilitation practice, which includes all levels and disciplines of staff working together, communicating treatment plans, and collaborating on a consistent basis as they provide care.

Medical Model

- Communication is more vertical than lateral
- Usually physician driven
- Approach effective when discipline is ordered as consult

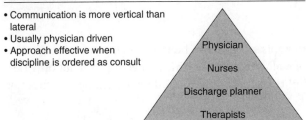

Physician
Nurses
Discharge planner
Therapists

FIGURE 5.1   The medical model.

Multidisciplinary Model

Professionals in the **multidisciplinary model** (Figure 5.2) usually work independently to accomplish discipline-specific goals. Sharing information and making decisions based on that information, these team members may not directly communicate with all team members regarding care planning (Albrecht, Higginbotham, & Freeman, 2001). Communication is more vertical than lateral, and team members do not usually participate in team conferences. Sheehan, Robertson, and Ormond (2007) note that members working independently often lack a common understanding of issues that could influence interventions. Therefore, this model is not seen as being as effective for rehabilitation programs as some others.

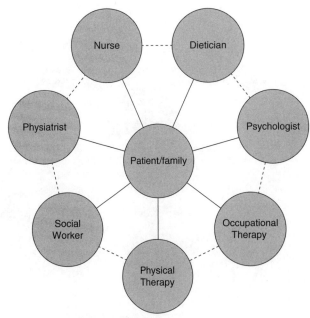

FIGURE 5.2   Multidisciplinary model.

An example of this model might be seen in an acute care setting when a physician orders physical therapy for ambulation education and occupational therapy to assess activities of daily living with a person who sustained a lower extremity fracture and sprained wrist as result of an accident. Each therapist would perform an assessment, treat according to their discipline, and document their interventions without any collaboration with other team members.

BOX 5.3   Don't Forget the Silent Team Member!!

Hovering in the background, but never far from the action, are the payers: managed care entities (Blue Cross/Anthem, United Health Care, Aetna, etc.), Medicare, and Medicaid. They review team documentation, either concurrently (managed care) or retrospectively (Medicare), and base hospital payment on outcomes achieved in a timely manner. The nurse case manager or utilization review nurse usually plays a pivotal role in keeping the team aware of the requirements and limitations of these "silent team members" as well as acting as an intermediary between the team and the payer.

Interdisciplinary Practice Model

The **interdisciplinary model** (Figure 5.3), which may also be referred to as an interprofessional model (Sheehan et al., 2007), uses a more collaborative approach. The key factor that makes this model different from the multidisciplinary model is that team members work together

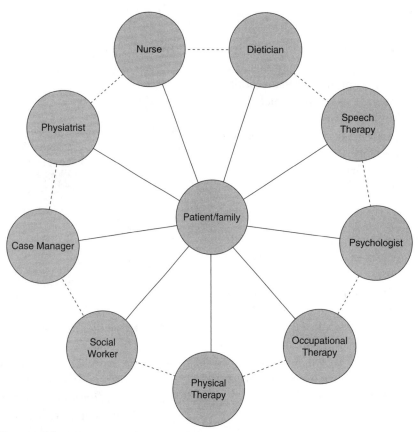

FIGURE 5.3 Interdisciplinary model.

in goal setting, treatment, decision making, and ongoing problem solving to ensure continuity of care and a more holistic approach (Albrecht et al., 2001). Patients and families are an integral part of the team. Communication between all members of the team is crucial to ensure all members, including the patient, are part of the decision and care planning process.

In comparing the two most common models (interdisciplinary and multidisciplinary), it can be seen that in rehabilitation settings the interdisciplinary approach is more effective because it allows for a more holistic, collaborative, and patient-focused approach. From the time of admission to discharge the patient and team work together to establish, evaluate, and accomplish mutually agreed on goals.

Transdisciplinary Model

In this model one team member is the primary provider (Figure 5.4). Guided by the other team members, the primary team member provides services to the patient. Team members are cross-trained in several areas besides their own specialty. Although the nurse may be the primary provider, a therapist who receives direction from other

therapists could also be the primary provider. Because of a blurring of roles, this model requires not only flexibility but willingness of all team members to function

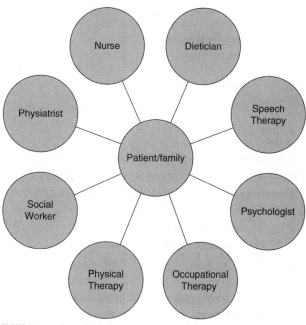

FIGURE 5.4 Transdisciplinary model.

in this framework (Mumma & Nelson, 1996). Nursing home facilities may use this model in their restorative care program. If a resident has a change in status, a therapist may be ordered to reevaluate a resident and make recommendations. It is then the nurses' responsibility to see that those interventions are incorporated into the resident's care plan and carried out on a daily basis.

For this model to be effective, staff must be cross-trained to perform any duties that are normally discipline specific so the patient receives appropriate treatment regardless of who is caring for the patient. This is time consuming and often presents a level of discomfort for team members to learn skills that were not included in their basic educational program. However, in some instances, for example with infants and children, this model can be an effective method to provide early intervention services, using a developmental approach to interventions versus discipline-specific approach.

BENEFITS AND CHALLENGES OF MODELS

Benefits of functioning in an effective IDT include increased continuity of services, collaboration toward goal achievement, shared understanding and problem solving between professionals, valuing of team members, and greater patient, family, and staff satisfaction (Sheehan et al., 2007). Although IDT functioning offers numerous benefits to the patient and family as well as their team members, studies have shown there can be challenges as well. According to Strasser, Falconer, and Martino-Saltzmann (1994), two challenge areas are conflicts regarding professional boundaries and defensiveness from team members who believe their professional judgment is being questioned. The tendency to function within the professional boundaries in which one was educated can lead to disciplinary silos and impede efforts toward collaborative thinking (Herbert et al., 2007).

Communication is a key factor in thinking and functioning collaboratively as a team, and discipline-specific language, or jargon, has been identified as a limiting factor when creating a well-functioning team. Nurses, like other disciplines, are educated within certain domains and have their own "language"; therefore, when we work with other members of the team there is potential difficulty in speaking with a unified, interdisciplinary voice. Bokhour (2006), in a study on communication in interdisciplinary team meetings, found that "**collaborative discussion**" occurs when team members step out of their discipline-specific framework and focus on patient's needs, allowing for a more open dialogue and exchange of ideas. Sheehan et al. (2007) found that more effective teams used inclusive language in their discussions. Other factors identified that can have an enormous impact on the success of a team include personality differences and emotional intelligence (McCallin & Bamford, 2007), addressed later in this chapter.

MEMBERS OF THE REHABILITATION TEAM

The interdisciplinary team consists of a number of disciplines and is dictated by the service needs of the patient. The core team for most inpatients in a rehabilitation setting includes

- Patient and family
- **Nurses:** registered nurses and licensed practical nurses
- **Advance practice nurses:** clinical nurse specialists and nurse practitioners
- **Physiatrists:** doctor of physical medicine and rehabilitation
- Therapists: **Physical** and **occupational therapists**, **speech-language pathologists**, recreational therapists, and respiratory therapists (as needed)
- **Psychologists**
- **Case managers** (some facilities will have related positions such as utilization review nurses, care coordinators, nurse navigators, MDS nurses, and coding specialist that may also be part of the team)
- **Social workers**
- **Dieticians**
- Chaplains

Depending on the size of the facility/organization and extent of services provided, patients may also receive services from vocational specialists, orthotists/prosthetists, biomedical engineers, and audiologists as needed. Additionally, alternative services, such as music and pet therapy, may be available.

Role of Team Members

Professional members of the team may function in several roles: as a care provider, patient advocate, or a coordinator of care. Larger interdisciplinary teams, common in most rehabilitation units or facilities, often include both a social worker/discharge planner and a case manager. Case managers are routinely seen as the coordinator of care and may share the role of team leader with the physician. Each member of the team brings with them discipline-specific expertise. Table 5.1 provides brief descriptions of each team member.

TABLE 5.1	Team Member Roles With Examples	
Discipline	**Primary Role in the Team**	**Examples of Collaboration With Other Team Members**
Physiatrist	Responsible for physical medicine and rehabilitation management of patient's care.	Often leads the team. Orders assessment and ongoing treatment in collaboration with team.
Staff nurse	Coordinates and provides day-to-day patient care. Educates patient/family regarding medical and health issues as well as skills needed to provide safe health care (i.e., catheterization skills, bowel programs, skin maintenance/wound management). Patient advocate.	Supports and coaches patients to practice newly learned skills. Cues them as needed. Provides feedback to therapists re: patient ability to follow through with skill and if there are cognitive, behavioral, or physical changes during the day that are impacting patient's ability to consistently perform on unit.
Physical therapist (PT)	Maximizes patient function by working with patients to improve gross motor skills. Focuses on mobility, including ambulation, balance, W/C skills, Provides modalities for pain management.	PT and OT work together to develop strength, balance, and teaching skills needed for ADLs. Patient works on W/C transfers, whereas OT incorporates what PT has taught patient to practice toilet transfers, and instructs patient on clothing management, personal hygiene.
Occupational therapist (OT)	Assist patient gain maximal function in areas of ADLs.	OT and PT collaborate to assist patient to become functional with all components of skills/ADLs.
Speech-language pathologist (SLP)	Evaluates and treats cognition, communication, swallowing disorders, and hearing deficits.	Communicates with team regarding patient communication needs, how to cue patient when learning an activity, impact of cognitive deficits on ability to learn and retain information. Communicates with team regarding feeding and swallowing disorders and works with physicians, nurses, and dieticians about appropriate food and liquid consistencies, compensatory strategies to maintain safe swallow.
Therapeutic recreation (TR)	Assists patients to reenter their community and helps patients adapt so they can enjoy leisure activities.	Incorporates what patient has learned from other disciplines to assist patient with community reentry and leisure activities in preparation for patient discharge.
Respiratory therapist (RT)	Evaluates and treats a patient's breathing, including assist of ventilation as needed.	Supports maintenance of respiratory status and prevention of complications related to inactivity. Works with PT to increase tolerance for increased mobility.
Neuropsychologist	Evaluates cognitive and behavior status, assists in the adjustment to illness/disability. Provides support to patient and family as they come to grips with issues related to illness/disability.	Works with team regarding cognitive and behavioral needs of patients, developing appropriate plans of care related to cognitive and behavioral management.
Case manager	Coordinates implementation of treatment plan, communicates insurance benefit information to patient/families and the team. Advocates for services. Acts as liaison between patient, hospital, and payer. Provides updated information to insurance companies. Coordinates optimal use of available benefits.	Coordinates team to look at patient days, status of insurance to assist in planning for discharge, and to keep members mindful of time allotted to accomplish goals

TABLE 5.1	Team Member Roles With Examples *(Continued)*	
Discipline	**Primary Role in the Team**	**Examples of Collaboration With Other Team Members**
Social worker/ discharge planner	Focuses on psychosocial support. Prepares patients and families for discharge. Identifies supportive services, resources needed after discharge. Links patient/family to community physicians, services, home health care, long-term care facilities, and medical equipment providers.	Communicates patient/family wishes regarding necessary services. Collaborates with team regarding patient's needs. Communicates status of services obtained. Works with case management in coordinating all written information that will go home with patient. Provides necessary information about patient to community providers to ensure continuity of care.
Dietician	Oversees patient's nutritional status and works with physician to provide necessary dietary requirements; provides patient/family education on diets.	Collaborates with team to adapt diet according to patient's needs. Monitors calories, labs as patient's needs change. Works with patient/family to provide foods of preference within dietary restrictions. Communicates nutritional status to team.
Advanced practice nurse (CNS /nurse practitioner)	Conducts comprehensive assessment. Integrates education, research, and consultation into clinical practice	Collaborates with nursing peers, interdisciplinary team, including physician, regarding evidenced-based practice. Integrates education, research and consultation into clinical practice.
Chaplains	Supports patients in their spiritual/religious practices. Provides encouragement and support.	Guides team to provide support while coping with illness/disability, consistent with patient's faith/beliefs.
Vocational services	Evaluates impact of illness/injury on vocation. Assists patients with adaptations to return to present vocation or retraining/education.	Communicates status of patient's vocational needs. Works with therapists to develop, adapt, or improve skills required for return to work or school.

ADLs, activities of daily living; CNS, Clinical Nurse Specialist; W/C, wheelchair.

Responsibilities of IDT Members

Well-functioning and effective team members need to understand their roles and responsibilities. Although roles are dictated partially by the discipline of each member, responsibility for an effective IDT falls on all team members. Members need to value and demonstrate a collaborative approach with patients, family, and other team members when setting goals, coordinating care, and providing education and discharge planning. Secrest (2007) describes a number of components required to have an effectively functioning team: trust, mutual respect, communication, coordination of care, knowledge, shared responsibility, and a commitment to each other. Box 5.4 provides additional information on IDT competence.

BOX 5.4	How to Achieve Team Competence

- Technical competence is the focus of most professional programs in health care.
- Both technical and team competence are critical to ensure safe patient care.
- Healthcare professionals who understand each other's roles and work together effectively provide higher quality care (Barnsteiner, Disch, Hall, Mayer, & Moore, 2007).
- Members of collaborative teams enjoy greater job satisfaction (Chaboyer & Patterson, 2001).

Freeman (2000) states there are three individual philosophies of teamwork that impact its role, comprehension, and communication: directive, integrative, and elective.

Those who have a directive philosophy view their role as a team leader. Persons with an integrative approach are often therapists, social workers, and nurses who view their role as upholding collaboration and being a team player. Those with an elective philosophy favor brief communications and work more autonomously. Differing philosophies among team members can contribute to turf issues and negatively impact attempts to have a cohesive and collaborative team. The responsibility of addressing any negatives within the team falls on each member of the team; often there are senior, more experienced team members who understand and practice the philosophy of interdisciplinary and collaborative care who will assume a leadership role to address issues. Characteristics of an effective team are discussed in the following section.

CHARACTERISTICS OF AN EFFECTIVE IDT

In rehabilitation one thing is certain: No one discipline and no single approach can provide the comprehensive services needed to facilitate recovery from complex injuries and mitigation of multiple deficits. However, in recent years empirical research has emerged identifying the well-functioning IDT as one of the determinants of improved functional gains for rehabilitation patients. Optimal outcomes require the integration of complex medical, financial, psychosocial, educational, and vocational resources across diverse specialties and multiple systems in a highly visible setting with patients and families involved at all levels (Strasser et al., 2008).

Rehabilitation can be a lengthy and often frustrating process. Rehabilitation professionals have the dual challenge of helping families remain hopeful while preparing them for scenarios that may be disappointing. At the same time, being part of an IDT can be exhilarating, with daily collaboration among skilled professionals implementing exciting and creative, evidence-based care.

Personal commitment to the team and a willingness to put notions about differing status of members aside are prerequisites of effective IDT membership. Collaborative discussion demands communication skill and an ability to transcend professional jargon, shed the expectation of physician dominance, and become comfortable with blurred professional boundaries. Negotiation skills and an appreciation and valuing of diversity and individual differences are desirable traits for IDT members.

IDTs can be somewhat fluid, with members entering and leaving, as personal and professional lives change. Ideally, senior members of the IDT will assist the group to process the changes in group dynamics that inevitably

follow alterations in team structure. During these times the group may experience an interruption in cohesiveness as members seek renewed commitment to the goals and purposes of the group. IDT members most likely to assist the group to understand these shifting dynamics are the psychologist, the clinical nurse specialist, and the nurse care coordinator (case manager) or social worker. The registered nurse is in an excellent position to prompt the team to refocus their shared commitment on the care of patients and families.

It is important that IDT members relinquish their perceptions of perceived professional boundaries and nurture a mutual respect for the value other members bring to the team. Even in teams highly skilled in working collaboratively, conflict is inevitable. However, if moments of conflict are viewed as opportunities to come together and achieve synergistic solutions, both the team and patients benefit. Well-educated professionals, taught to be assertive and think critically, will have conflicts. The key is to accept conflict as a natural outcome when creative energies collide and work to resolve it (Hall & Weaver, 2001). Box 5.5 provides keys to preparing for IDT membership.

BOX 5.5   How Do You Prepare for Membership on an IDT?

- Appreciate your own discipline and its unique contribution to rehabilitative care.
- As a student, seek every opportunity to observe and/or be part of an IDT.
- Do not be afraid to stretch outside the comfort zone of your own discipline.
- Participate in committees or groups that include other healthcare professionals.
- Experience with interdisciplinary collaborative practice as a student has been shown to be a determinant of positive attitudes about IDTs as students enter the job market (Florence, Goodrow, Wachs, Grover, & Olive, 2007).

TEAM COMPETENCE

Team competence derives from the ability of multiple disciplines to behave as a single system. Moving beyond task focus, IDTs are capable of achieving a level of team thinking and an environment of creative inquiry that exceeds what can be accomplished by individuals operating in professional silos.

Brookfield and Preskill (1999) describe habits of collaborative discussion inherent in interdisciplinary teams as "group talk," a blending of conversation, discussion, dialogue, and cooperation. Although group talk is part of team competence, it does not ensure effective team function. Group talk is only useful if team members recognize, identify, and share important clinical and psychosocial cues. Nurses, with 24-hour presence and accountability, are in a key position to enhance effective team function through the timely transfer of critical information (Miller, Riley, & Davis, 2009).

Equally important to the ability to recognize and communicate critical information is **emotional intelligence**, defined as "the ability to perceive emotions, to access and generate emotions so as to assist thought, to understand emotions and emotional knowledge, and to reflectively regulate emotions to promote intellectual growth" (Mayer & Salovey, 1997, p. 6). The concept of emotional intelligence, introduced by Daniel Goleman (1995), asserts that an effective team needs more than technical and clinical skills. Nurses, to maximize their contribution to the IDT, need to be aware of the role emotional intelligence plays in team function. Nurses will benefit from supplementing their technical education with training designed to refine interactional skills that emphasize increasing awareness of the impact of team diversity and individual personality differences on team working relationships.

Emotional intelligence is the quality that allows IDT members to engage in dialogue, transcend stereotypes, and collaborate to achieve synergistic solutions. Although little is known about nurse performance on IDTs (Institute of Medicine, 2003), studies by Glaser (1998) and McCallin (2001) support the notion that nurses' ability to develop cohesive relationships within the IDT is pivotal to their success.

Individual clinical performance skills (task training) and the behaviors necessary for effective IDT function should ideally be taught simultaneously and valued by the organizations and professionals delivering care. The skills that enable IDTs to effect change in process and outcomes need to be taught at the team level. Whether by interactive workshops, structured online training, or group education connecting outcome data to team interventions, hospital systems and the various entities delivering patient care must endeavor to demonstrate the value placed on competent IDT function.

The primary action of the IDT takes place in the team meeting and during IDT rounds. Whatever the arena, the themes of consensus, professional synergy, and fostering a learning culture are of major importance for the IDT to achieve team competence (Shaw, Walker, & Hogue, 2008). Commitment to consensus avoids reliance on discipline-specific knowledge and is demonstrated by team acceptance of different viewpoints and knowledge bases.

Professional synergy is realized when team members relinquish autonomy in favor of using resources available within the entire team. Becoming comfortable with "team-ness," described by Shaw et al. (2008) as the ebb and flow of teamwork, is a process. In the rehabilitation dance, team members, comfortable with the talents they bring to the IDT, allow members with expert knowledge to step in and guide the team when it is in the best interest of the patient.

IDT members have a responsibility to contribute to the learning culture of the team and should demonstrate the capacity to learn from other team members. Embracing knowledge transfer and reciprocity (professional–professional, professional–patient, patient–professional), IDT members avoid the pitfalls of rote performance: doing things the same way because that's the way they have always been done. Instead, there is an understanding that team function and patient outcomes can always be better.

IDTs have leadership but not necessarily one leader. Successful team relationships, forged in the midst of practice, allow leaders to emerge when their expertise is needed and then blend again into "team-ness." This is the dynamic nature of teams. Professionals on the IDT are accountable both as individuals and team members.

New team members benefit from mentorship to ease the transition from discipline-specific practice to an environment where collaboration is expected. The nurse considering becoming part of an IDT will want to inquire about orientation to the process and available education to enhance these skills.

The final, but perhaps most important, requirement for team competence is this: embracing the idea that the patient is not simply part of the IDT but the center of it. Healthy People 2020 (2009), a report detailing national health promotion and disease prevention agendas, defines one of the determinants of health as individual behavior and personal choice. Involving patients and families in decisions regarding their care, to the greatest extent possible, along with coordinated, concurrent education from all involved team members, is key for successful patient recovery.

EVALUATING TEAM EFFECTIVENESS

There is no one prescription for effective team development, and no one model that can be deployed with a guaranteed outcome. However, team function can be evaluated, both objectively and subjectively.

Objective data supporting team success can be found in the analysis of changes in functional independence measures that, when correlated with length of stay, speaks to rehabilitation program success and team efficacy. The Commission on Accreditation of Rehabilitation Facilities and The Joint Commission, in their accreditation surveys of program implementation and outcomes, look specifically at IDT function and, in fact, require IDT to be part of programmatic design (see Box 5.2).

Specific outcome measures, gleaned from length of stay, patient satisfaction, and return to productivity data, demonstrate team and individual effectiveness. When patients report satisfaction and show measurable improvement, IDT members experience enhanced job satisfaction. Mikan and Rodger (2005) describe effective teams as having a well-defined purpose, identifiable goals, good leaders, regular patterns of communication, and an environment of mutual respect—all qualities that can be observed and evaluated.

Effective teams also require an opportunity for team maintenance, often accomplished offline and separate from patient discussion. Taking time to reflect on teamwork successes or failures, appraise performance, and identify programmatic plans are hallmarks of a team that is proactive, not merely reactive. Effective teams design strategies based on data and best practice evidence and implement necessary program changes. Having a willingness to adjust to ever-evolving challenges is what ultimately defines effective teams.

CRITICAL THINKING

Read the two scenarios and answer the questions that follow by applying the material from this chapter.

Scenario 1

Sally is a 67-year-old married woman who was admitted to the rehabilitation unit after being hospitalized for left-sided ischemic stroke 4 days ago. Upon admission, the rehab nurse completed an admission assessment and initiated care planning. Later that afternoon, the physical therapist (PT), occupational therapist (OT), and speech-language pathologist completed their assessments with Sally. Sally's husband came in during the session with the PT and assisted Sally in answering questions.

On day 4 of Sally's stay the team (including PT, OT, nurse, physician, psychologist, case manager, and social

worker) convened for a conference to discuss her status, findings of their evaluations, and set up a plan of care and tentative discharge date. Each member of the team gave a report on their findings. The PT identified goals for mobility, the OT stated goals for activities of daily living, and the speech-language pathologist addressed swallowing and communication goals. The nurse addressed the status of Sally's bowel, bladder, and skin and stated goals for management. The team then chose a tentative discharge date. It was discussed that because Sally's husband was still working outside the home, Sally would need either to be fairly independent and able to be left alone for 7 to 8 hours a day or to have additional assistance in the home while he worked. Going to a long-term care facility was not an option Sally or her husband wanted to explore at this time. A psychosocial assessment completed by the social worker indicated that the home had five steps to enter but there were railings on both sides.

After the conference the case manager went to Sally's room to discuss plans for her stay and give her the tentative discharge date. The nurse case manager noted that the patient's managed care plan had authorized 7 days, but daily progress toward home discharge would be necessary.

Scenario 2

Bill is a 21-year-old man who sustained a C7–8 spinal cord injury as result of a motor vehicle accident. Once medically stable, he was transferred to a rehabilitation unit. Within 24 hours of admission the physician, nurse, therapists, dietician, case manager, and social worker had completed an assessment based on their discipline and role on the team. Bill attended his first conference with the team approximately 1 week after admission to discuss their findings, set goals, and develop a plan of care. The case manager shared what Bill and she had discussed related to the goals he wanted to accomplish while on the unit. The social worker shared that Bill's plan was to return home to his parent's house and that his parents were agreeable. House accessibility was also discussed. The PT and OT discussed what activities they had worked on the past week and future plans to help facilitate his ability to be as independent as possible and what changes would need to occur to make the house more accessible.

Bill expressed his concerns regarding bowel and bladder management, sharing he did not want his parents to have to do this unless absolutely necessary. The nurse, OT, and PT addressed Bill's present functional level and plans to further assess his ability to perform skills, including transfers and assistive devices.

The team discussed with Bill what goals could realistically be accomplished during his stay and together prioritized what goals should be focused on initially, stating that each week they would reevaluate his status and goals and make adjustments accordingly.

Exercises

1. Choose the scenario you believe has a functioning and effective IDT.
2. Identify the behaviors or actions that led you to your decision and what behaviors/actions were missing from the other scenario.
3. What evidence of collaboration did you find in the chosen scenario?
4. Compare and contrast the level of patient involvement in each scenario.
5. If you were the patient, which scenario would make you feel more involved in the decision-making process of your rehab stay? Why?
6. What strategies were used by each team to identify problems and set goals?
7. What advice would you give to the team not chosen to help them function more collaboratively?
8. Based on your answers, what type of team do you believe the other scenario depicted and why?

PERSONAL REFLECTION

- Have you ever been a member of an interdisciplinary team? Reflect on that experience. Was the patient a part of the team? Were any members of the team more dominant than others, and if so, why? Were team goals explicit? Were goals mutually established? Were the team goals accomplished?

- Which team members do you most associate with in your role as a rehabilitation nurse? Why?

- What type of model does your facility or organization use? Do you believe this is the most effective model for patient care?

- What is the one characteristic of an effective IDT that most describes the team with which you work?

- Think of one area that you personally could improve upon in your role as a rehabilitation nurse to help the team function more effectively.

REFERENCES

Albrecht, G., Higginbotham, N., & Freeman, S. (2001). Transdisciplinary thinking in health social science research: Definitions, rationale, and procedure. *Health Social Science: A Transdisciplinary and Complexity perspective, 4*, 78–89.

Barnsteiner, J. H., Disch, J. M., Hall, L., Mayer, D. & Moore, S. M. (2007). Promoting interprofessional education. *Nursing Outlook, 55*(3), 144–150.

Bokhour, B. (2006). Communication in interdisciplinary team meetings: What are we talking about? *Journal of Interprofessional Care, 20*(4), 349–363.

Brookfield, S. D., & Preskill, S. (1999). *Discussion as a way of teaching: Tools and techniques for democratic classrooms.* San Francisco: Jossey-Bass.

Chaboyer, W. P., & Patterson, E. (2001). Australian hospital generalist and critical care nurse's perceptions of doctor-nurse collaboration. *Nursing and Health Sciences, 3*(2), 73–79.

Florence, J. A., Goodrow, B., Wachs, J., Grover, S., & Olive, K. E. (2007). Rural health professions education at East Tennessee State University: Survey of graduates from the first decade of the community partnership program. *Journal of Rural Health, 23*(1), 77–83.

Freeman, L. C. (2000). Visualizing social networks. *Journal of Social Structure, 1*(1). Retrieved from http://www.heinz.cmu.edu/project/INSNA/joss/vsn.html

Gage, M. (1998). From independence to interdependence. Creating synergistic health care teams. *Journal of Nursing Administration, 28*(4), 17–26.

Glaser, B. G. (1998). *Doing grounded theory: Issues and discussions.* Mill Valley, CA: Sociology Press.

Goleman, D. (1995). *Emotional intelligence: Why it can matter more than IQ.* New York: Bantam Books.

Hall, P., & Weaver, L. (2001). Interdisciplinary education and teamwork: A long and winding road. *Medical Education, 35*(9), 867–875.

Healthy People 2020. (October 30, 2009). Retrieved from www.healthypeople.gov/hp2010

Herbert, C. P., Bainbridge, L., Bickford, J., et al. (2007). Factors that influence engagement in collaborative practice: How 8 health professionals became advocates. *Canadian Family Physician, 53*, 1328–1325.

Institute of Medicine. (2003). *Health professions education: A bridge to quality.* Washington, DC: National Academies Press.

Lewin, K. (1951). *Field theory in social sciences.* New York: Harper.

Mayer, J. D. & Salovey, P. (1997). What is emotional intelligence? In P. Salovey & D. Sluyter (Eds). *Emotional development and emotional intelligence: Implications for educators* (pp. 3–31). New York: Basic Books.

McCallin, A. (2001). Interdisciplinary practice—a matter of teamwork: An integrated literature review. *Journal of Clinical Nursing, 10*, 419–428.

McCallin, A., & Bamford, A. (2007). Interdisciplinary teamwork: Is the influence of emotional intelligence fully appreciated? *Journal of Nursing Management, 15*, 386–391.

Mikan, S. M., & Rodger, S. A. (2005). Effective health care teams: A model of six characteristics developed from shared perceptions. *Journal of Interprofessional Care, 19*(4), 358–370.

Miller, K., Riley, W., & Davis, S. (2009). Identifying key nursing and team behaviours to achieve high reliability. *Journal of Nursing Management, 17*, 247–255.

Mumma, C. M., & Nelson, A. (1996). *Rehabilitation nursing: Process and applications* (2nd ed., pp. 20–36). St. Louis, MO: Mosby.

Rogers, D. (1932). Teamwork within the hospital. *American Journal of Nursing, 32*, 657–659.

Rossen, E. K., Bartlett, R., & Herrick, C. A. (2008). Interdisciplinary collaboration: The need to revisit. *Issues in Mental Health Nursing, 29*, 387–396.

Rubenfeld, G. M., & Scheffer, B. K. (2010). *Critical thinking tactics.* Sudbury, MA: Jones and Bartlett Learning.

Secrest, J. (2007). Rehabilitation and rehabilitation nursing. In K. L. Mauk (Ed.), *The specialty practice of rehabilitation nursing: A core curriculum* (5th ed., pp. 2–12). Glenview, IL: Association of Rehabilitation Nurses.

Shaw, L., Walker, R., & Hogue, A. (2008). The art and science of teamwork: Enacting a transdiciplinary approach in work rehabilitation. *Work, 30*, 297–306.

Sheehan, D., Robertson, L., & Ormond, T., (2007). Comparison of language used and patterns of communication interprofessional and multidisciplinary teams. *Journal of Interprofessional Care, 21*(1), 17–30.

Strasser, D. C., Falconer, J. A., & Martino-Saltzmann, D., (1994) The rehabilitation team: Staff perceptions of the hospital environment, the interdisciplinary team environment, and interprofessional relations. *Archives of Physical Medicine and Rehabilitation, 75*, 177–182.

Strasser, D. C., Uomoto, J. M., & Smits, S. J. (2008). The rehabilitation team and polytrauma rehabilitation: Prescription for partnership. *Archives of Physical Medicine and Rehabilitation, 89*, 179–181.

CHAPTER 6

Nursing Roles

Donna Williams
Stephanie Davis Burnett

LEARNING OBJECTIVES

At the end of this chapter, the reader will be able to

- List various roles of a rehabilitation nurse.
- State at least three different settings in which rehabilitation nursing is practiced.
- Recognize benefits of certification in the specialty of rehabilitation.
- Discuss career options that advanced education can offer.
- Define competency in practice.
- Appreciate the patient advocacy role in rehabilitation nursing.
- Describe the effect of evidence-based practice on rehabilitation nursing roles.

KEY CONCEPTS AND TERMS

Advanced practice registered
    nurse (APRN)
Advocacy
Association of Rehabilitation
    Nurses (ARN)
Association of Rehabilitation
    Nurses Competency
    Assessment Test (ARN-CAT)
Care provider
Case manager
Certification

Certified rehabilitation
    registered nurse (CRRN)
Clinical nurse leader
Clinician
Competencies
Doctorate of nursing practice
Educator
Evidenced-based practice
Geriatric rehabilitation nurses
Home health care
    rehabilitation nurse

Liaison nurse
Licensed practical nurse/
    licensed vocational nurse
Life care plan
Managers
Pediatric rehabilitation nurse
Professional geriatric care
    manager
Rehabilitation nursing
Researcher

Nurses are central and often pivotal contributors to the multiprofessional rehabilitation team. With the growing population of older adults and of the disabled, the medical community has responded by increasing rehabilitation skilled nursing and acute facilities, which has increased the demand for more rehabilitation therapists and nurses within the healthcare community (Heinemann, 2008). Rehabilitation nurses practice in a variety of settings and assume a myriad of roles, as reimbursement and quality considerations has demanded an array of providers. Job titles may vary, but nursing roles use the foundations of nursing science as guiding principles for ethical practice.

The content in this chapter provides basic descriptions of rehabilitation nursing roles. For each role, the implications of education, competency, teaching, advocacy, and evidence-based practice are addressed. A case study is given for each role, with critical thinking questions and personal reflections to assist the reader with application of the chapter content.

> According to a landmark study by Audrey Nelson and colleagues (2007), a 6% increase in certified rehabilitation nurses was associated with a one day reduction in average length of stay.

CARE PROVIDER

Care provider is the most common role of the rehabilitation nurse involving direct care activities, such as assessment, technical, and physical care, and indirect functions, such as coordination of services and communication (Long, Kneafsey, Ryan, & Berry, 2002). Staff nurses and clinicians are two examples of those who provide direct patient care.

Educational Preparation and Certification

Nurses with various levels of education (associate, diploma, baccalaureate, masters, doctorate, or equivalent) may work as direct care providers, but each must be licensed by the board of nursing in the state where they practice. **Licensed practical nurses** and **licensed vocational nurses** also play an important role on the rehabilitation team under the supervision of the registered nurse in some settings. These nurse positions may be more prominent in long-term care facilities than in other settings, making it essential for these entry-level nurses to have some specialized education and training in rehabilitation. Some basic nursing programs offer limited experience in the rehabilitation arena, but few programs offer rehabilitation within the curriculum. Leaders in rehabilitation hope this will change and have made integrating rehabilitation into the nursing curriculum a part of the future strategic plan for the discipline.

Certification is "a professional recognition of skills in a specialty practice . . . developed and maintained by professional nursing organizations such as ANA [American Nurses Association] or ARN [Association of Rehabilitation Nurses]" (Secrest, 2007, p. 11). Certification in rehabilitation nursing is one means to validate to the public a nurse's specialized skills, knowledge, and abilities in the practice of rehabilitation nursing. Facilities with or seeking nursing clinical ladder programs and ANA's Magnet Recognition are frequently the "impetus" for healthcare organizations to promote certification, as demonstration of its commitment to professional nurse development (Watts, 2010, p, 52). According to a study by Nelson and colleagues (2007), certification in rehabilitation was inversely related to patient length of stay. Specifically, a 6% increase in certified rehabilitation nurses was associated with a one day reduction in length of stay.

Eligibility to seek certification in rehabilitation nursing includes a current, unrestricted registered nurse (RN) license and at least 2 years of rehabilitation nursing practice as an RN (or 1 year of experience and 1 year of advanced study in nursing) within the 5 years preceding examination. According to the **Association of Rehabilitation Nurses (ARN)**, certification is offered through the Rehabilitation Nursing Certification Board, a subsidiary of the ARN. Those successful in meeting the criteria and passing the certification exam earn the **certified rehabilitation registered nurse (CRRN)** credential (ARN, n.d.).

Work Settings and Job Descriptions

There are numerous work settings for the clinical or direct care provider. Settings may include but are not limited to acute hospitals with or without a rehabilitation designated unit, free-standing rehabilitation hospitals, skilled nursing facilities, long-term acute care hospitals, clinics, home health agencies, residential units or facilities, and others (see Chapter 3). Rehabilitation nurses are also valuable team members on units not focused on rehabilitation because they bring the rehabilitation philosophy of promoting expertise in self-care or self-directed care to the patient regardless of their diagnosis.

TEACHING AND ADVOCACY

Advocacy, or ethical "decisions and actions on behalf of patients" (ARN, 2008, p. 29) or "championing the needs and interests of another" (Hoeman, Duchene, & Vierling, 2008, p. 33), is a core concept in the practice of rehabilitation nursing in all settings and throughout the continuum of care. The Standards and Scope of Rehabilitation Nursing Practice prescribes the rehabilitation registered nurse to directly advocate for patients as well as assist them to develop skills to advocate for themselves, as rehabilitation patients typically are faced with societal barriers and inequalities (ARN, 2008).

Possessing the knowledge and skills to educate patients, families, other healthcare providers, and payors is basic to rehabilitation nursing practice (ARN, 2008). The opportunities for teaching patients and families are limitless. Each time there is an interaction with a patient or family member, there is an opportunity for informal or formal teaching. Teaching can occur through simple conversation or can be structured with any combination of teaching aids or resources. Teaching can also occur in a more structured setting with a planned program, including prearranged sessions or group learning activities. Because rehabilitation is a philosophical as well as a pragmatic approach to patient care, topics for teaching can include diagnoses, the plan of care, expected outcomes, medication management, independence and self-care skills (such as skin, gastrointestinal and genitourinary system management, and performance of activities of daily living), coping with disability, psychosocial and role changes, and health and wellness instructions (ARN, 2008). These topics are just a sample of those that can be addressed with patients and their families.

Evidence-Based Practice

DiCenso, Guyatt, and Ciliska (2005) defined evidence-based practice as "the conscientious, explicit, and judicious use of current best evidence" (p. 555) to make decisions and integrate clinical expertise and resources for the care of individual patients. **Evidence-based practice** involves identifying a burning clinical question and then through a defined process searching for relevant research, synthesizing the findings, and implementing them into nursing practice to increase the quality of patient care. The goal is to provide the highest quality and most cost-efficient nursing care with the best patient outcomes possible (Melnyk & Fineout-Overholt, 2011). Practice based on research findings is a process that includes the collection, interpretation, evaluation, and integration of valid, important, and current and past applicable research as well as clinical guidelines and other information resources. To correctly apply findings to practice, nurses must understand the concept of research and know how to accurately evaluate this research and the implications for practice. Rehabilitation nurses should have this knowledge to translate rehabilitation research into foundations for evidence-based rehabilitation nursing practice (ARN, 2004).

> *Evidence-based practice involves identifying a burning clinical question and then, through a defined process, searching for relevant research, synthesizing the findings and implementing them into nursing practice to increase the quality of patient care.*

Competencies

Competencies can clarify the core "essential skills, knowledge and personal characteristics" that are needed to meet the performance standard for a particular profession, job, or role (Baldwin, Clark, Fulton, & Mayo, 2009, p. 193). Before establishing competencies for performance, standards of practice were developed. Standards describe the nursing profession's responsibilities for which its practitioners are accountable and reflect the values and priorities of the profession (ANA, 2010). ARN first established standards in 1977 and revised them several times, most recently in 2008. ARN has also developed competencies in the field of rehabilitation and offers users

of their website the ability to assess their competencies online in 16 basic competencies.

The **Association of Rehabilitation Nurses Competency Assessment Test (ARN-CAT)** provides multiple-choice online tests, currently in 16 assessment areas: general rehabilitation, autonomic dysreflexia, communication, disability, dysphagia, gerontology and pediatric care management, musculoskeletal/body mechanics/transfer techniques, bowel and bladder management, neuropathophysiology (such as stroke, spinal cord injury, and traumatic brain injury), functional assessment, pain management, patient/family education, safe patient handling, sexuality, and skin care (ARN, 2010). The ARN-CAT can be used as a tool by nursing leadership to evaluate the proficiency of rehabilitation nurses (Secrest, 2007).

Defining Critical Thinking

Critical thinking involves applying skillful reasoning as a guide to belief or action (Melnyk & Fineout-Overholt, 2011). Critical thinking is purposeful, outcome directed, driven by need, and based on principles of the nursing process and scientific methods. It is guided by professional standards and ethics. Nurses apply critical thinking in their professional lives on a daily basis as they assess their patients, gather information, and determine courses of action based on their assessments, knowledge, experience, and standards and guidelines. Case Study 6.1 provides an example of how a direct care provider might use critical thinking skills to devise an appropriate nursing plan of care.

CASE STUDY 6.1

You have just come on the day shift to take over care of a 35-year-old patient with multiple trauma. He has been progressing with mobility and activities of daily living. The previous nurse reported sleep problems during the night shift. On assessment your patient is agitated and slightly disoriented. He is not able to tell you specifically why he is agitated but reports high pain levels. During the course of the conversation he tells you a previously unreported history of opiate use and problems with sleep and over-the-counter sleep aides.

Critical Thinking

1. What do you believe might be the problem?
2. What should your assessment include?
3. What resources do you have for your assessment in addition to the patient?
4. Is it possible there are multiple factors causing disorientation and agitation?

5. What might those factors be?
6. To make a change in the plan of care, what information have you considered to affect that change?

Personal Reflection

- How have you felt about your experience providing direct care to persons with disabilities or impairments?
- What difference do you believe you could make for a person with a disability or impairment?
- What appeals to you about a rehabilitation clinical position?
- How do you believe you could apply principles or rehabilitation nursing in settings other that a rehabilitation setting?

HOME HEALTH/HOME CARE NURSE AS BOTH ROLE AND PRACTICE SETTING

The **home health care rehabilitation nurse** is one example of a nursing position that denotes both a role and a setting for practice. The rehabilitation nurse in home health care acts as an advocate for clients and their families as they move from the hospital or facility to the home and the community, promoting autonomy and independence. The home care rehabilitation nurse coordinates the services provided by the interdisciplinary team of an agency and implements the plan of care that has been developed by the client, the physician, and the rehabilitation team to promote community reintegration. Here, the home care rehabilitation nurse functions as a clinical resource, care coordinator, advocate, direct care provider, teacher, consultant, and team member. These role components are discussed further later in this chapter. The home care nurse, using rehabilitation expertise, revises and develops individualized services for the client and the client's family or care giver.

NURSE LIAISON

The rehabilitation **liaison nurse** completes preadmission evaluations and arranges for admission of clients to services or programs along the rehabilitation continuum of care. The evaluation includes determining resources for the patient such as requirements or limitations of payer sources, regulations, and family and community resources. In the role of liaison, the rehabilitation nurse's ultimate aim is to "maximize client choice and autonomy and the enablement of independent living or optimal functioning within the client's own environment" (Long et al., 2002, p. 76). The liaison nurse may also perform activities and duties related to recruitment and in-service education.

Education Preparation and Certification

ARN recommends the nurse liaison hold licensure as an RN, preferably with a bachelor's degree in nursing from an accredited school, and a minimum of 2 years of clinical experience in the rehabilitation of chronically or catastrophically ill or injured individuals (ARN, 2004). Certification in rehabilitation nursing or a related specialty is recommended. Additionally, employers may require demonstrated expertise in assessment, analysis, decision making, time management, oral and written communication, and computer use. The nurse liaison should also have familiarity with the resources available for use in assessing regulations and the parameters of third-party reimbursement.

Work Settings and Job Descriptions

Nurse liaisons may work autonomously in outpatient settings or inpatient rehabilitation facilities. They may screen (assess) patients for acute or skilled settings, residential programs, day care, clinics, or in-home services. As a **clinician**, the nurse liaison may perform preadmission screening and clinical assessment to recommend the appropriate level of care. As an educator, the nurse liaison ensures that all patients are aware of rehabilitation programs and services. As consultant, facilitator, and negotiator the liaison assists with certification of the treatment plan, provides information, and negotiates rates, providing data regarding the outcome of the stay. The marketing role requires thorough knowledge of the facility, services, and outcomes. Relationships are developed with referral sources and clients sometimes through exhibiting or tours, as required. Good public relationships are always promoted, and the liaison collaborates with the team, client, and external sources to work toward the optimal outcome (ARN, 2003).

Teaching and Advocacy

Nurse liaisons are in a pivotal role to teach and advocate for rehabilitation and rehabilitation nursing. In the advocate role, the liaison works with the internal and external case manager/payer toward a cost-effective plan. Each time they are called to complete an assessment, nurses, patients, and facilities can be educated about the diagnoses, potential treatment options, prognosis for recovery, financial concerns, community resources, and discharge needs. While communicating with referral sources, nurse liaisons continue their roles as educators, informing patients, families, and professionals about programs and advocating for patient's welfare. Marketing can include networking with known referral sources, presenting programs, or seeking new referral sources. By offering information to the professional and lay community, the nurse liaison advocates for an informed community regarding rehabilitation and rehabilitation nursing. Those communities are then better prepared to consider options as situations of life present to family, friends, acquaintances, and other professionals.

Evidence-Based Practice

It is critical for the liaison nurses to remain abreast of current standards of care and evidence-based practice as they evaluate patients for programs. Remaining knowledgeable about best practices and outcomes, they will be prepared to make the appropriate decisions about patients they are considering for admission to a facility or a program. Additionally, as they interact with referral sources, other facilities, insurance companies, and the community, outcomes of evidence-based practice can be presented and rehabilitation will be promoted for those in need.

Competencies

Assessments, knowledge of standards of care, and expectations of outcomes are key components of the skill set of the liaison nurse. The liaison nurse can validate competency of assessment skills and knowledge of diagnoses and treatments through the ARN-CAT and by maintaining CRRN certification. With multiple different payer sources, the liaison nurse needs to maintain contact with those sources to facilitate the admission, appropriate treatment plan and length of stay, and best discharge plan. Case Study 6.2 provides an example of how the nurse liaison might use critical thinking skills to devise an appropriate plan of care.

CASE STUDY 6.2

You have a referral for the local hospital for a potential patient with a new bilateral below the knee amputation for the rehabilitation facility. You make arrangements to see the 65-year-old patient and gather his history. When you arrive the patient is agitated, though his diagnosis does not usually have cognitive sequelae. He is restrained in bed with a vest. You find that while the patient is appropriate physically for admission, he is homeless, has no insurance, and is a poor historian. There are not many medical records to review. Your facility prefers to know the discharge plan before admission.

Critical Thinking

1. Can you identify several problems?
2. How will you find resources to consider this man for rehabilitation?

3. Can you identify a team that might be able to assist with problem solving for this gentleman?

Personal Reflection

- How do you think about your assessment skills?
- Do you enjoy interacting with multiple people in a variety of settings (i.e., referral sources, marketing, and community)?

REHABILITATION NURSING ROLES ACROSS THE LIFE SPAN

Injury and disability is without age boundaries. Infants are born with neurological or orthopedic injuries that require specialized care, children and adolescents are injured or become ill, adults may develop disease processes or have accidents, and older adults are at high risk for both injury and disabling disease. Access to health care in these vulnerable groups is a major aspect where the role of the nurse can be involved. Rehabilitation nurses are in the unique position to assist patients across the life span to achieve or return to the highest independence level possible. The much debated Patient Protection and Affordable Care Act (P.L. 111-148) makes particular provisions concerning patient quality and outcomes. P.L. 111-148 proposes workforce development initiative through proposed loan, recruitment, and retention programs for pediatric specialty nursing students in particular and allocations for geriatric fellowship funding (Gallagher, 2010).

PEDIATRIC REHABILITATION NURSE

Pediatric rehabilitation nursing is the specialty practice committed to improving the quality of life for children and adolescents with disabilities and their families (ARN, 2003). Pediatric rehabilitation nurses must possess both rehabilitation specialty and generalist pediatric skills that integrate the developmental tasks of childhood, the effect of disability, and appropriate interventions to reach the desired outcomes as the patient's transition into adulthood occurs (Jackson, 2008).

Educational Preparation and Certification

An RN choosing to specialize in pediatric rehabilitation may do so following basic preparation. Nurses may gain experience in pediatrics through work experience and formal classes in pediatric care and pediatric rehabilitation. Pediatric rehabilitation nurses must have an in-depth knowledge of normal developmental theory and related assessment skills as well as knowledge of interventions, including therapeutic play activities that promote developmental milestones. CRRNs work with all age groups and bring their rehabilitation knowledge and practice to pediatric patients in rehabilitation. Two organizations, the Pediatric Nursing Certification Board and the American Nurses Credentialing Center, offer certification programs specifically in pediatric care to validate specialized knowledge and expertise in pediatric nursing beyond basic RN licensure (McClain, Richardson, & Wyatt, 2004).

Work Settings and Job Descriptions

Pediatric rehabilitation nurses may practice in a variety of settings that meet the needs of infants, children, and adolescents, such as acute inpatient rehabilitation facilities, day hospitals, medical day care programs, home health care services, outpatient facilities, and school settings (Jackson, 2008). Job descriptions may include delineation of the pediatric rehabilitation nurse as direct care provider and team member, a coordinator of care (including academic educational activities), and a leader and consultant for the team, patient and family, and others involved in the treatment plan. Pediatric rehabilitation nurses are involved in health teaching and promotion of developmentally appropriate care. They are also encouraged to maintain knowledge and competency in their practice and to evaluate their own skills and needs to advance their practice. As a research consumer the pediatric rehabilitation nurse may participate in research but also evaluates existing research and findings and integrates evidence into practice.

Teaching and Advocacy

As an advocate for the child/adolescent, the pediatric rehabilitation nurse promotes appropriate care for the patient to include the family's needs in the plan of care. Advocate is a primary role of the pediatric rehabilitation nurse involved in the care of vulnerable pediatric patients with developmental disabilities. The needs of this group are significant due to their cognitive and communication deficits and safety risks (Hertzberg, 2008). The pediatric rehabilitation nurse facilitates patient and family transition from facility or program to home, community, and school. The pediatric rehabilitation nurse teaches patients according to their developmental level as well as their diagnosis, the family, the hospital care team, and school personnel regarding the child's diagnoses and implications for care (Jackson, 2008). Additionally, education is offered to the community and specifically any interested individual about the needs of children with disabilities and their families.

Evidence-Based Practice

Evidence-based practice is a systematic approach to making "best practice" decisions. Clinically-based nurses who use evidence-based treatment approaches for the care of pediatric patients and their families seek to maximize clinical outcomes. Their efforts include collaboration and sharing of ideas and information among their peers, the team, and other nursing institutions/agencies and the community and program evaluation (Jackson, 2008). Research for best practice is supported by ARN and the Society of Pediatric Nurses for the purpose of conducting research related specifically to the care of children and their families (ARN, 2003).

Competencies

Pediatric rehabilitation competency begins with acquiring basic nursing education followed by specialty education and experience in both pediatrics and rehabilitation. Additionally, the ARN-CAT is one tool that can be used to assess the competence level of the **pediatric rehabilitation nurse**. This tool can be used to assess the proficiency of the nurse and direct further education needs. Case Study 6.3 provides an example of how the pediatric rehabilitation nurse might use critical thinking skills to devise an appropriate plan of care.

CASE STUDY 6.3

You are a pediatric nurse working in the community. Your patient is a 13-year-old girl who has been through rehabilitation for a lumbar spinal cord injury. She is at home and has returned to school where she was an exemplary student and well known and liked. She reports the first 2 days at school went well and on the third day she refuses to go and is reluctant to state why.

Critical Thinking

1. Can you identify the problem?
2. What information do you need?
3. After talking to your patient, who else do you need to gather information from?
4. How should critical thinking be used here?
5. Who should be involved in problem-solving strategies?

Personal Reflection

- How do you feel about caring for children that are ill, injured, or disabled?
- How would you advocate for a child returning to his or her home and community?
- What special needs do you see yourself fulfilling for children and their families?

GERIATRIC REHABILITATION NURSE/ GERIATRIC CONSULTANT

According to the Rehabilitation Nursing Scope of Practice, the rise in the number of elderly Americans has increased the need for rehabilitation (ARN, 2008). Gerontological rehabilitation nursing is the specialty practice that focuses on the unique requirements of elderly rehabilitation clients. According to the U.S. Department of Health and Human Services 2005 profile of older Americans, persons 65 years or older numbered over 36 million in 2004 and represented 12.4% of the nation's population, or one in every eight (n.d.). **Geriatric rehabilitation nurses** may be direct care providers, consultants or care/case **managers**, educators, researchers, or geriatric nurse practitioners, for example. Geriatric rehabilitation nurses may be especially valuable on units that do not focus on the geriatric population or rehabilitation, because they apply their knowledge and experience in the principles of rehabilitation and facilitate care of the elderly in any setting. The **professional geriatric care manager** is an experienced guide and resource for families of older adults and others with chronic needs and issues related to aging (National Association of Professional Geriatric Care Managers, n.d.)

Educational Preparation and Certification

Any nurse who has completed a basic nursing program may specialize in caring for the geriatric population, given the appropriate work experience. As with other specialties, after basic nursing there are specialized programs for education in the care of geriatrics. Research has indicated that nurses with further education in geriatrics provide improved care to older adults (Stierle, et al., 2006). Certified gerontological nurses are registered nurses who have met certain criteria and successfully passed a certification examination. Eligibility for the American Nurses Credentialing Center (ANCC) geriatric certification includes 2,000 hours of clinical practice and 30 hours of education in gerontological nursing. Advanced practice nurses, nurse practitioners (NPs), and clinical specialists may also be certified by ANCC at an advanced level. The CRRN certification addresses the elderly population for the clinical nurse. For those who are geriatric care managers, the National Association of Professional Geriatric Care Managers recognizes the following certifications: Care Manager Certified, Certified Case Manager, Certified Advanced Social Worker in Case Management, and Certified Social Work Case Manager.

Work Settings and Job Descriptions

There are many settings appropriate for gerontological rehabilitation nurse specialists. They are needed in any setting where the elderly population may be seen, including acute hospitals, long-term care facilities, nursing homes, and residential facilities and clinics. Nurses with a gerontological specialty attend to the unique needs of the aging population. Additionally, geriatric rehabilitation nurses use their expertise to "improve or maintain physical function with targeted interventions" (Lee & Higgins, 2008, p. 170) specific to the needs of the elderly.

Teaching and Advocacy

Both the clinical rehabilitation nurse and the professional geriatric case manager must attempt to involve the older person, to the greatest extent possible, in decisions that impact his or her life regardless of the determination of competence (National Association of Professional Geriatric Care Managers, n.d.). As an advocate, the gerontological rehabilitation nurse promotes the best interests of the elderly, strengthening autonomy and allowing personal decision making. This allows the person to remain as independent as possible and promotes retention of dignity (Mauk, 2010). The gerontological rehabilitation nurse focuses on teaching patients, families, and caregivers about risk factors that can be modified to decrease the risk of either having an illness or injury or decreasing the risk of complications associated with injury or illness, either acute or chronic.

With a focus on modifiable risk factors, education is also provided on health promotion. Nurses with this expertise also are responsible for teaching other nurses so that quality care, the highest possible functional level, healthy living, and autonomy are promoted for this population. The gerontological nurse teaches techniques or approaches to care that are specific to the aged or the aged with a specific acute or chronic illness or injury, keeping in mind that comorbidities may exist that affect response to illness or injury.

Evidence-Based Practice

The University of Iowa Gerontological Nursing Intervention Research Center, funded by National Institute of Nursing Research (NINR), provides opportunities that lead to research that improves the quality of life for older people. ConsultGeriRN.org is an online resource for nurses in clinical and educational settings. It is the evidence-based geriatric clinical nursing website of The Hartford Institute for Geriatric Nursing at New York

University's College of Nursing, College of Dentistry. *The Journal of Gerontological Nursing* and *Geriatric Nursing* are two examples of peer-reviewed journals that publish research for evidenced-based practice for the older population. GeroNurseOnline.org is the website of ANA that is a resource for nurses to link to research, trends and developments, and evidence-based practice and has links to nursing associations and geriatric websites (Box 6.1).

BOX 6.1   Helpful Geriatric Websites

http://www.hartfordign.org
John A. Hartford Foundation Institute for Geriatric Nursing with multiple links

http://www.hartfordign.org/resources/education/tryThis.html
Hartford Geriatric Nursing initiative "Try This" series with free downloadable tools

http://www.consultgerirn.org/
ConsultGeriRN has many helpful links to evidence-based geriatric nursing practice

http://consultgerirn.org/resources/geriatric_topics
Evidence-based geriatric protocols and topics written by geriatric nurse experts

http://www.ngna.org
National Gerontological Nursing Association

http://www.hartfordign.org/programs/niche/kit-protocols.html
NICHE: Nurses improving care for health system elders has links to practice protocols via National Clearinghouse Guidelines

http://www.americangeriatrics.org/
American Geriatrics Society (interdisciplinary)

http://www.aghe.org/site/aghewebsite/
Association for Gerontology in Higher Education (interdisciplinary)

http://www.gericareonline.net
Practicing physician education in geriatrics

http://www.geronurseonline.org
Official geriatric nursing website of the ANA

http://www.aacn.nche.edu/Education/Hartford/GNEC.htm
Geriatric Nursing Education Consortium

http://www.caremanager.org/
National Association of Professional Geriatric Care Managers

http://www.rehabnurse.org
ARN website; can find gerontological rehab nurse role description at this link

http://www.ncal.org/about/index.cfm
National Center for Assisted Living

http://www.medicare.gov/Publications/Pubs/pdf/10050.pdf
CMS publication: Medicare and You, 2008

Competencies

The education committee of the American Geriatrics Society has been involved in the research and development of competencies for those who care for older people. The National Association of Professional Geriatric Case Managers has developed standards of practice for professional geriatric care managers. Certification addresses core competencies of critical thinking, communication, assessment, and technical skills as well as the core nursing knowledge and age-based practice. Case Study 6.4 provides an example of how the geriatric nurse might use critical thinking skills to devise an appropriate plan of care.

CASE STUDY 6.4

Mr. and Mrs. Smith, both 82 years old, were involved in a motor vehicle accident. Mr. Smith was driving and was bruised and sore but had no other injuries. Mrs. Smith suffered a broken vertebra and several fractured ribs. Mr. Smith was seen in the emergency room and released. Mrs. Smith was discharged after several days. She received medication for pain and was to follow-up with her orthopedic physician. The Smith children live in another state and have asked a geriatric care manager to assist their parents.

Critical Thinking

1. Do you assume potential problems before meeting the Smiths?
2. Who will be your information resources?
3. What will your assessment include?
4. What are potential key concerns?
5. Who are your resources for considering how best to assist the Smiths?

Personal Reflection

- How do you feel about working with the aging population?
- What special encounters have you had with the elderly?
- How have you felt when teaching elderly patients and their families?

CASE MANAGER

Because the need for long-term management of resources in the care of the disabled has grown, the role of **case manager** has become invaluable in health care today. Case management is the "process of planning, organizing, coordinating, and monitoring the services and resources needed to respond to a person's healthcare needs" (ARN, 1998, p. 2). The Case Management Society of America's revised standards of practice for 2010 defines case management as a "collaborative process of assessment, planning, facilitation and advocacy for options and services to meet an individual's and family's health needs through communication and available resources to promote quality cost-effective outcomes" (Case Management Society of America [CMSA], 2010, p. 8). The ANA defines case management as a "dynamic and systematic collaborative approach to provided and coordinate healthcare services to a defined population. The process includes assessment, planning, implementation, evaluation and interaction" (Williams & McCollum, 2007, p. 413).

> Case management is the "collaborative process of assessment, planning, facilitation and advocacy for options and services to meet an individual's health needs through communication and available resources to promote quality cost-effective outcomes"
>
> (CMSA, 2009).

Educational Preparation and Certification

The CMSA recognizes licensed healthcare professionals as case managers: RNs at any level of educational preparation, physicians, physical therapists, occupational therapists, licensed social workers, and others (Borglund, 2008). CMSA recognizes over 20 specialties that case managers may be certified in, including the CRRN. Certification is offered through the Commission for Case Management Certification and the National Academy of Certified Case Managers, for example. CRRNs working as case managers are held to the standards and scope of practice of both case management and rehabilitation nursing.

Work Settings and Job Descriptions

Nurse case managers work in a variety of settings and job descriptions. Job titles may also vary in any given setting and with a range of necessary experience depending on the job criteria. Case managers may work for inpatient or outpatient facilities, insurance companies, clinics, school programs, and government programs or may be privately employed or self-employed. They may subspecialize within the role of case management. For example, some may work only with a workers' compensation system (namely, external case manager), or only as an internal case manager in a facility, or only private

pay case manager (namely, insurance case manager), or management of patients with catastrophic illness/injuries. Job descriptions vary by setting or employer, but the ultimate goal of the case manager is to facilitate the provision of high-quality, cost-effective services. Case managers are responsible for assessing patients in areas of diagnoses, resources (financial, physical, psychosocial, community), treatments rendered and expected, goals, and discharge plans from facilities, programs, or systems. They are responsible for communication, collaboration, negotiation, and conflict resolution.

Case managers may also function as life care planners. A **life care plan** is a projection of costs of medical and associated care over a person's lifetime. The plan involves a comprehensive assessment, data analysis, and research. These plans are used to identify costs in personal injury cases and insurance or reinsurance cases and may be used as tool to guide clients, family's healthcare plans, insurance expenditures, or settlement costs (Williams & McCollum, 2007).

Teaching and Advocacy

The case manager advocates for his or her patient/client for access to services within a system or community and coordinates those services. The approach should be patient/client centered with goals identified and agreed on with the cooperation of the patient, physician, team, family, payer, and others involved in the care plan or outcome goals. Case managers teach their patients/clients regarding their diagnoses, services available, obstacles to care, resources, and plans to achieve identified goals. Case managers also educate team members regarding resources, or lack of, and alternatives available to assist with attaining goals. Physicians may require education regarding resources or system guidelines, and payers may need education regarding diagnoses, expectations, and justification for treatment plans. Case managers are excellent resources to the community regarding access to services needed for various populations within the community (i.e., disabled children, the elderly, those with disabilities or impairments, or those needing assistance with activities of daily living).

Evidence-Based Practice

Case managers must work to document the value of their practice by analyzing outcomes to determine the most effective interventions that impact the quality and cost of care along the healthcare continuum. Borglund's

(2008) study on case management quality of life outcomes for adults with disability indicated limited correlation between type of case manager and quality of life outcomes, which also reflects the diversity and disparity across settings. However, the study recommends further nursing research that reflects the value of the nurse case manager's perspective of caring for the whole person, in addition to knowledge of availability and coordination of services (Borglund, 2008).

Competencies

Industry standards, professional codes of ethics, and standards of care are considered when developing competencies. Competencies may be developed by an organization for general expectations, but each facility or employer may also develop competencies based on their facility/program mission and goals as well as specific job descriptions with accountability detailed. Competencies allow case managers to self-assess their skill level, develop a course of action to attend to areas that need improvement, and as a validation tool.

Competencies may be based on the nursing process of assessing, planning, intervention, and evaluation and may also focus on such areas as screening, utilization review or management, discharge planning, coordination of care, advocacy, professional practice, and critical thinking. Case Study 6.5 provides an example of how the rehabilitation case manager might use critical thinking skills to devise an appropriate plan of care.

CASE STUDY 6.5

Mr. J. is a 50 year old who injured his back at work 10 years ago. He had back surgery that was unsuccessful in relieving his pain. He describes high pain levels and low function as well as depression and a sleep disorder. He is married but separated from his wife. Lab values indicate that liver function tests are elevated, and physicians have related the abnormal values to medications. He is on multiple opiates. He has developed hypertension and diabetes. During the course of assessment by an internist a hepatitis panel was run and was read as positive. Mr. J reports he probably contracted hepatitis while in the army. He has been disabled for a number of years and has Medicare but has not paid his annual deductible and has no other insurance for diagnoses not related to his back. He is afraid to know more information about the hepatitis.

Critical Thinking

1. What are some identified problems?
2. What other information do you need to consider?

3. Why is critical thinking needed in this case?
4. What resources will you contact?
5. Who will you problem solve with?

Personal Reflection

- Describe your abilities to gain a broad perspective on your patients.
- Are you interested in physical, psychosocial, financial, and environmental aspect of your patients? Why or why not?
- Explain how you see yourself as part of a team and describe the team.

MANAGER/ADMINISTRATION

A nurse leader in today's healthcare environment is faced with multiple and many times competing challenges related to human resource management, fiscal accountability, staff development, recruitment, retention issues, patient performance indicators, and quality outcomes (Hader, 2010; Stichler, 2006). The nurse administrator is responsible to oversee and influence the work of a defined environment or to manage the daily functions of a group, influencing the organization's shared vision among its staff (ANA, 2009). According to ARN's role description, the rehabilitation nurse manager is a "registered nurse holding primary accountability for the management of (a) rehabilitation unit(s) or area(s) within a healthcare institution, agency or ambulatory care setting and for services provided to recipients" (ARN, 2003, p. 2). Managers and administrators are essential roles for facilities and clinics. Nurse executives are multidimensional and multifaceted, requiring crucial skills in leadership, time management, communication, managing change, and resources (Stichler, 2006).

Educational Preparation and Certification

A bachelor's degree in nursing is usually the preferred basic preparation with certification in rehabilitation nursing for a rehabilitation nurse manager (ARN, 2003). However, in today's healthcare environment, with the baccalaureate degree discussed for entry into practice in the near future, an administrator should have a graduate degree or higher in nursing, management, policy, or administration. **Clinical nurse leaders** may fill this role in many geographical locations. Other places may prefer nurses with the **doctorate of nursing practice** degree, which also prepares nurses for system management. Focus on clinical management is most desirable to meet the demands of today complex workforce (ANA, 2009). Additionally, leadership development programs may be available and recommended to enhance leadership competency skills (Swearingen, 2009; Weston et al., 2008).

In addition to the specialty rehabilitation generalist credential, there are several credentials available specific for the nurse manager/leader/executive. In 2008 the American Association of Critical Care Nurses and the American Organization of Nurse Executives (AONE) launched the first certification examination specifically for certified nurse manager and leader role (American Association of Critical-Care Nurses, 2008). The board-certified nurse executive credential is available for nurses in mid-level administration positions, such as nurse manager, supervisor, director or assistant director of nursing, and other related teaching or consultant roles. The nurse executive advanced credential may be sought by nurse executive at the administrative or executive nursing administration level (ANCC, n.d.).

Work Settings and Job Descriptions

Generally, many work settings incorporate some form of administration or leadership position to ensure that the facility's program mission is accomplished. The term administrator or executive implies a responsibility for the overall facility or program or a specific area. Such an administrator may be responsible for finances, facility operations, nursing department, or all clinical areas. Additionally, there may be multiple layers of management, depending on the facility and departments. Rehabilitation nurse managers may have primary responsibility for implementing the mission, vision, policies, goals, and objectives of the organization and the nursing/clinical services within their area(s). Specific job tasks may include staff development, recruitment/retention efforts, unit staffing and scheduling, budgetary duties, management of physical resources, safety, goal setting for the area/department, and monitoring the progress of the goals to meet quality goals, regulatory accreditation requirements, and credentialing, such as the Joint Commission and Commission on Accreditation of Rehabilitation Facilities (ARN, 2003).

Teaching and Advocacy

Managers and administrators advocate for the staff as well as the patients in the work setting. Leaders advocate for staff by promoting developmental opportunities in both personal and professional arenas, which allows the staff to offer the best practice to their patients in a safe, knowledgeable environment and encourages them to advance professionally. The nurse leader advocates for the safety, protection, and rights of individual patients and nurses, the community, and the nursing profession (ANA, 2009). Additionally, the rehabilitation nurse manager and administrator "advocates for persons with chronic illness and/or disability by participation in the activities of professional organizations and the community" (ARN, 2003, p. 2).

Nurse leaders are an integral part of the nursing profession. The nurse administrator should embrace the concepts of ANA's Magnet Recognition Program®: transformative leadership, structural empowerment, exemplary professional practice, new knowledge, innovation, and improvement, and empirical evidence; these concepts are key to the organization's excellence in professional nursing practice (ANA, 2009). ARN has identified leadership as one of the core goal areas. Each nurse in the rehabilitation practice is also a leader, and current leaders must ensure that each nurse has the skills to be the leaders regardless of the setting and the audience. As such, beyond their direct management duties, there is a duty to educate the future leaders of the profession (ARN Leadership Taskforce, personal communication, 2010). Managers and administrators are responsible to see that educational opportunities are available to their staff in promotion of the advancement of rehabilitation nursing best practices.

Evidence-Based Practice

The rehabilitation nurse leader is responsible for promoting critical thinking and research activities and utilization among the staff to advance the profession and enhance outcomes (ARN, 2003). AONE established the AONE Institute for Nursing Leadership Research and Education to support nursing research. The program includes research seed grants to support research projects related to nursing administration practice and educational scholarships to support nurse executives, directors, and managers who are pursuing an advanced course of study in nursing leadership (AONE, 2010).

Competencies

Nurse executive or leadership competencies have been identified in the areas of leadership (interpersonal skills, analytical and critical thinking, conceptual, technical/ clinical skills, knowledge, and governance), problem solving, collaborating, management, learning and performance improvement, professionalism, planning, implementing and evaluating programs, business skills, and accountability (ANA, 2009; AONE, 2005). Nurse administration must use technology to enhance work flow and improve processes. They must be competent in legal and regulatory compliance practices and statutes, monitoring laws, and changes in professional and quality standards. They are accountable to uphold nursing standards, monitoring licensure and credentialing standards and to so protect the public and uphold the rights of nurses (ANA, 2009). Case Study 6.6 provides an example of how the rehabilitation nurse manager might use critical thinking skills to devise an appropriate plan of care.

CASE STUDY 6.6

Nurses on the rehabilitation unit are arguing about their schedules, their work loads, the patients, and the nursing assistants. Census and acuity have both been high for the last few weeks, and there have been multiple sick calls and float nurses coming to the unit. Because of increased tension and complaints, the nurse manager has handed out guidelines for behavior between workers.

Critical Thinking

1. What is the problem?
2. Whose problem is it?
3. What interactions should have occurred before this point?
4. What should the nurse manager do?

Personal Reflection

- What appeals to you about the role of a manager or administrator?
- Discuss your ability to gain consensus to identify and plan to meet goals.
- What business skills do you have that could assist a unit or facility/program to be successful?
- How do you feel when you must confront difficult tasks or people?

EDUCATOR

The rehabilitation nurse's role as an **educator** is multifaceted and involves a variety of functions in a "variety of settings to develop and maintain the competency of nurses who care for individuals and groups with physical

disability and chronic illness" (ARN, 1995, p.2). Using the nursing plan of care, the rehabilitation nurse educator is responsible for assessing the educational needs, developing a plan to meet the needs identified, and implementing a plan based on legitimate evidence followed by an evaluation of the desired outcomes and evaluating the goals accomplished (ARN, 1995). The role of the rehabilitation nurse educator may include program planner, instructor, record keeper, role model, patient advocate, team member, and nurse leader (ARN, 1995). Facility-based educators and educators in academic settings are discussed here.

Education and Certification

The role of nurse educator is a dual one: nurse and educator. This requires nurses to remain current in nursing practice developments in their chosen specialty (such as gerontology or rehabilitation) and also remain current in education theory and practice (Uys & Gwele, 2005). Preparation for rehabilitation educators may depend on the work setting. Minimum requirements for educators teaching in some healthcare facilities may range from associate degree to doctorate preparation, depending on the environment (i.e., skilled nursing facility or large academic medical center). Educators in nursing academic programs may have a range of basic and highest educational preparation (and certification), depending on the curriculum or program, again, ranging from associate degree to doctorate level preparation. Additionally, certification is offered through several credentialing bodies and academic programs may be required.

Work Settings and Job Descriptions

As previously mentioned, rehabilitation nurse educators may work in a variety of settings, healthcare or academic arenas, and provide education to other healthcare professionals, including nurses, the patient/family, or the public. They may be part of a consulting or interdisciplinary team member whose aim is to meet the educational needs of interdisciplinary staff members. The activities of the rehabilitation nurse educator may include orientation, staff development, continuing education, in-service education, student education, and patient education (ARN, 1995). Typically, educators for facilities (staff development) plan and teach classes geared to the need of the employee of the facility or program and possibly the community or referral sources. Nurse educators participate in orientation for facility employees or students or as consultant to other specialty areas. Rehabilitation nurse educators may be responsible for planning or teaching classes on topics to include diagnoses, treatment plans, team responsibilities, discharge planning, body mechanics, and so on. The rehabilitation nurse educator may also coordinate programs, collaborating with other nurses or disciplines internal or external to the facility/organization. Job descriptions may include elements related to program planning, dissemination of information, record keeper, role modeling, advocacy, clinical competency, collaboration, and leadership (ARN, 1995).

Rehabilitation nurse educators in academic settings may have some of the same basic job activities of program or curriculum planning, instruction, keeping records, role modeling, advocating, and leadership as they disseminate information, foster learning, and while monitoring and assessing student competency. Their job descriptions may include curriculum development and revision; providing didactic teaching and clinical teaching as well as research and publication. In addition, they may also choose to work in facilities as direct care providers to keep the clinical skills current (ARN, 1995).

Teaching and Advocacy

Rehabilitation nurse educators are advocates for their students, regardless of setting, as well as for patients. Educators promote best nursing practice, standards of care, and evidence-based practice so that those they are instructing or guiding will deliver that standard to the population with which they work. The Institute of Medicine report series on quality and safety of patient care and the workplace recognizes the implications for nursing educators. Nurse educators are central in advocacy for safety as they perform their primary function of educating the workforce and monitoring core competencies (Finkelman & Kenner, 2009).

Evidence-Based Practice

Nurse educators in either a clinical or academic setting have a primary responsibility to ensure that students are taught according to standards of care and best practice based on current evidence. Rehabilitation nurse educators must consider both those practice standards of generalist nursing practice as well as those for rehabilitation nursing practice. Promotion of evidence-based practice advances the knowledge and skill of rehabilitation nurses

and improves the outcomes and well-being of the population they serve.

Nursing education has evolved from its early days of hospital-based diploma programs into colleges and universities in response to the vision of nursing as a profession with its own unique body of knowledge. Nursing educators have been central to "produce professional nurses with a commitment to lifelong learning and to expanding scientific knowledge within the discipline" (Sullivan, 2010, p. 38). However, many nurse faculty members find it difficult to meet the demands of academia while maintaining their clinical skills. The clinical rotation for the typical nursing college program is 1 to 2 days per week in the clinical environment, which does not offer the new graduate a realistic view of the nursing experience. Therefore, based on evidenced-based approaches for transition, many institutions today are introducing strategies to extend orientation through nurse preceptor, practicums, and residency programs (Sullivan, 2010). Studies, such as those of the Institute of Medicine on quality and safety and medical errors, that of Dr. Patricia Benner of the Carnegie Foundation of nursing education for excellence, and the Quality and Safety Education for Nurses work of nursing educators at the University of Carolina at Chapel Hill led by Drs. Linda Cronenwett and Gwen Sherwood, have impacted the emphasis on the key role of current nursing education to improve quality, safety, and technology in health care (Finkelman & Kenner, 2009; Sullivan, 2010).

Competencies

The National League for Nursing (NLN) has developed eight core competencies and 66 related task statements for nurse educators. The *Core Competencies for Nurse Educators with Task Statements* (NLN, 2005) provide a framework to prepare the nurse educator and serves as a resource to transform and guide nurse educator scholarship and practice. These core competencies are as follows: facilitate learning, facilitate learner development and socialization, use assessment and evaluation strategies, participate in curriculum design and evaluation of program outcomes, function as a change agent and leader, pursue continuous quality improvement in the nurse educator role, engage in scholarship, and function within the educational environment (NLN, 2005). Case Study 6.7 provides an example of how the rehabilitation nurse educator might use critical thinking skills to devise an appropriate plan of care. The NLN offers a certification for nurse educator.

You are a nursing professor, teaching at your local university and the university hospital. You have students on several floors. They are in various levels of the program. Nurses on one floor are welcoming and act as mentors to students. On another floor, both the nurses and attendants are distant, uncommunicative, and do not like to wait for students when tasks need to be completed. You have spoken to the manager before having students assigned to the unit.

Critical Thinking

1. What is the problem?
2. Why is it a problem?
3. What are key issues?
4. Who will you consult for information on the problem?
5. How should critical thinking be used?
6. What problem-solving strategies should you and the unit manager use?

Personal Reflection

- How do you feel when you educate your patients and families?
- How do you feel when you present information to your peers?
- If teaching interests you, why?

RESEARCHER

Polit and Beck (2008) define nursing research as the "systematic inquiry" (p. 3) of evidence regarding issues important to nursing practice, education, administration, and informatics. The rehabilitation nurse **researcher** "focuses on the activities within the research and quality improvement domain . . . , develops and maintains the knowledge base for nurses who care for individuals/families and groups with physical disability and chronic illness" (ARN, 2004, p. 2). The Rehabilitation Nursing Research Agenda identifies four high priority areas for research: nursing and nursing-led interdisciplinary interventions, experience of disability and/or chronic health problems for individuals and family across the life span, rehabilitation in the changing health care system, and the rehabilitation nursing profession (Jacelon, Pierce, & Buhrer, 2007). "Research is needed to provide the evidence upon which to base practice . . . useful to rehabilitation nurses wherever they practice" (Jacelon et al., 2007, p. 23). Therefore, ARN, the rehabilitation nursing professional specialty nursing organization, supports research by offering annual grants to promote research

that affect rehabilitation nursing or the recipients of rehabilitation care through the Rehabilitation Nursing Foundation. Evidence-based practice is the cornerstone of practice excellence, used for the development of standards of practice and to influence policy and legislation impacting those with chronic illness and disability (Jacelon et al., 2007).

> "Research is needed to provide the evidence upon which to base practice . . . useful to rehabilitation nurses wherever they practice"
>
> (Jacelon, Pierce, & Buhrer, 2007, p. 23).

Educational Preparation and Certification

Nurses at all levels can be involved in research activities, and the number of those involved are increasing in number, as evidenced by the 2005 ARN member survey where 20% of the respondents identified themselves as researchers, compared with an earlier member survey in 1993 in which more than 40% reported not being involved with research at all (Jacelon et al. 2007). Rehabilitation nurses may be involved in research as principle investigators directly conducting new research or by replicating a study. Others may be involved in research and evidence-based activities in a variety of other ways, through journal club participation, conducting a quality or process improvement project in their setting to improve outcomes, participation in the facility's research or evidence-based practice committee/council, communicating research findings to peers through presentations, flyers, or posters aimed at educating staff on new evidence, or by writing or revising a hospital or policy or standard of practice (Miller & Bach, 2007). Rehabilitation nurse researchers are most likely educated at various levels ranging from the baccalaureate level, where students are introduced to the research process to the doctorate level where research application is a more integral part of the program.

Work Settings and Job Descriptions

Nurse researchers work in a variety of settings, such as academia, government, private sector, healthcare facilities or programs, or in private practice where they include research as part of their practice or business. In academe, nurse faculty members may be expected to engage in nursing scholarly activities that may include participating in research activities as part of their mandatory scholarly activities and publication to achieve or maintain tenure and promotion (ARN, 2004).

Teaching and Advocacy

The rehabilitation nurse researcher role is inherently consistent with the goal of rehabilitation nursing to improve nursing practice and patient outcomes. Through research and evidence-based practice, the researcher teaches and advocates the public regarding the specialty practice of rehabilitation nursing, for the care and needs of the disabled and chronically ill, and to promote the treatment of those with functional disabilities and chronic conditions, promoting health across the life span (ARN, 2008). Researchers can increase their roles of teacher and advocate through publication in peer-reviewed journals and publication for the general population (Miller & Bach, 2007).

Evidence-Based Practice

The rehabilitation nurse researcher is responsible for analyzing, interpreting, and disseminating findings through many sources, such as presentation, publication, or other media sources. The researcher in rehabilitation must synthesize the evidence for application and relevance to the setting and population and to evaluate the impact this evidence may have on practice (ARN, 2004).

Direct application of evidence-based practice does not elude the role of the nurse researcher. The nurse researcher must use current evidence-based strategies and technology to seek information. These strategies are evident in the work of the NINR, which is founded on an overall mission to facilitate research that promotes the health through collaborative research efforts to enhance communication and resources. Investigators of NINR focus on common areas of interest in disease management, health disparities, improving patient outcomes, or end-or-life care issues, for example (Grady, 2009). NINR has structured its research funding support in three stages: *nursing science*, which targets the emerging research of schools of nursing, supporting small to mid-level studies; *nursing centers of excellence*, designed for more experienced research investigators and institutions; and the *research program projects*, for large well-established collaborative research studies (Grady, 2009). This type of support brings together colleagues at many levels together who share a common research interest which increases opportunities. Case Study 6.8 provides an example of how the rehabilitation nurse researcher might use critical thinking skills to devise an appropriate plan of care.

CASE STUDY 6.8

You are an APRN at your facility and a major focus of your job description is improvement of nursing care and patient outcomes. Your facility participates in programs that indicate patient status on admission and discharge as well as patient satisfaction. The nurses come to you with concerns that patient evaluations are not accurate.

Critical Thinking

1. What information do you need to start a process to review their concerns?
2. Who are your resources?
3. Does anybody else in the facility have the same concern?
4. If others don't, does this mean there is no problem?
5. What effect could research on this topic have for your facility?

Personal Reflection

- What appeals to you about nursing/rehabilitation research?
- Do you have any ideas now about research that is needed in rehabilitation nursing?
- How do you feel about your writing and analysis skills?
- How do you feel about conducting literature reviews for relevant material related to a nursing problem?

ADVANCED PRACTICE REGISTERED NURSE

The **advanced practice registered nurse (APRN)** is an umbrella term used to describe those nurse roles of certified registered nurse anesthetist, certified nurse midwife, clinical nurse specialist (CNS), and NP (ANA, 2004). These roles are very distinguishable in many ways and yet share common core knowledge and skills. In the rehabilitation setting, two roles (CNS and NP) are the ones commonly seen and are discussed here. According to the *Standards and Scope of Rehabilitation Nursing Practice* (ARN, 2008), advanced practice rehabilitation registered nurses "possess and demonstrate advanced levels of expertise in providing, directing, managing, and influencing the care of rehabilitation patients" (p. 18).

Nurse Practitioner

NPs diagnose and treat a wide range of health problems while focusing on health promotion, disease prevention, health education, and counseling to management acute and chronic illness and diseases. NPs perform comprehensive assessments; order, conduct, supervise, and interpret diagnostic and laboratory tests; and order appropriate pharmacological and nonpharmacological treatments in collaboration with other healthcare professionals as appropriate and in accordance with state and federal standard (ANA, 2008).

Clinical Nurse Specialist

The CNS functions as a clinical expert in a specialty of nursing practice. The CNS designs, implements, and evaluates programs; provides expert knowledge and skill to the team; and serves as a mentor, educator, and researcher to advance evidenced-based nursing practice (American Association of College of Nursing, 2010). The CNS in the rehabilitation setting is the clinical expert and consultant within the specialty to manage health concerns of individual patients/families, populations, and staff through program development or through a more direct care role, performing health assessment, diagnosis, and providing pharmacological and nonpharmacological treatment as allowed by state, federal, or facility standards.

Educational Preparation and Certification

The APRN is a licensed RN who has acquired advanced specialized clinical knowledge and skills in a specialized area of care. The APRN is expected to hold a master's or doctorate degree and demonstrate a certain level of competence and certification according to state and federal mandates (ARN, 2004; ANA, 2008). Currently, there is no advanced practice certification in rehabilitation nursing. The CRRN-A credential, held by only a small number of APRNs in rehabilitation, was phased out in 2009. Therefore, APRNs in rehabilitation typically are trained and certified in another specialty area, such as practitioners in adult, family, gerontological, pediatric, and women's health; acute care; psychiatric-mental health; neonatal; occupational; and emergency care for example, and hold certification as a generalist in rehabilitation nursing.

According to the American Academy of Nurse Practitioners (2010), the entry-level preparation of the NP is at the graduate level. Didactic and clinical courses prepare nurses with specialized knowledge and clinical competency to practice in primary care, acute care, and long-term care. The doctor of nursing practice is considered to be a terminal practice doctorate degree and proposed for future programs preparing the CNS and NP. It is aimed at educating nurses "at the point of care and apply evidence-based practice and research to patient outcomes and quality of care" (Finkelman & Kenner, 2009, pp. 54–55).

Work Settings and Job Descriptions

Practice settings for the APRN are evolving and growing as more attention is focused on meeting the healthcare demands of this nation's citizens effectively and efficiently. In rehabilitation, the APRN's work or practice setting may include but may not be limited to inpatient facilities, outpatient clinics and physician offices, academic medical centers, long-term care and residential programs, insurance companies, private practice, ambulatory care and retail clinics, pharmaceutical companies, universities and colleges, and schools (ARN, 2004; ANA, 2008). The evolution of technology has impacted the delivery of APRN services to others. Telehealth or telemedicine technology has made delivery of services to remote settings possible and available to more communities. Healthcare clinics in large department stores and shopping malls, known as *retail clinics*, have provided a unique method of bringing health care to the area not only where people live but to where they shop.

Teaching and Advocacy

APRNs in rehabilitation provide essential information to individual patients regarding disease prevention and treatment and groups and championing for a positive learning environment. They advocate on behalf of the patient/family and for the nursing practice, advocating as a change agent and for social reform and policy changes. They advocate by pursuing leadership positions in professional organizations and in the community (Howard & Mauk, 2007).

This is a critical time for the APRN, most especially the NP, as our nation debates issues of quality, access, concern for patient safety, and delivery. As the demand for primary care providers increases, the role of the APRN will most assuredly grow. But, with this potential for growth, so grows the responsibility to teach, advocate, and effectively communicate to the public their role in health care and their capability to provide quality care (Mullinix & Bucholtz, 2009). By 2020 it is estimated that 85,000 additional practitioners will be needed, and expanding the use and independent practice of APRNs is being advocated to meet this need. One big proponent of advancing the role and autonomy of APRNs, however disguised as concern for patient safety, has come from the medical community. Calls from the American Medical Association insist that all patient care be directed or supervised by physicians rather than in collaboration between APRN and physicians, which has proven to result in safe and effective outcomes (Mullinix & Bucholtz, 2009).

APRNs in rehabilitation are responsible for teaching patients, families, interdisciplinary staff, physicians or other APRNs, and the community. The APRN must communicate to the patient/family the findings of any assessed risks, benefits, and expected outcomes of their healthcare treatment and plan. APRNs must participate in and communicate realistic goal setting and advocate ethically within the rehabilitation treatment team (ARN, 2008). Rehabilitation APRNs are involved in educating nursing students and other health professional students both in the clinical and academic setting of the unique care of rehabilitation patients and their families.

Evidence-Based Practice

Mullinix and Bucholtz (2009) performed a literature review of the NP role and quality patient outcomes. Through their review of multiple studies that compare patient satisfaction, health status, and clinical outcomes, they found that many studies were flawed and conducted either "by parties with an interest in advancing the practice of the NP, potentially biasing the study in favor of the NP . . . [and in] other studies appear to have been conducted with an inherent bias against the NP . . ." (p. 95). Yet, by a review of more rigorous studies, they concluded that the care provided by NPs resulted in higher quality care measures, such as diagnostic accuracy, comprehensive health history, resolution of illness and functional status, patient satisfaction, and compliance (Mullinix & Bucholtz, 2009). "Scientific underpinnings for practice" is one of the eight essentials of doctorate of nursing practice educational programs, as the APRN is expected to use and synthesize knowledge and current evidence, translating it into practice (Finkelman & Kenner, 2009).

The American Academy of Nurse Practitioners Research Department provides information on NP research and limited guidance for NPs and others interested in research about NPs and their practices. The National Organization of Nurse Practitioner Faculties also promotes participation and excellence in clinical scholarship. Rehabilitation nurses must use best practices, and NPs are held to the higher level of advanced practice nurses when caring for their patients. NPs develop clinical research questions and use the evidence from research to promote best practice (American Academy of Nurse Practitioners, 2010), which will result in more complete assessments and problem solving, accurate diagnoses, improved plans of care, and improved patient outcomes as well as increased job satisfaction.

Competencies

Competencies have been developed for APRNs in direct clinical practice; expert coaching and guidance; consultation; research; clinical, professional, and systems leadership; collaboration; and ethical decision making (Hamric, Spross, & Hanson, 2008).

The National Organization of Nurse Practitioner Faculties has adopted competencies for practitioners in adult, family, gerontological, pediatric, and women's health; acute care; psychiatric-mental health; and emergency care. Competencies are in management of patient health/illness status, NP–patient relationship, teaching-coaching function, professional role, managing and negotiating healthcare delivery systems, monitoring and ensuring the quality of healthcare practices, and cultural competence (National Organization of Nurse Practitioner Faculties, 2006).

As APRNs, CNSs have a responsibility of accountability to the public. Hence, the CNS core competencies were developed in 1995 by the National Association of Clinical Nurse Specialists validated in a 2005 national study. The core competencies are designed to articulate the underpinning of CNS practice and its difference from other advanced nurse roles. There are 75 core competencies covered in three domains or "spheres of influence": client (direct care clinical experts in diagnosis and treatment), nurse and nursing practice (practice based on evidence), and organization/system (contributing to health systems as a whole) (Baldwin et al., 2009; Goudreau et al., 2007). The full description of competencies can be found in the *Statement on Clinical Nurse Specialist Practice and Education* (National Association of Clinical Nurse Specialists, 2009). Competencies are tested in the certification process. Case Study 6.9 provides an example of how the rehabilitation CNS might use critical thinking skills to devise an appropriate plan of care.

CASE STUDY 6.9

Advance Practice Nurse Exercises

Personal Reflection

- How do you feel about further education?
- Do you believe experience before further education would enhance your practice? Why?
- Discuss your self-assessment of your analysis and critical thinking skills.

NP Case Study

You are working in an outpatient clinic were patients return for therapy and follow-up on medical care after discharge from the rehabilitation facility. A stroke patient has returned for speech and physical therapy and appears to have declined since the previous visit 4 days earlier. He is 3 weeks poststroke. Although he appears to be alert and oriented, the speech therapist reports he is having problems with attending to the session. The physical therapist has noted the same and also commented on reduced balance and poor endurance.

Critical Thinking

1. How will your assessment start?
2. What will it include?
3. Is there information you may need that is not immediately available in his chart?
4. Who will you talk to for further information?
5. How will you analyze the data you have collected?

Personal Reflection

- Do you see yourself practicing at the autonomous level of an NP? How?
- How do you believe an NP would function in a rehabilitation facility? A clinic? A physician office?

CNS Case Study

Nurses on your unit have questions about nursing practice related to transfers, falls, and restraints. They believe the hospital procedures do not adequately cover the safety of themselves or their patients.

Critical Thinking

1. What will your first actions be?
2. Who will you gather information from?
3. What other resources will you access?
4. Are there specific policy, procedures, or departments you will want to discuss?
5. Can this problem be resolved by critical thinking or are there other processes you will want to consider?

Personal Reflection

- What would lead you to become a clinical specialist?
- Do you find one area of rehabilitation more interesting than others?
- Do you see yourself as a resource to others? How?

SUMMARY

The role of the rehabilitation nurse is complex, overlapping, and, as demonstrated, multifaceted in the healthcare arena. The rehabilitation nurse's role is key in its partnership with the interdisciplinary team and central to the success of the rehabilitation program. The nurse brings unique education and knowledge of the specialty practice of rehabilitation, competent practice and leadership skills, founded in current evidence, while collaborating with and advocating for others, to achieve optimal outcomes for comprehensive rehabilitation care.

Opportunities for nurses in rehabilitation are almost endless, depending on the interest and self-motivation of the individual nurse. Nurses may enter the field of rehabilitation nursing knowing what area interests them most. Others may have an experience that excites them to pursue further knowledge and experience in a specific area. Not all nurses are automatic teachers, leaders, or researchers. Some nurses will want to further themselves as advanced practice nurses and some will be excellent direct caregivers. Likewise, some nurses will find the most satisfaction with pediatrics or the older population, and some will find they are most effective with a general population or a specific diagnosis. Regardless, all the roles listed here, and additional roles, are important services to the client population along the continuum of care and the continuum of life.

CASE STUDY 6.10

Mr. A is a 29-year-old who was involved in an altercation. He was hit in the head and then fell and struck his head on the sidewalk and became unconscious. He was taken to the local hospital, stabilized, and admitted to the ICU on a ventilator. After several weeks he is awake and alert and off the ventilator but still on a feeding tube. He is intermittently physically and verbally agitated and cannot be left alone. He is able to participate in therapy with the assistance of a nursing attendant.

Before injury he lived alone. His parents are elderly and live out of state. He worked part time at a local grocery store and has a minimal insurance policy.

1. As a direct care provider what are your concerns?
2. Identify three interventions for this patient regarding safety and discharge planning.
3. Who would you identify as the team for this patient?
4. Who are your resources?
5. As manager of the Brain Injury unit, what are your considerations in providing safe care to this patient?
6. As the clinical specialist, what are your opportunities for working with the staff and patient?
7. How will you determine a plan of care per evidence-based practice?
8. You are the case manager for this patient.
   a. Describe your interactions with the team.
   b. When will you start discussing the discharge plan and who are your resources?
   c. What information will you need to discuss Mr. A with his insurance company?
   d. What do you anticipate will affect the discharge plan?

CASE STUDY 6.11

Mr. B is an 80-year-old married man. His wife is 79. They have been married for 50 years and live independently. Two children live in the same town. Mr. B. has suffered a massive stoke and currently has left hemiplegia with neglect and impulsivity. He is 5'10" tall, weighs 200 pounds, has a history of coronary artery disease and diabetes, and has had the toes of his right foot amputated. His wife is healthy and is 5'1" and weighs 124 pounds.

1. As the nurse liaison, what should your assessment include?
2. What would be the goal of the rehabilitation admission?
3. As the direct care clinician, what are your concerns and how will your plan address those concerns?
4. What are topics for education and who should be included in the education?
5. Who should be included in the discharge plan?
6. What do you believe community resources are?
7. Who are the case managers that could be included in this case?
8. Who should the team members be for this patient and how will you communicate your concerns to the entire team?
9. As direct care provider, manager, or clinical specialist, do you believe this would be a good patient for a nursing student to care for? Why?

REFERENCES

American Academy of Nurse Practitioners. (2010). About NPs. Retrieved from http://www.aanp.org/AANPCMS2/AboutAANP/About+NPs.htm

American Association of Colleges of Nurses. (2010). The essentials of master's education for advanced practice nursing. Retrieved from http://www.aacn.nche.edu/Educatioin/pdf/MasEssential96.pdf

American Association of Critical-Care Nurses. (2008). AACN and AONE launch certified nurse manager and leader credential. *AACN News, 25*(11), 1.

American Nurses Association (ANA). (2004). *Nursing: Scope and standards of practice.* Silver Spring, MD: Author.

American Nurses Association (ANA). (2008). *Nursing administration: Scope and standards of practice.* Silver Spring, MD: Author.

American Nurses Credentialing Center (ANCC). (n.d.). *2008–2010 Testing information/certification application form: Nurse executive, advanced* [Brochure]. Baltimore: Author.

American Organization of Nurse Executives (AONE). (2005). AONE nurse executive competencies. Nurse leader (pp. 50–56). Retrieved from http://www.aone.org/aone/pdf/February%20Nurse%20Leader--final%draft--for%20web.pdf

American Organization of Nurse Executive (AONE). (2010). Retrieved from http://www.aone.org

Association of Rehabilitation Nurses (ARN). (n.d.).Certification: Eligibility criteria. Retrieved August 9, 2010, from http://www.rehabnurse.org/certification/criteria.html

Association of Rehabilitation Nurses (ARN). (1995). *The rehabilitation nurse educator: Role description* [Brochure]. Glenview, IL: Author.

Association of Rehabilitation Nurses (ARN). (2003). *The rehabilitation nurse manager: Role description* [Brochure]. Glenview, IL: Author.

Association of Rehabilitation Nurses (ARN). (2004). *The rehabilitation nurse researcher: Role description* [Brochure]. Glenview, IL: Author.

Association of Rehabilitation Nurses (ARN). (2008). *Standards and scope of rehabilitation nursing practice.* Glenview, IL: Author.

Association of Rehabilitation Nurses (ARN). (2010). Rehabilitation nursing. Retrieved from www.rehabnurse.org

Baldwin, K. M., Clark, A. P., Fulton, J., & Mayo, A. (2009). National validation of the NACNS clinical nurse specialist core competencies. *Journal of Nursing Scholarship, 41*(2), 193–201.

Borglund, S. T. (2008). Case management quality-of-life outcomes for adults with a disability. *Rehabilitation Nursing, 33*(6), 260–267.

Case Management Society of American (CMSA). (2010). *Standards of practice for case management* (revised). Little Rock, AK: Author.

DiCenso, A., Guyatt, G., & Ciliska, D. (Eds.). (2005). *Evidence-based nursing: A guide to clinical practice.* St. Louis, MO: Mosby.

Finkelman, A., & Kenner, C. (2009). *Teaching IOM: Implications of the IOM reports for nursing education* (2nd ed.). Silver Spring, MD: American Nurses Association.

Gallagher, R. M. (2010). Quality is not an irreconcilable difference *Nursing Management, 41*(8), 18–20.

Goudreau, K. A., Baldwin, K., Clark, A., et al. (2007). *A vision of the future for clinical nurse specialists.* Prepared by the National Association of Clinical Nurse Specialists. Harrisburg, PA: NACNS.

Grady, P. A. (2009). The NINR research centers program. *Nursing Outlook, 57*(2), 113–115.

Hader, R. (2010). Numbers don't tell the whole story. *Nursing Management, 41*(8), 6.

Hamric, A, Spross, J., & Hanson, C, (2008). *Advanced practice nursing* (4th ed.). Philadelphia: W.B. Saunders

Heinemann, A.W. (2008). State of the science of postacute rehabilitation: Setting a research agenda and developing an evidence base for practice and policy. An introduction. *Rehabilitation Nursing, 33*(2), 82–87.

Hertzberg, D. L. (2008). Rehabilitation nursing care of people with intellectual/developmental disabilities. In S. P. Hoeman (Ed.), *Rehabilitation nursing: Prevention, intervention, & outcomes* (4th ed., pp. 610–631). Naples, ME: Mosby.

Hoeman, S. P., Duchene, P. M., & Vierling, L. (2008). Ethical and legal issues in rehabilitation nursing. In S.P. Hoeman (Ed.), *Rehabilitation nursing: Prevention, intervention, & outcomes* (4th ed., pp. 30–44). Naples, ME: Mosby.

Howard, C. J., & Mauk, K. L. (2007). Stroke. In K. L. Mauk (Ed.), *The specialty practice of rehabilitation nursing: A core curriculum* (5th ed., pp. 156–182). Glenview, IL: ARN.

Jacelon, C. S., Pierce, L. L., & Buhrer, R. (2007). Revision of the rehabilitation nursing research agenda. *Rehabilitation Nursing, 32*(1), 23–30.

Jackson, D. F. (2008). Pediatric rehabilitation nursing. In S.P. Hoeman (Ed.), *Rehabilitation nursing: Prevention, intervention, & outcomes* (4th ed., pp. 632–654). Naples, ME: Mosby.

Lee, J., & Higgins, P. A. (2008). Predicting posthospital recovery of physical function among older adults after lower extremity surgery in a short-stay skilled nursing facility. *Rehabilitation Nursing, 33*(4), 170–177.

Long, A. F., Kneafsey, R. Ryan, J., & Berry, J. (2002). The role of the nurse within the multi-professional rehabilitation team. *Journal of Advanced Nursing, 37*(1), 70–78.

Mauk, K. L. (2010). *Gerontological Nursing: Competencies for Care.* Sudbury, MA: Jones and Bartlett Publishers.

McClain, N., Richardson, B., & Wyatt, J. S. (2004). A profile of certification for pediatric nurses. *Pediatric Nursing, 30*(3), 207–211.

Melnyk, B.M., & Fineout-Overholt, E. (2011). *Evidence-based practice in nursing & healthcare: A guide to best practice* (2nd ed.). Philadelphia: Lippincott Williams & Wilkins.

Miller, E. T., & Bach, C. A. (2007). Research and evidence-based practice. In K. L. Mauk (Ed.), *The specialty practice of rehabilitation nursing: A core curriculum* (5th ed., pp. 433–447). Glenview, IL: ARN.

Mullinix, C., & Bucholtz, D. P. (2009). Role and quality of nurse practitioner practice: A policy Issues. *Nursing Outlook, 57*(2), 93–96.

National Association of Clinical Nurse Specialists. (2009). Core practice doctorate clinical nurse specialist (CNS) competencies. Retrieved from http://www.nacns.org/LinkClick.aspx?fileticket=AADJmIZ7EaM%3d&tabid=36

National Association of Nurse Practitioners Faculties. (2010). Competencies for nursing practitioners. Retrieved from http://www.nonpf.com/displaycommon.cfm?an=1&subarticlenbr=14

National Association of Professional Geriatric Care Managers. (n.d.). What is a professional geriatric care manager? Retrieved from http://www.caremanager.org/displaycommon.dfm?an=1&subarticlenbr=76

National League for Nursing (NLN). (2005). Core competencies of nurse educators with task statements. Retrieved from http://www.nln.org/facultydevelopment/pdf/corecompetencies.pdf

Nelson, A., Powell-Cope, G., Palacios, P., Luther, S. L., Black, T., Hillman, T., Christiansen, B., Nathenson, P., & Gross, J. C. (2007). Nurse staffing and patient outcomes in inpatient rehabilitation settings. *Rehabilitation Nursing, 32*(5), 179–202.

Polit, D. F., & Beck, C. T. (2008). *Nursing research: Generating and assessing evidence for nursing practice* (8th ed.). Philadelphia: Lippincott Williams & Wilkins.

Secrest, J. (2007). Rehabilitation and rehabilitation nursing. In K. L. Mauk (Ed.), *The specialty practice of rehabilitation nursing: A core curriculum* (5th ed., pp. 2–12). Glenview, IL: ARN.

Stichler, J. F. (2006). Skills and competencies for today's nurse executive. *AWHONN Lifelines, 10*(3), 255–257.

Stierle, L. J., Mezey, M., Schumann, M. J., Esterson, J., Smolenski, M. C., Horsley, K. D., et al. (2006). Professional development. The Nurse Competence in Aging initiative: encouraging expertise in the care of older adults. *American Journal of Nursing, 106*(9), 93–4, 96.

Sullivan, D. T. (2010). Connecting nursing education and practice: A focus on shared goals for quality and safety. *Creative Nursing, 16*(1), 37–43.

Swearingen, S. (2009). A journey to leadership: designing a nursing leadership development program. *Journal of Continuing Education in Nursing, 40*(3), 107–112.

U.S. Department of Health and Human Services, Administration on Aging. (n.d.). A profile of older Americans: 2005. Retrieved from http://assets.aarp.org/rgcenter/general/profile_2005.pdf

Uys, L. R., & Gwele, N. S. (2005). *Curriculum development in nursing: Process and innovation.* New York: Routledge.

Watts, M. D. (2010). Certification and clinical ladder as the impetus for professional development. *Critical Care Nursing Quarterly, 33*(1), 52–59.

Weston, M. J., Falter, B., Lamb, G. S., et al (2008). Health care leadership academy: A statewide collaboration to enhance nursing leadership competencies. *Journal of Continuing Education in Nursing, 39*(10), 468–472.

Williams, D., & McCollum, P. (2007). Rehabilitation nursing and case management. In K. L. Mauk (Ed.), *The specialty practice of rehabilitation nursing: A core curriculum* (5th ed., pp. 412–420). Glenview, IL: ARN.

ONLINE RESOURCES

Agency for Health Research and Quality: www.ahrq.gov

American Academy of Nurse Practitioners: www.aanp.org

American Association of College of nursing: www.aacn.niche.edu

American Geriatrics Society: www.americangeriatrics.org

American Nurses Association: www.nursingworld.org

ANA GeroNurse Online: www.geronurseonline.org

American Nurses Credentialing Center: www.nursecredentialing.org

Association of Nurse Executives: www.aone.org

Association of Rehabilitation Nurses: www.rehabnurse.org

The Center for Nursing Advocacy: www.nursingadvocacy.org

Gerontological Nursing Interventions Research Center: www.nursing.uiowa.edu

Hartford Institute for Geriatric Nursing: www.consultgeriRN. org

National League for Nursing: www.nln.org

National Association of Clinical Specialists: www.nacns.org

National Organization of Nurse Practitioner Faculties: www. nonpf.com

National Nursing Staff Development Organization: www.nnsdo. org

National Institute of Nursing Research: www.ninr.nih.gov

Society of Pediatric Nurses: www.pedsnurses.org

CHAPTER 7

Improving Nutritional Status and Swallowing

Reatha Collinsworth

LEARNING OBJECTIVES

At the end of this chapter, the reader will be able to

- Describe nutritional needs over the life span.
- Name tools used to assess nutritional condition.
- Discuss how nutrition impacts or is affected by certain rehab conditions.
- Identify patients at risk for dysphasia and its diagnosis and treatment.
- Recognize complications of parenteral and enteral feeding routes.
- Explain the importance of interdisciplinary management of nutritional needs.

KEY CONCEPTS AND TERMS

Absorption	Low-density-lipoprotein (LDL)	Percutaneous endoscopic
Albumin	cholesterol	gastrostomy (PEG) tube
Amino acids	Macronutrients	Percutaneous endoscopic
Anabolism	Malnutrition	jejunostomy tube
Anorexia nervosa	Metabolism	Polyunsaturated fatty acids
Basic nutrients	Micronutrients	(PUFA)
Bulimia	Monounsaturated fatty acids	Polysaccharides
Catabolism	(MUFA)	Prealbumin
Cholesterol	Nasogastric (NG) tube	Triglyceride
Disaccharides	Nonessential proteins	
Hydrogenated	Nutrients	

The incidence of **malnutrition** in hospitalized patients can range from 30% to 50%, with even more patients at risk. Complications from poor nutrition can lead to increased morbidity, mortality, length of stay, and expense (Charney & Malone, 2009). Good nutritional management can prevent complications and/or improve outcomes. Registered dietitians or nutritionists are the experts who provide the best resource for nutritional management, but when this resource is not available, rehabilitation nurses may play a more important role in this area. The rehabilitation setting is likely to serve patients with the gamut of nutritional needs or conditions. It is incumbent on the rehabilitation nurse to understand nutrition, know nutritional needs of specific rehabilitation conditions, to be able to assess nutritional condition, and to respond appropriately.

> *Micronutrients are substances needed for metabolism. Included are vitamins, vitamin-like substances, minerals, and elements that are essential for survival. Vitamins are divided into water soluble and fat soluble.*

BASIC NUTRITION

Three classes of **nutrients** are needed by humans: protein, carbohydrates, and fats. **Micronutrients** (vitamins, minerals, and trace elements) are also needed for growth and maintenance. Protein is a source of **amino acids**, necessary for the body to build and repair its tissues. Osmotic pressure is maintained by adequate protein levels, and protein is a component of antibodies and enzymes. Essential proteins are those the body cannot synthesize and must be present in the diet. **Nonessential proteins** are those that can be manufactured by the body. Sources of all essential amino acids include eggs, meat, poultry, dairy products, and certain combinations of grains, beans, legumes, nuts, and seeds such as corn and beans. Each gram of protein provides about 4 kcal and provides a greater level of satiety than fats or carbohydrates. The recommended dietary allowance for protein is 0.8 g/kg of body weight per day (U.S. Department of Health & Human Services, 2005).

Anabolism is the process of storing or using protein for tissue building. Conversely, **catabolism** is the breaking down of protein for use as energy when needed, via the Krebs cycle. Protein is the only **macronutrient** that contains nitrogen and the body is said to be in positive nitrogen balance in anabolism and in negative nitrogen balance when catabolism is occurring. During catabolism nitrogenous wastes (urea, uric acid, ammonia, and creatinine) result; thus, protein may be restricted in hepatic or renal failure. Great demand for protein occurs in times of growth or when there is need for repair, as in burns or trauma. Protein ingestion beyond anabolic need is stored as glycogen or fat.

After mechanical digestion in the mouth, pepsin, hydrochloric acid, and rennin in the stomach begin protein digestion. Then, pancreatic and intestinal enzymes in the small intestine complete the process, and **absorption** takes place in the small bowel.

The body's main source of energy is from carbohydrates (providing about 60% of the caloric need for most adults), the main source of vitamins and minerals and the only source of fiber. Carbohydrates get their name from the elements that make up its molecule, carbon, oxygen, and hydrogen.

Carbohydrates can be grouped into simple (mono- and **disaccharides**) and complex (**polysaccharides**). Simple carbohydrates can be further broken down into the monosaccharides, which include glucose, fructose, and galactose, and the disaccharides, which include maltose, sucrose, and lactose. Simple carbohydrates are easily digested and are often present in the diet as sweeteners added to processed foods and beverages. The complex carbohydrate molecule consists of starch and cellulose and is obtained from fruits, vegetables, whole grains, and beans. Starch is the main dietary source of carbohydrate.

Lipids are found in both plant and animal sources and are needed by the body as an energy source to provide fatty acids and the fat-soluble vitamins A, D, E, and K. Lipids also enhance the flavor of food. Fat, at 9 kcal/g, provides the highest energy density of the three major nutrient groups. Three classes of fat occur naturally: saturated, **monounsaturated fatty acids (MUFAs)**, and **polyunsaturated fatty acids (PUFAs)**. An unsaturated molecule of fat has a double bond between two carbon atoms. In a saturated fat one of those bonds is between the two carbon atoms and one is with a hydrogen atom, thus the term **hydrogenated**. Oleic acid is the most common form of MUFA. It is found in canola and olive oil, peanuts, pecans, and avocados. The diet of the Mediterranean region is rich in legumes and MUFA-rich oils. Conforming to this diet can reduce platelet activity and may also reduce cardiac events (Peckenpaugh, 2010).

Saturated fats, which are primarily from animal sources, are usually solid at room temperature and contribute to increases in **low-density-lipoprotein (LDL) cholesterol**, or harmful cholesterol. Adding hydrogen to unsaturated fat can change the configuration to trans fatty acid, which is useful to extend the life of certain foods. However, trans fatty acid has gained attention as an unhealthy fat, which can raise LDL cholesterol. Trans fats are found in partially hydrogenated vegetable oils, margarine, and many snack foods such as cookies and chips. Careful reading of food labels can help in avoiding this undesirable fat.

Cholesterol is a lipid compound found exclusively in animal tissue. It can be ingested or produced by the body. The body requires cholesterol to produce certain hormones, cell walls and bile acids for digestion. **Triglyceride** is a chemical name for fats in the body or in food. It consists of three fatty acids and a glycerol molecule.

Mechanical and chemical digestion of fat begins in the mouth with lingual lipase and continues in the stomach with gastric lipase and in the duodenum, with most absorption taking place in the proximal small bowel. The recommendation is that no more than 20% to 35% of calories be from fat (U.S. Department of Health & Human Services, 2005).

Consuming healthy fats such as PUFAs and MUFAs can help to favorably manage lipid levels. PUFAs include omega 3 and omega 6 fatty acids. Omega 3 fatty acids can decrease serum triglycerides, platelet aggregation, and inflammation—highly desirable for cardiac health. Total cholesterol, LDL cholesterol, and high-density-lipoprotein cholesterol can be lowered by PUFAs.

Omega 6 (linoleic acid), which is a precursor of prostaglandins and is a component of cell membranes, cannot be synthesized by the body and must be provided by the diet (Hark & Morrison, 2003). Linoleic acid is found in corn, canola, safflower, and sunflower oils.

TABLE 7.1	Water-Soluble Vitamins		
Vitamin	**Sources**	**Function**	**Deficiency**
B1, thiamine	Pork, beef, liver, whole grains	Normal growth, heart, nerve and muscle function	Beriberi, GI and CNS symptoms, CHF
B2, riboflavin	Meat, dairy, grains	Normal growth and energy	Glossitis, stomatitis skin eruptions
B3, niacin	Meat, dairy products, eggs nuts, grains	Energy, growth, skin health	Pellagra, anorexia, skin problems, confusion
B5, pantothenic acid	Fish, poultry organ meat, egg, legumes, whole grains	Energy release from carbohydrates, fats, and protein	Natural deficiency not known to exist
B6, pyridoxine	Fish, poultry, meat, soy, fortified grains, fruit	Amino acid metabolism protein synthesis, heme synthesis	Anemia, irritability, convulsions, neuritis
B12	Meat dairy, shellfish, eggs	Synthesis of heme, myelin sheath formation	Neuropathy pernicious anemia due to lack of intrinsic factor
Vitamin C	Citrus, tomatoes, melons leafy dark leafy vegetables	Collagen synthesis, iron metabolism	Scurvy
Folic acid	Fruits, vegetables, fortified grains	Needed by rapidly growing tissue, metabolism of amino acids	Fetal neural tube defects, macrocytic anemia, GI problems
Biotin	Egg yolk, soy, peanut butter, mushrooms	Needed for synthesis of fatty and amino acids and purines	Alopecia, nausea, vomiting, dermatitis depression, lethargy Deficiency is rare

CHF, congestive heart failure; CNS, central nervous system; GI, gastrointestinal

MUFA, found in canola or olive oil, peanuts, pecans, and avocados, can lower LDL cholesterol without lowering high-density-lipoprotein cholesterol and can help to lower triglycerides.

Micronutrients are substances needed for **metabolism**. Included are vitamins, vitamin-like substances, minerals, and elements that are essential for survival.

Vitamins are divided into water soluble and fat soluble (Table 7.1 and Table 7.2). Minerals provide structure for the body and help regulate bodily processes. Included are calcium, phosphorus, potassium magnesium, sodium, chloride, and sulfur. Trace elements are zinc, iron, copper, selenium, manganese, cobalt molybdenum, iodine, and fluoride, among others (Figure 7.1).

TABLE 7.2	Fat-Soluble Vitamins		
Vitamin	**Sources**	**Function**	**Deficiency**
Vitamin A Retinol	Organ meats, egg yolks Fortified milk and fish	Eye health, epithelial cell health, bone growth, immunity	Night blindness, dry eye, increased susceptibility to disease
Vitamin D Cholecalciferol	Fortified milk, sun exposure, fatty fish	Bone health, calcium and phosphorus metabolism	Ricketts Osteoporosis
Vitamin E	Vegetable oils and seeds	Antioxidant, healthy cellular membranes	Muscle weakness, hemolysis, ataxia, poor vision Deficiency is rare
Vitamin K	Synthesized by intestinal flora, green leafy vegetables	Needed to produce several clotting factors Bone development	Coagulopathy

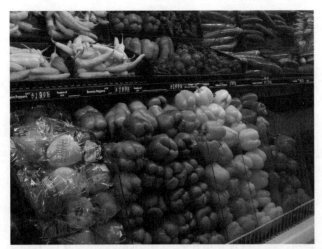

FIGURE 7.1   Eating a variety of foods helps promote balanced nutrition.

WATER

Life cannot be sustained without water. Approximately 45% to 75% of our body weight is water (Peckenpaugh, 2010), which is held in intracellular and extracellular compartments. Water is needed as a solvent for all electrolytes and for other substances. Body temperature is regulated by evaporation of water from the skin. Circulating throughout the body, water transports nutrients, electrolytes, and bodily secretions to all cells of the body and carries away waste. Movement of internal organs and joints require lubrication provided by water.

ALTERED NUTRITIONAL STATES

Undernutrition

When overall intake of nutrients is severely limited, loss of lean body mass and wasting occurs. Marasmus is just one of three types of serious protein-energy malnutrition. The other two forms include kwashiorkor and marasmic kwashiorkor (Rabinowitz, Gehri, Paolo, & Wetterer, 2009). These conditions are more commonly seen in children after weaning age in developing countries. Babies and small children have a higher need for protein and are thus more commonly affected. The child may have generalized edema or a bloated stomach (with kwashiorkor), whereas limbs may appear wasted. Undernutrition may result from not being able to obtain or consume enough or proper types of food, high bodily requirement, rapid excretion of nutrients, or inability to absorb and metabolize nutrients.

Another common malnutrition state is anorexia. The client with **anorexia nervosa** has an altered body image.

Seeing herself or himself as fat (regardless of evidence to the contrary), food intake is sharply curtailed. A weight of less than 85% of that expected for height defines anorexia (Nix, 2009). The condition can lead to malnutrition, damage to vital organs, and even death.

Eating binges and purging are characteristic of **bulimia**, but with bulimia weight is often normal. Excessive exercise, laxative use, appetite suppressants, and diuretic medications may be used by bulimic and anorexic clients. Both conditions are more likely to improve with psychological/psychiatric and nutritional intervention.

Most commercial oral supplements can provide complete nutrition, but these supplements are meant to provide kilocalories and nutrients *in addition* to those consumed at meals. Often, these supplements are administered as between-meal drinks. Oral supplements are not usually used for tube feedings.

Overnutrition

The incidence of obesity in the United States has reached epidemic proportions over the last 30 years. As many as two-thirds of adults are overweight, and half of that number are considered obese. Nearly 20% of children are overweight (National Center for Health Statistics, 2006). As obesity increases so does the risk of serious diseases such as heart disease, hypertension, type 2 diabetes, sleep apnea, stroke, arthritis, and some cancers and is associated with increased mortality (Katz, 2008). The impact of obesity is not limited to health issues. The condition has increased the national health bill by a staggering $75 billion per year, 9% of the total healthcare bill (Harper, 2006; Katz, 2008). This figure does not include the cost of health-related absenteeism.

The obese client also suffers psychologically, with a negative body image, poor self-esteem, and social prejudice. The obese are more likely to live at the poverty level and have fewer opportunities in life than persons of lesser weight (Katz, 2008). With many factors impacting weight gain (e.g., sedentary lifestyle, genetics, poor food choices, psychological issues, social and family dynamics), there is no easy solution to the problem of obesity. Stores, books, magazines, and television commercials are filled with offerings of new diets, pills, workout gadgets, and prepackaged diets that promise to remove that fat for a price. When energy intake exceeds body needs, the excess is stored as fat. Often, a fad diet will recommend restriction of a specific nutrient; however, each nutrient provides something the body needs, and limiting a single nutrient is not wise.

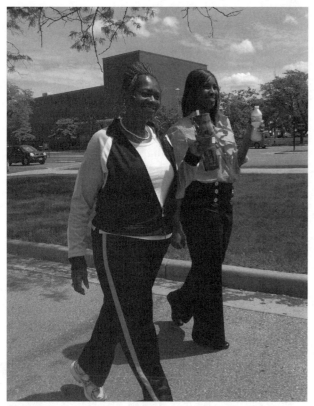

FIGURE 7.2 Exercise and hydration are important parts of weight management.

Much has been written about diets, but the strongest support in the literature (Katz, 2003) calls for a well-balanced diet consisting of fruits and vegetables, whole-grain cereals, lean protein, and restriction of sugar, refined starches, and some fats along with an exercise program. Weight reduction requires motivation (Figure 7.2), determination, and a willingness to change habits and lifestyle. Some tools to support changes are setting reasonable goals, keeping a food/exercise diary, preplanning menus and shopping lists, and enlisting support from family, friends, or a weight loss group. Dietary and psychological counseling may also be helpful in many cases.

> *Much has been written about diets, but the strongest support in the literature (Katz, 2003) is for a well-balanced diet consisting of fruits and vegetables, whole-grain cereals, lean protein, and restriction of sugar, refined starches, and some fats along with an exercise program.*

ASSESSMENT

The Joint Commission (2010) requires that all patients admitted to acute care have nutritional screening and,

when indicated, an in-depth nutritional assessment is performed. Many nutritional screens are available and usually consist of a few short questions about unintended, recent weight loss and appetite. When a problem is identified by screening, a full nutritional assessment should follow, by a dietitian if possible.

The nutritional assessment uses both objective and subjective data to include history; admitting diagnosis; other medical, surgical, or psychiatric problems; medication use and history; food and drug allergies; food preferences, intolerances, and aversions; diet history; and cultural and religious needs. Anthropometric and laboratory data also provide important information. No single nutritional indicator should be relied on to provide an accurate picture of the nutritional condition.

Height and Weight

Anthropometric data are measurements of the body's fat and muscle mass and can be found in Charney and Malone (2009).

1. Current height and weight compared with ideal body weight:
   Males: 106 lbs for first 5 feet and 6 lbs for each inch thereafter
   Females: 100 lbs for the first 5 feet and 5 lbs per inch thereafter
   Add or subtract 10% for small or large frame
2. Ideal body weight adjustments for frame size, amputation, and spinal cord injury:
   For amputations, decrease as follows:

   | Hand, 0.7% | Forearm and hand, 2.3% | Entire arm, 5% |
   | Foot, 1.5% | Below knee, 5.9% | Leg, 16% |

   For spinal cord injury or paraplegia decrease by 10% to 15%
   Quadriplegia decrease by 15% to 20%
3. Body mass index can be determined by the following equation:
   Weight (kg) ÷ height (m^2) × 100 or weight (lbs) ÷ height (inches^2) × 100

   Weight classifications appear in Box 7.1.

Laboratory Values

Laboratory tests are a valuable adjunct to other assessment methods. Protein, prealbumin, albumin, and transferrin provide values needed to assess protein-calorie

BOX 7.1   Weight Classifications by BMI

	BMI	Obesity Class
Underweight	<18.4	
Normal	18.5–24.9	
Overweight	25–29.9	
Obesity	30–34.9	I
Moderate obesity	35–39.09	II
Extreme obesity	≥40	III

BMI, body mass index.

malnutrition. **Prealbumin** is reflective of protein intake within a few days previous to the test, whereas protein and **albumin** have a longer half-life, reflecting protein intake as much as a month earlier. Albumin levels in the average adult should be 3.5 to 5.0 g/dL. Decreased albumin has been associated with negative rehabilitation outcomes, especially in older adults.

Transferrin is needed to transport iron, is also more sensitive to recent changes, and may indicate protein-calorie malnutrition. Testing can be done when iron and electrolyte (sodium, potassium, calcium) deficiency is suspected. Box 7.2 provides a summary of laboratory values.

BOX 7.2   Important Nutritional Values

Test	Normal Range (Adults)
Protein	6.4–8.3 g/dL
Albumin	3.5–5 g/dL
Prealbumin	16–40 mg/dL
Transferrin	200–400 mg/dL
Hemoglobin	14–18 g/dL males, 12–16 g/dL females
Hematocrit	42%–52% males, 37%–47% females
White blood cell count	5,000–10,000 mm^3
Blood urea nitrogen	10–20 mg/dL
Creatinine	3.5–5mEq/L
Sodium	136–145 mEq/L
Potassium	3.5–5 mEq/L
Glucose	70–109
HbA$_{1c}$	4–8%

Source: From Charney and Malone (2009).

NUTRITIONAL NEEDS IN SPECIFIC REHABILITATION SITUATIONS

Cardiovascular Disease and Stroke

The leading cause of death in the United States continues to be cardiovascular disease. It is estimated that lifestyle changes could result in a significant reduction in incidence of cardiovascular disease (Chuive, McCullough, Sacks, & Rimm, 2006). Modifications such as exercise, diet, blood pressure control, weight management, and smoking cessation are crucial to improving disease rate and are the essential components of patient education.

Diet has been linked to heart disease since the 1930s when food shortages due to the Great Depression were observed to reduce the incidence of cardiovascular events (Katz, 2008). Atherogenesis, the growth of plaque in blood vessels, begins with fatty deposits in coronary arteries caused by serum lipid levels and oxidation. Progression of the lesions is affected by hypertension, hyperinsulinemia, oxidation, and inflammation, all modifiable by diet (Katz, 2008).

Control of atherogenesis can be assisted by following a heart-healthy diet that includes weight reduction, reduced fat intake (or consumption of healthy fats), and inclusion of high antioxidant foods. Reduction in total fat limits the amount of lipid available for deposit in blood vessels. Adding soluble fiber to the diet is another way to reduce LDL cholesterol. The National Cholesterol Adult Treatment Panel (National Institutes of Health, 2001) recommends at least 5 to 10 g of fiber per day. Foods rich in dietary fiber include dried beans, oatmeal, cereal bran, citrus fruits and Brussels sprouts. Fiber forms a gelatin-like substance in the bowel that removes bile acids before they can be reabsorbed.

Weight control is a necessary component of a heart-healthy diet because excess weight tends to increase LDL cholesterol, blood pressure, and the likelihood of type 2 diabetes, all of which contribute to atherosclerosis and are serious risk factors for heart disease. Adult Treatment Panel III guidelines for cholesterol appear in Box 7.3.

Neurological Conditions

A common thread in neurological conditions such as Parkinson's disease, cerebrovascular accidents, multiple sclerosis, spinal cord injury, and head injury is the rehabilitation diagnosis of mobility impairment. When the body is less active it is subject to a number of problems, including weight gain, pressure ulcers, thrombi, pneumonia, urinary tract infections, loss of bone mass, and constipation. Good dietary management can prevent

BOX 7.3 Adult Treatment Panel III Guidelines for Cholesterol			
	Desirable Range	Elevated	High
Total cholesterol	<200	200–239	>240
HDL cholesterol	40–59	>60	
LDL cholesterol	<100	100–159	>160
Triglyceride	<150	150–199	200–499

HDL, high-density lipoprotein.

many of these issues. Many neurological conditions have nutritional guidelines that generally recommend maintaining a healthy weight, eating a well-balanced, high fiber diet, and getting a good fluid intake (Box 7.4). Dysphagia is seen in many neurological conditions as well. Dysphagia is discussed in the next section.

Spinal Cord Injury

During the acute and post acute phase of spinal cord injury nutritional demands are often elevated, due to catabolism, but caloric needs decrease as the body adjusts to a decreased mobility pattern. Ideal body weight is lower for spinal cord injured patients who do not walk. For tetraplegia the ideal body weight should be reduced 10% to 15% and for paraplegia, reduced by 5% to 10% (Charney & Malone, 2009). Because calcium loss is common after spinal cord injury, it may be necessary to reduce calcium intake if intake is high.

Parkinson's Disease

Falls are a common problem with Parkinson's patients due to gait abnormalities as well as from orthostatic hypotension. Adequate calcium and vitamin D intake helps to reduce the likelihood of fractures with falls.

BOX 7.4 Web Resources With Information on Nutrition for Various Disorders
Paralyzed Veterans Association www.pva.org
Parkinson's Disease Foundation www.pdf.org
Multiple Sclerosis Society www.mssociety.org

High fiber and adequate fluid intake helps to manage the constipation problems that many Parkinson's patients experience. Vitamin B6 and protein may limit the effectiveness of levodopa, so supplements of B6 and foods fortified with it should be monitored. Treatment of Parkinson's with levadopa is improved when the medication is taken at a time of day when protein intake is lower (Peckinpaugh, 2010). Frequency and severity of tremors can drive up the need for calories, and with chewing, swallowing, self-feeding deficits malnutrition can be seen with this diagnosis. Several small meals per day provided at times when optimal medication benefit is achieved can improve intake.

Stroke

Strokes often comprise a large percent of admissions to rehabilitation units, and these patients can have numerous reasons for poor nutritional condition. Preexisting malnutrition, dental problems, loss of appetite, depression, impaired ability to feed, visual or cognitive deficits, and swallowing difficulties can place this population at risk. Poor nutrition places this patient at higher risk for pressure ulcers and falls with injury as well. Proper nutrition is vital for recovery after stroke. In one study, patients with severe strokes who were tube fed for more than 25% of their stay in rehabilitation demonstrated greater increases in total motor and cognitive Functional Independence Measure (FIM) scores and greater improvement in severity of illness by discharge (James et al., 2005).

For those who can take nutrition orally (which is the preferred route) a screening to rule out dysphagia and monitored feeding should help ensure adequate intake. The speech pathologist evaluates chewing ability and safe swallowing. Monitoring of the patient can be done by nursing staff and/or dietitians to identify many of the above issues as well as to note type and amounts of foods and fluids taken or any change in eating pattern.

No educational program for preventing strokes can be complete without stressing the importance of dietary interventions. Many strokes occur as a result of the same process that causes atherosclerosis and heart attacks and can be modified by food choices. Hypertension is an important risk factor leading to stroke, with diet playing a key role in its control. A diagnosis of diabetes also places one at risk for a stroke, and diabetic control relies strongly on diet. Intake of fruits and vegetables is emerging as an important preventative measure for stroke (Katz, 2008).

Traumatic Brain Injury

An increase in metabolism is often seen in brain injury due to the injury itself or resultant seizures. The victim may be unable to consume the needed calories and protein for tissue repair or may have intolerance to ingested food. Depending on severity of injury, the traumatic brain injured patient may be unconscious or may have an endotracheal tube or dysphagia. It may become necessary to use enteral or parenteral feeding to provide needed nutrients. Cook, Peppard, and Magnuson (2008) recommend starting enteral nutrition within 48 hours to prevent depletion of fat and protein stores. The Brain Trauma Foundation (2007) recommends full caloric replacement by the 7th day after injury.

Surgery or Trauma

The body undergoing surgery or trauma can reach a high level of stress. If surgery is elective, there is time for evaluating nutrition and correcting problems. When surgery is emergent or trauma occurs, protein–calorie stores can be depleted. Protein is needed for tissue repair, including bone, and higher carbohydrate intake is needed to provide energy and spare protein. Adequate protein levels are needed to maintain osmotic pressure, prevent edema and shock, and to keep the immune system healthy. The B vitamins, vitamin C and K, as well as adequate minerals such as iron and zinc are also needed.

Inadequate absorption may result from surgeries, illnesses, or injuries involving the digestive tract. These patients require continued monitoring by dietitian and nurse. Stomach surgery can result in dumping syndrome. A solution of high osmolarity quickly enters the duodenum, pulling water from circulation and causing shock-like symptoms. Following the prescribed dietary plan can help prevent dumping syndrome.

Burns

Burns can induce a hypermetabolic state and can range from mild to life threatening depending on the depth of burn, percentage of body surface affected, and age of the victim. Children and the elderly are at more risk from burns. High-risk burn cases are usually managed at a burn center, and nutritional management is crucial to survival.

Nix (2009) identifies three stages of nutrition care for burn patients:

Stage 1 During the first 24 hours after the burn, massive amounts of water, electrolytes, and protein are lost. Cells dehydrate as water is drawn out along with potassium. Therapy is initiated with intravenous solutions that replace fluid and electrolytes. With good management, fluid loss usually stabilizes after 2 or 3 days. Continued vigilance is needed to maintain the delicate balance between dehydration and fluid overload.

Stage 2 This phase begins about 1 week postburn. Protein needs for wound healing and immune function increase. The need for calories, vitamins A and C, and zinc also is higher. Nutrition may be provided by parenteral or enteral route, and amount is based on weight and area of burn.

Stage 3 During this follow-up phase, continued nutritional support is important to support surgeries for grafting or reconstruction and reconditioning the body.

Pressure Ulcers

Many reversible factors impact development and healing of pressure ulcers: immobility, incontinence, dependence in self-care, chewing/swallowing problems, and poor nutritional intake/choices. For clients at risk, the National Pressure Ulcer Advisory Panel (2009) has recommended the following:

- Each individual at risk for pressure ulcers should be screened and assessed for nutritional status in every setting.
- Each individual with nutritional risk and pressure ulcer risk should be referred to a registered dietitian and if needed to a multidisciplinary nutrition team.
- For those who have developed a pressure ulcer, screening and assessment of nutritional status should be done on admission, with each condition change, or when pressure ulcer closure is not observed and provision of adequate calories, protein, vitamins, and fluids. A dietitian's involvement in the care of this client helps to ensure adequate dietary support. Equally important is nursing monitoring of intake and tolerance of diet.

DYSPHAGIA AND SWALLOWING PROBLEMS

The act of swallowing occurs many times a day and is so automatic we give no thought to the process. Swallowing is in fact a complex process that requires an intricate coordination of muscles nerves, reflexes, and many levels of sensory and motor control in the brain. Five of the 12 cranial nerves are involved in the act of swallowing: trigeminal (V), facial (VII), glossopharyngeal (IX), vagus (X), and hypoglossal (XII). Nerves work with the multiple facial, jaw, and throat muscles and tongue to swallow successfully. Impairment of motor or sensory function at any level can result in poor swallowing and can even be life threatening.

Neurological events or conditions (e.g., stroke, multiple sclerosis, amyotrophic lateral sclerosis, Parkinson's disease, or head injury) should alert the rehabilitation nurse that a swallowing problem may exist (Box 7.5). A chart review should include notation of neurological conditions; surgery, radiation, or burns on or around the head or neck; current nutritional condition; history of pneumonia; invasive procedures (e.g., endotracheal or percutaneous endoscopic gastrostomy tube insertion); and medications that could affect appetite or swallowing.

BOX 7.5   Nursing Diagnoses and Commonly Associated Disorders in Rehabilitation Clients

Imbalanced nutrition: less than body requirements
  Renal disease
  Stroke
  Diabetes
  Frailty
  Functional debility
  Cognitive impairment
Imbalanced nutrition: more than body requirements
  Obesity
  Heart disease
  Diabetes
  Impaired swallowing
  Stroke
  Parkinson's disease
  Multiple sclerosis
  Amyotrophic lateral sclerosis
  Myasthenia gravis
  Guillain-Barré syndrome
  Post-polio syndrome
  Traumatic brain injury or brain tumor
  Patients who are fatigued
Deficient knowledge
  Could be any disease process, depending on patient and caregiver

---

BOX 7.6   Signs and Symptoms of Swallowing Problems

Choking
Coughing
Multiple swallows
Clearing the throat
Moist sounding voice after eating or drinking
Eyes watering
Breathing difficulties or exacerbation of asthma
Increased temperature
Runny nose after meals

On physical exam, the general appearance of nutritional state, level of cognition, mobility, and how the client is receiving nutrition (oral, intravenous, tube) should be noted. Check cranial nerves for deficits. Observe for wet or raspy voice, expressive aphasia, drooling, facial asymmetry, somnolence, coughing, choking, prolonged feeding, and whether or not assistance is needed with feeding. Box 7.6 gives signs and symptoms of swallowing problems.

The sedating effects of some central nervous system medications may cause dysphagia. Dryness of the mouth can result from taking diuretics or anticholinergics, leading to impairment of bolus movement in the mouth and pharynx. Patients with drug-induced xerostomia (mouth ulcers) can have difficulty chewing and swallowing and can even have loss of appetite. Guidance for medication assessment in patients with swallowing disorders can be found at www.pbm.va.gov.

The varied literature on dysphagia divides swallowing into anywhere from three to six phases. The four phases described by Daniels and Huckabee (2008) are discussed here.

1. *Preoral:* Preparing to eat is affected by level of hunger, seeing, smelling and anticipating the taste of food, saliva production, and hydration. Neurological/cognitive deficits, pain, or distraction may affect the ability to pay attention or interpret sensory data, and cueing may be needed.

2. *Oral:* This is the phase in which the food or liquid is taken into the mouth, chewed, and mixed with saliva. The lips close to retain the bolus, and the tongue and jaws move the food around to facilitate mixing with saliva. When the bolus is ready, breathing may stop just before or just after the transfer on the bolus into the oropharynx, vocal cords close, the

tongue pushes the bolus posteriorly against the palate, and it is transferred into the oropharynx. Oral transfer usually takes less than 1 second.

3. *Pharyngeal:* The nasopharynx is sealed off with the retraction of the soft palate, the larynx closes and elevates along with the hyoid bone, the upper esophageal sphincter opens, the base of the tongue retracts, and the posterior pharyngeal wall contracts. This phase also take approximately 1 second. Exact coordination of these events is needed for a safe and successful phase.

4. *Esophageal:* Both the upper and lower esophageal sphincters are closed at rest to prevent escape of stomach contents, but both open as the bolus enters the esophagus. Muscles of the esophagus begin peristaltic movements that send the bolus to the stomach. Transit time varies from 8 to 20 seconds. Swallowing difficulties at this stage can consist of esophageal strictures that keep the bolus in the esophagus and increase aspiration risk. It should be noted that great variability in the events of each phase can occur depending on the consistency, taste, and amount of food; age of subject; and whether or not cueing is needed.

Once a concern exists that safe swallowing could be compromised, the nurse or speech pathologist should do a bedside screening.

Standard Bedside Evaluation

1. Evaluate the client's cognition, posture, voice quality, and saliva control.
2. The client is offered a small amount of water, usually 1 teaspoon.
3. Follow with a larger amount if the smaller amount is swallowed safely.

Videofluoroscopy

Videofluoroscopy is a visual radiological recording of each phase of the swallowing event and the most widely used tool to diagnose dysphagia. Also known as the modified barium swallow, this test can identify the exact location, cause, and extent of the problem and help guide the treatment plan. The client, seated or standing at the x-ray machine, swallows a variety of textures of food as the x-ray image of the action is videotaped. The speech language pathologist and radiologist can then determine where problems are with the patient's swallowing. The results of the barium swallow assist the speech therapist in determining the diet for the patient and what consistencies of foods and liquids he or she can safely swallow.

ENTERAL NUTRITION

Enteral nutrition is given when a person cannot safely eat in the usual manner by mouth. Nutritional supplements are delivered by nasogastric tube or through a surgically inserted tube into the stomach or sometimes another portion of the gut. Use of the gut to process nutrients helps to preserve its integrity, and at least 100 cm of functioning gut is needed for absorption.

Feeding Tubes

In acute care settings patients are often unable to eat due to dysphagia, aspiration, cognitive impairments, endotracheal tubes, tumor or other obstruction, facial/throat/stomach injury or condition, surgery, or burns and thus tube feeding may be initiated. With feeding tubes controlled amounts of nutrients, fluids, and medications can be provided to prevent malnutrition and dehydration or to maintain medication administration.

A tube inserted through the nose into the stomach (**nasogastric or NG tube**) is the most common feeding tube and is typically used on a short-term basis. Placement should be confirmed via x-ray before initial use and should be checked before each use.

For those patients requiring tube feeding for a longer period of time, a gastrostomy tube may be used. The typical gastrostomy tube is inserted directly into the stomach in the operating room under sterile conditions and general anesthesia. This is a more costly procedure that involves more risk to the patient. The tube is secured with sutures, which pose an additional infection hazard. Today, the **percutaneous endoscopic gastrostomy (PEG) tube** is the preferred type for long-term enteral nutrition. The PEG tube is inserted using endoscopy that requires only local anesthetic and conscious sedation. Via endoscopy, the physician is able to visualize the ideal placement for the tube. Once this place is determined, the light from the fiberoptic scope is shone from the inside of the stomach out toward the skin, where it is marked on the outside. The scope is then removed, but a guidance tube (or guide wire) is left in place. The PEG tube is then inserted through the mouth of the patient and threaded down the esophagus via the guidance tube to the stomach, where a stab wound has been made in the marked spot on the skin. The tube is then pulled out through this small stab wound, with the larger bulb-type end remaining inside the stomach taut against the stomach wall. A T-bar or triangular type of plastic bumper on the outside against the patient's abdominal skin held secure the tube against the stomach wall. The guide wire is also removed. The entire procedure is relatively fast (less than 30 minutes). No sutures are present, and the tube is held in place as a fibrous tissue forms around the bulb-like end of the tube in the stomach over 1 to 2 weeks (Easton, 1999). Newly inserted tubes are often taped to the abdomen. PEG tubes provide the added benefit of safe use within several hours of placement (Bankhead et al., 2009). Skin checks are particularly important, because the main complication of PEG tubes is infection at the insertion site.

A **percutaneous endoscopic jejunostomy tube** is surgically placed through a stab wound from the outside directly into the jejunum. Placement may be for long-term nutrition support, for emptying of the stomach after surgery, or if an NG tube is not tolerated. Percutaneous endoscopic jejunostomy tube placement is used with patients at risk for recurrent aspiration of tube feeding or those at risk for impaired gastric motility, such as head trauma. The percutaneous endoscopic jejunostomy tube is an expensive and difficult procedure and associated with a higher incidence of tube occlusion and dislodgement.

Complications of Tube Feeding

Tube feeding is a common and usually safe procedure, but complications can occur. Diarrhea is the most common, and its causes could include antibiotics or sorbitol-containing products, altered bacterial flora, formula composition, contamination, or infusion rate. Use of a hyperosmolar solution can cause increased fluid in the intestines, resulting in diarrhea. Table 7.3 provides information about choosing formulas. Aspiration, alterations

TABLE 7.3 Guidelines for Formula Selection	
Patient Factors	**Formula Factors**
Age	Osmolality
Diagnosis	Renal solute load
Associated nutritional problems	Caloric density and viscosity
Nutritional requirements	Nutrient composition: type and amount of cholesterol, fat, and protein
Gastrointestinal function	Product availability and cost

Source: Julie Daniel, R.D.L.D. (personal communication, June 22, 2010)

in drug absorption and metabolism, and fluid/electrolyte imbalances may also occur.

Care of the Client Receiving Tube Feeding

Prevention of diarrhea can sometimes be accomplished by good hand washing and use of clean technique to prevent contamination. Once opened, solutions should be discarded per facility policy, usually after 24 hours. Care is taken to use prescribed amounts of solution and water and infused at the prescribed rate. The physician and/or dietitian may be consulted if diarrhea continues.

To limit the risk of aspiration with gastric feeding, raise the head of the bed at least 45 degrees during feeding and for 1 hour after. If possible, place the patient in a sitting position for a more normal eating patterns. Although there is not strong research evidence for preferring one administration method over another in general (e.g., continuous, intermittent, or bolus feeding), one expert guideline panel concluded that, "A gradual change from continuous to cyclical delivery should be considered in patients requiring parenteral nutrition for more than 2 weeks" (National Collaborating Centre for Acute Care, 2005, p. 11). Gastric residuals should be checked regularly, and the client should be monitored for tolerance of the feeding.

NG tube placement is verified before feeding by aspirating stomach contents if possible and by auscultation over the epigastric area, as a few milliliters of air is injected into the feeding tube. Vomiting or coughing could dislodge NG tubes, requiring an x-ray to verify tube position. Rehabilitation nurses should be familiar with their unit's policy on checking tube placement and monitoring feeding tubes.

Fluid, electrolytes, and weight should be monitored, with a dietitian if possible. The tube should be checked daily for leakage or signs of infection. Mouth care is needed at least daily.

PARENTERAL NUTRITION

Parenteral nutrition is the delivery of **basic nutrients** intravenously and is reserved for those who are unable to meet nutritional requirements or those who should not take nutrition via the gastrointestinal system. Some indications for parenteral delivery include bowel or accessory gastrointestinal organ surgery or disease, when nutrient need exceeds what can be obtained via gastrointestinal tract (e.g., in burns), and when bowel rest is needed (e.g., Crohn's disease or ulcerative colitis).

The peripheral route (arm vein) can be used for dilute, short-term (less than a week) nutrition. For long-term, more concentrated solutions, the superior vena cava, via the subclavian vein, can be accessed in the shoulder area or with a catheter (such as a PICC line) threaded through an arm vein. Parenteral insertion sites should be inspected frequently for catheter dislodgement, redness, or swelling. Temperature, intake and output, blood chemistry, and weight are also important to monitor. The facility's protocol should be followed when monitoring these devices.

NUTRITION ACROSS THE LIFE SPAN

The foundation for good nutritional status begins during pregnancy. Increased amounts of protein are needed for the rapid tissue growth that is occurring in mother and baby. An increased rate of metabolism during pregnancy drives the need for additional energy as well as the need to spare protein for use in tissue building. Caloric intake should be balanced to meet the energy needs of mother and baby without causing excessive weight gain. Total normal average weight gain during pregnancy is approximately 29 lbs. The standard recommendation is for increase of approximately 340 kcal/day during the second trimester and 450 kcal/day for the third trimester (Nix, 2009). Vitamin supplements are often prescribed to ensure intake of adequate micronutrients, especially vitamin D for bone growth and folate to prevent neural tube defects. The need for energy and nutrients continues during breastfeeding along with additional fluid needs, up to 3 L/day, to produce milk (Nix, 2009).

Growth continues to be rapid during infancy and childhood, keeping energy needs high. Protein, calcium, and iron are critical during this period, and supplements may be needed in some cases. Preferences for certain foods develop, and risk for adult obesity can be identified from the body mass index. Because infants and toddlers have higher percentages of body weight as water, the risk of dehydration is greater when intake is limited or if there is increased loss of fluid as in diarrhea or vomiting. In addition to the usual nutritional assessment tools, head circumference is monitored and growth charts (available from the Centers for Disease Control and Prevention, http://www.cdc.gov/GROWTHcharts) are used as guidelines to assess normal growth.

Adolescence is a time of growth spurts, which usually start earlier in girls than boys, requiring more nutrients. Fast foods or snacks may take precedence over good nutri-

tion choices. Preoccupation with body image is common at this age, and that focus may result in an eating disorder. Use of alcohol may begin. Sexual maturity occurs during teen years, and additional zinc may be needed for healthy development. For teen girls menstrual flow, when heavy, can result in iron losses, and a pregnancy at this time places added demands for nutrition on girls whose own nutrition may be marginal.

Good eating habits can be developed in adulthood that can prevent many health problems in later years. Eating and drinking habits have been implicated in 6 of the 10 leading causes of death (heart disease, cancer, stroke, diabetes, arteriosclerosis, and liver disease) as well as debilitating disorders like osteoporosis and diverticulosis (Mauk, 2010). Adulthood can also be a stressful time. The time demands of starting and sustaining a family, career, and educational development can make the use of fast foods or skipping meals tempting. The basal metabolic rate declines 1% to 2% per decade and more rapidly at midlife (Nix, 2009); thus, caloric consumption needs to be lower to sustain a healthy weight. It continues to be important to make food choices that are nutrient dense along with exercise to maintain a healthy weight.

The geriatric patient presents a special challenge in nutritional management because of multiple physical, psychological, and social issues. The older adult often presents with poor nutrition, which can be a contributing factor in the incident leading to need for rehabilitation. Multiple comorbidities, pain, polypharmacy, cognitive impairment, depression, and limited or ineffective social support systems are factors that may contribute to a less than optimal nutritional state. Limited finances or transportation may impair ability to obtain food. Poor eyesight/cognition, low energy level, and lack of appropriate facilities may limit the ability to prepare food. Decreased sense of smell, taste, poorly fitting dentures, or missing teeth can cause the older adult to eat less or choose foods of lower nutritional value.

Chronic diseases become more prevalent in the elderly, often negatively impacting appetite and nutritional state. These conditions frequently result in increased amount and kinds of medication, which can affect cognition, appetite, and hydration, interfering with optimal nutrition. As the individual ages, muscle and bone mass, along with range of motion, decreases, affecting balance and agility. Rehabilitation patients often need increased calories for wound healing and due to increased expended energy.

The aging gastrointestinal system is less able to absorb nutrients, and production of digestive enzymes and saliva is reduced. The gag reflex becomes weaker, increasing aspiration risk, and the incidence of dysphasia is much higher in this group. Slowed motility of the bowel can lead to constipation. Some elderly may rely on laxatives and mineral oil, leading to impaired absorption of fat-soluble vitamins. For an older adult undergoing rehabilitation, good nutritional assessment and management is vital to an optimal outcome.

INTERDISCIPLINARY MANAGEMENT

Many disciplines may have input into ensuring optimal nutrition for their client. The rehabilitation nurse has the advantage of observing the patient take nourishment and is often doing the feeding or setting up enteral feedings. Being with the patient 24 hours a day offers the advantage of observing for problems with eating or tolerating food. Table 7.4 gives some general guidelines for the interdisciplinary team about improving nutritional status in rehabilitation patients.

Assessing and prescribing the appropriate diet, monitoring, teaching, and ensuring nutritional progress is the forte of the dietitian (Figure 7.3). Physical and occupational therapists assist in strengthening, positioning, assessing cognitive function, and providing adaptive equipment to facilitate independence in eating. Swallowing problems are identified and treated by the speech pathologist to ensure the safest intake of nutrients. Safe swallowing protocols are suggested by the speech therapist. Table 7.5 provides some guidelines to promote safe swallowing.

TABLE 7.4   General Guidelines for the Improving Nutritional Status
• Check the client's plate or tray to make certain the proper diet has been provided. Be sure that liquids are thickened to the prescribed consistency.
• Give cues to patients who are self-feeding to go slowly. Mealtimes should never be rushed.
• Make certain that the client's adaptive equipment is clean and available for each meal.
• Consult with the occupational therapist if it appears that modifications in adaptive feeding utensils may be needed.
• Obtain weights regularly. Report weight loss to the physician, and follow up with the nutritionist.
• Ask patients about favorite foods, likes, and dislikes. Try to provide culturally appropriate foods within dietary restrictions.
• Make community dining a pleasant experience through a clean, well-kept, home-like environment. Background music and ambience can make mealtime more appealing.
• Assist with setting up the meal (e.g., opening difficult containers, etc.) for patients who are learning to feed themselves.
• Consider seating those at risk for swallowing problems at a certain table where they can be more closely monitored by a staff member.
• Assess client's fatigue level, because this can interfere with having enough energy for mealtimes.
• Offer choices, however small, if the patient has difficulty with decision making or cannot feed him- or herself.
• Closely monitor for signs or symptoms of dysphagia.
• Give positive reinforcement of patient attempts toward self-feeding.

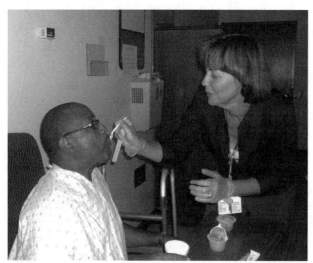

FIGURE 7.3   Persons with dysphagia may need to follow specific steps for safe swallowing.

The physiatrist or nurse practitioner monitors and manages medical and rehabilitation progress. Finding community resources such as meal delivery, communal dining programs, or home assistance in obtaining and preparing food can be accomplished by the social worker. When the need arises, other disciplines may also add value to treatment.

Problems are more readily identified and solved when working as a team. If one can imagine each team member providing their care without input from any of the others, it becomes clear that the optimal outcome for the patient will not be achieved. Interdisciplinary care is truly a case of the whole being greater than the sum of the parts.

TABLE 7.5   Guidelines to Promote Safe Swallowing for Persons With Dysphagia

- Follow the swallowing guidelines prescribed by your speech therapist. (In the event that no specific guidelines are available, implement general guidelines as discussed in this chapter or other procedures such as the supraglottic technique.)
- Avoid water, milk products, and other thin liquids. Thin liquids are easily aspirated. Milk products can thicken secretions. Thicken liquids to a nectar-like consistency (or consistency specified by the speech therapist).
- Be patient. Allow time to eat. Remember that the retraining of swallowing muscles is a gradual process.
- Sit up when eating meals or drinking fluids. Sitting up straight in a chair, when possible, is preferred. Continue to sit up at least 45 minutes to an hour after meals.
- Eating smaller meals five to six times per day may be helpful in decreasing fatigue levels while promoting good nutrition.
- Avoid use of straws unless otherwise instructed by the speech therapist.
- For those with difficulty swallowing liquids, taking small amounts by teaspoon or half teaspoon may be recommended.
- Try using smaller amounts of food at a time.
- Alternate solids and liquids.
- Use adaptive equipment as instructed by the occupational therapist.
- Family members can assist the patient with head control or lip closure if needed.
- Place food on the unaffected side of the mouth where the patient can sense it and manipulate it more effectively.
- Be sure to inspect the mouth, or instruct the patient to use a mirror, to be sure food or medication was swallowed and not pocketed.
- Stroking the sides of the trachea and neck can help stimulate a swallow response.
- The client may need to verbal cues about swallowing.
- Have suction equipment available for an emergency.

TEACHING PATIENTS AND FAMILIES ABOUT NUTRITION

The nutrition treatment plan is not complete without giving the client the tools needed to maintain good nutritional health. An initial learning assessment includes determining ability to learn. Cognitive deficits need to be addressed, such as providing glasses or hearing aids or using large-print visuals. If there is indication of memory loss, the information may need to be repeated, in writing, or be provided to the closest relative or friend.

Timing teaching episodes with readiness to learn helps to ensure compliance. For instance, the person who has just had a stroke is often receptive to hearing about a low sodium diet to assist with management of hypertension. Also, teaching should be attempted at a time when the client is rested, has no treatment or therapy scheduled, and is not under any unusual stress or distraction.

Age, cultural and religious beliefs, and educational level should also be considered. The eating habits of teenagers may be influenced by peer pressure or time constraints of school activities. The elderly may have cognitive impairments or need more time to absorb information provided. Food is a focal point of many cultural events and religious practices. Learning your client's practices ahead of time and making your lessons consistent with them will be beneficial (see Case Study 7.1). Likewise, determine literacy level before teaching. It would be most embarrassing to provide the learner with written material only to learn that he or she never learned to read.

Learning styles differ from person to person and may be visual, auditory, interactive, or tactile. With this in mind, providing a variety of written material, discussions, videos, and hands-on activities will help address the individual need. Chapter 13 provides detailed information about educating patients and families.

CASE STUDY 7.1

Mrs. Norris, a 92-year-old Mexican-American patient with myasthenia gravis, was noted to have a poor oral intake at breakfast each morning as a result of swallowing difficulties. She was admitted on a pureed diet from the nursing home. The student nurse caring for Mrs. Norris also noted that she did not participate as well during her 8:30 A.M. physical therapy session as she did later in the day. On examination of her medication schedule, it was found that Mrs. Norris' medication dose of Mestinon was being given at 8:00 A.M. but had a 30- to 60-minute onset of action period.

Questions

1. What action should the nursing student take?
2. What team members might be helpful in addressing this issue?
3. What small changes could be made in the medication regimen that might promote better nutrition for Mrs. Norris?

Teaching Topics

Education is part of the process of improving the client's self-care ability. Basic nutritional needs, weight loss or gain, calculating body mass index, and information on nutritional needs of specific conditions (e.g., heart health, diabetes, and surgery) are some good starting points. Your patient's diagnosis can be used as a guide to providing useful nutrition information to him or her, but there are other useful topics that may not come to mind immediately. Reading food labels; care, storage, and preparation of food to prevent contamination; or how to find food recalls can also be taught.

SUMMARY

The impact of good nutrition on rehabilitation outcomes cannot be overemphasized. The well-nourished client will be stronger, can regain function more quickly, and will be less likely to develop complications. More and more we are learning that the foods we choose impact our ability to stay well and have a good quality of life. This knowledge can be used to benefit not only our clients but ourselves as well.

WEB EXPLORATION

1. Visit the American Society for Parenteral and Enteral Nutrition (ASPEN) at www.nutritioncare.org
2. Browse the Dietary Guidelines for Americans at www.health.gov/dietaryguidelines/dga2005/document
3. Examine the Food Guide Pyramid from the U.S Dept of Agriculture, Center for Nutrition Policy and Promotion at www.mypyramid.gov

CRITICAL THINKING

1. Visit the guideline on enteral feedings at www.guidelines.gov. What levels of evidence exist for the various aspects of this type of nutritional therapy?
2. Compare the above guideline summary with the one found at www.guidelines.gov. How are these guidelines the same? How are they different?
3. We have all been in environments that were not conducive to learning. Think back to a time when you were in a class that was too hot, too cold, too dark, too noisy, the speaker was inaudible, the visuals were too far away or too small, and seating was poorly arranged (hopefully not all at the same time!). Discuss how these environmental issues could interfere with your teaching sessions.
4. Compare the benefits of a PEG tube over the NG tube. Why is the PEG tube used in the long term instead of the NG tube?

PERSONAL REFLECTION

- Imagine you have had a severe stroke and are unable to eat as usual. What fears might you have about an NG tube? A PEG tube? What would be your goals? What would be your greatest challenges? How would food be different to you?
- Have you ever cared for a person with a PEG tube? How did you feel about giving medications, food, and fluids through the tube? What problems, if any, did you encounter?
- In many societies food is important to local culture. For a person who is unable to eat food orally, how does this change other aspects of their lives?

RECOMMENDED READINGS

Grundy, S. M., Cleeman, J. I., Bairey-Mertz, C. N., Brewer, H. B., Clark, L. T., Hunninghake, D. B., Pasternak, R. C., Smith, S. C., & Stone, N. J. U. for the Coordinating Committee of the National Cholesterol Education Program. (2004). Implications of recent clinical trials for the National Cholesterol Education Program Adult Treatment Panel III guidelines. *Circulation, 110*(2), 227–239.

Hark, L., & Morrison, G. (2003). *Medical nutrition and disease: A case based approach.* Malden, MA: Blackwell.

Kruizenga, H. M. (2004). Development and Validation of a hospital screening tool for malnutrition: The short nutritional assessment questionnaire (SNAQ). *Clinical Nutrition, 24*(1), 75–82.

Lim, A. (2008). A pilot study of respiration and swallowing integration in Parkinson's disease. *Dysphagia, 23*(1), 76–81.

Perry, L. (2001). Screening swallowing function of patients with acute stroke: Part one. *Journal of Clinical Nursing, 10*(4), 463–473.

REFERENCES

Bankhead, R., Boullata, J., Brantley, S., Corkins, M., Guenter, P., Krenitsky, J., et al. (2009). Enteral access devices: Selection, insertion, and maintenance considerations. In A.S.P.E.N. enteral nutrition practice recommendations. Retrieved September 1, 2010, from http://www.guidelines.gov/content.aspx?id=14716&search=tube+feedings#Section420

Brain Trauma Foundation. (2007). Management of severe traumatic brain injury. *Journal of Neurotrauma, 24*(1), S1–S95.

Charney, P., & Malone, A. (2009). *ADA pocket guide to nutrition assessment* (2nd ed.). Chicago: American Dietetic Association.

Chiuve, S., McCullough, M., Sacks, F., & Rimm, E. (2006). Healthy lifestyles factors in the primary prevention of coronary heart disease among men: Benefits among users and nonusers of lipid-lowering and antihypertensive medications. *Circulation, 114*(2), 160–167.

Cook, A., Peppard, A., & Magnuson, B. (2008). Nutrition considerations in traumatic brain injury. *Nutrition in Clinical Practice, 23*(6), 609.

Daniels, S., & Huckabee, M. (2008). *Dysphagia following stroke* (pp. 43–49). Grand Rapids, MI: Plural Inc.

Easton, K. L. (1999). *Gerontological rehabilitation nursing.* Philadelphia: W.B. Saunders.

Harper, M. (2006). The hidden cost of obesity. Retrieved September 1, 2010, from http://www.forbes.com/business/2006/07/19/obesity-fat-costs_cx_mh_0720obesity.html

James, R., Gines, D., Menlove, A., Horn, S., Gassaway, J., & Smout, R. (2005). Nutrition support (tube feeding) as a rehabilitation intervention. *Archives of Physical Medicine Rehabilitation, 86*(12 suppl 2), 82–92.

The Joint Commission. (2010). Patient care standard 01.02.03, element of performance 7. Retrieved from www.jointcommission.org/Post_PatientCenteredCareStandardsEPs_20100609.pdf

Katz, D. L. (2003). Pandemic obesity and the contagion of nutritional nonsense. *Public Health Review, 31*(1), 33–34.

Katz, D. L. (2008) *Nutrition in clinical practice: A comprehensive, evidence-based manual for the practitioner.* Philadelphia: Lippincott Williams & Wilkins.

Mauk, K. (2010). *Gerontological nursing: Competencies for care* (2nd ed.). Sudbury, MA: Jones and Bartlett.

National Center for Health Care Statistics. (2006). *Health, United States, with Chartbook on trends in health of Americans.* Hyattsville, MD: U.S. Government Printing Office.

National Collaborating Centre for Acute Care. (2005). Nutrition support in adults: Oral nutrition support, enteral tube feeding and parenteral nutrition. Retrieved September 1, 2010, from http://www.guidelines.gov/content.aspx?id=8739&search=tube+feedings#Section420

National Institutes of Health. (2001). Adult Treatment Panel guidelines at a glance. NIH publication no. 01-3305. National Institutes of Health; National Heart and Lung Institute. Retrieved September 1, 2010, from www.nhlbi.nih.gov/guidelines/cholesterol/atglance.htm

National Pressure Ulcer Advisory Panel. (2009). *Prevention and treatment of pressure ulcers: Clinical practice guidelines.* Retrieved September 1, 2010, from www.npuap/org

Nix, S. (2009). *Williams' basic nutrition & diet therapy.* St. Louis, MO: Mosby

Peckenpaugh, N. (2010). *Nutrition essentials and diet therapy* (11th ed.). St. Louis, MO: Saunders.

Rabinowitz, S., Gehri, M., Di Paolo, E. R., & Wetterer, N. M. (2009). Marasmus. Retrieved September 1, 2010, from http://emedicine.medscape.com/article/984496-overview

U.S. Department of Health & Human Services. (2005). *Dietary guidelines for Americans.* Retrieved September 1, 2010, from http://www.health.gov/dietaryguidelines/dga2005/document

CHAPTER 8

Maintaining Skin Integrity

Paula M. Anton

LEARNING OBJECTIVES

At the end of this chapter, the reader will be able to

- Identify persons at risk for impaired skin integrity.
- Recognize the major layers and function of the skin.
- Describe the stages of wound healing.
- Identify aspects of risk, skin, and wound assessment.
- State interventions for prevention of pressure ulcers.
- List the principles of wound healing.
- Describe dressings and topical treatments of wounds.
- Explain how topical treatments meet the goals of topical wound treatments.

KEY CONCEPTS AND TERMS

Bony prominences	Incontinence-associated	Necrotic (devitalized)
Braden Scale for Predicting	dermatitis	Norton scale
Pressure Ulcer Risk	Inflammatory phase	Pressure ulcers
Chronic wounds	Interdisciplinary team	Prevention
Complication	Maceration	Proliferative phase
Debridement	Maturation phase	Risk
Exudate	National Pressure Ulcer	Skin integrity
Hospital-acquired conditions	Advisory Panel (NPUAP)	Wound healing
Incontinence		

Maintaining **skin integrity** of rehabilitation patients is imperative for many reasons. **Pressure ulcers** are a persistent problem in rehabilitation, causing prolonged lengths of stay, increased reliance on extended-care facilities, increasing cost of care, altering function, and impacting lifestyles of patients and families. Pressure ulcers are a significant problem across all healthcare settings in the United States. Annually, 2.5 million patients are treated in acute care facilities for pressure ulcers (Ayello et al., 2009).

The cost to treat this **complication** is staggering. As of fiscal year 2007 the average cost per case paid by the Centers for Medicare & Medicaid Services (CMS) was over $43,000 (Ayello et al., 2009). Reddy, Gill, and Rochon (2006) estimate the net cost for caring for pressure ulcers at over $11 billion each year. Furthermore,

pressure ulcer incidence has been strongly tied to nursing care quality both in the United States and abroad (Chaboyer, Johnson, Hardy, Gehrke, & Panuwatwanich, 2010; Welton, 2008).

As a result of the huge cost and quality implications, in 2008 CMS included pressure ulcers as one of the hospital-acquired conditions that will be reimbursed differently in the future (CMS, n.d.). The CMS ruling caused hospitals to reevaluate their prevention strategies for pressure ulcers (Armstrong et al., 2008; Welton, 2008). Ayello et al. (2009) also point out that in addition to the economic and quality implications, pressure ulcer incidence has great legal implications for healthcare facilities. Prevention is the key to managing the skin of all patients.

AT RISK POPULATIONS

In rehabilitation patients, pressure ulcers are a major complication, but pressure ulcer rates in persons with disabilities varies in the literature and across the country. For spinal cord injury patients alone, between 24% and 59% will have a pressure ulcer at some time during their lifetime (Klipp, Spires, & Anton, 2002). Other rehabilitation populations, such as stroke, orthopedic, head injury, amputation, multiple sclerosis, burn, parkinsonism, and cancer, are prone to conditions that increase **risk** for skin breakdown. These conditions can include spasticity, presence of infection, diabetes mellitus, hematopoietic abnormalities (thrombocytopenia, neutropenia, and anemia), immunosuppression, and renal failure, among others. These same conditions frequently are the factors that delay healing in the same populations (Klipp et al., 2002). Pressure ulcer prevention is the key to maintaining skin integrity and begins with identification of risk in a patient and continues with the use of interventions to prevent pressure ulcer formation. Additionally, patients benefit from early identification of pressure-related skin problems and early treatment.

SKIN ANATOMY AND PHYSIOLOGY

It is important for the rehabilitation nurse to have a basic understanding of the anatomy and physiology of the skin, the types and classifications of wounds, the **wound healing** process and the phases of wound healing (Preston, Tebben, & Johnson, 2008). This knowledge allows the nurse to recognize and understand the factors that cause loss of skin integrity and complicate or delay wound healing.

It is important for the nurse to recognize and understand basic skin anatomy. The skin is made up of three layers. The outermost layer of the skin is the epidermis. The epidermis is made up of five sublayers called stratums. Its primary function is to act as a physical barrier to the outside. It protects the body from desiccation and prevents microorganisms from penetrating the body. The second layer is the dermis. It contains blood vessels, hair follicles, lymphatic vessels, sebaceous glands, and sweat glands. This layer is tough and elastic, containing fibroblasts that help to synthesize and secrete collagen and elastin to give the skin strength and elastic recoil. The basic function of the dermis is to provide strength, support, blood, nutrients, and oxygen to the skin. The final skin layer is the subcutaneous tissue composed of fat and connective tissue and carries major blood vessels, nerves, and lymphatic vessels. The major function of the subcutaneous layer is to provide insulation (Wysocki, 2007).

The skin is a body organ, in fact, the largest organ of the body, and overall provides six vital functions to the body. Skin provides protection against the outside world, keeping moisture in the body and keeping bacteria and other organisms out. It carries nerves to regulate sensation, allowing the person to feel pain, pressure, and sense temperature changes. Skin provides thermoregulation to assist in body temperature control. Waste products are eliminated through the skin. Vitamin D is synthesized in the skin, and this impacts metabolism. Finally, skin has aesthetic functions. It is the most common way the organism (person) is identified—through recognition—and it has a role to play in the psychological well-being of the individual. Scarring, for example, can trigger social reactions resulting in emotional responses of the individual (Maklebust & Sieggreen, 2001; Preston et al., 2008).

Types of Wounds

Webster's online dictionary defines a wound as "an injury to the body (as from violence, accident, or surgery) that typically involves laceration or breaking of a membrane (as the skin) and usually damage to underlying tissues" (2010). Rehabilitation nurses are concerned about and manage wounds of many etiologies in the patient population. Aside from pressure ulcers, the rehabilitation population may experience diabetic foot ulcers related to pressure or to their footwear and arterial ulcers related to peripheral vascular occlusive disease. Patients may experience venous stasis ulcers related to reduced venous return of blood and dependent edema. Patients may be under treatment for burns and/or traumatic wounds.

Because of **incontinence** issues in such rehabilitation patient populations as stroke and brain injury, **incontinence-associated dermatitis** is a significant problem in rehabilitation nursing. Therefore, pressure ulcers and incontinence-associated dermatitis are the types of wounds most often seen in the rehabilitation population, and the rehabilitation nurse must be able to manage these skin issues.

Factors That Influence Skin Integrity

Pressure ulcers are caused by unrelieved pressure on soft tissue between bony prominences and the sitting or lying surface. Pressure is the principle cause of pressure ulcers. An extended period of time in any one position exerts pressure over bony prominences at specific pres-

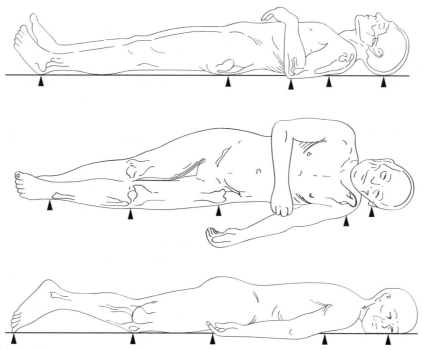

FIGURE 8.1   Pressure points while supine, prone, and sidelying.

Source: From *Pressure Ulcers: Guidelines for Prevention and Nursing Management*, by Joann Maklebust and Mary Sieggreen. Springhouse, Pennsylvania: Springhouse. Copyright 1991 by Lippincott, Williams and Wilkins. Used with permission.

sure points in various positions, creating tissue ischemia (Maklebust & Sieggreen, 2001). Shear, friction, and persistent moisture also cause this type of tissue damage. Figures 8.1 and 8.2 illustrate the areas of the body most prone to pressure ulcers (pressure points). Gravitational forces, improper positioning or repositioning, and improper sitting in bed or chair cause pressure to be exerted over bony prominences, creating a pressure gradient. This can cause shearing injury of soft tissue (Figure 8.3).

Pressure ulcer risk is described by Braden and Bergstrom (1989) as a combination of extrinsic factors (moisture, friction, and shear) and intrinsic factors (nutrition, age, and arteriolar pressure) that impact tissue tolerance to pressure and pressure factors such as mobility, activity, and sensory perception. Other factors such as immuno-suppression, smoking, presence of infection, and certain disease states also influence skin integrity and response to pressure. Table 8.1 provides more information on these factors.

The most effective way to reduce the incidence of pressure ulcers is to address these factors by specific interventions (Bergstrom, Braden, Kemp, Champagne, & Ruby, 1996). The most important factor is the presence of pressure. Priebe, Martin, Wuermser, Castillo, and McFarlin (2003) maintain, as do many practitioners in

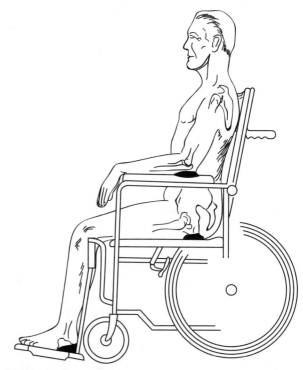

FIGURE 8.2   Pressure points while sitting.

Source: From *Pressure Ulcers: Guidelines for Prevention and Nursing Management,* by Joann Maklebust and Mary Sieggreen. Springhouse, Pennsylvania: Springhouse. Copyright 1991 by Lippincott, Williams and Wilkins. Used with permission.

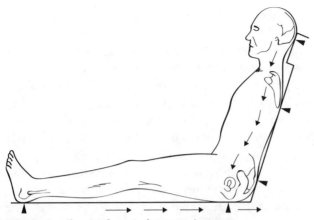

FIGURE 8.3   **Shearing forces on bony prominences.**

Source: From *Pressure Ulcers: Guidelines for Prevention and Nursing Management*, by Joann Maklebust and Mary Sieggreen. Springhouse, Pennsylvania: Springhouse. Copyright 1991 by Lippincott, Williams and Wilkins. Used with permission.

the wound care area, that to have a pressure ulcer there must be pressure, and if there is no pressure, there will be no pressure ulcer.

Wound Healing

There are three phases of wound healing: inflammatory, proliferative, and maturation. The first phase is the **inflammatory phase**, which is characterized by edema, erythema, hyperemia, and pain. In this phase (after hemostasis is achieved) white blood cells migrate to the area, each type with a different role to clean up the wound. At this time the wound walls itself off from the host to prevent infection. Growth factors begin to enter the area to stimulate tissue growth. This phase lasts from 4 to 6 days. The **proliferative phase** is the phase in which the defect is filled. Granulation tissue is generated. For this

TABLE 8.1 Factors That Influence Skin Integrity	
Tissue Tolerance Factors	**Explanations**
Extrinsic factors:	
Moisture	Moisture suggests the degree to which a patient is exposed to moisture from such sources as incontinence, perspiration, and body fluid drainage. The number of times linen and clothing must be changed can give a good indication of the impact of moisture.
Friction	Friction is mechanical force of skin moving against a support surface such as body parts dragging across the mattress when the patient is boosted to the head of the bed.
Shear	Shear is injury caused when skin remains stationary while the underlying tissue shifts, such as when the patient slides down in bed and the underlying tissue drags against the bone while the skin sticks to the mattress (see Figure 8.3).
Intrinsic factors:	
Nutrition	Nutrition entails the ability of the body to take in the nutrients necessary to meet the caloric needs of the patient.
Age	Extremes of age (very young and very old) represent differences in integument that can be associated with increased risk for skin breakdown and issues with healing.
Arteriolar pressure	Vascular insufficiencies affect the ability of the body to perfuse tissue.
Spasticity	Spasticity can influence blood flow through the affected tissues.
Infection	Infection increases the metabolic needs of the body.
Immunosuppression Disease states	Disease states such as diabetes, renal failure, immunosuppression, and hematopoietic abnormalities influence the ability of the system to produce cells needed to mediate tissue regeneration and growth.
Pressure Factors	
Mobility	Mobility is the ability and motivation to make changes in position and to maintain these changes. Can the patient turn, and will the patient stay in the turned position long enough to relieve pressure over another bony prominence?
Activity	Activity refers to the frequency and duration (distance) of ambulation. During walking, pressure is removed from all vulnerable skin surfaces and transferred to the soles of the feet.
Sensory Perception	Sensory perception denotes the patient's level of consciousness and the ability to detect cutaneous sensation, such as ability to respond to pain in a meaningful way.

Source: From Bryant (2000). Bryant & Clark (2007), and Preston, et al. (2008).

to occur collagen is produced to generate the matrix on which the granulation tissue fills in. Wound edges begin to contract. This phase lasts generally from 4 to 24 days or longer. The **maturation phase** is the last phase of wound healing, and this is when the wound epithelializes and matures. At this time the wound matures, scar forms, and the wound contracts or remodels. The skin increases in tensile strength to approximately 80% of its original strength. This phase can last from about 21 days to 2 years.

Most pressure ulcers and other types of wounds (such as vascular ulcers and neuropathic ulcers) that are caused by an underlying pathology (such as pressure with other risk factors) go on to become **chronic wounds**. Features of chronic wounds include protracted phases of healing, lysis of cells before remodeling occurs (cellular senescence), deficiency of growth factor receptor sites, reduced fibrin and growth factor production, and high level of enzymes in the wound. These factors in addition to host factors such as ischemia, malnutrition, and comorbidities (diabetes, renal disease, etc.) slow the rate of healing of the wound (Bryant & Nix, 2007).

ASSESSMENT

History and Physical Examination

The history and physical examination provides valuable information on the underlying conditions that will increase risk for pressure ulcer development. In addition, this information provides invaluable data to assist the interdisciplinary team (physician, nurse, occupational and physical therapists, dietician, social worker, rehabilitation psychologist, and discharge planner/utilization review specialist) to plan the care of a patient with wounds. This information should be widely shared.

Risk Assessment

The **National Pressure Ulcer Advisory Panel (NPUAP)** and the European Pressure Ulcer Advisory Panel (2009), along with regulatory agencies and other groups with specific interest in wound care and healing, recommend a risk assessment should be performed on all patients at admission to the healthcare facility and regularly as often as required based on individual need. Frequency of risk assessment is generally set based on the type of facility. The NPUAP–European Pressure Ulcer Advisory Panel recommendation (2009) goes on to state that the assessment should include assessments of activity and mobility, with individual consideration of nutrition fac-

tors, factors affecting tissue perfusion and oxygenation, skin moisture, age, friction and shear, sensory perception, general health status, and body temperature In most cases the nurse should use a systemic risk assessment for pressure ulcer formation such as the **Braden Scale for Predicting Pressure Ulcer Risk** (Bergstrom, Braden, Boynton, & Bruch, 1995) or the **Norton scale** (Norton, 1996). Current recommendations do not specifically state which risk assessment scale should be used.

The Braden Scale for Predicting Pressure Ulcer Risk is the most commonly used scale, and consists of six subscales that are scored from 1 to 3 or 4 points. The subscales are as follows (Bergstom et al., 1995):

1. *Sensory perception:* This is the ability to respond meaningfully to pressure-related discomfort based on level of consciousness and ability to detect cutaneous sensation
2. *Moisture:* This is the degree to which the skin is exposed to moisture from such sources as incontinence of urine or stool, perspiration, or wound drainage.
3. *Activity:* This is the frequency and duration (distance) of ambulation.
4. *Mobility:* The ability and motivation to change and control body position.
5. *Nutrition:* This is the usual food intake pattern of food taken by mouth, intravenously, by total parenteral nutrition, or tube feedings, measured by amount of protein intake each day and the quantity of food intake per meal.
6. *Friction and shear:* The extent to which the skin drags on the sheets while in bed, either by sliding down in bed or by pulling the patient up in bed, and the extent to which the bone shears the overlying tissue when the patient is moved in bed or in the chair.

The subscale scores are totaled to give a score ranging from 4 to 23. Many studies have been done to recommend at which score a patient can be said to be at risk, but the risk score remains elusive. Pieper (2007) suggests that examination of individual subscales of the Braden scale is a reasonable way to look at risk.

The Norton scale tests five parameters: physical condition, mental state, activity, mobility, and incontinence. Each parameter is rated from 1 to 4, based on the extent to which a problem exists in the parameter. The scale has been tested well, but mostly for the geriatric patient. Generally, a score of 12 or less indicates high risk for pressure ulcer formation, but other studies indicate 12 is too low (Pieper, 2007).

Skin Assessment

The NPUAP and European Pressure Ulcer Advisory Panel (2009) recommend a skin assessment should be a part of the skin care policy in all healthcare settings. In general, a nurse should perform a systematic skin assessment at least once per day in the inpatient rehabilitation setting (Pieper, 2007) The nurse should be looking for signs of blanching, edema, induration, and discoloration (redness or deeper color). The assessment should include all **bony prominences** and areas where medical devices rest on the skin. Frequency of skin inspection should be individualized. For example, for the wheelchair-bound individual, a skin inspection of pressure points from sitting should be done when the patient is put to bed after a day in his or her wheelchair.

Pressure Ulcer Assessment

In the event a pressure ulcer is identified, the wound assessment is extremely important for treatment decisions. The assessment includes the anatomical location of the wound, including the bony prominence. The size of the wound in centimeters is measured as on a clock, with 12:00 being the head, and 6:00 being the feet. Depth is measured using a cotton-tipped applicator in the deepest part of the wound and then measured against the measuring device. Undermining and tracking is measured under the skin, again with cotton-tipped applicator, measured against the measuring device, and documented as on the location of a clock. For example, "3 cm undermining from 9:00 to 11:00" indicates undermining on the upper left quadrant as the nurse looks at the wound.

Wound characteristics and drainage amount and character are documented. The wound-base tissue type is important for discerning whether debridement is needed. Viable tissue in the base could be granulation tissue, muscle, subcutaneous tissue, fascia, bone, or epithelialization. Nonviable tissue such as yellow, brown, gray, or black slough or eschar might also be seen. Wound exudate can be creamy, tan, yellow, green, purulent, sanguineous, serous, and serosanguineous, and amount of exudate can indicate presence of infection or high bacterial load.

Wound edges can be epithelializing if the wound is healing or rolled if the wound is chronic. Periwound skin assessment provides assistance in determining the state of wound healing. Inflammation might indicate infection. **Maceration** can indicate excess drainage of the wound,

so a more absorbent dressing may be needed, and desiccation can indicate need for an emollient or protective topical preparation on the periwound skin.

Other assessment aids include photography, planimetry, wound tracings, stereophotogrammetry, and wound molds of alginate or foams. Most of these methods require specialized training and are time consuming and difficult to perform. Photography is gaining popularity, but caution must be taken because there are also drawbacks. The NPUAP and the Wound, Ostomy and Continence Nurses Society neither recommend nor discourage photography as an assessment tool. Both organizations recommend that organizations have guidelines for wound photography that include the following:

- Informed consent
- Who takes the photographs, when, and under what conditions
- Type of camera (digital versus other)
- Patient identifiers
- File maintenance and storage
- Under what conditions and how photography is released to the family.

Photography techniques are beginning to be found in the literature, with recommendations for techniques that maximize accurate imaging for wound assessments recently published. These studies measure the accuracy of wound photographs for staging of pressure ulcers remotely (Baumgarten et al., 2009; Rennert, Golinko, Kaplan, Flattau, & Brem, 2009).

Nutrition assessment is a necessary assessment in patients with pressure ulcers. The nurse monitors weight changes over time, food intake, and laboratory studies such as complete blood count, transferrin levels, general chemistry for serum protein, and albumin and prealbumin levels for signs of protein-calorie malnutrition. (See Chapter 7 for more information on nutrition assessment.) Consultation with a dietician is advisable to determine if the patient is able to eat enough to maintain his or her health and heal a pressure ulcer (Edwards, 2001; Preston et al., 2008).

Pressure ulcers are classified by a standardized system called "staging" in which the amount or layers of tissue involved is described. Staging does not describe all features of a wound but is a description of the depth of the wound. In 2007 the NPUAP published the results of a consensus panel that clarified earlier versions of the staging system. Table 8.2 provides pressure ulcer staging descriptions.

TABLE 8.2   Staging Pressure Ulcers

Example	Stage
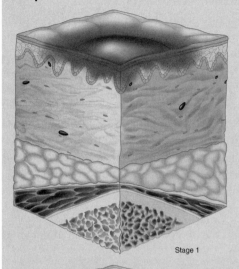 Stage 1	**Stage I:** Intact skin with non-blanchable redness of a localized area usually over a bony prominence. Darkly pigmented skin may not have visible blanching; its color may differ from the surrounding area. The area may be painful, firm, soft, warmer, or cooler as compared with adjacent tissue. Stage I may be difficult to detect in individuals with dark skin tones.
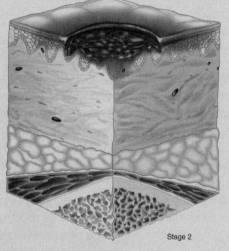 Stage 2	**Stage II:** Partial thickness loss of dermis presenting as a shallow open ulcer with a red pink wound bed, without slough. May also present as an intact or open/ruptured serum-filled blister. Presents as a shiny or dry shallow ulcer without slough or bruising. This stage should not be used to describe skin tears, tape burns, perineal dermatitis, maceration, or excoriation.
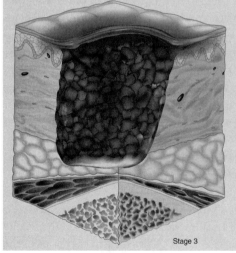 Stage 3	**Stage III:** Full-thickness tissue loss. Subcutaneous fat may be visible but bone, tendon, and muscle are not exposed. Slough may be present but does not obscure the depth of tissue loss. May include undermining and tunneling. The depth of a stage III pressure ulcer varies by anatomical location. The bridge of the nose, ear, occiput, and malleolus do not have subcutaneous tissue, and stage III ulcers can be shallow. In contrast, areas of significant adiposity can develop extremely deep stage III pressure ulcers. Bone/tendon is not visible or directly palpable.

TABLE 8.2   Staging Pressure Ulcers *(Continued)*

Example	Stage

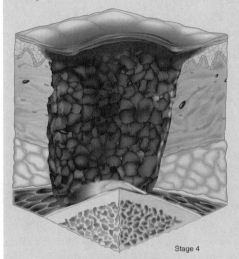

Stage 4

Stage IV:

Full-thickness tissue loss with exposed bone, tendon, or muscle. Slough or eschar may be present on some parts of the wound bed. Often include undermining and tunneling.

The depth of a stage IV pressure ulcer varies by anatomical location. The bridge of the nose, ear, occiput, and malleolus do not have subcutaneous tissue, and these ulcers can be shallow. Stage IV ulcers can extend into muscle and/or supporting structures (e.g., fascia, tendon, or joint capsule), making osteomyelitis possible. Exposed bone/tendon is visible or directly palpable

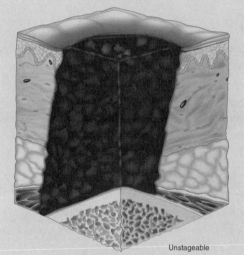

Unstageable

Unstageable:

Full-thickness tissue loss in which the base of the ulcer is covered by slough (yellow, tan, gray, green or brown) and/or eschar (tan, brown or black) in the wound bed.

Until enough slough and/or eschar is removed to expose the base of the wound, the true depth, and therefore stage, cannot be determined. Stable (dry, adherent, intact without erythema or fluctuance) eschar on the heels serves as "the body's natural (biological) cover" and should not be removed.

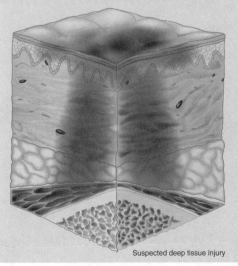

Suspected deep tissue injury

Suspected Deep Tissue Injury:

Purple or maroon localized area of discolored intact skin or blood-filled blister due to damage of underlying soft tissue from pressure and/or shear. The area may be preceded by tissue that is painful, firm, mushy, boggy, warmer, or cooler as compared with adjacent tissue.

Deep tissue injury may be difficult to detect in individuals with dark skin tones. Evolution may include a thin blister over a dark wound bed. The wound may further evolve and become covered by thin eschar. Evolution may be rapid exposing additional layers of tissue even with optimal treatment.

Source: NPUAP and European Pressure Ulcer Advisory Panel (2009).

NURSING STRATEGIES

Pressure Ulcer Prevention

Prevention is the most important nursing strategy that can be used to maintain skin integrity. For prevention strategies to be successful, they must focus on the specific risk factors the nurse is trying to mitigate. Areas of focus for pressure ulcer prevention include nutrition, the mechanical loading and support surfaces, moisture/incontinence, friction, shear, mobility, and activity. Within these areas, interventions focus on improving overall health through adequate nutrition and minimizing the effects of moisture, pressure, friction, and shear on the tissues through skin care, redistribution of pressure, positioning, and pressure relief.

> *Recent studies suggest that interventions for pressure ulcer prevention should be individualized to the patient based on the specific risk factors identified in the risk assessment (Arnold, 2003; Catania et al., 2003; Tannen et al., 2010).*

Studies suggest that interventions for pressure ulcer prevention should be individualized to the patient based on the specific risk factors identified in the risk assessment (Arnold, 2003; Catania et al., 2003; Tannen et al., 2010). Some suggest that the risk scale results influence the prevention interventions that nurses choose, further strengthening the notion that the care of the patient should be tied to the identified risk factors (Magnan & Maklebust, 2009).

Table 8.3 presents the most common risk factors (Arnold, 2003; NPUAP, 2010) and possible activities for the care of patients based on prevention guidelines (Ackley & Ladwig, 2006; NPUAP, 2010; U.S. Department of Health and Human Services, Public Health Service, Agency for Healthcare Research and Quality, 1992). Although the risk assessment scales do not replace clinical judgment, they can *supplement* clinical judgment in identification of specific risk factors in need of intervention.

Wound Care

In many cases in spite of careful pressure ulcer prevention, some do occur. In addition, many patients arrive at

TABLE 8.3 Nursing Interventions by Risk Factors	
Risk Factors	**Activities**
Limited sensory perception	Turn every 1–2 hours.
Decreased activity	Facilitate small shifts in body weight frequently.
Decreased mobility	Use pillows under calves to keep heels and bony prominence off the bed.
	Consider pressure-reducing bed surfaces for bed-bound individuals and, for chair-bound individuals, sitting surfaces.
	Avoid "donut" type devices to sacral area,
	Facilitate pressure relief activities for chair-bound individuals.
Skin exposed to moisture	Remove excess moisture from skin resulting from perspiration, wound drainage, and fecal or urinary incontinence.
	Apply protective barriers such as creams, or use moisture-absorbing pads.
	Consider fecal incontinence device.
	Moisturize dry, unbroken skin.
Inadequate nutrition	Weigh patient at appropriate intervals.
	Ensure adequate dietary intake.
	Monitor recorded intake for nutritional content and calories.
	Monitor nutritional indices (e.g., prealbumin, albumin).
	Determine with dietitian the number of calories and type of nutrients needed to meet nutrition requirements.
Friction	Minimize friction and shear sources.
Shear	Position head of bed < 30 degrees elevation or at 90 degrees for sitting unless necessary for medical condition.
	Use trapeze and/or lifting sheets to facilitate movement.

Source: From Ackley & Ladwig (1993) and NPUAP and European Pressure Ulcer Advisory Panel (2009).

the rehabilitation unit with pressure ulcers present. The interdisciplinary team is often faced with pressure ulcers and other wounds to manage. Because there are many ways to manage wounds and most of these are generally acceptable and successful, an organized approach to wound treatment is advisable. A strict adherence to "favorite" products and modalities can result in frustration and conflict among team members. Bryant (2000) and Rolstad and Ovington (2007) join other experts (Ayello & Cuddigan, 2004; Maklebust & Sieggreen, 2001; NPUAP & European Pressure Ulcer Advisory Panel, 2009) to propose specific principles of wound management to achieve wound healing (Box 8.1).

1. *Reduce or eliminate causative factors.* Wounds will not heal if the cause is not eliminated or controlled. For example, mechanical forces (pressure, friction, and shear) must be managed by pressure-relieving interventions such as turning, specialized mechanical loading, and support surfaces (pressure-relieving mattresses, beds, and wheelchair cushions). It is important to remember that wounds cannot heal if pressure is not removed or significantly reduced (Maklebust & Sieggreen, 2001). Another causative factor is circulatory impairment. The patient should be seen by a vascular specialist if circulation is compromised. Edema is a factor that must be controlled, especially in wounds of the extremities. In the setting of foot ulcers, referral to an orthotist for pressure-relieving devices is helpful.

2. *Provide systemic support for wound healing.* Optimization of the body system includes providing nutritional and fluid support, preventing or eliminating edema, and controlling systemic conditions that affect wound healing. Nutrition and fluid support can be achieved by providing the nutrients recommended by the dietician. Raising extremities above the level of the heart can assist with edema, and adding an edema specialist to the interdisciplinary care is advisable in extreme cases. Management of systemic conditions including spasticity, infection, diabetes, and renal failure is paramount. Diseases resulting in or caused by immunosuppression, as well as immunosuppression related to medications such as chemotherapy and corticosteroids, must be minimized. One strategy to mitigate the effect of medications is to wean the patient to the lowest possible dose of the immunosuppressing drug.

3. *Maintain the appropriate wound environment.* Bryant (2000) and Rolstad and Ovington (2007) identify goals of topical therapy of wounds that must be addressed for a wound to heal without complications or recurrence:

- Cleanse the wound. Sources agree that wounds must be cleansed at each dressing change (Maklebust & Sieggreen, 2001; NPUAP & European Pressure Ulcer Advisory Panel, 2009; Rolstad & Ovington, 2007). However, with the large number of chemical wound cleansers and antiseptics available on the market, contradicting opinion persists as to what solutions should be used to cleanse wounds. Atiyeh, Dibo, and Hayek (2009), Drosou, Falabella, and Kirsner (2003), Fernandez and Griffiths (2010), and NPUAP and European Pressure Ulcer Advisory Panel (2009) add to the body of evidence (Foresman, Payne, Becker, Lewis, & Rodheaver, 1993; Hellewell, Major, Foresman, & Rodeheaver, 1997) that cleansing wounds should be done using saline or portable water. The inclination of clinicians to abandon simple wound-cleansing solutions for the newer chemical cleansers has not borne out in independent research. Also, the most recent Cochrane review (Fernandez a& Griffiths, 2010) refutes the claims by some that tap water increases infection and gives evidence that it may even decrease infection of wounds.

- Remove necrotic tissue. Wounds do not heal when **necrotic** (also called **devitalized**) tissue is present, so wound **debridement** is the process by which the wound bed is prepared for healing. Debridement is the process by which this debris is removed from the wound, thus preparing the wound bed for granulation and eventual closure. Devitalized tissue is best removed once it has demarcated from the live tissue surrounding it. If the wound is debrided too soon, there is greater chance of removing live tissues or leaving necrotic tissue. For this reason, eschars are often removed only after they soften and begin to pull away from the surrounding tissue. Debridement is usually accomplished over time, beginning with primary or initial debridement followed by maintenance debridement. Think of this as keeping the wound in a constant state of readiness for closure. The wound should demonstrate improvement within 2 to 4 weeks of optimal treatment (Ayello & Cuddigan, 2004). There are four basic categories of debridement; surgical, mechanical, chemical, and autolytic.

> *The wound should demonstrate improvement within 2 to 4 weeks of optimal treatment (Ayello & Cuddingan, 2004).*

In surgical debridement the clinician uses instruments, usually scissors, scalpels, and forceps, to remove necrotic tissue from the wound. Although surgical debridement is generally the fastest, it is also the most painful. It may require systemic analgesics and/or local anesthetics as well as postprocedure pain control. Because bleeding can occur, this is not the best method for patients with clotting disorders or on anticoagulants. This type of debridement can be a selective method in which only necrotic tissue is removed (but in this case usually considerable necrotic tissue remains) or nonselective in which the necrotic tissue and viable tissue are removed. Situations such as a fulminating wound infection with sepsis or necrotizing fasciitis require rapid surgical debridement.

In mechanical debridement force is used to remove necrotic tissue. This can include irrigation, pulse lavage, whirlpool, or removal dressings with saline, topical antibiotics, or antiseptics. These methods can cause pain at the time of treatment (episodic pain), requiring premedication before the treatment. Mechanical debridement is generally nonselective because both nonviable and viable tissue are removed during the treatment. Wet to dry dressings are the most frequently prescribed method of mechanical debridement.

> *Use of a 35-mL syringe with a 19-gauge angiocatheter delivers 8 psi impact pressure, which is within the recommended range for mechanical wound debridement.*

Controversy exists over which solutions to use for wet to dry dressings. Saline is safe. Agency for Healthcare Research and Quality guidelines present data to suggest that antiseptic solutions such as povidone iodine, sodium hypochlorite, hydrogen peroxide, and acetic acid damage fibroblasts. Some clinicians reason that these products can be used in infected wounds. They cite that preventing spread of infection takes priority over protecting the few viable cells surviving in the hostile environment of an infected wound. More research is being done in animal models in which this issue is being studied more closely, but it is widely recommended that gauze dressings cause increased nursing workload, increased pain, and wound desiccation.

Wound irrigation is a form of mechanical wound debridement. Studies show that irrigation at pressures from 4 to 15 psi (pounds per square inch) impact pressure (amount of pressure delivered to the wound) is desirable to remove debris and bacteria from wounds. Researchers found that the bulb syringe provides 2.0 psi impact pressure and may not be adequate to remove necrotic tissue. Some irrigation devices can deliver impact pressures as high as more than 50 psi. Pressures higher than 15 psi may drive bacteria into the wound or cause damage to the soft tissues. Pulse lavage devices are made for wound irrigation and can deliver a range from 6 to 12 psi impact pressure. Use of a 35-mL syringe with a 19-gauge angiocatheter delivers 8 psi impact pressure.

Chemical debridement is a method of debridement that uses topical enzymes to remove necrotic tissue by breaking down and dissolving the devitalized tissue. This type of debridement is less painful than mechanical, but premedication may be required to remove the dressings, and some patients experience a stinging sensation at application of the debriding agent. Older versions of enzymes are nonselective and do not distinguish between viable and nonviable tissue. However, the newer generations of enzymatic debriding agents are selective, only recognizing devitalized tissue in the wound bed.

Autolytic debridement uses occlusive or semiocclusive dressings that retain moisture (such as hydrocolloids or transparent films) over the wound and allow the natural wound fluids that contain natural proteolytic enzymes to digest and liquefy necrotic tissue. It is generally nonpainful and the most selective mode of debridement. Autolytic debridement can soften a dry eschar for easier surgical, mechanical, or enzymatic debridement later. This process usually requires multiple dressing applications over days or weeks. It requires monitoring for signs of infection such as increased pain, odor, inflammation, and cellulitis, which requires a faster method of debridement.

Debridement of wounds by fly larvae (maggots) can be considered a form of debridement that works by mechanical and chemical means. Researchers have studied maggots for over 100 years, with renewed interest in the 1990s. The therapy was approved by the U.S. Food and Drug Administration for wound care in January 2004. Maggots secrete a mixture of proteolytic enzymes that break down and liquefy necrotic tissue, which they then ingest from the wound. These enzymes are neutralized in healthy tissue, so they do not harm the granulation tissue. The maggot also secretes chemicals with antimicrobial properties. These chemicals are able to combat wound infections caused by antibiotic-resistant strains of bacteria. This could become a major indicator for maggot use in wound care in the future. This is a quick, relatively painless, and very selective form of debridement (Sherman, 2002, 2009), but thorough patient and family teaching regarding the process is essential.

- Maintain a moist wound surface. Cells require a physiological environment in which to grow and reproduce. Maintaining (or, if needed, adding moisture to) the wound environment is essential to the healing wound. This is done by adding saline, wound gels, or other topical preparations to the wound to ensure sufficient moisture for healing without macerating the wound.

- In wounds with depth, such as stage 3 or 4 pressure ulcers, deep vascular ulcers, open surgical wounds, or deep diabetic foot ulcers, dead space must be obliterated. This is done by filling the wound to level of skin with dressing material such as absorbent fillers or gauze. Dead space provides an area in which fluid can collect, providing an environment for bacterial growth and causing maceration. The nurse must take care to avoid over-packing the wound, which can cause additional damage to the wound from pressure.

- For wounds with **exudate**, an important goal is to absorb the excess. To prevent pooling of exudate in the wound, absorptive dressing materials are used in the wound. Excess exudate in the wound causes maceration, thereby destroying granulation tissue, and provides a medium for bacterial growth.

- Protect the wound from infection and treat systemic infections. One role of the topical dressing is to prevent excessive invasion of the wound from external organisms. It is also necessary to treat infection present in the wound and the host to

BOX 8.1	Goals for Wound Therapy
Cleanse the wound
Remove necrotic tissue
Maintain moist wound surface
Obliterate dead space
Absorb excess exudate
Protect from infection
Provide thermal insulation
Protect the healing wound

Source: From Bryant (2000), Maklebust & Sieggreen (2001), and Ayello & Cuddigan (2004).

decrease energy expenditure and reduce the immune response of the host.

- Provide thermal insulation. It is important to maintain physiological body temperature within the wound. Loss of warmth from the wound during dressing changes and from evaporation of fluids from the wound can impede cellular functions essential for cell growth.

- The mechanical function of the wound dressing is to protect the healing wound. It is also essential to protect surrounding skin from the moisture and adhesives used in wound dressings.

Topical Treatment

Dressings and other topical agents are the component of wound care that gets the most discrimination and attention. Choice of dressings should be based on the condition of the wound bed, the condition of the surrounding skin, and the goals for wound therapy. Once the wound is cleansed and the decision on preparation of the wound bed is made, the selection of dressing gets under way. Usually, the goal is to maintain a moist wound environment, and then the decision evolves from that point based on the needs of the wound, goals of the patient, ability of the caregivers, and cost to the patient of the intervention. The type of dressing used for any wound is likely to change over time as the needs of the wound changes, but it is generally recommended to allow a treatment time to work before changing the regimen. Usually, 2 weeks is enough time to evaluate the effectiveness of a dressing choice (Bryant, 2000; Bryant & Nix, 2007).

Dressing materials with descriptions, indications, cautions, and uses are presented in Table 8.4. Although not exhaustive, this table gives a good starting point for the nurse who is faced with a wound problem. It is

TABLE 8.4   Types of Dressings

Product Classification and Common Brands	Description	Indications for Usage	Disadvantages	Recommended Use Change Frequency
Hydrocolloid	An occlusive, adhesive wafer that contains hydroactive particle to maintain/create a moist wound environment and promote autolysis	• Superficial or partial-thickness wounds • Shallow full-thickness wounds • Wounds with light to moderate exudate • To enhance autolytic debridement on wounds with eschar, slough, or fibrinous debris in wound bed	• Not recommended for wounds with heavy exudate, sinus tracts, or infections • May tear fragile periwound skin	• Every 3–7 days and PRN as it becomes saturated with drainage
Composite dressing	An adhesive polyurethane foam dressing consisting of a nonabsorbent wound contact fabric with a dehydrated hydrogel layer and a foam backing	• Partial-thickness and full-thickness wounds • Exudative wounds • Wounds that macerate when using hydrocolloid	• Not recommended for dry wounds • Nonocclusive	• Can remain in place up to 7 days • Change when it becomes saturated with drainage
Transparent film	A clear, adherent nonabsorbent dressing that is permeable to oxygen and water vapor	• Superficial, partial-thickness wounds • Wounds with little or no exudate	• No ability to absorb wound drainage • May macerate periwound skin due to trapping of wound drainage	• Two to three times weekly or PRN for trapped wound drainage
Barrier wipes	Non–water soluble, clear, copolymer protective barrier film	• Protection of periwound skin from stripping, maceration, and irritation from wound exudate • Protection under tape and other adhesive products • Increases adherence of hydrocolloid and thin film dressings	• Cannot be seen on the skin	• Daily or with dressing changes
Nonadherent moist	Loose mesh gauze impregnated with oil emulsion petroleum blend	• Full thickness wound when adherence of dressing is contraindicated • Allows free drainage of exudates	• Requires secondary dressing	• Daily or with dressing changes
Petrolatum gauze	Fine mesh gauze impregnated with petrolatum	• Partial-thickness and full-thickness that have minimal to no drainage • Abrasions • Superficial leg ulcers • Skin tears	• Requires secondary dressing	• Daily or with dressing changes

TABLE 8.4   Types of Dressings *(Continued)*

Product Classification and Common Brands	Description	Indications for Usage	Disadvantages	Recommended Use Change Frequency
Nonadherent gry	Nonstick material over absorbent cotton pad	• Partial-thickness and full-thickness that have moderate drainage	• Requires secondary dressing	• Daily or with dressing changes
Gauze	Woven gauze made of 100% cotton	• Partial and full-thickness wounds • Can be used to pack wounds • Can be used as an outer dressing	• Must be changed at least daily	• Minimum daily or as ordered
Gauze rolls	Woven gauze made of 100% cotton	• Partial and full-thickness wounds • Can be used to pack wounds • Can be used as an outer dressing	• Must be changed at least daily	• Minimum daily or as ordered
Foam	An absorptive, nonadhering, sponge-like polymer dressing	• Partial and full-thickness wounds with minimal to moderate exudate • As a secondary dressing for wounds with packing	• Not recommended for dry wounds • May macerate periwound skin	• Daily and PRN for increased drainage
Dressings/pads	Consists of a nonwoven layer and fluff filler for absorbency	• An outer dressing for highly exudative wounds		• With dressing changes
Absorbent sponges All purpose sponges	Nonwoven polyester/rayon blend sponge	• An outer dressing for smaller wounds with mild exudate • Applying topical creams and ointments • Prepping skin • Cleaning	• Not for use on open wounds or for packing wounds	• With dressing changes
Packing strips	All-natural, sterile 100% cotton fine-mesh gauze Antiseptic impregnated variety contains iodine	• For packing small wounds and wound tracts or fistulas • Antiseptic packing strips can be used in wounds with infectious or purulent drainage	• Antiseptic variety contains betadine-toxic to fibroblasts • Take care not to overpack the wound; use as a wick in tracts or fistulas	• With dressing changes, daily, or more
Hydrogel	Water-based gel dressing with some absorptive properties	• Partial-thickness and full-thickness wounds • Burns • Open blisters • Radiation skin damage	• Costly • Requires secondary dressing	• Every 12–24 hours

(Continued)

TABLE 8.4	Types of Dressings			
Product Classification and Common Brands	Description	Indications for Usage	Disadvantages	Recommended Use Change Frequency
Wound gel	Water-based gel with aloe	• Partial-thickness and full-thickness that dry out with saline packing alone	• Limited moisture absorption • May adhere to the wound bed if it dries out between dressing changes • Requires secondary dressing • Some patients experience stinging	• Every 12–24 hours
Calcium alginate	A nonwoven, highly absorptive dressing made from seaweed	• Partial and full-thickness wounds with moderate to heavy exudate	• Requires secondary dressing • Not recommended for dry wounds	• Every 12–24 hours and PRN for heavy drainage

Source: From Bryant (2000). Bryant & Clark (2007), and Preston, et al. (2008).

always advisable to consult the manufacturers' recommendations for use of the dressing and for dressing change frequency. New dressing products are introduced from time to time, and it is important for the nurse to recognize that many newer products may be new brands of older dressing products and that the evidence for efficacy of new products should always be studied. Table 8.5 describes topical wound medications, descriptions, and use.

Care of incontinence-associated dermatitis involves keeping the skin clean and dry and using barrier creams and pastes to protect the irritated skin from urine and stool and from friction forces. Moisture barrier creams and zinc oxide pastes generally protect the skin well and enhance healing of the cracked, open, and weepy skin of incontinence-associated dermatitis (Nix & Haugen, 2010).

Other Treatment Modalities

Other treatment modalities are available for wound healing in a variety of settings. One such modality, for example, is hydrotherapy. Hydrotherapy is usually provided by wound care physical therapists in the therapy department. Physical therapy provides wound care that includes whirlpool and pulse lavage irrigation for mechanical debridement of wounds. They also provide other physical therapy modalities (e.g., electrotherapy) that are helpful in the healing process. Wounds that benefit from hydrotherapy include wounds that require serial debridement and vigorous wound cleansing.

Several forms of energy have been proposed for the management of pressure ulcers and other chronic wounds. These therapies are grouped under the heading of biophysical treatments and include electrical stimulation, ultrasound, electromagnetic spectrum, and phototherapy treatments such as infrared radiation, ultraviolet light, and laser. With these modalities energy is delivered via medical devices, and it is important to consider whether or not the devices are approved by regulatory agencies and deemed safe.

Oxygen therapies for treatment of chronic wounds include hyperbaric oxygen in which oxygen is delivered under pressure to the wound area, and topical oxygen in which oxygen is applied directly to the wound. The evidence is not strong for the use of topical oxygen therapies.

Negative pressure wound therapy is a treatment that has been in use for over 10 years and has provided beneficial for enhancing granulation and closure of some pressure ulcers. It uses a dressing, either foam or gauze impregnated with antiseptic, covered with an occlusive layer and attached to a suction device. This type of therapy is best used to clean granulating wounds without osteomyelitis in the wound bed.

Other topical modalities such as biological dressings (synthetic and live cell–derived skin graft products) and

TABLE 8.5 Topical Agents

Product Classification Brand (Generic) Names	Description	Indications for Use	Contraindications	Considerations and Use
Antibiotic cream Silver sulfadiazine	Topical antibacterial agent containing silver, 10 mg/G. Prevents and treats infection, enhances healing. Softens eschar by adding moisture to the wound.	Second- and third-degree burns. Partial to full-thickness wounds.	Hypersensitivity to silver, sulfonamides or any component of the product. Not to be used on premature infants or newborns.	Fully cleanse the wound with soap and water, water, or saline at each dressing change to remove all traces of previous silver sulfadiazine. To apply: Impregnate dry gauze with the cream and apply to a clean wound. Change the dressing two times daily. May alternate one silver sulfadiazine dressing per day with one saline dressing per day. May macerate the wound.
Antibiotic cream Mafenide acetate	A soft, white, nonstaining, water-miscible anti-infective cream for topical administration to burn wounds.	Second- and third-degree burns. Partial to full-thickness wounds. Diffuses through devascularized areas (penetrates eschar).	Hypersensitivity to mafenide or any component of the product. It is not known whether there is cross-sensitivity to other sulfonamides.	Use the same as silver sulfadiazine.
Enzymatic debriding agent Collagenase	Collagenase is a proteolytic enzyme derived from fermentation of *Clostridium histolyticum*. It has the ability to digest collagen in necrotic tissue. Collagen in healthy tissue or in newly formed granulation tissue is not attacked.	For debridement of necrotic tissue and slough in acute and chronic wounds.	Infection. Hypersensitivity to any component of the product. Inactivated by detergents, hexachlorophene, acid solutions and antiseptics containing heavy metal ions. Does not penetrate dry eschar.	Cleanse the wound with water or saline before applying collagenase. Apply collagenase once per day and follow with dry gauze or saline-moistened gauze if the wound is dry. May apply antibiotic powder to the wound before collagenase to control bacterial load.
Growth hormone	Contains platelet-derived growth factor, which is part of the body's natural healing process. Delivers the growth factor directly to the ulcer.	Enhances formation of granulation tissue and promotes wound healing in diabetic foot ulcers in the presence of documented adequate perfusion. Occasionally used in the treatment of pressure ulcers.	Hypersensitivity to any component of the product including parabens. Not to be used in wounds closed by primary intention. Highly costly.	Apply only once per day, after cleansing the wound with water or saline. Apply a very thin layer of gel, then pack the wound with saline-moistened gauze. Change the saline-moistened gauze 12 hours later (every 12-hour dressing changes).

(Continued)

TABLE 8.5	Topical Agents			
Product Classification Brand (Generic) Names	**Description**	**Indications for Use**	**Contraindications**	**Considerations and Use**
Silver-impregnated dressing	A silver antimicrobial barrier dressing consisting of a rayon/polyester nonwoven core laminated between an upper and lower layer of silver-coated high density polyethylene mesh.	Partial and full-thickness wounds that are not improving with common silver preparations such as silver sulfadiazine.	Hypersensitivity to any component of the product.	The silver impregnated dressings are changed every 3–7 days, depending on brand. Must moisten with sterile water (do not use saline), cut the dressing to the size of the wound, and cover with a secondary dressing. Must keep moist with sterile water at all times. Avoid contact with electrodes and conductive gels during electronic measurements.
Antibiotic ointments Mupirocin calcium	Mupirocin calcium is an antibiotic available in a cream or petrolatum base.	Partial-thickness wounds such as broken blisters, abrasions, burns on the head and face.	Hypersensitivity to any component of the product.	Mupirocin calcium is effective against MRSA. Apply two to three times per day. Avoid the eye area.
Antibiotic ointments Triple antibiotic	Various antibiotic preparations and combination products in a petrolatum base (ointment).	Partial-thickness wounds such as broken blisters, abrasions, burns on the head and face.	Hypersensitivity to any component of the product.	Apply two to three times per day.

Source: From Bryant (2000). Bryant & Clark (2007), and Preston, et al. (2008).

growth factors (platelet-derived growth factors) are newer treatments that have had varied success in the treatment of pressure ulcers. The evidence for efficacy of these dressings for pressure ulcers is not strong. However, there is some utility for use of these products in other types of chronic wounds such as diabetic foot ulcers.

Surgical closure of pressure ulcers is attempted when a wound is refractory to traditional treatments. A surgeon (usually a plastic and reconstructive surgery specialist) is consulted for reconstruction options. Before surgery the patient and the wound are optimized, osteomyelitis treatment is completed, and the patient's ability to comply with treatment recommendations and seating recommendations is assessed. The surgeon designs a surgical flap (usually a myelocutaneous flap) that fills the wound defect with minimal tension. An adjacent site is chosen to

preserve future reconstructive options. Once the surgery is performed, the patient requires an extended period of recovery in which pressure on the flap is prevented while it adheres and heals. Subsequently, the patient is moved out of bed, and gradually sitting is reintroduced and the flap's tolerance to pressure is assessed.

Pain Management

Pressure ulcers and their treatment can be painful, and pain management during wound dressing changes and wound care is important. Patients experience several types of pain for various causes. The can have nociceptive (acute) pain, which is the normal processing of pain signals. Neuropathic pain can also be experienced in wounds, the result of nerve damage or malfunctioning. Visceral pain refers to pain in body organs and is not typically associated with wound pain. Somatic pain originates from bone, muscles, skin, and connective tissue. Sometimes pain can be a mixture of nociceptive and neuropathic factors (Krasner, Shapshak, & Hopf, 2007).

Causes of wound pain include intrinsic causes or background pain, pain that is usually there even when the wound is not being disturbed. The most common cause of pain is incidental pain, which is pain related to movement and activity. Procedural pain is associated with manipulation of the wound such as debridement, dressing changes, or application of devices over the wound (Krasner et al., 2007).

The role of the nurse in pain management is to assess pain, individualize the plan of care, administer pain interventions, and evaluate effectiveness of the interventions. Pain should be assessed using a reliable and valid pain scale that is appropriate for the patient. For example, an adult patient who is able to rate his or her pain is able to use a numerical pain scale, but a child may not understand the numerical scale and may be better assessed using a nonverbal pain rating scale. Wound pain should be treated as chronic and/or acute pain as appropriate. Long-acting pain medications are appropriate for intrinsic pain, which tends to be chronic. Breakthrough pain and preprocedural pain are best treated with short-acting pain medications, topical analgesics, and some nonpharmacological interventions such as positioning. Some researchers have studied other nonpharmacological interventions such as meditation during invasive procedures such as wound care and debridement (Astin, 2004). After pain is treated, the nurse reassesses pain using the valid reliable pain scale and adjusts interventions as appropriate.

EDUCATION

Staff Education

Staff education includes prevention, assessment, and treatment of pressure ulcers and other wounds. Nurses, assistive personnel, and the **interdisciplinary team** have responsibilities for aspects of skin maintenance and need to be educated. Information should be presented at the appropriate level and in various styles to ensure the outcomes of pressure ulcer prevention and skin integrity.

Patient and Family Education

Education of the patient and family should emphasize the care of the rehabilitation patient over the life cycle and in levels of care across the continuum. The most

---

BOX 8.2   Web Exploration

Visit these information sites for more information about wound care and pressure ulcers:

National Pressure Ulcer Advisory Panel:
   http://www.npuap.org

Wound Ostomy and Continence Wound Society:
   http://www.wocn.org

Wound Care Education Institute:
   http://www.woundconsultant.com

---

important aspect on which to educate is prevention. Education should be presented at an education level that is appropriate for the individual.

SUMMARY

Preventing skin breakdown and maintaining skin integrity are important rehabilitation goals. Taking appropriate preventative actions early in the rehabilitation process can save the client from complications that bring serious negative health outcomes. Wound care and management is a complex issue for rehabilitation nurses and physicians, and is influenced by many factors as were discussed in this chapter. Educating clients, their families, and caregivers about the importance of prevention of skin breakdown and/or treatment for wound healing is essential to promote better client outcomes.

CRITICAL THINKING

1. You have a 31-year-old male patient who has bilateral ischial pressure ulcers. He is athletic and strong. His favorite hobby is playing wheelchair basketball. He tells you he gets out of his big-wheeled truck by swinging on the door as it opens and landing in his wheelchair several feet below. What would you tell him about this activity and its impact on his pressure ulcers?

2. What role could you envision advanced practice nurses playing in wound care within a long-term care facility? In a wound care clinic? In home health care? In underserved communities? In the plastic surgeon's office or practice? How would the role of the nurse practitioner differ from the clinical nurse specialist in each of these settings? How might they be similar? You may need to review Chapters 3, 5, and 6 to answer these questions.

PERSONAL REFLECTION

- How would you handle a situation in which a patient refuses to allow you to turn him every 2 hours?
- Have you ever had a family member or a friend who had a pressure ulcer? What is your thought on the cause of the wound? Did you feel angry with healthcare providers because of the pressure ulcer?
- Think about older adults living in a typical nursing home setting. Why is this population more at risk for developing pressure ulcers and skin problems?
- Imagine that you are a 98-year-old widow living alone and with decreased sensation in your legs due to peripheral artery disease and diabetes. What would you do to prevent skin breakdown and pressure areas? What would you do if you developed a red spot that didn't go away?

CASE STUDY 8.1

Mr. B. is a 75-year-old man recently admitted for spinal cord injury rehabilitation. On admission the nurse learns that he had surgery to repair an abdominal aortic aneurism and had the complication of spinal cord ischemia. His level of cord injury is T-11. A few days after surgery the nursing notes indicate and the family verifies that the patient had a "bruise" on his sacrum. You check the area and find a black area, not well demarcated from the surrounding skin, with edema, warmth, and swelling in the surrounding skin (Figure 8.4). His nutrition status

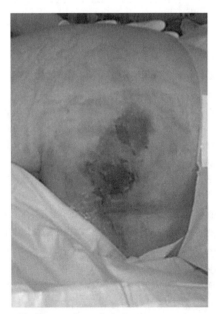

FIGURE 8.4   Mr. B's wound on admission.

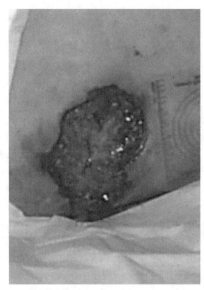

FIGURE 8.5   Mr. B's wound immediately after surgical debridement.

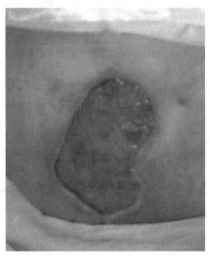

FIGURE 8.6   Mr. B's wound after one month of treatment. It is clean and granulating, a healing pressure ulcer.

is poor. He is eating less than half of his meals, has lost 20 pounds, and his prealbumin level is 18.

Plastic surgery is consulted and comes to debride the pressure ulcer. Figure 8.5 shows the wound immediately after debridement. The wound is treated with local wound care, and after 1 month the wound is clean and granulating, a healing pressure ulcer (Figure 8.6).

Questions

1. What stage is the pressure ulcer in Figure 8.4? Why?
2. What topical medications might be used on this wound after debridement and why?

3. What dressing would you use with the topical medication you chose?

4. Does he need a nutrition consultation?

RECOMMENDED READINGS

Bradeis, G. H., Berlowitz, D. R., & Katz, P. (2001). Are pressure ulcers preventable: A survey of experts. *Advances in Skin and Wound Care, 14*(5), 244–248.

Centers for Medicare & Medicaid Services (CMS). (2008). Medicare program: Proposed changes to the hospital inpatient prospective payment systems and fiscal year 2009 rates; proposed changes to disclosure of physician ownership in hospitals and physician self-referral rules; proposed collection of information regarding financial relationships between hospitals and physicians. Proposed rule. Federal Register 73:23550. Retrieved August 15, 2010, from http://edocket.access.gpo.gov/2008/pdf/08-1135.pdf

Hoeman, S. P. (Ed.). (2008). *Rehabilitation nursing: Process, application and outcomes* (4th ed.). St. Louis, MO: Mosby.

Russo, C.A., Steiner, C., & Spector, W. (2008). Hospitalizations related to pressure ulcers among adults 18 years and older, 2006. HCUP Statistical Brief #64. December 2008. Retrieved August 15, 2010, from http://www.hcup-us.ahrq.gov/reports/statbriefs/sb64.pdf

REFERENCES

Ackley, B. J., & Ladwig, G. B. (2006). *Nursing diagnosis handbook: A guide to planning care* (7th ed.). St. Louis, MO: Mosby.

Armstrong, D. G., Ayello, E. A., Capitulo, K. L., Fowler, E., Krasner, D. L., Levine, J. M., et al. (2008). New opportunities to improve pressure ulcer prevention and treatment: Implications of the CMS inpatient hospital care present on admission (POA) indicators/hospital-acquired conditions (HAC) policy. *Journal of Wound Ostomy and Continence Nursing, 35*(5), 485–492.

Arnold, M. (2003). Pressure ulcer prevention and management: The current evidence for care. *AACN Clinical Issues, 14*(3), 411–428.

Astin, J. A. (2004). Mind-body therapies for the management of pain. *Clinical Journal of Pain, 20*(1), 27–32.

Atiyeh, B. S., Dibo, S. A., & Hayek, S. N. (2009). Wound cleansing, topical antiseptics and wound healing. *International Wound Journal, 6*(6), 420–430.

Ayello, E. A., Capitulo, K. L., Fife, C. E., Fowler, E., Krasner, D. L., Mulder, et al. (2009). Legal issues in the care of pressure ulcer patients: Key concepts for health care providers. *Journal of Palliative Medicine, 12*(11), 995–1008.

Ayello, E. A., & Cuddigan, J. E. (2004). Conquer chronic wounds with wound bed preparation. *The Nurse Practitioner, The American Journal of Primary Health Care, 29*(3), 8–27.

Baumgarten, M., Margolis, D. J., Selekof, J. L., Moye, N., Jones, P. S., & Shardell, M. (2009). Validity of pressure ulcer diagnosis using digital photography. *Wound Repair and Regeneration, 17*(2), 287–290.

Bergstrom, N., Braden, B., Boynton, P., & Bruch, S. (1995). Using a research-based assessment scale in clinical practice. *Nursing Clinics of North America, 30*(3), 539–551.

Bergstrom, N., Braden, B., Kemp, M., Champagne, M., & Ruby, E. (1996). Multi-site study of incidence of pressure ulcers and the relationship between risk level, demographic characteristics, diagnoses, and prescription of preventive interventions. *Journal of the American Geriatrics Society, 44*(1), 22–30.

Braden, G., & Bergstrom, M (1989). A conceptual schema for the study of the etiology of pressure sores. *Rehabilitation Nursing, 14*(5), 258.

Bryant, R. A. (2000). *Acute and chronic wounds* (2nd ed.). St. Louis, MO: Mosby.

Bryant, R. A., & Clark, R. A. (2007). Skin pathology and types of damage. In R. A. Bryant & D.P. Nix (Eds.), *Acute and chronic wounds: Current management concepts* (3rd ed., pp 100–129). St. Louis, MO: Mosby.

Bryant, R. A., & Nix, D. P. (Eds.). (2007). *Acute and chronic wounds: Current management concepts* (3rd ed.) St. Louis, MO: Mosby.

Catania, K., Huang, C., James, P., Madison, M., Moran, M., & Ohr, M. (2003) PUPPI: The Pressure Ulcer Prevention Protocol Interventions. *AJN: American Journal of Nursing, 107*(4), 44–52.

Centers for Medicare & Medicaid Services (CMS), Centers for Disease Control and Prevention. (n.d.). Medicare program: Listening session on hospital-acquired conditions in inpatient settings and hospital outpatient healthcare-associated conditions in outpatient settings, December 18, 2008 [transcript]. Retrieved August 15, 2010, from http://www.cms.gov/HospitalAcqCond/Downloads/HAC_Listening_Session_12-18-2008_Transcript.pdf

Chaboyer, W., Johnson, J., Hardy, L., Gehrke, T., & Panuwatwanich, K. (2010). Transforming care strategies and nursing-sensitive patient outcomes. *Journal of Advanced Nursing, 66*(5), 1111–1119.

Drosou, A., Falabella, A., & Kirsner, R. (2003). Antiseptics on wounds: An area of controversy. *Wounds, 15*(5), 149–166

Edwards, P. A. (Ed.). (2001). *The specialty practice of rehabilitation nursing: A core curriculum* (4th ed.). Glenview, IL: Association of Rehabilitation Nurses.

Fernandez, R., & Griffiths, R. (2010). Water for wound cleansing. *Cochrane Database of Systemic Reviews, 5.*

Foresman, P. A., Payne, D. S., Becker, D., Lewis, D., & Rodheaver, G. T. (1993). A relative toxicity index for wound cleansers. *Wounds, 5*(5), 226–231.

Hellewell, T., Major, D., Foresman, P., & Rodeheaver, G. (1997). A cytotoxicity evaluation of antimicrobial and non-microbial wound cleansers. *Wounds, 9*(1), 1–20.

Klipp, D. A., Spires, M. C., & Anton, P. A. (2002). Pressure ulcers: Prevention and care. In C. M. Brammer & M. C. Squires

(Eds.), (pp. 699–704). *Manual of physical medicine & rehabilitation.* Philadelphia: Hanley & Belfus.

Krasner, D. L., Shapshak, D., & Hopf, H. W. (2007). Managing wound pain. In R. A. Bryant & D.P. Nix (Eds.), *Acute and chronic wounds: Current management concepts* (3rd ed., pp. 100–129). St. Louis, MO: Mosby.

Magnan, M.A., & Maklebust, J. (2009). Braden Scale risk assessments and pressure ulcer prevention planning: What's the connection? *Journal of Wound Ostomy and Continence Nursing, 36*(6), 622–634.

Maklebust, J., & Sieggreen, M. (Eds.). (2001). *Pressure ulcers: Guidelines for prevention and management* (3rd ed.). Springhouse, PA: Springhouse Corp.

Merriam-Webster Online Dictionary. (2010). Wound. Retrieved August 15, 2010, from http://www.merriam-webster.com/dictionary/wound

National Pressure Ulcer Advisory Panel (NPUAP). (2007). Pressure ulcer stages revised by NPUAP. Retrieved August 15, 2010, from http://www.npuap.org/pr2.htm

National Pressure Ulcer Advisory Panel (NPUAP). (2010). Updated staging system. Retrieved August 15, 2010, from http://www.npuap.org/resources.htm

National Pressure Ulcer Advisory Panel (NPUAP) & European Pressure Ulcer Advisory Panel. (2009). Prevention and treatment of pressure ulcers: Quick reference guide. Washington DC: National Pressure Ulcer Advisory Panel.

Nix, D., & Haugen, V. (2010). Prevention and management of incontinence-associated dermatitis. *Drugs and Aging, 27*(6), 491–496.

Norton, D. (1996) Calculating the risk: Reflections on the Norton scale. *Advances in Wound Care, 9*(6), 38.

Pieper, B. (2007). Mechanical forces: Pressure shear and friction. In R. A. Bryant & D.P. Nix (Eds.), *Acute and chronic wounds: Current management concepts* (3rd ed., pp 205–234). St. Louis, MO: Mosby.

Preston, M., Tebben, C., & Johnson, K.M. (2008). Skin integrity. In S. P. Hoeman (Ed.), *Rehabilitation nursing: Process, application and outcomes* (4th ed., pp. 258–280). St. Louis, MO: Mosby.

Priebe, M. M., Martin, M., Wuermser, L. A., Castillo, T., & McFarlin, J. (2003). The medical management of pressure ulcers. In V. W. Lin (Ed.), *Spinal cord medicine: Principles and practice* (pp. 567–589). New York: Demos Medical Publishing.

Reddy, M., Gill, S. S., & Rochon, P.A. (2006). Preventing pressure ulcers: A systematic review. *Journal of the American Medical Association, 296*(8), 974–984.

Rennert, R., Golinko, M., Kaplan, D., Flattau, A., & Brem, H. (2009). Standardization of wound photography using the wound electronic medical record. *Advances in Skin & Wound Care, 22*(1), 32–38.

Rolstad, B. S., & Ovington, L. G. (2007). Principles of wound management. In R. A. Bryant & D.P. Nix (Eds.), *Acute and chronic wounds: Current management concepts* (3rd ed., pp. 391–426). St. Louis, MO: Mosby.

Sherman, R. A. (2002). Maggot versus conservative debridement therapy for the treatment of pressure ulcers. *Wound Repair and Regeneration, 10*(4), 208–214.

Sherman, R. A. (2009). Maggot therapy takes us back to the future of wound care: New and improved maggot therapy for the 21st century. *Journal of Diabetes Science and Technology, 3*(2), 336–344.

Tannen, A., Balzer, K., Kottner, J., Dassen, T., Halfens, R., & Mertens, E. (2010). Diagnostic accuracy of two pressure ulcer risk scales and a generic nursing assessment tool: A psychometric comparison. *Journal of Clinical Nursing, 19*(11–12), 1510–1518.

U.S. Department of Health and Human Services, Public Health Service, Agency for Healthcare Research and Quality (AHRQ), formerly AHCPR. (1992). *Pressure ulcers in adults: Prediction and prevention.* AHCPR Publication No. 92-0050. Washington, DC: Author.

U.S. Department of Health and Human Services, Public Health Service, Agency for Healthcare Research and Quality (AHRQ), formerly (AHCPR). (1995). *Treatment of pressure ulcers.* AHCPR Publication No. 95-0652. Washington, DC: Author.

Welton, J. M. (2008). Implications of Medicare reimbursement changes related to inpatient nursing care quality. *Journal of Nursing Administration, 38*(7–8), 325–333.

Wysocki, A. B. (2007). Anatomy and physiology of skin and soft tissue. In R. A. Bryant & D. P. Nix (Eds.), *Acute and chronic wounds: Current management concepts* (3rd ed., pp. 39–55). St. Louis, MO: Mosby.

CHAPTER 9

Bowel and Bladder Management

Jill Rye
Kristen L. Mauk

LEARNING OBJECTIVES

At the end of this chapter, the reader will be able to

- Understand the physiological structures of the bowel and bladder.
- Describe three main types of neurogenic bladders.
- Discuss bladder management strategies for rehabilitation patients.
- State causes, signs, and symptoms of autonomic dysreflexia.
- Identify the components of a bowel management program.
- Recognize three main types of neurogenic bowel function.
- Name strategies for preventing constipation.

KEY CONCEPTS AND TERMS

Areflexic	Incontinence	Parasympathetic
Autonomic dysreflexia	Internal urethral sphincter	Reflexic
Bladder	Kidney	Sphincter
Constipation	Micturition reflex	Stress incontinence
Defecation	Mitrofanoff	Suprapubic triggers
Detrusor	appendicovesicostomy	Transient incontinence
Detrusor sphincter dyssynergia	Neurogenic	Transurethral sphincterotomy
Evacuation	Neurogenic bladder	Uninhibited bladder
External urethral sphincter	dysfunction	Urethra
Functional incontinence	Overflow incontinence	Urge incontinence

Many patients in rehabilitation experience bowel and bladder changes related to their disease or condition. The ability to manage altered bladder and bowel function is an important aspect of rehabilitation nursing. Alterations in bladder and bowel management can be a barrier to community discharge. Failure to establish a continent elimination program has a serious negative impact on community reintegration. Knowledge of normal bladder and bowel function as well as disruption of function is a key skill for the rehabilitation nurse.

URINARY TRACT ANATOMY

The urinary tract is the body system responsible for elimination of water-soluble waste. Two **kidneys** are located in the retroperitoneal space in the upper abdomen. Each kidney contains greater than 1 million nephrons. These nephrons contain capillaries, the glomerulus, proximal convoluted tubule, loop of Henle, and finally the distal convoluted tubule, which empties into a collecting tubule (Figure 9.1). Each kidney receives approximately one-eighth of all cardiac volume via the renal artery. Each kidney filters materials such as electrolytes, glucose, water, and small proteins that are reabsorbed in the proximal tubule. Urine volumes are controlled by antidiuretic hormone to ensure fluid volumes are maintained. The **bladder** capacity of an adult bladder is approximately 400 to 500 mL (Dains, Ciofu, Baumann, & Scheibel, 2003).

The urine formed by the nephrons collects in the renal pelvis. From there urine moves into the ureters.

In an adult each ureter is approximately 30 cm long. Each ureter enters the bladder obliquely on the posterior aspect of bladder wall. The bladder consists of smooth muscle fibers that form the **detrusor** muscle. Urine exits the bladder via the **urethra**. The urethra extends from the bladder to the outside of the body. The **sphincter** muscles control excretion of the urine from the bladder through the urethra. The **internal urethral sphincter** is a ring of smooth muscle located where the urethra and bladder meet. The **external urethral sphincter** is made of striated muscles and is under voluntary muscle control. The female urethra is 3 to 4 cm long and the male urethra is 18 to 20 cm. This difference in urethral length accounts for one of the reasons females tend to get more bladder infections than males.

The bladder and internal urethral sphincter are innervated by **parasympathetic** fibers of the autonomic nervous system. The nerves follow the blood supply through the sacral levels of the spinal cord. The reflex arc required to void is stimulated by mechanoreceptors that respond to the bladder stretching. These receptors sense bladder fullness and send messages to the sacral level of the spinal cord when the bladder fills. When the bladder has 250 to 300 mL of urine, the person feels the urge to void, but the urge can be inhibited or facilitated by impulses from the brain, resulting in voluntary urinary control (McCance & Huether, 2006). During normal voiding, the bladder contracts and the internal sphincter relaxes by activating the spinal reflex arc. This is known as the **micturition reflex**. Voluntary control of voiding can be adversely affected by a number of neurological conditions such as stroke or multiple sclerosis (MS). The pudendal nerve exits the spinal cord at S2–4 and controls the skeletal muscles of the external sphincter and pelvic muscles that support bladder function (Mauk, 2007).

URINARY TRACT PATHOPHYSIOLOGY

Urinary **incontinence** is defined as the involuntary leakage of urine. It can happen due to psychological, pathological, anatomical, or physiological factors that result in obstruction or bladder irritability or as a result of neurological problems (e.g., MS, Parkinson's disease). Both **transient incontinence** (often reversible) and neurogenic bladder dysfunction (more chronic) are discussed in the following sections.

There are three major tracts through which the brain and spinal cord communicate about the bladder: the cortical regulatory, dorsal column, and lateral spinothalamic. The names indicate their location within the nervous system. The cortical regulatory tract in the spinal cord assists with voluntary control. The dorsal column tract signals filling and distention. The lateral spinothalamic tract senses pain and temperature. An

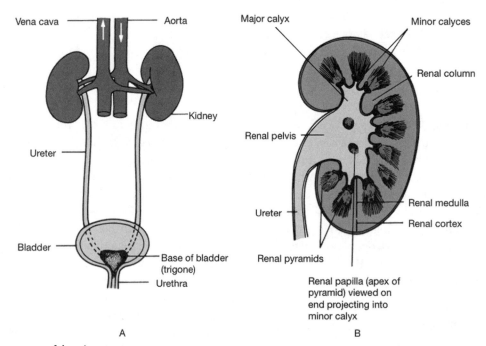

A   B

FIGURE 9.1   Components of the urinary system.

Source: Crowley, Introduction to Human Disease, (2004)

TABLE 9.1   Factors Contributing to Incontinence in the Older Adult Rehabilitation Client
Immobility, functional impairment
Urinary tract infection
Medications
Neurogenic bladder dysfunction
Poor behavioral adjustment
Cognitive deficits
Decreased bladder capacity
Delirium
Dementia
Rectal impaction
Lack of caregiver support
Environmental barriers
Anxiety
Caffeine or other bladder irritants
Depression

interruption in any one or all of these tracts results in **neurogenic** bladder dysfunction.

Transient Incontinence

Urinary incontinence is a common, especially in older adults. There are many causes (Table 9.1). The U.S. prevalence in women is 26% during reproductive years and 30% to 40% in postmenopausal women. Approximately 15% to 30% of elderly women living in the community experience incontinence, and 8% to 22% of men living in the community also may experience incontinence. Up to 50% of individuals living in long-term care may be incontinent (Dains et al., 2003). Incontinence often leads to complications with recovery, including being associated with falls with fracture (Brown, Vittinghoff, Wyman, Stone, Nevitt, Ensrud, & Grady, 2000) and negative patient outcomes.

Incontinence is categorized by the impairment: stress incontinence, urge incontinence or overactive bladder, overflow incontinence, and incontinence from reversible causes. Urinary incontinence in older adults is associated with some serious complications such as delirium and falls (Brown et al., 2000). Many of these types of incontinence can be helped or reversed with a combination of medical and behavioral therapies (discussion follows). Gross (2003) stated that 80% of urinary incontinence could be helped by appropriate treatment and management. Transient causes of urinary incontinence are shown in Table 9.2

Leakage of urine with coughing, sneezing, laughing, or other activity is called **stress incontinence**. It occurs in most often in women who have had multiple children. The cause is weakness at the base of the bladder and urethra due to pelvic floor relaxation.

Urge incontinence is a sudden and strong sensation to void without the ability to delay urination. It is caused by hyperactivity or hypersensitivity of the bladder. An overactive detrusor muscle is triggered when disorders of the brain override the central inhibitory centers and do not prevent contractions of the muscle (Dains et al., 2003).

Overflow incontinence happens when the bladder is overdistended with underactive or acontractile detrusor muscle activity. Synergistic urinary sphincter relaxation is lost and the bladder detrusor muscle contracts, or there is bladder outlet or urethral obstruction. Sphincter weakness can occur from a damaged urethra, damage to the nerves controlling the urethra, or due to pelvic floor muscle relaxation.

When causes are not physiological in nature, the term **functional incontinence** may be used. Persons who might otherwise have bladder control may be incontinent because of the inability to reach the toilet in time. Causes of this could include obesity, distance to the toilet, use of adaptive equipment to ambulate to toilet (such as a walker or splint), or a cluttered environment that stands in the way of the bathroom. Mixed incontinence occurs when the incontinence is a result of several anatomical, physiological, or functional factors (Dains et al., 2003; Diebold, Fanning-Harding, & Hanson, 2010).

Anatomical incontinence can result from an obstruction in the lower urinary tract. A common cause of anatomical obstruction is **detrusor sphincter dyssynergia**. This phenomenon is the result of lack of synchrony between the detrusor muscle and the external sphincter. Usually, these muscle groups work in synergy to allow the bladder to empty (Abrams et al., 2002; Karsenty, Reitz, Wefer, Boy, & Schurch, 2005). In dyssynergia, smooth muscle found in the urethrovesical junction does not funnel urine during bladder emptying. A large prostate gland can also be a form of anatomical obstruction. This can be caused by acute inflammation, benign prostatic enlargement, or prostate cancer. The urethra is narrowed by the large prostate gland, causing difficulty initiating the urine stream. Scarring in the urethra can cause narrowing. This scarring can be caused by infection, injury, or surgery. Severe pelvic organ prolapse in women can cause bladder outlet obstruction. A cystocele can reach or protrude past the vaginal opening (McCance & Huether, 2006).

TABLE 9.2	Transient Causes of Urinary Incontinence
The mnemonic DIAPPERS has been established to list common causes of transient incontinence.	

Common Causes	Rationale
Delirium/dementia	Altered cognitive functioning interferes with the ability to recognize the need for toileting or respond in a timely manner.
Infection	The urinary frequency and urgency associated with symptomatic UTI may lead to urinary incontinence.
Atrophic vaginitis/ urethritis	Decreased estrogen in women results in thin, dry, friable vaginal and urethra mucosa.
Psychological	Depression may interfere with an individual's motivation and desire to perform activities of daily living or attend to continence. Anxiety or fear that leakage will occur may contribute to frequency difficulties controlling urge.
Pharmacological agents	Inadequate management of acute or chronic pain can interfere with the ability to attend to toileting needs. Narcotics, a component of many pain management regimens, can lead to constipation and fecal impaction that obstructs the bladder neck, leading to urine retention, overflow incontinence, and urgency. Narcotics can also decrease bladder muscle contraction resulting in urine retention, incomplete bladder emptying, increased risk for UTI, and overflow incontinence. Many medications have adverse or unintended side effects that may directly impact bladder function, bladder relaxation, urinary sphincter relaxation or obstruction, cognitive status (awareness of an effective response to need to void), or urine production. Polypharmacy increases the risk for adverse drug effects and drug interactions.
Endocrine disease	Metabolic conditions (hyperglycemia, hypercalcemia, low albumin states, diabetes insipidus) associated with polyuria increase fluid load on the bladder and increase the risk for urge and stress incontinence.
Restricted mobility	Limited ability to move about interferes with the ability to reach a toilet in time to prevent leakage.
Stool impaction	Overdistention of the rectum or anal canal can obstruct the bladder neck, leading to urine retention, overflow incontinence, and urgency.

Source: Resnick, 1985.

Neurogenic Bladder Dysfunction

Neurogenic bladder dysfunction describes a variety of lower urinary tract disorders caused by disease or disruption of neurological function. A cerebrovascular accident, brain injury, or brain tumor may cause neurogenic detrusor overactivity; this can cause uncontrolled or premature contraction of the detrusor muscle. These contractions cause urgency or leakage. Lesions that affect the spinal cord or nerves (such as spinal cord injury [SCI], transverse myelitis, or Guillian-Barré syndrome) are generally associated with the loss of bladder sensation and the loss of coordination between the detrusor and urethral sphincter and urethral sphincter muscles. An acontractile detrusor does not contract even when the bladder fills or there is a desire to urinate. This can occur after damage to the lumbosacral spine or cauda equina damage (McCance & Huether, 2006). Although there are several different types of bladder problems seen in the rehabilitation patient, three major types are discussed here: uninhibited, reflexic, and areflexic.

Uninhibited

Persons with this kind of bladder have a lesion or interruption somewhere along the cortical regulatory tract. **Uninhibited bladder** is associated with problems in the brain. This type of bladder function is common with stroke, brain injury, Parkinson's disease, Alzheimer's disease, cerebral palsy, and MS.

The person with uninhibited neurogenic bladder function may experience sensation but lack of voluntary control. The characteristics of this type of bladder include urgency, frequent bladder contractions, complete emptying (unless other complications are also present), and nocturia. The reflex arc (at S2–4) is intact, but there is an upper motor neuron problem, and because the cortical regulatory tract is related to voluntary control, incontinence is expected. Bladder capacity is decreased because involuntary voiding occurs before the usual level of fullness is reached. However, nursing treatment including scheduled voiding, monitoring fluid intake, and habit retraining is highly effective. Medications are available to assist with bladder or sphincter control until proper patterns are developed.

Reflexic

Persons with **reflexic** bladder control have an intact reflex arc, which can be stimulated to assist with voiding. A reflex neurogenic bladder occurs when there is an interruption to the ascending sensory tract above the S2–4 level. This can also be referred to as suprasacral, spastic, or central neurogenic bladder. Patients with this problem may include those with SCI, trauma, infection, MS, or tumors above the sacral level.

Persons with this type of bladder lack sensation to void. This causes the classic symptoms of urinary retention and large residual amounts of urine in the bladder. Nursing interventions center on emptying the bladder at regular intervals through intermittent catheterization and using **suprapubic triggers** to stimulate spontaneous voiding via the intact reflex arc. Examples of suprapubic triggers include tapping over the pubic area, squeezing

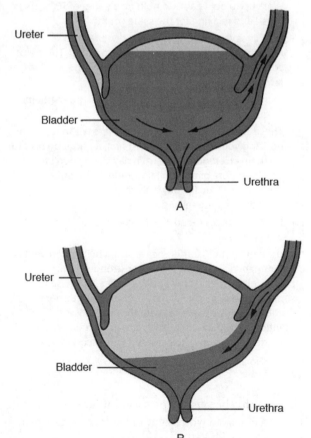

FIGURE 9.2   Vesicoureteral reflux.

Source: Crowley, Introduction to Human Disease, (2004)

the glans penis, stroking the thigh, pulling the pubic hair, or running water over the pubic area. These activities may stimulate the voiding reflex; however, many patients with reflexic bladders still need to perform intermittent catheterization and cannot solely rely on suprapubic triggers. Reflex voiding is recommended only for males who meet certain criteria (Consortium of Spinal Cord Medicine, 2006).

Areflexic

As the name suggests, in the **areflexic**, or autonomous, bladder there is damage to the reflex arc This lower motor neuron disorder produces a flaccid, atonic bladder because of injury to the S2–4 segments. Patients have involuntary voiding, no sensation, and overflow incontinence. This includes persons with sacral SCI (many of those with paraplegia), inflammation of the spinal cord, diabetes (in some cases), and other trauma to the cauda equina area. Nursing treatment of the areflexic bladder is aimed at avoiding fullness, because reflux can occur (even after one episode) and damage the renal structures (Figure 9.2). The Credé and Valsalva maneuvers are also used at times, along with intermittent catheterization to empty the bladder.

NURSING INTERVENTIONS

The goal of any bladder management program is to develop predictable, effective patterns of elimination (Mauk, 2007). The main purpose of bladder management is to empty the bladder of urine and prevent infection or potential complications. To achieve these goals, a combination of bladder training, behavior modification, and medications may be needed, with the least invasive effective method used. Bladder management must also fit with the patient's lifestyle (Mauk, 2007).

Bladder management programs are initiated after urodynamic studies are completed. The patient should be involved in designing a bladder management program that will work for him or her. A thorough assessment should be made. Table 9.3 gives a summary of the components of a basic evaluation for urinary function.

Bladder Training

Several different techniques can be used to facilitate bladder retraining for those with transient incontinence or uninhibited neurogenic bladder. Pelvic floor exercises (also known as Kegel exercises) are useful in many conditions to help strengthen the muscles used to prevent leakage of urine. A sample of instructions for patients

TABLE 9.3 Assessment of Urinary Function in Those With Neurogenic Bladder
History
Medical diagnosis and comorbidities, neurological, genitourinary
Explore symptoms of incontinent episodes
Assess risk factors for UI or other bladder dysfunction and complications
Review medications for contributing side effects
Physical examination
Should include general, abdominal, rectal, pelvic (women), prostate/genital (men)
Postvoid residual (if problems), preferably through bladder scan
Urinalysis (add culture and sensitivity if needed or infection suspected)
Urodynamic studies

on the proper way to perform these exercises appears in Box 9.1.

Some patients have better outcomes with certain approaches than with others. For example, adults with head injury have been well managed with a combination of fluids, scheduled voiding, and positive reinforcement (Grinspun, 1993). Stroke patients that are alert and oriented may have more success with traditional scheduled voiding than those who have cognitive problems, including disorientation and memory loss (Consortium for Spinal Cord Medicine, 2006; Owen, Getz, & Bulla, 1995). Elderly institutionalized patient seem to experience less incontinence with a prompted voiding approach. Thus, rehabilitation nurses should be flexible and alert to the unique needs of each person.

Intermittent Catheterization

Intermittent catheterization is a technique to empty the bladder by inserting a flexible tube into the bladder and draining the urine. This is used for persons who cannot voluntarily empty the bladder, such as persons with SCI. The catheter does not remain in the bladder, but the patient performs self-catheterization several times per day to empty the bladder. Clean technique is used by the patient, while sterile technique is used by health professionals during the hospital and rehabilitation stay (Consortium for Spinal Cord Medicine, 2006). In patients who have repeated infections, sterile catheters may be used. Intermittent catheterization can also be taught to a family member or caregiver if the patient is unable to

---

BOX 9.1 Client Teaching: Pelvic Floor Muscle Exercises (Kegel Exercises)

The purpose of these exercises is to help strengthen the muscles that support the bladder and surrounding structures. By exercising them as you would any other muscle group, you can make them stronger and learn to control them voluntarily. Learning how to squeeze the urethra closed by tightening those muscles when needed can help decrease incontinence.

- Locate the correct pelvic floor muscles. This is done most easily by sitting on the toilet and beginning to urinate. Stop the stream of urine. Think about drawing in and lifting up the rectal/anal sphincter muscle. Even if you cannot completely stop the urine stream but it slows down, you are using the right muscles. Practice this several times.
- The buttocks should not tense when performing these exercises. Your abdomen should not be moving when you do this either. If they do, go back to the toileting exercise and practice locating the correct muscles again.
- Do not hold your breath when doing these exercises.
- To perform a Kegel exercise, squeeze the pelvic floor muscles and hold for a slow count of 2. Then relax the muscles for a slow count of 2. This is one repetition. Work up to being able to hold for a count of 10 (at the most) and relaxing for the same count
- Do this several times per day by dividing into 15 repetitions each: lying, sitting, and standing. This helps condition your body to reacting in different positions, as it may feel differently.
- If unable to do 15 exercises at a time, do fewer, but more frequently.
- These exercises can be done anywhere without anyone noticing you are doing them. At first, it might be best to do them at a regular time each day so you don't forget, such as before or after meals. Gradually incorporate them more often in your daily routine, such as riding to work or watching television.
- Don't get discouraged. It will take time to develop muscle strength.

You should notice a difference in your ability to prevent incontinence as these muscles get stronger. When the urge is felt to void, sit still and use a Kegel exercise to suppress the urge until you can get to the bathroom. Combining these exercises with the other things mentioned by your nurse, such as a habit training and fluid management, should help control your incontinence.

Source: From Diebold et al. (2010), Easton (1999), and Stevens (2008).

---

perform this because of physical limitations. However, the decision as to which type of bladder management to use must consider all factors.

Bladder volumes, or urine output obtained from intermittent catheterization, should not exceed 500 mL

(Consortium for Spinal Cord Medicine, 2006). If volumes are higher than this, bacteria will grow and the person is more apt to acquire a urinary tract infection (UTI). The patient should be taught to perform intermittent catheterization more frequently and monitor intake and output more carefully. Patients should not be encouraged to decrease fluid intake solely for the sake of being able to do intermittent catheterization less often for convenience, because this also can contribute to an increase in UTIs.

> Rehabilitation nurses are encouraged to address bowel and bladder function as one of the major aspects of rehabilitation nursing care.

For those with areflexic bladders, a technique called Credé can be used to help with emptying by applying pressure with the blade of one hand to the lower abdomen above the pubic area. The Consortium on Spinal Cord Medicine's (2006) clinical practice guidelines states the following: "consider the use of Credé and Valsalva for individuals who have lower motor neuron injuries with low outlet resistance or who have had a sphincterotomy" (p. 22). Credé is performed when gentle external pressure may assist with bladder elimination. Likewise, the Valsalva maneuver is a technique that uses the abdominal muscles with the diaphragm to push down on the bladder to promote emptying. This is useful when the bladder is flaccid and does not have the ability to contract, or when the bladder can contract but cannot empty completely. This technique would not be used for persons with the complication of detrusor sphincter dyssynergia (discussion follows).

Indwelling Catheters

Generally, indwelling catheters should be removed as soon as possible in the rehabilitation program (Stevens, 2008). Catheters should be removed early in the morning so the patient's voiding ability can be monitored throughout the day and toileting can be initiated. Indwelling catheters are associated with higher rates of bladder infection than intermittent catheterization, so this is not the preferred method for bladder management in the long term. However, an indwelling urinary catheter may be the most practical and effective means of urinary emptying for the patients with poor hand function, high fluid intake, no caregiver assistance, and lack of success with other types of programs (Consortium on Spinal Cord Medicine, 2006). If an indwelling catheter is the preferred method, it should be changed about once per month.

The patient or caregiver will need to be instructed about cleansing the area around the tube, measuring intake and output, signs and symptoms of bladder infection, what to do if the catheter becomes plugged, proper anchoring of the catheter, and so on.

A suprapubic catheter may be an alternative to an indwelling catheter or intermittent catheterization. This catheter is placed into the bladder through an incision in the lower abdomen above the pubic bone. This catheter can be removed in the future if the patient's condition changes, and the opening will close in 1 to 2 days (Consortium for Spinal Cord Medicine, 2006).

Botulinum toxin (Botox) injection may be an option for patients with detrusor sphincter dyssynergia. This chemical can be used to relax the urinary sphincter. The Botox is injected into the sphincter, and it takes about a week for the medicine to show effect. The Botox effects last about 3 to 6 months. Alpha blockers and anticholinergic medications may also be effective to manage bladder issues (Consortium for Spinal Cord Medicine, 1999, 2006).

Surgical procedures may be needed to manage neurogenic bladder problems. **Transurethral sphincterotomy** procedure makes an incision in the urinary sphincter. This is used for males who have detrusor sphincter dyssynergia. The goal is to decrease the pressure in the bladder and allow it to empty more completely. The cutting of the sphincter muscle allows for more effective drainage and decreased bladder infections. The bladder may shrink after SCI or become overactive. Bladder augmentation may be needed to expand the capacity of the bladder. This is done by surgically graphing a segment of the small intestine, stomach, or other tissue to the bladder. The goal is to decrease leaking and protect the kidneys from becoming damaged (Consortium for Spinal Cord Medicine, 2006).

A continent urinary diversion is a surgical procedure that bypasses the bladder by creating an internal pouch or pseudo-bladder. The ureters are connected to this new pouch either attached to the patient's urethra or to a stoma created in the lower abdomen (Consortium for Spinal Cord Medicine, 2006). The **Mitrofanoff appendicovesicostomy** is a surgical procedure that creates a stoma in the lower abdomen using a length of intestine or the appendix. This stoma, usually located at the umbilicus, can be used for intermittent catheterization in those with neurogenic bladder (Hsu & Shortliffe, 2004). This procedure may allow for greater independence for those who previously may have relied on a caregiver for intermittent catheterization.

COMPLICATIONS OF BLADDER DYSFUNCTION

Many complications are associated with neurogenic bladders, as well as with incontinence due to other causes. Some of these can be life-threatening, and some occur more frequently in the older population.

Detrusor Sphincter Dyssynergia

This type of dysfunction results from asynchrony of the sphincters. As the detrusor contracts, the sphincters do not relax. This results in a poor urine stream, large residual urine amounts, and an increased incidence of UTIs. Treatment may include medications such as diazepam (Valium), dantrolene sodium (Dantrium), or baclofen (Lioresal), which decrease the spasticity of skeletal muscles, promoting relaxation of the external urinary sphincter. (Valium should be used with extreme caution in older adults.) With detrusor sphincter dyssynergia, performance of the Valsalva or Credé maneuvers is contraindicated, because this could cause damaging reflux. Such complications occur commonly with SCI.

Hydronephrosis or Reflux

When obstruction occurs, whether from stricture, congenital malformation, or an overdistended bladder, reflux of urine from the bladder into the kidneys can occur, causing hydronephrosis. This is a complication to which persons with neurogenic bladder must be constantly alert, particularly those prone to overflow. Patients with SCI are particularly at risk. Intake and output should be monitored, and urodynamic studies should be done routinely. Medications such as bethanechol (Urecholine) increase bladder tone and contractions of the bladder. Oxybutynin chloride (Ditropan) relaxes smooth muscles through antispasmodic properties. Persons with urinary retention and incomplete emptying often have high urine volumes. If patients forget to catheterize or allow too much urine to accumulate in the bladder, reflux can result in permanent renal damage (Figure 9.3)

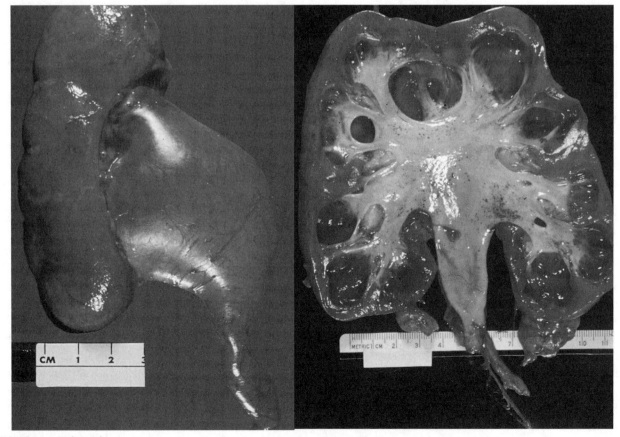

FIGURE 9.3   Hydronephrosis.

Source: Photo courtesy of Leonard V. Crowley.

Urinary Tract Infection

Infections related to bladder dysfunction are common. Those with SCI or diabetes and the elderly are at greatest risk. Women are more at risk of UTIs than men because of a shorter urethra. Indwelling catheters are a major source of infection, both from contamination during insertion and from continued exposure of the bladder to bacteria that can come from the catheter. UTIs remain a major cause of death in persons with SCI. Prevention of UTI is of prime concern and can be accomplished through adequate fluid intake and regular emptying of the bladder.

Calculi

Older rehabilitation patients who experience immobility are particularly at risk for development of kidney or bladder stones. With inactivity, calcium can leave the bone and can be displaced elsewhere. Although most stones are passed spontaneously, calculi cause extreme pain and discomfort. Some experts believe that decreasing calcium and phosphorus in the diet reduces the chance of calculi development. Increasing fluids to 3,000 mL/day and promoting weight-bearing activities should reduce the person's risk.

Signs and symptoms of calculi include pain that appears as dull flank pain or irritation that moves and radiates, depending on the location of the stone. Nausea, vomiting, and elevated pulse and blood pressure can also result. For elders with sensory damage, pain may not be felt so the nurse must rely on other signs such as sweating, bladder spasms, or blood in the urine to detect this problem. Diagnostic studies can confirm presence and location of calculi. Treatment can center on increasing the acidity of the urine to prevent stone formation, forcing fluids, restricting calcium, surgery, or ultrasonic disintegration.

Autonomic Dysreflexia

This is an acute medical emergency that requires prompt treatment. Autonomic dysreflexia, or hyperreflexia, is most often seen in persons with cervical SCI, but it occurs in 48–90% of those with SCI at or above T-6 level and four times more frequently in males (Dittmar, 1989; Campagnolo, 2009). Usually occurring within the first 6 months after injury, this complication of neurogenic bladder can be seen even years after injury.

Autonomic dysreflexia is caused when stimuli sent to the brain via the spinal cord cannot reach the message center. Sensory receptors in the S2–4 region are stimulated, sending impulses to the brain. Because these are blocked, the stimuli continue and the impulses build, producing a reflex arteriolar spasm through the autonomic nervous system. This leads to arteriole vasoconstriction and elevated blood pressure, with massive vasodilatation to the heart and the brain. Once the brain centers have detected an elevation in blood pressure, the brain decreases the heart rate and dilates smaller vessels in an attempt to compensate. Efferent impulses from the sympathetic ganglia of the spinal cord dilate blood vessels above the lesion, resulting in flushing and sweating and a continued rise in blood pressure. Blood vessels from the lower body are constricted, causing pallor and "goose flesh."

These mechanisms cause the clinical signs and symptoms seen in autonomic dysreflexia. If unrecognized and allowed to continue, these physiological changes can result in systolic blood pressures as high as 300 mm Hg. Stroke and coma or death can occur.

Causes of this disorder center around the S2–4 sites or below. The most common cause is a distended bladder, as in cases in which a person with SCI and an areflexic bladder may have skipped a catheterization. A kinked or blocked indwelling catheter in the bladder may also be a common cause. Impaction that distends the rectum, genital stimulation, urological or gynecological procedures, sexual intercourse, gallstones, pressure sores, pregnancy, and rapid emptying of an overdistended bladder are other common causes (Campagnolo, 2009). For the older rehabilitation patient, bladder distention and impaction are the two most likely stimuli.

The rehabilitation nurse should be alert to the signs and symptoms of autonomic dysreflexia because it is a life-threatening condition (Table 9.4). The patient presents with hypertension, bradycardia, flushing, redness of the face, a blotchy neck, and perspiration of the skin above the level of injury. Complaints include a pounding headache and blurred vision.

As with most complications in rehabilitation, prevention is the best treatment. Bladder fullness must be avoided in patients, especially those with complete lesions above the T-6 level. A reliable bowel program will help prevent constipation. Treatment is directed at relieving the causing stimuli (Table 9.5) and lowering the blood pressure. There are some immediate actions the nurse can take toward managing the hypertensive crisis. The head of the bed should be raised immediately to take advantage of orthostatic hypotension. Tight clothing should be loosened. The nurse should

TABLE 9.4   Signs and Symptoms of Autonomic Dysreflexia

Hypertension (based on baseline blood pressure)

Bradycardia (relative to patient's baseline)

Red face; blotchy skin on face and neck

Flushing and perspiration above the level of injury

Pounding headache

Blurred vision

Nasal congestion

Pallor or goose flesh below level of lesion

Cardiac dysrthymias

Complaints of anxiety, nervousness

Nausea

BOX 9.2   Web Exploration

There are excellent evidence-based clinical practice guidelines for the management of autonomic dysreflexia. Review this site:

Paralyzed Veterans of America & Consortium for Spinal Cord Medicine. Acute management of autonomic dysreflexia: Individuals with spinal cord injury presenting to healthcare facilities at http://www.guidelines.gov/content.aspx?id=2964&search=autonomic+dysreflexia#Section420

be aware of the patient's baseline vital signs. The average blood pressure for a quadriplegic may be 90/60 mm Hg while sitting, and not all patients will present with such obvious hypertension in early stages. If symptoms are present, check blood pressure. Many persons with T-6 lesions and above run a lower blood pressure of between 90 and 110 mm Hg systolic (Paralyzed Veterans of America & Consortium for Spinal Cord Medicine, 2001). Even a rise of 20 to 40 mm Hg above baseline can signify elevation of blood pressure. The aged individual may show less of a rise in blood pressure than a person in his or her twenties. Box 9.2 gives Web links to clinical practice guidelines for the management of autonomic dysreflexia.

TABLE 9.5   Common Causative Factors of Autonomic Hyperreflexia

Bladder distention or fullness

Kinked or blocked catheter tubing

Impaction or rectal distention

Genital stimulation

Urological or gynecological procedures

Rapid emptying of the bladder

Pressure sores

Pregnancy and delivery

Pain

Fractures or trauma

Other (less commonly reported): ingrown toenails, tight shoes or clothing

BOWEL ANATOMY

The digestive system is made up of the mouth, esophagus, stomach, small intestine, large intestine, rectum, and anus. Its function is to break down ingested food, prepare it for use by the body's cells, provide body water, and eliminate waste. Ingested food is broken down by the mouth by chewing and moves to the stomach where it is churned and mixed by stomach acids and enzymes. It moves into the small intestine where biochemicals and enzymes secreted by the liver and pancreas break the food down into absorbable proteins, carbohydrates, and fats. The nutrients pass through the walls of the small intestine into blood vessels and lymphatics that deliver it to the liver for storage or processing. Substances not absorbed in the small intestine are transported to the large intestine where fluids continue to absorb. Fluid waste travels to the kidneys and is eliminated via urine. Solid wastes continue on to the rectum and are eliminated through the anus. When fecal matter enters the rectum, stretch receptors send a message to the brain that the bowel needs to be emptied. In a person without neurogenic problems, inhibitory reflexes allow inhibition of the need to defecate until a suitable place is found.

The function of the digestive system is under autonomic nervous system control, except for chewing, swallowing, and **defecation** of solid waste. The autonomic innervation is both sympathetic and parasympathetic and is controlled by centers in the brain mediated at networks of nerve fibers in the gastrointestinal walls (McCance & Huether, 2006).

NEUROGENIC BOWEL CHARACTERISTICS AND TREATMENTS

Any disruption of the nerve impulses to the bowel interrupts the normal process of elimination. Damage to the brain or the spinal cord can disrupt the awareness or sensation to empty the bowel as well as the muscle strength to evacuate the stool. A bowel program is a plan to help regain control of bowel function. The requirements for the formation of normal stool and bowel function include adequate fiber in the diet, adequate fluid, general activity and mobility, and upright position (Consortium for Spinal Cord Medicine, 2010).

Similarly to neurogenic bladder function, three main types of neurogenic bowel function are discussed here: uninhibited, reflexic, and areflexic. Table 9.6 provides a summary of these three bowel types. The rate of bowel incontinence is unknown, but constipation is often more of a problem with most rehabilitation patients. The stigma with bowel incontinence may be greater than with bladder incontinence because of odor and more difficulty hiding the problem.

Uninhibited

This bowel function is seen in those with lesion above C-1 or those that occur in the brain. Bowel sensation and reflex activity are intact, but the brain does not have the same control over inhibitory processes that prevented incontinence before. Uninhibited neurogenic bowel function is often associated with stroke. Stroke patients are typically able to regain bowel function more quickly than bladder function. Suppository use may be needed initially, but natural means should be the goal for a long-term bowel program with stroke survivors. Other patients with this type of function include those with head injury, dementia, Parkinson's disease, and MS. Characteristics of this type of bowel function may include involuntary stools, a lack of awareness of need to defecate, urgency, smearing, **constipation** (more than 3 days with no bowel movement), impaction, hypoactive bowel sounds, and decreased sphincter control (Easton, 1999). Treatment includes establishing a consistent schedule for toileting, managing controllable factors, and using suppositories and/or other medications as needed. Most of these patient experience good success with regaining bowel control.

TABLE 9.6	Summary of Three Main Types of Neurogenic Bowel		
Type	**Associated Diagnoses**	**Traits**	**Treatment**
Uninhibited	Stroke	Urgency	Managing controllable factors
	TBI	Incontinence	Toileting schedule
	Brain tumor	Smearing	Suppositories, PRN
	MS	Constipation	
	Parkinson's disease	Intact reflexes	
	Alzheimer's disease	Hypoactive bowel sounds	
		Decreased awareness of need	
		Lesions above C-1	
Reflexic	SCI	Incontinence	Bowel program
	SC tumors	Loss of urge	Digital stimulation
	SC infarct	S2–4 intact	Suppository
	Quadriplegia	Empties automatically	
	MS	Impaired external sphincter control	
	Trauma	Lack of voluntary control	
	High thoracic paraplegics	Damage above T12–L1	
Areflexic	Spina bifida	Incontinence	High fiber diet
	Cauda equina injury	Sensory loss of need to defecate	Valsalva maneuver
	Diabetes	Flaccid external sphincter	Manual removal
	Intervertebral disk problem	Leakage of stool	Suppository
	Trauma to S2–4	Damage below T12–L1	
	Paraplegia		

Reflexic

As the name suggests, in this type of bowel function the defecation reflex (located around S2–4) remains intact. Persons with this problem have an upper motor neuron disorder. This may be due to spinal tumors, infarct, SCI, or lesions (as with MS). Characteristics of reflexic bowel function include loss of urge to defecate, incontinence, automatic emptying, and impaired external sphincter control. Most persons with quadriplegia fall into this category and may require a caregiver to assist with the bowel program. Nursing management include capitalizing on the intact reflex for defecation. Digital stimulation, use of gravity, and promoting all natural means of bowel management are used. Digital stimulation is done by gently inserting a lubricated gloved finger into the rectum and rotating the finger in a circular motion. This should be done for 20 seconds to no more than 1 minute. The digital stimulation relaxes and opens the external anal sphincter to allow the stool to completely empty. It is important to monitor the amount, consistency, and color of the results. Digital stimulation is contraindicated in certain patients, including those with cardiac problems.

Areflexic

The autonomous bowel is caused by injury to the lumbosacral cord and spinal root. This lower motor neuron disorder results from damage to the sacral segments that control the reflex for defecation. Persons with this type of bowel function include those with spina bifida, cauda equina injury, diabetes, or SCI with paraplegia. Traits seen include recurring and frequent incontinence, a flaccid external sphincter that results in leakage of stool, and the sensory loss of the need to defecate (Gender, 1996). This is often the most difficult bowel problem to manage. Treatment includes strict adherence to a bowel program, plenty of fiber and fluids in the diet to maintain a firm stool and prevent diarrhea, use of suppositories and manual removal of stool, and the Valsalva maneuver to promote defecation (if not contraindicated).

General Guidelines

Before devising a bowel program, the nurse should perform a thorough assessment. This should include a history noting previous bowel patterns, dietary habits (Folden et al., 2002), history of constipation, diagnosis, and medical problems. A physical examination should include at least assessment of the person's functional status and abilities and abdominal, rectal, oral, and neurological function.

The goals of a bowel program are that it be realistic, predictable, convenient, inexpensive, and as natural as possible (Mauk, 2005). There are many fancy products

on the market that claim to help with bowel control. In reality, a program must be fitted to the person's unique needs and abilities to maintain it. All natural means should be tried first. Those with spinal injury will probably have a more complex routine than those recovering from a stroke. Many factors affect a person's ability to manage his or her own bowel program, including loss of muscle tone, cognitive ability, functional ability, dexterity, ability to transfer to the toilet, and environmental barriers (Easton, 1999). Each of these components should be addressed.

To establish a bowel pattern after damage to the spinal cord requires a planned bowel program. Table 9.7 gives principles of starting a bowel program. To begin the process, a time of day is scheduled for planned **evacuation** of the bowel. The time should be established at the same time daily or every other day. It is best to position the patient upright on a toilet or commode. To ensure consistent results from a bowel program, it is important to monitor the diet, fluid intake, and medications. Adequate fiber intake and fluids can ensure the bowel maintains a consistent pattern. The minimum daily recommended fiber is 15 g, which should be gradually increased to 20 to 35 g/day (Folden et al., 2002). Fluid intake should be 500 mL/day greater than is recommended for the general public (Consortium for Spinal Cord Medicine, 2010).

Preventing Constipation

Difficulties with a bowel program may include chronic constipation. This could include infrequent small or hard stool or no stool for several days. This can enlarge the descending colon and result in dependence on laxatives or enemas. Diarrhea or frequent liquid stools may also occur (Mauk, 2007). Chronic constipation is the most common bowel disorder (Folden et al., 2002). Box 9.3 provides a Web link to an excellent practice guideline for management of constipation in adults.

TABLE 9.7   Principles of Starting a Bowel Program

Complete a thorough history and physical

Start with a clean bowel

Try all natural means first: Remember the first 5 components!

Know the mechanism of suppository use: choose most appropriate type

Change only one program component at a time and give it a few days to work before making additional changes

Avoid enemas when possible (and use least caustic type when needed to cleanse bowel before program begins)

Avoid bedpans

BOX 9.3   Web Exploration

Consider these practice guidelines for the management of constipation in adults (2002) available at http://www.rehabnurse.org/pdf/BowelGuideforWEB.pdf. You can download the 51-page document for free. This clinical practice guideline provides excellent in-depth information about the problem and current treatment recommendations.

TABLE 9.8   Medications That May Contribute To Constipation

Medication/Purpose	Example
Analgesics	Tylenol with Codeine
Anticholinergics	Cogentin
Anticonvulsives	Dilantin
Antidepressants	Ludiomil, Elavil
Antiparkinsonians	Levodopa
Antihypertensives	Diuril, Aldactone
Diuretics	Lasix
Opiates	Morphine, codeine
Iron supplements	Feosol
Muscle relaxants	Lioresal

Several factors are key to preventing constipation: diet, fluids, timing, activity, positioning, and medication (if needed) (Mauk, 2005). The diet should include foods high in fiber such as popcorn, root vegetables, fruits and fruit juices (such as apples and prunes), and nuts (but take care for those with swallowing problems). Twenty-five to 35 grams of fiber per day is recommended to prevent constipation. Increase fluids to 2 L per day if possible. This may not be realistic for older adults. Water is the best fluid for constipation prevention. Use the person's premorbid bowel habits to begin with when choosing the best time for toileting; if this does not work try the first 5 to 15 minutes after breakfast to take advantage of the gastrocolic reflex. Persons should be encouraged to promptly respond to the urge to defecate. Increase activity, especially walking. Activity stimulates more normal bowel action than being in bed. Get persons up and mobile. Immobility is a common cause of constipation. Positioning the patient upright on the toilet or commode and providing for privacy and time for defecation also help to promote good bowel habits. Finally, evaluate medications that could be contributing to constipation (Table 9.8) as well as those that could be useful in managing it (Mauk, 2005; Smith & Newman, 1989).

Medications

Medications may be necessary at first to maintain bowel elimination. Use when needed, but try all natural means first (as above). Choose the most appropriate and effective medication while continuing to modify the natural components of the program. A goal for most stroke survivors is to be medication free for bowel management and to use natural means (Venn, Taft, Carpenter, & Applebaugh, 1992). Persons with SCI may require long-term use of medications and/or suppositories.

Oral medications may include bulk laxatives, hyperosmotics, lubricants, saline preps, stimulants, and softeners. Bulk formers soften the stool by drawing water into the fecal mass. The person needs an adequate fluid intake for these to be effective. Do not give with warm water, because this can contribute to blockage in the gut. Examples include Fibermed and Metamucil. Hyperosmotics facilitate transit in the gut by stimulating peristalsis. A common example is lactulose. This is effective for many older adults in long-term care facilities. A common lubricant example is mineral oil (but this not recommended for persons with dysphagia), but this is used less often than the other classes for rehabilitation patients. Saline preparations provide osmotic effect that stimulates motility; they are effective and often used in bowel preps for diagnostic testing. Saline preparations work quickly and should mainly be used for acute constipation, not long term. Examples include Milk of Magnesia and magnesium citrate. Stimulants help with peristalsis for those with trouble moving the stool into the rectum, but they can cause cramping. Senna and Dulcolax are common examples. Stool softeners work by drawing in emollients and fats to the fecal mass. The person needs to drink 1 to 2 liters of fluid per day for effectiveness. The most commonly used is Colace.

Suppositories provide rectal medication for relief of constipation. The typical suppository takes 15 to 60 minutes to melt in the rectum and produce results, and it must be placed against the rectal mucosa to be effective. Choose suppositories carefully. Glycerin suppositories tend to be milder than others. Dulcolax suppositories are stronger and may cause cramping but are often used in bowel preps because they are effective. Ceo-Two is a suppository that is placed in warm water until it bubbles and then is inserted. Do not use lubricant (this inactivates it) with this type. Mini-enemas such as Therevac and Enemeeze already are solutions (Mauk, 2005). These work faster than waxy suppositories, but care must be taken not to cause trauma to rectal tissues when inserting the end of the tube before squeezing in the medication.

SUMMARY

Discussion of bowel and bladder function is taboo in many societies. This may contribute to a patient's reluctance to talk about problems with constipation or incontinence. Rehabilitation nurses are encouraged to address bowel and bladder function as one of the major aspects of rehabilitation nursing care, encouraging patients that there are many strategies that assist them to return to a more "normal" pattern.

CRITICAL THINKING

1. Visit www.pva.org to find the best practices for bladder and bowel care. This website provides links to clinical practice guidelines developed by the Consortium for Spinal Cord Medicine.
2. Learn about the Americans with Disabilities Act to review the law that ensures people with disabilities have wheelchair access to public restrooms.
3. Does the place where you work ever provide services for patients with autonomic dysreflexia? If so, what protocol is followed for an episode?
4. For patients with SCI, bladder management can be a challenge. How would you proceed if you were responsible for teaching a male patient with a complete C-6 injury to perform self-catheterization?

CASE STUDY 9.1

Jane is a 21-year-old woman who experienced a T-5 complete SCI as a result of a water skiing accident. Previously an active young single woman, she expresses anxiety about how to manage her bowel and bladder programs. She currently is learning how to perform self-catheterization five times a day, and she does have difficulty with bowel constipation. Her usual blood pressure is 94/60. During therapy she begins to complain of a headache and has redness and sweating of her face and upper chest. The physical therapist calls you to check on her and you note that Jane is complaining of blurred vision, nasal congestion, and a pounding headache.

Questions

1. Using evidence-based practice guidelines, what should be your first action?
2. What is the most likely problem that Jane is having based on the information given?

3. After assessing her blood pressure, the nurse finds it to be 160/96. What does this suggest? What should the nurse do next?
4. What are the most likely causes of this problem? What are other possible causes?

PERSONAL REFLECTION

- Have you helped a patient to establish a bladder or bowel program? What skills are needed to help manage their care?
- How difficult do you think it would be to have a caregiver assist you with emptying your bladder or assist with bowel elimination?
- Have you eve assisted a person in a wheelchair use a wheelchair accessible public restroom? How easy or difficult was it? What barriers were encountered?

RECOMMENDED READINGS

Borrie, M. J., Campbell, K., Arcese, Z. A., Bray, J., Labate, T., & Hesch, P. (2001). Urinary retention in patients in a geriatric rehabilitation unit: Prevalence, risk factors, and validity of bladder scan evaluation. *Rehabilitation Nursing, 26*(5), 187–191.

Burgio, K. L., & Burgio, L. D. (1986). Behavioral therapies for urinary incontinence in the elderly. *Clinics in Geriatric Medicine, 2*(4), 809–827.

Consensus Conference. (1989). Urinary incontinence in adults. *Journal of the American Medical Association, 261*(18), 2685–2690.

Consensus Conference: Urinary Continence Guideline Panel. (1992). Urinary incontinence in adults. AHCPR Publication No. 92-0038. Rockville, MD: U.S. Department of Health and Human Services.

Fantl, J. A., Newman, D. K., Colling, J., et al. (1996). Urinary incontinence in adults: Acute and chronic management. Clinical practice guideline No. 2. AHCPR Publication No. 96-0682. Rockville, MD: U.S. Department of Health Care Policy and Research.

Fonda, D., Benvenuti, F., Cottenden, A., DuBeau, C., Kirshner-Hermanns, R., Miller, K., et al. (2002). Urinary incontinence and bladder dysfunction in older persons. In P. Abrams, L. Cardozo, S. Khoury, & A. Wein (Eds.), *Incontinence: Proceedings from the second international consultation on incontinence*. Plymouth, UK: Health Publication.

Godfrey, H. (2008). Older people, continence and catheters: Dilemmas and resolutions. *British Journal of Nursing, 17*(9), S4–S11.

Godfrey, H., & Hogg, A. (2007). Links between social isolation and incontinence. *British Journal of Nursing, 1*(3), S1–S8

Hajjar, P. R. (2004). Psychosocial impact of urinary incontinence in the elderly population. *Clinical Geriatric Medicine, 20*(3), 553–564

Lekan-Rutledge, D. (2004). Urinary incontinence strategies for frail elderly women. *Urologic Nursing, 24*(4), 281–283, 287–302.

Mueller, N. (2004). What the future holds for incontinence care. *Urologic Nurse, 24*(3), 181–186.

Newman, D. K. (2002). *Managing and treating urinary incontinence.* Baltimore, MD: Health Professions Press

Skoner, M. M. (1994). Self-management of urinary incontinence among women 31 to 50 years. *Rehabilitation Nursing, 19*(6), 339–343.

Tunis, S. R., Norris, A., & Simon, K. (2000). *Medicare coverage policy decisions. Biofeedback for treatment of urinary incontinence* (#CAG - 00020). Washington, DC: Health Care Financing Administration.

Urinary Continence Guideline Panel. (1992). *Urinary incontinence in adults.* AHCPR Publication No. 92-0038. Rockville, MD: U.S. Department of Health and Human Services.

REFERENCES

Abrams, R., Cardozo, L., Fall, M., Derek, F., Rosier, P., Ulmsten, U., et al. (2002). The Standardization of terminology of lower urinary tract function: Report from the standardization sub-committee of the international continence society. *Neurourology and Urodynamics, 21*, 167–178.

Brown, J. S., Vittinghoff, E., Wyman, J. F., Stone, K. L., Nevitt, M. C., Ensrud, K. E., et al. (2000). Urinary incontinence: Does it increase risk for falls and fractures? *Journal of the American Geriatrics Society, 48*, 721–725.

Campagnolo, D. (2009). Autonomic dysreflexia in spinal cord injury. Retrieved August 15, 2010, from http://emedicine.medscape.com/article/322809-overview

Consortium for Spinal Cord Medicine. (1999). *Neurogenic bowel: What you should know.* Clinical Practice Guidelines. Washington, DC: Paralyzed Veterans of America.

Consortium for Spinal Cord Medicine. (2006). *Bladder management for adults with spinal cord injury: A clinical practice guideline for health care providers.* Washington, DC: Paralyzed Veterans of America.

Consortium for Spinal Cord Medicine. (2010). *Bladder management following spinal cord injury: What you should know.* Clinical Practice Guidelines. Washington, DC: Paralyzed Veterans of America.

Dains, J. E., Ciofu Baumann, L., & Scheibel, P. (2003). *Advanced health assessment and clinical diagnosis in primary care* (2nd ed.). St. Louis, MO: Mosby.

Diebold, C., Fanning-Harding, F., & Hanson, P. (2010). Management of common problems. In K. L. Mauk (Ed.), *Gerontological nursing: Competencies for care* (pp. 454–528). Sudbury, MA: Jones and Bartlett Publishers.

Dittmar, S. (1989). *Rehabilitation nursing: Process and application.* St. Louis, MO: C.V. Mosby.

Easton, K. L. (1999). *Gerontological rehabilitation nursing.* Philadelphia: W. B. Saunders.

Folden, S., Backer, J. H., Gilbride, J. A., Maynard, F., Pires, M., Stevens, K., et al. (2002). *Practice guidelines for the management of constipation in adults.* Glenview, IL: Rehabilitation Nursing Foundation.

Gender, A. R. (1996). Bowel regulation and elimination. In S. Hoeman (Ed.), *Rehabilitation nursing: Process and application* (pp. 452–475). St. Louis, MO; Mosby-Year Book.

Gross, J. C. (2003). Urinary Incontinence After Stroke: Evaluation and behavioral treatment. *Topics in Geriatric Rehabilitation, 19*(1), 60–83.

Grinspun, D. (1993). Bladder management for adults following head injury. *Rehabilitation Nursing, 18*, 300–305.

Hus, T. H. S., & Shortliffe, L. D. (2004). Laparoscopic Mitrofanoff appendicovesicostomy. *Urology, 64*(4), 802–804.

Karsenty, G., Reitz, A., Wefer, B., Boy, S., & Schurch, B. (2005). Understanding detrusor sphincter dyssynergia: Significance of chronology. *Journal of Urology, 66*(4), 763–768.

Mauk, K. (Ed.). (2007). *The specialty practice of rehabilitation nursing* (3rd ed.). Glenview, IL: Association of Rehabilitation Nurses.

Mauk, K. (2005). Preventing constipation in older adults. *Nursing 2005, 35*(6), 22–23.

McCance, K. L., & Huether, S. E. (2006). *Pathophysiology: The biologic basis for disease in adults and children* (5th ed.). St. Louis, MO: Elsevier Mosby.

Owen, D. C., Getz, P. A., & Bulla, S. (1995). A comparison of characteristics of patients with completed stroke: Those who achieve continence and those who do not. *Rehabiltiation Nursing, 29*(4), 197–203.

Paralyzed Veterans of America & Consortium for Spinal Cord Medicine. (2001). *Acute management of autonomic dysreflexia: Individuals with spinal cord injury presenting to health-care facilities.* Washington, DC: Paralyzed Veterans of America.

Resnick, N. M. & Yalla, S. V. (1985). Management of Urinary Incontinence in the Elderly. *New England Journal of Medicine, 313*, 800-804.

Resnick, B. (1993). Retraining the bladder after catheterization. *American Journal of Nursing, 93*(11), 46–49.

Smith, D., & Newman, D. (1989). Beating the cycle of constipation, laxative abuse, and fecal incontinence. *Today's Nursing Home, 4*(4), 12–13.

Stevens, K. A. (2008). Urinary elimination and continence. In S. P. Hoeman (Ed.), *Rehabilitation nursing: Prevention, intervention, & outcomes.* (pp. 334–368). St. Louis, MO: Mosby Elsevier.

Venn, M. R., Taft, L., Carpenter, B., & Applebaugh, G. (1992). The influence of timing and suppository use on efficiency and effectiveness of bowel training after a stroke. *Rehabilitation Nursing, 17*(3), 116–120.

CHAPTER 10

Promoting Mobility and Function

Sharleen Koenig
Joseph Teixeira
Elizabeth Yetzer

LEARNING OBJECTIVES

At the end of the chapter, the reader will be able to

- Discuss at least five effects of immobility on the body.
- List three principles of using proper body mechanics.
- List three differences between the different assist levels.
- Describe what specific activities comprise the self-care portion of activities of daily living and what general activities comprise instrumental activities of daily living.
- Describe three ways adaptive equipment can allow clients with physical impairments to perform activities of daily living and instrumental activities of daily living at a higher level.
- Articulate the significance of the safe patient handling movement.

KEY CONCEPTS AND TERMS

Active range of motion	Functional independence	Mechanical lifts
Activities of daily living (ADLs)	measure (FIM)	Mobility
Adaptive equipment	Functional mobility	Passive range of motion
Assistive device	Gait belt	Prior level of function
Berg Balance Scale	Instrumental activities of daily	Safe patient handling
Current level of function	living (IADLs)	Static balance
Dynamic balance	Levels of assist	Transfers
Dynamic gait index	Manual muscle test	

Mobility is the ability to move spontaneously and independently within the environment and to do purposeful activities such as caring for one's self. **Functional mobility** is the ability to move from one position in space to another and includes bed mobility, transfers, ambulation, wheelchair mobility, stairs, and driving (Association of Rehabilitation Nurses & Rehabilitation Nursing Foundation, 2006, p. 20).

The loss of mobility may be through disease, trauma, illness, or inactivity (Cournan, Kautz, & Conrad, 2007). The results of immobility have deleterious effects on all body systems and include muscular atrophy and contractures; orthostatic hypotension and deep vein thrombosis; glucose intolerance and negative nitrogen balance;

pneumonia and atelectasis; dehydration and constipation; urinary tract infections and stones; sensory deprivation, disorientation, and depression; and skin breakdown. Prevention of the effects of immobility is one of the goals of the rehabilitation team.

Physical and occupational therapists help to improve a person's overall mobility, function, and therefore independence as much as possible. Devices are often used to facilitate activities of daily living (ADLs) because many clients must compensate for loss of certain abilities and/or overall function over time.

In this chapter we review tools to assess mobility, goals and interventions to maintain the client's mobility and to prevent the effects of immobility, safe patient handling concepts, fall risk assessment and fall prevention, principles of body mechanics, the use of adaptive equipment and assistive devices, and the nursing diagnoses associated with immobility.

ASSESSMENT

Various tools are used to perform an initial assessment or a reassessment. Therapists document each objective test performed and use these assessments to mark progress and to determine rehabilitation goals.

Functional Scales

The **functional independence measure (FIM)** is commonly used throughout the rehabilitation world as a measurement of disability. The FIM is an 18-item instrument graded on a nominal 1 to 7 scale in terms of how much assistance a person needs regarding tasks ranging from ambulation and tub/shower transfers to communication and bladder management. Levels of function range from "complete independence (rating of 7)" to "total assistance (rating of 1)" (Uniform Data System for Medical Rehabilitation, 1997a, p. 1).

Levels of assist (Table 10.1) refer to the amount of assistance required for the client by a helper. Otherwise stated, it is the amount of effort expended by the person assisting the client. The FIM levels also use these terms, but the FIM goes into much greater detail about the definition of each category and the assist needed. Assist

levels can be used for more narrative descriptions and for those who are not fully aware of the FIM.

Another functional scale is the WeeFIM (Uniform Data System for Medical Rehabilitation, 1997b). This scale has been adapted for pediatric populations (Counan et al., 2007).

Physical Indicators

Physical therapists assess a person's range of motion, muscle strength, balance, coordination, and endurance as part of the initial evaluation. These indicators should continue to be reassessed throughout the course of therapy to look for marks of progress. **Active range of motion** refers to the extent of movement within a given joint that the person can perform solely on his or her own. How far a person can, for example, raise his or her own arm overhead gives the therapist an idea of the client's active range of motion. A person may be limited in his or her active range of motion because of muscle/joint tightness, pain, and/or muscle weakness. **Passive range of motion**, conversely, consists of the therapist moving a joint while the client is relaxed.

A **manual muscle test** is used to isolate each muscle group to check the strength of a muscle. Manual muscle tests are graded on a scale of 0 to 5, ranging in the ability to lift the muscle against the pull of gravity or hold against maximal resistance (Table 10.2).

Gait is also evaluated, if applicable, during the initial assessment. Inquiring about a person's **prior level of**

TABLE 10.1	**Levels of Assist**
Level	Explanation
Total assist	Client performs 0–25% of task; client may require the help of more than one person; also referred to as a dependent transfer.
Maximum assist	Client gives 25% of the effort while the helper performs majority of the work.
Moderate assist	Client gives 50% of the effort; about equal effort of the client and the helper.
Minimal assist	Client gives 75% of effort.
Contact guard assist	No physical assistance is needed; however, helper is physically touching the client for steadying or guiding purposes, or in case client loses balance.
Stand by assist	Helper is standing near the client with hands up and ready in case physical assistance becomes needed.
Supervision	Verbal instruction may be required; safety concerns are still present, so supervision of the task, even at a distant, is needed.
Modified independent	Client requires an assistive device or extra time to complete a task.
Independent	Client able to perform task safely, without any instruction or assistance.

Source: From Uniform Data System for Medical Rehabilitation (1997a).

TABLE 10.2		Manual Muscle Test
Rating		**Explanation/finding**
5	Normal	Maximum resistance, unable to "break" the client from test position
4+		Moderate to strong resistance
4	Good	Moderate resistance
4–		Less than moderate resistance
3+		Minimal resistance: "two-finger" pressure
3		Holds test position against gravity but unable to tolerate any additional pressure
3–	Fair	Incomplete ROM against gravity
2+		Moves through 50% or less of ROM against gravity, or holds against resistance in gravity-eliminated position
2	Poor	Full ROM in gravity-eliminated position
2–		Incomplete ROM in gravity-eliminated position
1	Trace	Palpable or observable muscle contraction, muscle twitch
0	Zero	No contraction

ROM, range of motion.

Source: From O'Sullivan (2001).

function in terms of ambulation ability can lead to more realistic goals to work on in therapy. Depending on the client's **current level of function**, a client can be assessed for gait for the first time in the parallel bars or by using a front-wheel walker and progressed accordingly.

Transfer ability is another significant component of the assessment. **Transfers** refer to the ability to move one's body from one position in space to another. Transfers include going from the wheelchair to the bed, toilet, or tub bench. Transfers can also be a walking transfer. The ability to walk, turn around, and sit onto a chair is called a chair transfer.

Balance can be determined by either direct observation or through special tests during the assessment process. With the client seated on the bed, does he or she lean off to one side or is he or she able to sit unsupported safely? **Dynamic balance**, as opposed to **static balance** (balance while being still), refers to the ability to maintain balance with movement or perturbations. For example, to assess dynamic sitting balance one can assess if assistance is needed to maintain balance while donning a shirt or during a manual muscle test. Or, a therapist can simply apply resistance to a person's chest, shoulder, and back and see if the person can maintain sitting balance. Standing balance is assessed in a similar way.

Standardized balance tests are used to test more specific elements of balance. The **Berg Balance Scale** and **Dynamic Gait Index** are examples of these tests that act as a predictor of falls in the elderly. These tests assess and score different facets of balance such as weight shifting, reaching, transferring from one chair to another, and stepping over obstacles (discussed in the section Falls: Risk Assessment and Prevention).

Coordination is also assessed, especially in those with neurological insults such as stroke. Finger-to-nose and heel-to-shin tests are commonly used to assess for any over/undershooting and/or slow, clumsy movements. The ability to tap one's foot rapidly on the floor or supinate/pronate hands on one's lap is another way to assess for any neurological dysfunction.

Socioeconomic and Perceptual Factors

A commonly asked question on any initial evaluation is about the client's living situation and social support. Whether a person lives alone in a two-story home or with a supportive family in a single-story home can make significant difference in terms of goal setting and discharge planning.

FALLS: RISK ASSESSMENT AND PREVENTION

Falls in the rehabilitation setting result from many factors. Clients may have a knowledge deficit related to the use of equipment, the effects of their disease processes, the side effects of medications, or safety techniques. They often have impaired mobility and are not able to do activities as before. There may be cognitive impairments, so they are unable to judge safety needs and to prevent injury. Sensory deficits such as seen with stroke or brain injury affect proprioception so clients may be unable to recognize where the body is in space. Impairments with vision, hearing, and speech reduce their ability to see safety hazards, hear or understand safety instructions, or to ask for help. There are environmental factors related to being in a strange place. Unmet elimination needs or urinary incontinence may cause the client to attempt to walk to the bathroom without assistance. Fatigue from therapy may influence their judgment in ambulating safely (Dale, 2007). In addition, two medications are associated with higher fall incidence in older adults: benzodiazepines and antiepileptic drugs (Gray-Micelli, 2007). See Box 10.1.

When the client is admitted to the rehabilitation unit, a fall risk assessment should be performed. The safety assessment should include age, mobility, sensation, cogni-

BOX 10.1   **Web Exploration**
Check out the Nursing Standard of Practice Protocol for Falls at http://consultgerirn.org/topics/falls/want_to_know_more

tive and language abilities, perceptual abilities, emotional status, medications for interactions and side effects, and history of falls and injuries. Gray-Micelli (2008) adds to this safety assessment the factors of functional disabilities and use of assistive devices, gait and balance, and comorbidities such as dementia, hip fracture, diabetes, Parkinson's, arthritis, and depression.

If the client falls while on the rehabilitation unit, a postfall assessment should be completed as soon as any significant injury is ruled out. Gray-Micelli, (2008) identifies the following as part of the postfall assessment: patient or witness description of the fall; circumstances of the fall such as location, time of day, activity, and significant symptoms; review of underlying illness and medications; assessment of functional, sensory, and psychological status; environmental conditions; and risk factors for falling. The admission assessment and the postfall assessment must be documented according to facility policies.

Assessment of fall risk is an essential component in physical therapy and nursing (Table 10.3). As mentioned earlier, there are various tests to assess a person's balance and mobility. The Berg Balance Scale is one of the most popular tests that grade function and mobility tasks on a four-point scale. Assistive devices such as walkers and canes are not allowed. There is a maximum score of 56, and anything less than 46 points means the person tested is a fall risk. Examples of items assessed include ability to stand unsupported, transfer from one chair to another, picking up an object off the floor, and standing on one leg (O'Sullivan, 2001).

The Dynamic Gait Index is a test that acts as a predictor for falls. It assesses a person's ability to walk with changing task demands, such as walking while turning the head horizontally, stepping over obstacles, and going up and down stairs. A score of less than 19 (out of a possible 24) means that a person is at risk for falls. This test is usually performed for patients already walking on their own, and an assistive device may be used (O'Sullivan, 2001).

Prevention of Falls

Prevention of falls is an important component of rehabilitation. Preventative measures are discussed in the

TABLE 10.3   **Risk Factors for Falls in Rehabilitation**
Advanced age
Diagnosis of stroke or brain injury, especially with left weakness/right brain damage (due to impulsivity and lack of safety awareness)
Impaired physical abilities (such as poor balance, abnormal gait, hemiplegia)
Altered mental state (such as delirium, dementia, dizziness, sleep disorders, psychiatric diagnoses)
Altered elimination patterns (such as incontinence, urgency, frequency, nocturia)
Cognitive/sensory impairments (such as impaired memory, poor judgment, visual or hearing impairment, aphasia, neglect)
Altered proprioception
Medications that affect fluid balance or sensorium (such as diuretics, narcotics, sedatives, antidepressants, benzodiazepines, and antiepileptics)
History of drug or alcohol abuse
Other psychological factors (such as denying fall history, hesitation to ask for assistance)

next section. Using gait belts and advanced planning are key to preventing falls. Table 10.4 lists ways to promote a safe environment, whether in rehabilitation or the client's home. Clients and family members should be taught these principles before discharge.

> *Monitor the effects of medications that could cause dizziness or poor balance, especially benzodiazepines and antiepileptics in older adults.*

Communication, proper documentation, and team work are vital in the prevention of falls. A disconnect can occur and potential progress is inhibited when nursing staff do not know of what a client is functionally capable. For example, if a client is able to get out of bed with supervision in therapy but the nursing staff automatically assists the client out of bed, the staff is not allowing the client to become as independent as possible. Written and verbal communication especially needs to take place if a client has any cognitive deficits and poor safety awareness or judgment. If a client is unsafe using a walker yet the client has his or her personal walker in his room, this must be communicated to the rest of the staff.

Prevention of falls includes the facility protocols for a falls prevention program. A multidisciplinary plan of care to prevent falls should be developed and communicated. The staff should have written procedures describing

TABLE 10.4	Safety/Fall Prevention Strategies

Install hand rails in the bathroom and along stairs. Mark stairs with brightly colored tape if needed.

Arrange the bedroom and kitchen so that the person can reach commonly used household items.

Remove all throw rugs or uneven flooring.

Use two knobs in the shower for singular hot and cold to better control extremes in temperature.

Install lower tubs or tubs with a side door for safer transfer.

Obtain adaptive equipment to facilitate ADLs (such as shower chairs, rolling commodes, tub benches, reachers, walkers, etc.).

Arrange furniture to avoid clutter of walkways.

At home, be careful of small animals and children, who can accidentally cause a person to lose balance.

Monitor the effects of medications that could cause dizziness or poor balance, especially benzodiazepines and antiepileptics in older adults.

Use nonskid, appropriate footwear.

Lock wheelchair, bed, commode, and shower brakes before transfers.

Be sure clothing is hemmed well above the shoes.

Ensure that sufficient light is available at night to light paths to the bathroom.

Be sure that position changes occur slowly, especially lying to sitting or rising to avoid/minimize orthostatic hypotension.

Place needed items near the bedside.

Have a call system on the unit and one at home as needed (such as a bell or whistle).

Consider the installation and use of a system such as the Lifeline, especially for those living alone.

Keep emergency numbers close to the phone.

Lower medicine cabinets to wheelchair level (if needed).

Use nonslip mats in shower or tub.

actions when a client falls. The incidence of falls and of client injury should be monitored. Continuous quality improvement criteria should be incorporated into the falls prevention program. The Joint Commission (2009) lists National Patient Safety Goal 9 as reducing the risk of harm resulting from falls. Elements of performance for this goal include assessment of the client's risk for falls, implementation of interventions to reduce falls, education of staff and client on fall reduction strategies, and the evaluation of the effectiveness of fall reduction activities. The outcome indicators are to decrease number of falls and decrease the number and severity of fall-related injuries.

TABLE 10.5	Example of Client Goals for Physical Therapy	
Goal-setting	**Example**
Prior level of function	Pt. was modified independently using a single-point cane for both household and community ambulation.
Current level of function	Pt. requires minimal assistance with ambulation 100 feet using a front-wheel walker.
Short-term goal in 2 weeks	Pt. will be modified independently with ambulation using a front-wheel walker for 150 feet.
Long-term goal in 1 month	Pt. will be modified independently using a single-point cane for 300 feet.

GOALS

Rehabilitation is a form of treatment that keeps client goals in mind. Reimbursement from insurance companies will not occur if goals are not accurately written and met. Short- and long-term goals are made after first assessing the client (Table 10.5). Therapy is not performed merely for maintenance but rather for progress. Again, insurance companies will not pay to keep a patient in the hospital or on rehabilitation services if documentation does not reveal that a person is benefiting from therapy. The most ideal goal is to return the patient back to his or her prior level of function, although that may not always be possible. Figure 10.1 provides a simplified example of a client going through physical therapy, with associated goals.

INTERVENTIONS

Principles of Body Mechanics

Using proper body mechanics is vital for both the protection of one's self and for the protection of the client. Not only will it reduce one's risk for serious injury to the lower back or shoulder, for example, but it allows nurses and therapists to be most efficient by having the mechanical advantage when attempting to transfer a patient. Protection of oneself leads to the protection of others, while maximizing the caregiver's ability to continue helping clients for years to come.

Three principles of body mechanics are as follows (O'Sullivan 2007):

1. Pushing is safer than pulling. Pushing allows you to use your legs, chest, and arm muscles, but pulling only leaves your low back acting as the fulcrum, leading to serious injury.

DATE OF ADMISSION: 3/12/2010

DATE OF EVALUATION: 3/14/2010

DIAGNOSIS: Deconditioning

PERTINENT HISTORY/PRECAUTIONS: 83-year-old male, admitted for urinary tract infection, now with resulting impairments in mobility.

PMH includes: PVD, CAD, diabetes, HTN, hyperlipidemia, left TKR in 1999

SUBJECTIVE: Pt. reports "feeling real weak. I can't walk. I've been in bed way too long." Pt. has no current complaints of pain. He reports having one fall in the last year. He states his mobility began to decline a few weeks ago until he finally got admitted a couple days ago.

Social history: Pt. lives with family in two-story home with 3 steps to enter with unilateral rail; tub shower

Prior level of function: Pt. was a community ambulatory using a rollator walker; independent with all ADLs

Current level of function: Pt. wheelchair-bound and dependent with all ADLs

OBJECTIVE

Strength (MMT):

Bilateral Upper Extremity: gross 4/5

Bilateral Lower Extremity: gross 4–/5 except, left quads 3–/5

Range of Motion:

UEs: WFL

LEs: WFL except for L quads secondary to strength deficits

Functional Assessment:

Bed mobility:

Rolling: modified independent using bedrail

Supine-to-sit: minimal assist using bedrail

Transfers:

Wheelchair ßàbed: moderate assist (modA) squat pivot transfer

Sit-to-stand: modA using FWW

Locomotion:

Ambulation: modA using FWW 50 ft.

Balance (static/dynamic):

Sitting: Good/Fair

Standing: Poor/Poor

General Cognitive and Communication: alert and oriented x 3

ASSESSMENT AND GOALS:

Patient very motivated to start therapy and get stronger.

Short-term goals in 1 week:

1. Patient will be able to perform supine-to-sit with minA without bedrail.

2. Patient will be able to transfer from wheelchair to bed with minA squat pivot.

3. Patient will be able to ambulate with a minA using FWW 100 ft.

Long-term goals in 2 weeks:

1. Pt. will be independent with supine-to-sit without bedrail.

2. Patient will be able to perform a walking transfer to the bed with supervision using a FWW.

3. Patient will be able to ambulate 150 ft. with supervision using FWW.

PLAN: lower extremity strengthening, bed mobility training, gait, transfer, and balance training, family/caregiver training as needed; discharge patient home with family at a supervised level in two weeks

FWW, front wheeled walker; WFL, within functional limits; modA, moderate assistance; minA, minimum assistance; PMH, past medical history; PVD, peripheral vascular disease; CAD, coronary artery disease; HTN, hypertension; TKR, total knee replacement, MMT, manual muscle testing; UE, upper extremity; LE, lower extremity

FIGURE 10.1   Example of physical therapy evaluation.

2. Keep the load close. Whether you are attempting to lift an object or a person or providing passive range of motion exercises, the activity needs to be performed as close to your own body as possible. Avoid reaching and extending your arms out, especially if any type of weight is involved.

3. No bending and twisting, or reaching and twisting. Both bending and twisting motions make for poor body mechanics. The coupled motions of bending and reaching *while* twisting is all the more harmful, with possible risk of straining muscles, wearing down the vertebral joints, increasing pressure in the vertebral discs, and even breaking down of the ligaments in the spine.

Bracing your abdominal muscles before any activity can serve to protect your back. Therapists and nurses should keep a wide base of support, using their legs to do the lifting rather than their back and arms. Think of maintaining a long spine from the base of your skull to the tailbone.

An example of transferring a patient from the bed to the wheelchair can involve the following. Once the patient is seated at the edge of the bed, take a low stance with feet wider than hip width. Knees are bent into a squat position with trunk upright, spine straight. Brace the abdominals *before* assisting the client to stand up. To avoid twisting when assisting the client to sit down into the chair, think about moving *with* the patient by pivoting your feet and squaring yourself up to the patient and the chair. Lower the client into the chair by bending your legs as the client bends his or her knees in order to sit.

Using a Gait Belt

Gait belts are plastic or cloth straps that wrap around the patient to promote safety if the patient were to lose his or her balance. The gait belt is positioned around the patient's waist, closest to his or her center of gravity. This is around the belt line, not under the arms. For women, be certain the belt is placed under the breasts, close to the waist. Gait belts are used to help guide transfers and promote safety during ambulation. They are considered a safety device. A therapist or nursing staff can potentially injure (e.g., subluxation or dislocate) a client's shoulder by grabbing, lifting, or pulling under the client's arm to move him or her. Failure to use a gait belt or transfer belt can result in patient falls, injury, and subsequent lawsuits (see Case 10.1).

Gait belts are also commonly used for assist during transfers because the belts provide a handle to help

---

CASE STUDY 10.1

Mrs. Smith is a 76-year-old patient in acute rehabilitation for functional debility that resulted from a long hospital stay for pneumonia and other medical complications. One evening Mrs. Smith used her call light and expressed an urgent desire to use the bathroom. The nursing assistant, wishing to assist the patient quickly to the toilet, did not apply the gait belt as was the unit protocol and appropriate measure chose by the rehabilitation team. After ambulating a few steps, Mrs. Smith suddenly fell forward, apparently fainting. The patient's gown the nursing assistant was holding onto tore and Mrs. Smith fell, sustaining a concussion and a serious laceration to her forehead that required sutures. Because the assistant had not applied the gait belt, she had no way to assist the patient safely to the floor or otherwise prevent injury during a fall. Mrs. Smith suffered unnecessary injuries and emotional distress, and the hospital and nursing assistant were open to liability for the accident.

Questions

1. How could this accident have been prevented?
2. What should the nursing assistant have done?
3. Why couldn't the nursing assistant determine whether or not to use the gait belt in that situation?
4. How would you have handled this same situation?

---

move a client. Gait belts should be used whenever staff members are working with a client for the first time, up until the patient proves to be safe and independent and is no longer in need of a gait belt.

Basic Types of Transfers

There are various types of transfers. For example, patients may transfer from wheelchair to bed using lateral scoot (with or without sliding board), squat pivot, stand pivot, or a walking transfer:

1. A lateral scoot transfer involves a person scooting sideways on his or her bottom by barely lifting the pelvis off the sitting surface.
2. A squat pivot involves a transfer in which the person does not come all the way into full standing and just pivots his or her feet in order to sit on another chair, toilet, or bed. This may also be called a modified stand-pivot transfer.

3. A stand pivot involves a person standing all the way up and then adjusting the feet before sitting back down.

4. A sliding board is used for a person to laterally scoot, because it acts as a bridge from one sitting surface to another. A person may use a sliding board if he or she requires a maximum assist to transfer or can transfer on his or her own but does not have the leg strength to stand up to transfer. Persons with amputation often use sliding boards or similar bridge devices to transfer from one surface to another.

5. A walking transfer is simply a transfer performed while walking, versus, for example, from a wheelchair level. A walking transfer can be performed while using an assistive device such as a front-wheel walker or without such a device. A walking transfer assesses the ability for the client to safely walk to the destination, turn around, and sit safely onto the new sitting surface.

The physical therapist assists patients/clients to learn what type of transfer is most appropriate and safest based on a variety of factors such as those mentioned above during the initial assessment. The patient's ability to transfer may improve with rehabilitation, so he or she may use different transfers throughout his recovery. The therapist and rehabilitation nurse work with the patient and family to learn the most appropriate way to safely transfer.

SAFE PATIENT HANDLING

The incidence of injuries to professionals that is associated with patient handling in rehabilitation is high. Nursing is consistently ranked as one of the top 10 professions experiencing work-related musculoskeletal injury (Nelson, 2005). "Patient handling and movement tasks are physically demanding, performed under unfavorable conditions, and are often unpredictable in nature. Patients offer multiple challenges including variations in size, physical disabilities, cognitive function, level of cooperation, and fluctuations in condition" (Nelson & Baptiste, 2004, p. 3).

Although team members may not agree on a **safe patient handling** protocol, particularly a "no lift" policy, there are benefits of safe patient handling. These include decreased injury to workers, increased safety and comfort for patients, decreased chance for litigation related to injuries, decreased lost work and wages due to injury, and decreased workers' compensation claims (Nelson, Harwood, Tracey, & Dunn, 2008). Team members are encouraged to discuss current research and evidence-based practice guidelines to establish mutually acceptable policies for patient handling.

Mechanical Lifts

Mechanical lifts are used for clients who are too dependent or heavy to safely transfer manually. Lifts use a sling and harness to lift the client off of the bed or wheelchair, either by a hand crank (manual Hoyer lift) or hydraulics (mechanical) using a button. Lifts are also useful because it only takes one person to transfer a person rather than a whole team of nurses. Although research studies have shown mixed results when studying the use and benefits of technology, mobile mechanical lift devices have been shown to decrease worker injury (Nelson & Baptiste, 2004).

Safe Lift Protocols

Both client and staff safety are important when assisting the client with ADLs and with transfers and ambulation. Using safe lift protocols reduces the incidence of injuries to clients and to staff (Association of Rehabilitation Nurses & Rehabilitation Nursing Foundation, 2006). See Box 10.2. In 2005 the Association of Rehabilitation Nurses, American Physical Therapy Association, and the Veterans Health Administration published a white paper with "the mutual goals of improving safety of patients during handling and movement tasks; safety of care providers during patient handling and movement tasks; and communication between interdisciplinary team members regarding safe patient handling" (Nelson, Tracey, Baxter, Nathenson, Rosario, Rockefeller, & Joffe et al, 2004, p. 80). The work of this committee was incorporated by the Association of Rehabilitation Nurses (2008) into a five-part safe patient handling tool kit that includes the business case for safe patient handling, how to conduct a risk assessment, myths and facts about safe patient handling in rehabilitation, selection of equipment, and therapeutic use of safe patient-handling equipment.

Safe patient handling training for schools of nursing curricular materials was developed by the National Institute for Occupational Safety and Health, Veterans Health Administration, and American Nurses Association (Wa-

BOX 10.2	Web Exploration

Explore the Association of Rehabilitation Nurses Competencies Assessment Tool on Safe Patient Handling at www.rehabnurse.org. See how many questions you can answer correctly.

ters, Nelson, Hughes, & Menzel, 2009). The curricular materials provide evidence-based training information for students and instructors, algorithms for safe handling in moving both regular weight and bariatric patients, and an assessment criteria and care plan for safe patient handling. The goal of the program is to assist students to apply content in a clinical setting. A Web-based training program is also available from www.cdc.gov.

Promoting Ambulation

The communication between the client, the therapist, and the nursing staff is paramount in promoting safe ambulation. The basic techniques of ambulation and safety precautions are taught by therapists. The progress of the client in ambulating and using assistive devices needs to be communicated to the nursing staff. The nursing staff should be involved in monitoring that the client uses safe techniques and the correct use of any assistive devices when not in therapy. All staff should be aware that changes in the client's medical condition, effects of medications, and fatigue will affect the client's ability to safely ambulate.

As the name states, **assistive devices** are devices that assist a person in the ability to walk or perform other ADLs. Examples of these are front-wheel walker, pick-up walker, hemi-walker, large-based quad cane, small-based quad cane, single-point cane, axillary crutch, Lofstrand (also known as forearm) crutches, and rollator walker. The therapist evaluates clients and instructs them in the safe use of assistive devices.

Oxygen Therapy

Physical therapists treat many patients that have to rely on oxygen. A pulse oximeter is often used during therapy sessions to make sure the patient is receiving enough oxygen, especially before, during, and after exercise or walking. Breathing techniques, such as pursed-lip breathing, and cues, such as "slowly breathe in through the nose, and out through the mouth" or "smell the roses, blow out the candles," are used to facilitate greater oxygen consumption and to reduce shortness of breath. The nurse should be notified if a patient's oxygen saturation falls below 90%.

Adaptive Equipment

At some point a healthcare provider may discover, either through a client's report, a formal evaluation, or treatment, that a client does not have adequate physical ability to perform certain important **activities of daily living (ADLs)** such as feeding, grooming, bathing, upper and lower extremity dressing, and toileting, also known as self-care. This lack of ability may be temporary or permanent, but in many cases adaptive equipment can be used to improve the client's ability to engage in their ADLs, as well as performing employment duties and the more complex **instrumental activities of daily living (IADLs)**, which include activities that may be more cognitively challenging or require more mobility, such as writing checks, shopping, housekeeping, and many other purposeful life tasks.

Adaptive equipment is designed to help compensate for a client's limitations in strength, range of motion, mobility, dexterity, speech, and other skills most of us take for granted. If a client cannot reach far enough, there is equipment that extends that reach. If a client does not have a strong or steady grasp, there is equipment that makes that grasp more secure. If a client's vision is poor, there is equipment to improve sight or make what they are looking at easier to see. If a client lacks the dexterity to manipulate small items, such as pens, pencils, nail clippers, buttons, or keys, there is relatively simple equipment that is designed to take the place of the hand and/or fingers.

Other examples of adaptive equipment include grab bars, Versaframes (a frame that mimics arm rests of a chair but is attached to a toilet), tub benches and shower chairs, and assistive devices. If a client in unable to move any part of his or her body below the neck, there is equipment that allows the client to control his or her environment, such as lights, phone, television, computer, and doors, through speech, head movements, or even blinking.

The price and complexity of adaptive equipment varies significantly. When a client's hands are impaired by conditions such as arthritis, burns, or spinal cord injury, a simple button hook or zipper pull, sometimes made up of nothing more than a handle and a curved piece of wire and costing as little as 5 or 6 dollars, can be irreplaceable in allowing a client to independently put on a shirt or jacket. Also, a client whose hands shake or are weak may find it difficult or impossible to write checks to pay bills, hold the tools used to maintain a garden, perform other IADLs, or even their employment duties. But adaptive writing aids, built up or weighted handles, and other devices or modifications can provide a very inexpensive solution to the problem. However, an environmental control unit, which helps weakened or paralyzed clients control many different household devices, such as doors, lights, televisions, adjustable beds, and the phone to contact caregivers and emergency response, may cost thousands of dollars.

The general public is usually unaware of the type of adaptive equipment available or even that such equipment exists. An experienced occupational therapist can be helpful in determining what adaptive equipment is needed. There is not only different equipment to perform a wide range of different tasks, but there are sometimes many different choices of adaptive equipment, even very different sizes, designs, prices, that do the same things. An experienced therapist should be familiar with general types of adaptive equipment for many different problems but should also know about different types of the same equipment so the client gets the most and easiest use from the equipment. Also, because a piece of adaptive equipment, like any tool, usually requires some amount of training to use effectively and safely, an experienced therapist can provide that service.

Use of Safety Devices

Safety devices are used to protect patients from harm and may be used proactively as in the case of quick-release belts (for those who get up without assistance and are a high risk for falls), low beds and floor mats for those who roll out of bed, or various types of alarms. Restraints should be used only when the client is a danger to him- or herself or to others (Mauk & Lehman, 2007) and then at the least restrictive level possible, with proper documentation and frequent reevaluation. Aside from active physical restraints such as wrist and ankle straps, mittens, and pillows, there are also passive restraints that can be used. These include bed or chair alarms that activate when a client gets off the bed or wheelchair. Bed rails also act as a restraint. Hand splints such as those made or ordered by an occupational therapist secondarily act as restraints because they restrict motion.

Physical restraints must have appropriate doctor's orders. There are several reasons for a person to be put into restraints: if the person is a fall risk with extremely combative or agitated behaviors that pose a danger to himself or others, or to prevent pulling out lines such as nasogastric tube or tracheostomy tube. From an ethical viewpoint one cannot take away another's freedom to move unless he or she is a danger to oneself or to others. Regulations for residents in long-term care facilities are more strict, requiring limits on the physical and chemical restraints. The staff should know the restraint policy of their facility.

REHABILITATION NURSE'S ROLE

The rehabilitation nurse is a member of the rehabilitation team that works with the client and family. The nurse's role includes, but is not limited to, the following:

- Assessing the client, perhaps before the client is admitted to the rehabilitation unit, and frequently reevaluating the client's progress toward the rehabilitation goals.
- Preventing complications such as skin breakdown, contractures, infections, and falls, which would delay the client's progress.
- Reinforcing the knowledge and skills the client and family are taught by the rehabilitation team.
- Assisting the client and family with meeting their psychosocial needs and developing coping skills.
- Participating as a member of the rehabilitation team in assessing client's needs, developing a plan of care (goals) with the client and family, assisting the client and family to meet the goals, evaluating the client's progress, and revising the plan of care as the client's needs, knowledge, and skills change. See Box 10.3.

BOX 10.3   Web Exploration

Association of Rehabilitation Nurses Competencies Assessment Tool (CAT), Safe Patient Handling www.rehabnurses.org

Berg Balance Scale www.fallssa.com.au/documents/hp/ Berg_Balance_Scale.pdf www.aahf.info/pdf/Berg_Balance_Scale.pdf

Dynamic Gait Index web.missouri.edu/~proste/tool/ Danamic_Gait_Index.rtf

Introduction to Manual Muscle Testing, created by Occupational Therapy Students, University of New England youtube.com/watch?v=RyEK_QBSemQ

Manual Muscle Testing Procedures (2007) http://wwwniehs.nih.gov/research/resources/callab/ imacs/docs/act

National Guidelines Clearing House http://www.guideline .gov

Safe Patient Handling Tool Kit (2008). Association of Rehabilitation Nurses www.rehabnurses.org http://www.ohcow.on.ca/resources/handbooks/ patient_handling/patient_handling.htm

NURSING DIAGNOSIS, OUTCOMES, AND INTERVENTIONS

There are several nursing diagnoses related to mobility, immobility, and risk for falls. These include knowledge deficit, impaired physical mobility, activity intolerance, and risk for falls or injury.

Knowledge deficit is the absence of information or skills for management of disability, absence of skills for using assistive devices, or lack of knowledge of safety techniques. A primary outcome when addressing knowledge deficits is that the client and family can use the information and skills taught by nursing and therapist to improve mobility. Interventions include the following:

- Assess client's level of mobility using standardized measures.
- Set mutual goals and evaluate progress.
- Reinforce teaching in the use of adaptive equipment and techniques.

Impaired physical mobility is the inability of the client to move within the environment. Expected outcomes are prevention of the hazards of immobility and that the client will incorporate prevention measures into daily self-care activities. Nursing interventions include the following:

- Use of activities to prevent skin breakdown as turning, pressure relief.
- Develop bowel and incontinence programs if necessary.
- Provide adequate fluid intake.
- Assess for signs of venous thrombus.
- Educate on prevention of postural hypotension.
- Encourage social interactions.
- Encourage deep breathing and coughing to clear bronchial secretions.
- Provide or supervise range of motion exercises (Cournan et al., 2007).

Activity intolerance occurs when there is a lack of strength and endurance to carry out ADLs. The nurse writes desired outcomes, such as "the client will pace self to do ADLs" or "the client will use energy conservation techniques and adaptive equipment to adapt the environment to meet needs." Nursing interventions for activity intolerance are as follows:

- Assist client in learning techniques for energy conservation.

- Encourage use of rest periods between periods of activity.
- Encourage use of adaptive devices for ADLs and ambulation.
- Build exercise endurance by increasing activity in small increments over time.

Risk of falls or injuries is due to changes in mobility and balance. Rehabilitation nurses express outcomes such as "the client will use knowledge and skills to prevent falls and identify the risk of falls." Interventions are as follows:

- Teach evaluation of situation for environmental hazards.
- Encourage use of adaptive equipment for safe ambulation.
- Reinforce safety instruction for transfer techniques, gait training, and use of mobility devices.
- Assist the family to evaluate situations at home and in the community for safety problems and determine actions to prevent accidents (Dale, 2007).

SUMMARY

This chapter reviewed tools that can be used to assess the client's mobility. Goals, interventions, and techniques to prevent the effects of immobility were discussed. Principles of body mechanics to prevent injury to staff and clients include those set forth in the new safe patient handling movement that is sweeping the country. Resources for fall risk assessment and prevention and safe patient handling should be incorporated in rehabilitation nursing practice. Increased communication between staff members may be needed to come to a consensus on safe patient handling in rehabilitation. The role of the rehabilitation nurse in mobility for the client with immobility issues is essential.

CRITICAL THINKING

1. Name at least five effects of immobility on the body systems.
2. What are five nursing interventions to prevent the effects of immobility? Which of these would be most useful in the following clients: those with stroke, brain injury, multiple trauma, spinal cord injury?
3. Discuss the protocol for identifying and reporting client falls at your facility. Share this with a peer.

4. Describe activities that comprise activities of daily living and instrumental activities of daily living. Which of these would be most affected for a person with multiple sclerosis or Parkinson's disease?

5. Using the information about the client from Figure 10.1, develop a nursing care plan for the client.

PERSONAL REFLECTION

- Look around where you are sitting right now. What safety hazards to you see for the average, able-bodied person? What safety hazards do you see for persons with an altered gait? Using a wheelchair? A cane or walker? How would a change in the environment make it safer for a person with a disability?

- Evaluate the place where you work or go to school. What are the strengths and weaknesses related to safety in that environment? How would you need to change the surroundings to accommodate those with various disabilities?

- If you suddenly lost the ability to walk, what would be the your most significant goals, both long term and short term? How would you achieve them? What role would therapy play in that plan?

REFERENCES

Association of Rehabilitation Nurses. (2008). Safe patient handling tool kit. Retrieved September 10, 2010, from www.rehabnurse.org

Association of Rehabilitation Nurses & Rehabilitation Nursing Foundation. (2006). *Evidence-based rehabilitation nursing: Common challenges and interventions.* Glenview, IL: Author.

Cournan, M., Kautz, D., & Conrad, B. (2007). Physical healthcare patterns and nursing interventions. In K. Mauk (Ed.), *The specialty practice of rehabilitation nursing: A core curriculum* (5th ed., pp. 109–115). Glenview, IL: Association of Rehabilitation Nurses.

Dale, K. (2007). Health maintenance and management of therapeutic regimens. In K. Mauk (Ed.), *The specialty practice of rehabilitation nursing: A core curriculum* (5th ed., pp. 73–78). Glenview, IL: Association of Rehabilitation Nurses.

Gray-Micelli, D. (2007). *Fall risk assessment for older adults: The Hendricks Fall Risk II model.* New York: Hartford Foundation for Geriatric Nursing.

Gray-Micelli, D. (2008). Preventing falls in acute care. In E. Capezuti, D. Zwicker, M. Mezey, & T. Fulmer (Eds.), *Evidence-based geriatric nursing protocols for best practice* (3rd ed., pp. 161–198). New York: Springer.

Joint Commission on Accreditation of Healthcare Organizations. (2009). *2010 National Patient Safety Goals, 29*(10), 30. Retrieved September 10, 2010, from www.jointcommission.org

Mauk, K., & Lehman, C. (2007). Gerontological rehabilitation nursing. In K. Mauk (Ed.), *The specialty practice of rehabilitation nursing: A core curriculum* (pp. 365–382). Glenview, IL: Association of Rehabilitation Nurses.

Nelson, A. (2005). Strategies to improve patient and healthcare provider safety in patient handling and movement tasks. *Rehabilitation Nursing Journal, 30*(3), 80–83.

Nelson, A., Harwood, K. J., Tracey, C. A., & Dunn, K. L. (2008). Myths and facts about safe patient handling in rehabilitation. *Rehabilitation Nursing, 33*(1), 10–17.

Nelson, A. L., & Baptiste, A. (2004). Evidence based practices for safe patient handling and movement. *Online Journal of Issues in Nursing, 19*(3), 3. Retrieved September 10, 2010, from www.nursingworld.org/ojin/topic25/tpc25)3htm.

Nelson, A., Tracey, C. A., Baxter, M. L., Nathenson, P., Rosario, M., Rockefeller, K, et al. (2004). Improving patient and health care provider safety. Retrieved September 10, 2010, from http://www.apta.org

O'Sullivan, S. (2001). Assessment of motor function. In S. O'Sullivan & T. Schmitz (Ed.), *Physical rehabilitation assessment and treatment* (4th ed., pp. 196–197). Philadelphia: F.A. Davis.

O'Sullivan, S., & Siegelman R. (2007). Musculoskeletal physical therapy. In S. O'Sullivan & T. Siegelman (Eds.), *National physical therapy examination review & study guide* (pp. 66–67). Evanston, IL: International Educational Resources.

Uniform Data System for Medical Rehabilitation. (1997a). *Functional independence measure.* Buffalo, NY: University of Buffalo.

Uniform Data System for Medical Rehabilitation. (1997b). *Functional independence measure for Children.* Buffalo, NY: University of Buffalo.

Waters, T., Nelson, A., Hughes, N., & Menzel, N. (2009). Safe patient handling training for schools of nursing. Retrieved September 10, 2010, from www.cdc.gov/niosh/docs/2009-127

White, J. D. (2001). Musculoskeletal assessment. In S. O'Sullivan and & T. Schmitz (Eds.), *Physical rehabilitation, assessment and treatment* (pp. 120–144). Philadelphia: F.A. Davis.

CHAPTER 11

Enhancing Cognition, Communication, and Behavior

Jeffrey E. Evans
Dana Hanifan

LEARNING OBJECTIVES

At the end of this chapter, the reader will be able to

- Identify cognitive impairment that might be expected from injury to specific areas of the brain.
- Compare speech and language disorders.
- Distinguish between several types of memory.
- List several therapeutic strategies that staff can use to assist patients with impairment in memory, in executive control, and in communication.

KEY CONCEPTS AND TERMS

Affect	Delirium	Lethargic
Agitation	Dementia	Metacognition
Anergia	Disorientation	Obtunded
Anosagnosia	Distractibility	Perseveration
Aphasia	Dysarthria	Pragmatics
Apraxia	Encoding	Rancho Los Amigos scale of
Attention	Hemispatial inattention	cognitive recovery
Cognition	Hyperkinesia	Somatosensation
Confabulation	Impulsivity	Somnolent
Consciousness	Insight	Stuporous

In the interdisciplinary rehabilitation setting, enhancing cognition, communication, and behavior is a team responsibility. The team's familiarity with common impairments is important in improving the effectiveness of each patient's rehabilitation. In the first section of this chapter ways in which knowledge of neuroanatomy helps us anticipate patients' deficits is discussed. In the second section, common impairments are described, and strategies for helping patients with their deficits are also discussed. In the final portion of the chapter, management strategies are presented in greater depth.

NEUROANATOMY AND FUNCTION

Left Cerebral Hemisphere

Whereas the body's sensory and motor functions are controlled by the cerebral hemisphere opposite to the body part in question, control of language is largely a function of the left hemisphere. Specifically, in over 90% of right-hand–dominant people and close to 80% of left-hand–dominant people the left hemisphere is dominant for language. This embodies both one's ability to express through words and symbols as well as to comprehend speech or writing. In most cases a patient who experiences aphasia is likely to have had discrete neurological damage to the left cerebral hemisphere, typically a stroke, a focal tumor, or open head injury (e.g., a gun shot wound) (Love & Webb, 1992).

Within the left side of the brain are various structures that lead to specific behaviors and, thus, impairments when they are damaged. Conversely, knowing a patient's cluster of impairments allows insight into the location of the lesion.

Right Cerebral Hemisphere

Whereas the left hemisphere typically serves use of language and other symbols (such as numbers), the right hemisphere serves functions of global awareness, visual-spatial abilities, and attention. As described above, right hemisphere lesions often result in impaired attention to the left side of space, but the right hemisphere also serves more general vigilance and awareness of the "big picture." By big picture we refer to the patient's own situation, including insight into deficits, the rationale for medical and rehabilitation procedures, for mobility, and other safety restrictions.

Lateralization of lesions to the left or right hemisphere is only one indication of the behavior and deficits that can be expected from neurological damage. For example, the degree to which a lesion is anterior versus posterior also implies what behavior is to be expected. In another example, in the realm of speech and language, persons with anterior lesions of the left hemisphere, specifically in the frontal, anterior temporal, and anterior parietal lobes, may exhibit predominant deficits in verbal expression, resulting in a nonfluent pattern and often word finding difficulty. Their ability to comprehend spoken language is often superior to their ability to verbally express language. Conversely, posterior lesions, such as those in the superior temporal region, posterior extension to the parietal lobe, and the angular gyrus, result predominantly in comprehension deficits. Verbal output would be characterized as fluent but jargon-like (also referred to as empty speech). For example, a person with a superior temporal lobe insult may be unable to respond "yes" to the question "are you a man?" Rather, he may produce jargon that is unintelligible. In addition, the auditory comprehension feedback loop (the means by which we comprehend our own speech) is disrupted so patients may be unaware of their deficits or may be perceived as disinterested, or almost euphoric.

Anterior versus posterior lesion location implies that different cognitive deficits may be emphasized. In general, lesions that are anterior are associated with executive cognitive functions such as planning, organizing, coordinating, and multitasking, including the generation of language as discussed above. Lesions that are posterior are generally associated with perceptual functions, such as vision, hearing, spatial perception, and tactile sensation, including the comprehension of language. It should be emphasized that these are generalizations, but they can be useful in anticipating patients' needs and vulnerabilities.

COMMON IMPAIRMENTS IN REHABILITATION PATIENTS

Consciousness, Attention, and Executive Control

Consciousness is defined, simply, as awareness. **Attention** is the ability to focus awareness to accomplish a particular task. Executive control has several facets but most generally involves the ability to allocate attention and to plan, organize, and monitor one's behavior to achieve particular goals. The term **metacognition** is often used synonymously with executive control.

Levels of Consciousness

It is useful to distinguish among several levels of consciousness because they can vary with the effects of illness, fatigue, and medication. When a patient is alert, he or she has the ability to notice changes in the environment, and so alertness is necessary for responsiveness. When a patient is not alert, he or she may be unconscious, **obtunded**, **stuporous**, or merely **lethargic** or **somnolent**. Although these terms have their own definitions (Box 11.1), they are sometimes used interchangeably and sometimes incorrectly. To avoid ambiguity, it is important to report the patient's level of alertness with a *"specific statement of what the patient did in response to particular stimuli"* (Blumenfeld, 2002, p. 644). Beyond alertness, the ability to sustain attention is necessary for memory, problem solving, and higher cognitive functions, as discussed in the following sections.

> *". . . it is important to report the patient's level of alertness with a* specific statement *of what the patient did in response to particular stimuli" (Blumenfeld, 2002, p. 644).*

Confusion and Disorientation

The terms confusion and **disorientation** are also often used interchangeably (Anthoney, 1994). Disorientation typically refers to impaired sense of person, place, time,

---

BOX 11.1 Definitions of Commonly Used Terms

Affect: Feeling or emotion.

Agitation: Extreme emotional disturbance.

Anergia: Lack of energy resulting in reduced initiation.

Anosagnosia: Lack of knowledge or insight into one's own illness, injury, or medical condition.

Aphasia: The disturbed capacity to interpret and express conventional, meaningful symbols and is not attributable to dementia, sensory loss, motor dysfunction, or psychopathology.

Attention: Focused awareness.

Cognition: Mental processes of knowing and thinking.

Confabulation: Providing a spurious answer to a question, rather than admitting lack of knowledge.

Consciousness: Awareness.

Delirium: An acute confusional state often due to medication, environmental, toxic, or metabolic factors.

Dementia: A diffuse decline in cognitive functioning usually resulting from neurodegeneration and especially affecting memory, executive functions, visuospatial functioning, and processing speed.

Disorientation: Reduced awareness or confusion with respect to person, time, place, and reason or purpose.

Distractibility: Inattention, in which focus is drawn away by environmental or other stimuli.

Dysarthria: Impairment in speech as a result of reduction in muscle strength, speed, range of motion, and/or coordination.

Hemispatial inattention: Inability or reduced ability to attend to one side of space and of the body (called "neglect").

Hyperkinesia: Abnormally increased motor function or activity.

Impulsivity: Acting quickly, without prior thought.

Insight: Understanding the inner nature of things.

Lethargic: Slow in behavior.

Obtunded: State of reduced consciousness.

Perseveration: Inappropriate or ineffective repetition of behavior or speech.

Pragmatic (behavior): Behavior that is appropriate and purpose-driven.

Rancho Los Amigos scale of cognitive recovery: An evaluation tool created by the Rancho Los Amigos National Rehabilitation Center that describes stages of recovery typically seen after a brain injury.

Somatosensation: Bodily sensation and perception.

Somnolent: Sleepy.

Stuporous: State of reduced consciousness.

Unconscious: Not conscious.

Verbal apraxia: Impairment in the motor programming needed to produce speech and can occur in the absence of an apparent reduction in muscle strength.

---

and reason (for being in the hospital/facility). Orientation is commonly tested by questions such as, "What is your name?," "How old are you?," "Where are you?," "What is the name of this place?," "What is the town or city?," "What is the date (year, month, day)?," "What time is it?," and "Why are you here?". When a person is alert and fully oriented, he or she is often referred to as oriented times four, or A&O × 4 (person, place, date/time, and reason). Nurses more commonly report a patient or resident being oriented × 3 (e.g., to person, place, and date/time). It is not unusual for patients who are unable to generate correct answers on their own to be able to respond correctly when given choices. That is, these patients may be better at recognizing a correct choice than at recalling it without a cue. Accordingly, as patients recover, they may begin to recognize correct answers before being able to produce them on their own. In addition, with recovery often comes the ability to independently apply strategies to remain oriented. Examples include searching for a wall clock or recalling a recent event in an attempt to find the correct time.

Disorientation is sometimes accompanied by general confusion, that is, lack of clear knowledge about "what is going on." More often, there are specific points of confusion such as who visited, when they visited, or even if they visited. Patients can also be confused about the identity of persons or about the motives or intentions of people, including staff whose routine care or attempts at assistance may be misinterpreted. Therefore, besides overlapping with impaired memory, confusion and disorientation can result in fear and suspiciousness and can even mimic psychiatric symptoms such as paranoia. Finally, in some cases disorientation and confusion are accompanied by confabulation, in which a patient inappropriately incorporates elements of his history into his current situation. An example is of the veteran who reports on his military experiences as if they are happening currently and who might believe he is in a field hospital because he sees the medical helicopters coming and going outside his window. **Confabulation** is therefore a function of impaired recall for what is actually happening day to day and an attempt to construct an account of what is going on by using information that is actually recalled but is out of the current context.

Delirium

Delirium is an acute confusional state most commonly caused by metabolic or toxic disorders, including medication side effects (Blumenfeld, 2002). Delirium can be exacerbated by the diminishment of orienting cues associated with the low light of evening ("sun-downing") or monotonous environments ("ICU psychosis"). Behaviorally, delirium appears as confusion and inattention and can be accompanied by anxiety and agitation. Considering a patient's medications and hospital environment is helpful in distinguishing delirium from other forms of cognitive impairment (see Case Study 11.1).

CASE STUDY 11.1

A 55-year-old man sustained a severe traumatic brain injury in an assault. In acute rehabilitation he was alternately somnolent and agitated, crying and holding his head. The staff was concerned that he was depressed, and an order was obtained for an antidepressant (a selective serotonin reuptake inhibitor). His agitation increased, and it was determined that he was delirious, caused by excess serotonin. Discontinuing the selective serotonin reuptake inhibitor returned him to his previous state of agitation, which resolved with time and with addition of other medications used to treat extreme anxiety and unstable mood.

Distractibility

Patients with impaired attention and executive control often experience **distractibility**. Distractibility can present as difficulty hearing all that is said, staying on task, or participating in organized activities such as therapeutic exercises and activities of daily living (ADLs). It is common for patients to be distractible in a hospital environment where ambient noise and the sounds of human activity are heightened. Simple strategies like closing doors and maintaining quiet can be effective in helping patients keep their focus. Distractibility, along with impulsivity (see Case Study 11.2), is sometimes the clearest indicator of cognitive impairment in patients with right hemisphere lesions who otherwise may function well enough to compensate for impaired memory or visuospatial difficulties. (See the following sections for typical combinations of deficits depending on lesion location.)

CASE STUDY 11.2

A 59-year-old woman with a right hemisphere ischemic stroke (with left hemiparesis but minimal cognitive impairment) was being taught to give her own heparin injections before discharge from the hospital. Her husband was also present to learn the procedure, and her mother and sister-in-law were in the room helping to pack for the trip home. Although trying to focus on the nurse's teaching, the patient's attention was repeatedly drawn to other activities in the room and noises in the hallway, to the point that the nurse was concerned that the patient was not learning. Asking family members not involved in the teaching to leave the room temporarily and shutting the door were successful strategies in helping the patient focus on the task.

Perseveration

Perseveration refers to the inability, or simply to the difficulty, of switching attention from one idea or response to another. It is a deficit in mental flexibility that can result in fixating on a topic of conversation, a word, or an action. For example, while performing ADLs in the morning, a perseverative patient may brush her teeth several times or she might not stop combing her hair until directed to do so. Sometimes patients perseverate between settings or between contexts, for example, continuing behaviors from a bedside occupational therapy session after the session is over when the nurse is trying to help them move on to the next task. Perseveration is a failure of executive control that normally allows for switching from one task to another. It differs from forgetting in that a simple reminder may not be effective in facilitating a switch in behavior. Rather, the perseverative person may have to be actively redirected to the desired behavior. For example, the nurse might say, "We're finished with that now Ms. Smith, and it's time to take your medication" (while removing the hairbrush or other objects associated with the occupational therapy session just completed).

Hemispatial Inattention (Neglect)

One of the most striking symptoms of brain dysfunction is **hemispatial inattention**. Most common in stroke, it is seen typically in damage to the right hemisphere, where it is called left neglect. Just as injury to a hemisphere causes sensory and motor dysfunction on the opposite side of the body, the ability to orient and pay attention to the side opposite the lesion is diminished. The "neglect syndrome" is far more common and more severe with damage to the right than to the left hemisphere. This is due to the special role of the right hemisphere is processing spatial cognition—the ability to attend and perceive and to manipulate information on the layout and pattern of objects in one's field of view, including parts of one's own body. Neglect, however, can involve not only visual-spatial attention but also movement, **somatosensation** (tactile sensation and proprioception), and even hearing. In severe cases of left neglect, the entire sensory field to the left of midline can subjectively cease to exist for the patient.

In appearance, a patient with left neglect often displays a right head turn or gaze preference and, at least in the acute stage, has difficulty moving head and eyes to the left of midline. When addressed from his left side the patient is likely to be unaware that someone is speaking. When food is put in front of him, he may eat only the food on the right half of the tray. He might also dress only the right side of his body. Neglect of the right side due to left hemisphere injury is also sometimes seen but, again, is less severe than left neglect and usually consists of slowed responses or of missing visual details on the right.

Helpful interactions with a patient who has left neglect include reminders to look to the left and setting up the environment to encourage left field scanning and object manipulation, including addressing the patient from the left. For remediation of reading and writing, speech-language pathologists have developed strategies of colorful markers or anchors on the left side of a page that encourage patients to orient to the left. Even the orientation of a patient's bed in relation to the door of the hospital room can be therapeutic. For example, depending on the patient's condition, having a door on the left that opens out onto the hallway of the unit can provide stimulation that encourages attention to the neglected side. Of course, not all arrangements or interactions with a "neglect patient" need to be for the purpose of treating the neglect. For example, there are times when working on the patient's intact right side is preferable for logistic reasons. An example is helping a patient get ready for a therapy appointment when time is short. Another example is a teaching situation, when it is important to maximize the patient's attention.

It is important to note that a patient with neglect usually experiences a more general impairment in visuospatial functioning; that is, she may have generally distorted visual perception affecting accuracy of locating objects in space, of judging objects in relation to each other, or of hand–eye coordination. Interestingly, these patients can also display difficulty attending to the left side of objects that are located in the right visual field.

Speech and Language

The terms speech and language are interrelated and refer to the global act of communication. However, the two terms are not interchangeable and encompass different modalities of communication. Speech refers to the motor act of expressing our language through verbal means. Speech is characterized via the physiological subsystems of respiration, phonation (voicing), resonance (how the air is moving through the oral, throat, and nasal cavities), articulation, and prosody (the use of rate, stress, and intonation to further characterize the utterance). The foundation of speech begins with one's ability to use respiratory musculature to support pressure to move the vocal folds. Movement of the vocal folds creates a distinct voice as they come together in a formation to create sound waves. The air used to create the vocal fold closure then resonates through the throat, oral, and nasal cavities. The articulators (e.g., lips, teeth, tongue, and palate) move in various positions to form specific speech sounds and can only be distinct via a sufficient amount of resonated air. The subsystems of respiration, phonation, resonance, and articulation are then made unique through one's ability to use varied intonation, inflection, stress, and emphasis on specific words (Zemlin, 1988).

Individuals can experience an impairment in their speech as a result of either an organic (a known physical) or functional (no known physical) cause. Most common causes of motor speech disorders in the rehabilitation patient arise from a neurological event such as a stroke, head injury, tumor, or aneurysm. The site of the brain's lesion determines the type of motor speech disorder one sustains (Darley, Aronson, & Brown, 1975).

There are two types of motor speech disorders: **apraxia** and the **dysarthrias**. Apraxia refers to impairment in the motor programming needed to produce speech and can occur in the absence of an apparent reduction of muscle strength. Apraxia of speech results in deficits of articulation and prosody. Errors are highly inconsistent yet most often occur with complex (lengthier) words. A primary behavioral characteristic of a verbal apraxia (or apraxia of speech) is struggling or groping. Apraxia often coexists with other linguistic pathology due to the specific area of the brain injured (Wertz, LaPointe, & Rosenbek, 1991).

The different types of dysarthrias are identified based on their specific clustered motor speech features and the area of the brain's pathology (Duffy, 1995) (Table 11.1).

TABLE 11.1	The Dysarthrias		
Type	**Site of Lesion**	**Common Etiologies**	**Distinguishing Features**
Flaccid	Neuromuscular junction of final common pathway; lower motor neuron	Myasthenia gravis; brainstem stroke; Guillian-Barré; muscular dystrophy	Breathy voice; nasal emission; hypernasality; articulatory distortion
Spastic	Bilateral upper motor neuron, cortical involvement	Multiple infarcts; TBI; encephalopathy	Strained, strangled voice, slow rate, low pitch
Ataxic	Cerebellar control circuit	Friedrich's ataxia, vascular disease	Irregular articulatory breakdown; excess and equal stress; dysprosody
Hypokinetic	Basal ganglia control circuit	Parkinson's disease; subcortical stroke	Bursts of rapid speech; hypophonia; phoneme repetition; masked face
Hyperkinetic	Basal ganglia control circuit	Huntington's disease; toxic/metabolic; vascular disease	Forced inspiration, expiration; strained voice; variable rate; prolonged phonemes; vocal tremor; excess and equal stress
Unilateral upper motor neuron	Upper motor neurons	Unilateral stroke; lacunar infarcts	Mild, acute, temporary; imprecise articulation; strained voice; slow rate
Mixed spastic and flaccid	Both upper and lower motor neurons	ALS (Lou Gehrig's disease)	Strained, breathy voice; hypernasality; imprecise articulation; slow rate

ALS, amyotrophic lateral sclerosis; TBI, traumatic brain injury.

Source: From Darley, et al. (1975).

Dysarthria is not an impairment of language but rather is an impairment of speech.

> *A speech-language pathologist is trained in evaluating, identifying the differential diagnosis, and treating the individual with motor speech disorders or aphasia.*

Discrete language disorders, or focal language disturbances, are synonymous with the term aphasia. **Aphasia** is an impairment of language functions after brain damage. Specifically, it is the disturbed capacity to decode (interpret) and encode (formulate, express) conventional, meaningful symbols (Table 11.2). Aphasia is not attributable to dementia, sensory loss, motor dysfunction, or psychopathology (Sarno, 1981). However, with brain injury one often has motor speech disorders that coexist with aphasia. Aphasia can be manifested in disorders of auditory comprehension and/or verbal expression as well as reading comprehension and/or written expression. As in dysarthria, there are classical types of aphasia that correlate with the site of brain lesions.

A speech-language pathologist is trained in evaluating, identifying the differential diagnosis, and treating the individual with motor speech disorders or aphasia. Making the distinction between speech and language disorders can be a challenge, especially because the disorders often coexist. Determining the difference between motor speech disorders (e.g., the dysarthrias, apraxia) and aphasia involves motor speech examination, language evaluation, the specific speech features, and the patient's reaction to his or her difficulties.

Memory

Memory is the mental function most commonly affected by damage to the brain. There are several types of memory, and they are differentially vulnerable to the affects of injury or illness.

Types of Memory With Respect to Time

How long a person is able to retain information is an important practical consideration and has led to familiar categories of memory with respect to time, such as "short-term memory," "long-term memory," and "working memory." (For an authoritative reference on the neuropsychology of memory, see Squire & Schachter [2003].) Where one category of memory ends and the next begins

TABLE 11.2	The Aphasias		
Type	**Site of Lesion**	**Major Characteristics**	**Differential Diagnosis**
Global	Typically left* hemisphere, middle cerebral artery territory	Impairments in all modalities of comprehension and expression	Nonfluent; impaired auditory comprehension; impaired repetition
Broca's	Posterior-inferior left frontal lobe (Broca's area)	Agrammatic syntax, word-finding problems, poor naming, slow labored output	Nonfluent; impaired repetition; adequate auditory comprehension
Wernicke's	Posterior superior temporal gyrus (Wernicke's area)	Jargon, neologisms, empty speech, unaware of errors, normal melodic contour	Fluent; impaired auditory comprehension; impaired repetition
Conduction	Left arcuate fasciculus, supramarginal gyrus	Literal paraphasias, word repetition better than speech production	Fluent; impaired repetition; adequate auditory comprehension
Anomic	Left temporal-parietal cortex	Word-finding difficulty	Fluent; adequate repetition; adequate auditory comprehension
Transcortical motor	Anterior-superior to Broca's area	Agrammatic, stuttering, spontaneous output, near-normal repetition	Nonfluent; good repetition; adequate auditory comprehension
Transcortical sensory	Temporal-parietal border zone	Echolalia, poor naming	Fluent; good to excellent repetition; impaired auditory comprehension

*The left hemisphere is usually dominant for language, especially in right-handed people.

Source: From Goodglass, H., & Kaplan, E. (1972). *The assessment of aphasia and related disorders.* Philadelphia: Lea and Febinger.

is less important in clinical work than in general functional descriptions, which follow:

- *Working memory:* The retention and manipulation of information for several seconds, such as keeping a phone number in mind for the time it takes to dial it or completing mental arithmetic.
- *Short-term memory:* Sometimes called immediate memory, short-term memory refers to retention of information over a period of seconds to minutes. A patient with impaired short-term memory may forget when the nurse enters her room why she had pressed the call light. A helpful response by the nurse in this case is to suggest possible reasons for the patient using the call light: Did it have to do with the bathroom, for example. Patients with impaired short-term memory are likely to o recognize the reason when told to them, even if they cannot recall it on their own. Short-term memory is the type of memory most frequently affected by damage to the brain.
- *Long-term memory:* Sometimes called delayed memory, long-term memory refers to retention of information for minutes or hours. Long-term memory includes the patient recalling what he had for breakfast hours earlier or what he did in his last therapy appointment. A therapeutic response in this situation

is to provide the patient with multiple-choice cues of what he might have had for breakfast with the goal of stimulating memory through recognition. (For an authoritative source for strategies of cognitive rehabilitation, see Sohlberg & Mateer [2001].)

- *Remote memory:* This type includes memory for information and events that took place days ago, such as the history of the current illness. Remote memory can refer to a time period of weeks or months in the past. Reminding the patient of what led to his or her hospitalization can, through repetition, aid recovery of remote memory.
- *Autobiographical memory:* This type refers to memory for biographical information and events such as the year of high school graduation, description of a childhood home, details of medical history, and so forth. Encouraging the family to provide family pictures, for example, can help the patient regain orientation to his or her own life.

Types of Memory With Respect to Content

We remember information, such as names and phone numbers; events, such as what happened in physical therapy earlier in the day; and procedures, such as how to steer a wheelchair. Each of these types of information—

details, events, and procedures—is processed by a different memory system in the brain; furthermore, they not equally vulnerable to the illnesses and injuries that cause memory impairment:

- *Declarative memory:* Memory for detailed information such as names, phone numbers, timing and doses of medications, instructions for home exercises, and so on. Such information is typically in the form of words and numbers; impaired declarative memory is most easily remediated by compensatory strategies such as keeping notes and lists and cueing, such as thinking through the letters of the alphabet when trying to retrieve a name.
- *Episodic memory:* Memory for events (episodes) such as the happenings of the day, for example, what happened in therapy, if someone came to visit, or if a change was made in the therapy schedule. (The name of the visitor and the details of the schedule change are part of declarative memory.) Who told the patient of the schedule change is considered part of episodic memory and is called "source memory." Episodic information is often in the form of visual images. Impaired episodic memory can also be remediated by compensatory strategies such as note and list making; however, because episodic memory is often visually represented in the mind, patients are advised to think backward, or "rewind the video tape" of their memory, to get at past events.
- *Procedural memory:* Memory for procedures such as dressing, driving an automobile, or propelling a wheelchair. Procedures typically have a motoric component, and as they are learned they become increasingly automatic and unconscious. For example, once driving a car is learned, one does not have to "think about" how to do it. Procedural memory is often preserved, even when declarative or episodic memory is severely impaired. In rehabilitation, much of compensating for a new physical disability involves revising memory for everyday procedures, such as ambulating, in addition to possibly learning new procedures such as operating a wheelchair. Repetition is the usual route to learning a new procedure.

Other Memory Concepts Useful in Rehabilitation

Recall, also referred to as free recall or retrieval, refers to the act of remembering on one's own, without the aid of external hints or cues. Recall can be more or less spontaneous, or it can involve strategies for "finding" the information to be remembered, as mentioned above. For example, a patient might use the strategy of thinking back to when she was instructed to use a sliding board in order to remember how to use it now. Regarding orientation, a patient may mentally review the events of the day to estimate the current time. Teaching memory strategies is an important part of cognitive rehabilitation.

- *Recognition:* The ability to recognize implies intact **encoding** and is the ability to know the correct answer when presented with a list of alternatives or with less direct cues that merely point to the answer. An example in a patient with impaired orientation is to ask "is this 1989, 2010, or 2001?" A less direct cue is to say "the year is two-thousand. . . ." Intact recognition means that the information is encoded, or stored, in memory and may be activated by the appropriate hint or cue. This is different from recall, which is the ability to find what is encoded without a cue. Successful encoding requires adequate attention to the material to be remembered. With adequate attention, information becomes part of a network of related memories. The information is therefore activated and recalled when related cues are encountered.
- *Carryover:* The ability to apply information or a procedure in a context other than the one in which it was learned. Carryover can refer to time, that is, being able to execute a stand-pivot transfer today that was first learned yesterday. Carryover can also refer to situation; that is, being able to transfer from wheelchair to toilet as well as bed to wheelchair. These examples involve procedural memory. An example of carryover of declarative memory is the patient's ability to recall details of her exercise program at home as well as in the hospital or clinic. Carryover can also refer to the ability to translate instructions given verbally, into the appropriate actions.

Insight and Judgment

Insight and judgment are closely related to memory, attention, and executive control as well as to each other. Having insight is having the ability to see the ""big picture," that is, especially, to understand how one's deficits impact independent functioning.

Anosagnosia (Impaired Knowledge of Deficits)

Patients with **anosagnosia** have diminished insight into their own illness, in particular into their physical and cognitive deficits (Prigitano & Schachter, 1991). They appear to be unaware of, indifferent to, or in some cases in denial of their disabilities. Anosagnosia differs from denial, however, in that it is a form of cognitive impairment—an inability to appreciate what is going on (in the sense of the "big picture") as opposed to an emotionally driven defense (e.g., not wanting to know because it is too painful).

Abstract Versus Concrete Thinking

To have insight one must be able to perceive and think about one's situation in the abstract (in general) rather than merely being stuck in a single, concrete situation. Abstract thinking means having perspective and therefore the potential to correct or modify a situation to make it better. Insight, therefore, gives a patient the necessary awareness to seek out and participate in rehabilitation.

Verbal Versus Performative Judgment

A patient may be able to talk about her illness or disability and appear to have the necessary understanding to follow medical advice and to participate in rehabilitation, while being unable to put that apparent verbal understanding into action. The proof of functional insight is in what the patient does, not necessarily in what she says.

Impulse Control

Impulsivity and Anergia

Impulsivity is a common behavioral symptom after traumatic brain injury, stroke, and other illnesses that involve the brain. By definition, impulsivity involves initiation of an action apparently without thought and in which the action is unwise, inappropriate, or dangerous. A common example in rehabilitation is attempting to transfer from a wheelchair before first checking that the brakes are locked. Impulsivity is distinguished from normal spontaneity in which initiation may occur quickly but the action is appropriate and the person is in control.

Conversely, **anergia** is another symptom of brain involvement that denotes an impairment of initiation in which the patient begins an action either slowly or not at all. An example is the patient who requires external cueing to move through the steps involved in a familiar ADL such as brushing his or her teeth.

Impaired initiation and impulsivity are both common after injuries to the frontal lobes; impulsivity is also frequently seen in right hemisphere disease. Impulsivity can be a direct result of injury to the brain, in which inhibitory mechanisms are eliminated or reduced. It can also be a secondary result of diminished insight into deficits (anosognosia), in which the patient lacks sufficient knowledge of his or her situation and thus neglects to take necessary precautions before acting. An example is the patient with hemiparesis who "forgets" he needs assistance to ambulate and sustains a fall.

Agitation, Restlessness, and Hyperkinesia

On the acute rehabilitation service, **agitation** is most often associated with a stage in recovery from traumatic brain injury—level IV of the **Rancho Los Amigos scale of cognitive recovery**. Level IV, the "agitation stage," is often reached after a patient's awareness has increased but before he or she is able to focus attention on one thing at a time and to screen out irrelevant or interfering stimuli. Patients in level IV are overwhelmed, confused, and frequently frightened due to lack of cognitive control over their perceptions and over their own thoughts (Table 11.3). The agitated patient, then, is disorganized and may appear desperate to escape from his or her situation, including from the hospital room and from staff in attendance. Helpful staff responses to patient agitation include reducing stimulation (e.g., dimming lights, limiting people in the room, reducing extraneous noise) and determining stimuli that are calming to the patient (e.g., favorite music, certain visitors) (for additional helpful strategies, see below).

Restlessness is sometimes mistaken for agitation. An important difference is that whereas the agitated patient is disturbed by internal and external stimuli, the restless patient just cannot seem to get comfortable. Although pain and physical discomfort can certainly contribute to agitation, they are a principal cause of restlessness. General hyperarousal (e.g., jitteriness or jumpiness) can also contribute to restlessness and must be distinguished from anxious mood states frequently associated with agitation.

Hyperkinesia is a descriptive term that simply means an excess of movement—more movement or more rapid movement than is appropriate or necessary for the situation. Agitated and restless patients often exhibit hyperkinesias, as do patients with neurological conditions such as Huntington's disease.

Affect and Mood

In the realm of emotion and emotional expression, **affect** refers to the appearance of emotion in a person's tone of voice, facial expression, and other nonverbal behavior. Normal affect is usually referred to as broad in range, which means the patient is able to express a range of feelings spontaneously and appropriately. Flat affect can be a pathological result of brain injury or illness: The voice is monotone, the face expressionless. In brain injury or

TABLE 11.3	Rancho Los Amigos Levels of Cognitive Functioning	
Level	**Description**	**Suggestions for Stimulation**
I: no response	Unresponsive to any stimulus	Brief, frequent time with family and friends
II: generalized response	Inconsistent but stereotyped reaction to stimuli	Talk in normal voice; brief, frequent time with family and friends
III: localized response	Inconsistent but specific reactions to stimuli; starts to follow simple commands; vague awareness of self/body	Minimize distractions; encourage purposeful responses
IV: confused, agitated	High activity; bizarre, non-purposeful behavior; may be euphoric or hostile	Limit visitors and stimulation; bring in family pictures; allow as much movement as is safe
V: confused, inappropriate, nonagitated	Follows commands more consistently; severe memory impairment; poor initiation; highly distractible	Orient frequently; repeat information as needed
VI: confused, appropriate	Consistently follows simple directions; goal-directed; responds appropriately to discomfort	Repeat information; help start and continue activities; encourage daily therapy participation
VII: automatic, appropriate	Appropriate, oriented, but robot-like; superficial awareness of condition; carryover of new learning; poor judgment	Help with decision-making, problem-solving, safety; encourage participation in therapy
VIII: purposeful, appropriate	Alert, oriented, carries over, physically independent; may fatigue easily and have low stress tolerance	Involve in complex tasks; initiate vocational rehab

Source: From Los Amigos Research and Educational Institute (1990).

illness flat affect can result from injury of the brain's ability to initiate, control, and modify verbal and facial expression. In addition to brain injury, extreme cases of depression can cause affect to be flat, as can responses to drugs or medications. As such, flat affect can also be a symptom of delirium. Restricted affect is not normal but is not entirely flat: Spontaneity is reduced, and affect is "restricted to" a narrow range dictated by the person's situation and predominant mood.

Mood is the underlying emotional state that contributes to affect, for example, depressed, anxious, or a combination of the two. Although affect is of shorter duration and more variable (like the weather), mood is "sustained and pervasive" (like climate) (Zuckerman, 2005). Depression and anxiety are complex mood states that can be more or less biologically based and more or less reactive to a patient's current situation. Both have affective, cognitive, and behavioral facets (for lists of typical signs and symptoms see Zuckerman, 2005).

Social Behavior

Impulse control is central to getting along with others; however, brain injury can induce other impairments that affect the pragmatics of social behavior, including deficits of perception, abstract thinking, empathy, and speech/language. (For an authoritative reference on social neuroscience, see Caccioppo et al. [2007].) **Pragmatics** with regard to social behavior refers to the ability to act in ways that are appropriate and socially acceptable. Deficits in the pragmatics of behavior often result from impaired perception or judgment. For example, persons with traumatic brain injury often have difficulty understanding others or perceiving their intentions, especially when meanings are subtle, indirect, or unexpected as in irony, sarcasm, or humor. Consider the social disadvantage of the patient who is unable to distinguish humor from an insult or who perceives a friendly smile as a sneer.

From the staff point of view, getting to know a patient's sensitivities is essential to a therapeutic relationship. In addition, behavior that may have been premorbidly automatic—politeness or taking turns when speaking, for example—may require, after injury, weeks or months of therapy to regain. The task of acute staff in such instances is simply to remind patients of what is appropriate, without badgering them; acute staff members are also central to helping families interact appropriately and therapeutically with their injured family member.

A common patient presentation that is challenging for many staff is sexually inappropriate behavior. This is most often an issue between male brain-injured patients and female staff, although is not uncommon behavior of female patients. Most often, such behavior ranges from suggestive remarks or gestures to inappropriate touching. In the extreme such behavior can be harassing but rarely is it assaultive, by most definitions. In addition to patients touching staff inappropriately, a patient can touch himself inappropriately, for example, in public. The latter is seen most often during early stages of cognitive recovery when awareness of surroundings is limited and impulsivity may be more severe.

The goal of staff responses in instances of inappropriate sexual behavior is to reduce and eventually eliminate the behavior. Although best practices in these situations are not always clear-cut, the response should be appropriate to the infraction, because both under- and over-reaction can reinforce rather than reduce the undesirable behavior. Examples of generally effective staff responses vary from redirection of attention, for example, changing the subject or changing the activity, to verbal limit setting in which the patient is told that his behavior is inappropriate and what appropriate behavior would be. In more extreme situations the patient may have to be restrained. Staff should never hesitate to recruit other staff for assistance or for discussion of their responses to specific incidents.

A NOTE ABOUT DEMENTIA

Dementia results from degenerative diseases such as Alzheimer's disease, frontotemporal degeneration, and Parkinson's disease, among others. Behaviorally, dementia refers to a diffuse decline in cognitive functioning that especially affects memory, executive functions, visuospatial functioning, and processing speed. Patents have impaired learning, disorientation, diminished insight and judgment, and slowed mental and physical capacities. In more advanced cases, confusion, hallucinations, delusions, and other mental and emotional symptoms can result. At the extreme, dementia results in loss of control over bodily functions and in death, often from pneumonia or other secondary infections.

Because dementing conditions are degenerative and prominently affect the ability to learn, rehabilitation programs that involve restoration of function through learning, applying new strategies, and carrying over compensatory behaviors are of limited effectiveness. Still, mild degrees of dementia are sometimes encountered as a comorbidity in rehabilitation patients; distinguishing between the cognitive manifestations of dementia, delirium, depression (the 3 Ds), and the patient's primary

illness or injury is an important task of the rehabilitation team.

When you encounter a new patient whose cognitive or affective presentation seems out of the ordinary and cannot be explained by a known stroke or other brain injury, it is likely that one of the 3 Ds is involved. To determine what might be involved, remember the following:

- Delirium is typically caused by medication, metabolic derangement, infection, or environment and is usually reversible when the cause is determined.
- Dementia is typically of longer duration, and family usually describes cognitive or behavioral changes they have noticed over the past months or years. However, sometimes the decline at home has been so gradual or has not been discussed within the family that only after sensitive questioning by the team will it become fully a part of current treatment and posthospital planning.
- Depression can show itself affectively, cognitively, and behaviorally. Affectively the patient may appear sad, anxious, or both. Behaviorally the patient may be slowed in his or her responses, thoughts, and movements. Cognitively, the patient may have difficulty sustaining attention—with possible affects on memory—and may have pessimistic, hopeless, or helpless thoughts.

Consulting with other team members is especially useful to know if the patient's presentation varies or is the same across contexts and helps to distinguish among the 3 Ds.

BOX 11.2   **Web Exploration**
Visit the following websites for more information about speech, language, and cognitive deficits.
American Academy of Physical Medicine and Rehabilitation: *www.aapmr.org*
American Congress of Rehabilitation Medicine: www.acrm .org
American Speech-Language-Hearing Association: www.asha.org
American Stroke Association: *www.strokeassociation.org*
Brain Injury Association USA: *www.biausa.org*
National Academy of Neuropsychology: *www.nanonline .org*

STRATEGIES FOR MANAGING THE REHABILITATION PATIENT

Communication

It is critical as a member of the rehabilitation team to identify and implement strategies to optimize communication. The patient benefits more from the daily therapy routine if there is an appropriate level of rapport with his or her team members. Simple conversation and daily reorientation as needed are important rapport-building skills.

Using compensatory strategies to optimize daily interactions and global rehabilitation experiences are necessary for the patient as well as members of the rehabilitation staff. Basic strategies of listening, rewording, reviewing the patient's needs/wants, and asking for clarification when needed are essential. Staff members need to understand the patient's level of hearing, vision, and cognitive abilities. It is equally important to inquire into the patient's educational background, occupation, and premorbid ADLs. In doing this, the rehabilitation team member can adjust his or her style of communication, speaking rate, and grammar according to the needs of the patient. For example, it is essential to use a slow rate of speech and simple grammar in the case of a patient with a language deficit. The team member's ability to modify the therapy environment is also critical in ensuring success at various cognitive and communicative levels. Examples include turning off the television/radio, selecting a private versus semiprivate room, or having familiar pictures available in the case of a patient with a motor speech disorder, aphasia, agitation or confusion, or an attention impairment.

In some instances, staff members need to explore augmentative or alternative means to communicate with the patient. Nurses may need to consult with the patient's speech-language pathologist to learn about effective low-technology options (e.g., writing, letter board, picture board) or more advanced technology, such as speech-generated computer devices.

Memory

Many individuals receiving rehabilitative therapies experience memory difficulties. Causes of those difficulties can include attention deficits, encoding deficits, retrieval deficits, as well as other psychological, social, or behavioral factors. It is the primary role of the staff member to implement effective memory strategies and to ensure the strategy is used across the team to further enhance carryover of information taught. Many patients have daily log books or memory books that outline specific therapy tasks completed as well as daily logging of such meaningful events as visitors, television shows viewed, time of therapies, and time to take medication.

SUMMARY

Rehabilitation nurses are frontline administrators who ensure the patient and the rest of the team (everyone from the transporter to the therapists to the physician) are using the same compensatory system. As mentioned earlier, frequent reorientation and recall of daily tasks should be a part of each staff member's daily responsibilities to enhance the patient's ability to remember and learn from his or her rehabilitation program. Case Study 11.3 allows

---

CASE STUDY 11.3

A 24-year-old man was admitted with a severe traumatic brain injury after a motor vehicle accident. The patient was initially comatose and progressed through several levels of consciousness while on the acute care service. He was transferred to the inpatient rehabilitation service as he entered level IV of the Rancho Los Amigos scales of cognitive functioning. As he became more verbal, he was also found to have a severe spastic dysarthria, resulting in highly unintelligible verbal output. His agitation presumably escalated as a result of his inability to intelligibly make his needs and wants known. His family became increasingly frustrated trying to cope with his behavior.

Questions

1. Describe levels of consciousness the patient might have experienced before coming to the rehab service.
2. What is the Rancho Los Amigos scales of cognitive functioning and how might it apply to the patient's behavior and progression toward recovery?
3. How should the rehabilitation staff modify the patient's environment to ensure his comfort and safety?
4. Given his severe dysarthria, what alternative modes of communication can be used to assess the patient's orientation and pain level?
5. How could each member of the rehabilitation team (e.g., nursing, family member, physician, physical therapist, occupational therapist, psychologist, speech-language pathologist) contribute to the care and safety of a patient with agitation?
6. What strategies can the nurse use to help improve the patient's orientation and daily recall?

the reader to apply and synthesize the information from this chapter.

CRITICAL THINKING

1. If you notice a change in (a) your patient's affect or (b) your patient's cognition, how would you assess the cause and decide whether to consult with the physician or one of the therapists?
2. Consider the various types of aphasia listed in Table 11.2. Which type(s) have you seen most commonly in patients or nursing home residents? Which type do you believe would be the most frustrating for the patient? The most difficult to treat? Require the most assistance from speech therapy?
3. What is the role of the speech therapist in your facility/practice? After reading this chapter, with which additional areas can you see a speech therapist assisting the nursing staff?

PERSONAL REFLECTION

- If you have a friend or family member who has suffered from a neurological illness or injury affecting the brain (such as a stroke or traumatic brain injury) it can increase your understanding of your patients and their families to reflect on your own experience, thoughts, and feelings. Helpful tools for reflection include writing about your experience or discussing it with a friend or colleague.
- Have you ever had a family member or friend experience a neurological injury that resulted in impaired communication, cognition, or both? How did you interact with that person? How did you support the other family members or friends as they tried to cope with the event?

RECOMMENDED READINGS

Beaumont, J. G. (2008). *Introduction to neuropsychology*. New York: Guilford Press.

Bourgeois, M. S. (1991). Communication treatment for adults with dementia. *Journal of Speech and Hearing Research, 34,* 831–844.

Devinsky, O., & D'Esposito, M. (2004). *Neurology of cognitive and behavioral disorders*. New York: Oxford Press.

Dworkin, J. P. (1991) *Motor speech disorders: A treatment guide*. St. Louis, MO: Mosby Year Book.

Frattali, C., Bayles, K., Beeson, P., Kennedy, M. R., Wambaugh, J., & Yorkston, K. M. (2003). Development of evidence-based practice guidelines: committee update. *Journal of Medical Speech-Language Pathology, 11*(3), ix–xviii.

Halper, A. S., Cherney, L. R., & Miller, T. K. (1991). *Clinical management of communication problems in adults with traumatic brain injury*. Gaithersburg, MD: Aspen.

High, W. M., Sander, A. M., Struchen, M. A., & Hart, K. A. (2005). *Rehabilitation for traumatic brain injury*. New York: Oxford Press.

Shearer, W. M. (1979). *Illustrated speech anatomy*. Springfield, IL: Charles C. Thomas.

Tomoeda, C. K., & Bayles, K. A. (1990). The efficacy of speech-language pathology intervention: Dementia. *Seminars in Speech and Language, 11*(4), 311–318.

Ylvisaker, M., Feeney, T. J., & Urbanczyk, B. (1993). A social-environmental approach to communication and behavior after traumatic brain injury. *Seminars in Speech and Language, 14*(1), 74–87.

Yorkston, K. M., Spencer, K., Duffy, J., Beukelman, D., Golper, L. A., Miller, R., et al. (2001). Evidence-based practice guidelines for dysarthria: Management of velopharyngeal function. *Journal of Medical Speech-Language Pathology, 9*(4), 257–274.

REFERENCES

Anthoney, T. R. (1994). *Neuroanatomy and the neurologic exam*. Boca Raton, FL: CRC Press.

Blumenfeld, H. (2002). *Neuroanatomy through clinical cases*. Sunderland, MA: Sinauer.

Caccioppo, J. T., Amaral, D. G., Blanchard, J. J., Cameron, J. L., Carter, C. S, Crews, D., et al. (2007). Social neuroscience: Progress and implications for mental health. *Perspectives on Psychological Science, 2*(2), 99–123.

Darley, F. L., Aronson A. E., & Brown, J. R. (1975). *Motor speech disorders*. Philadelphia: W.B. Saunders.

Duffy, J. R. (1995). *Motor speech disorders: Substrates, differential diagnosis and management*. St. Louis, MO: Mosby Year Book.

Goodglass, H., Kaplan, E., & Barresis, B. (2001). *The assessment of aphasia and related disorders* (3rd ed.). Philadelphia: Lippincott Williams & Wilkins.

Love, R. J., & Webb, W. G. (1992). *Neurology for the speech-language pathologist*. Boston: Butterworth-Heinemann.

Prigitano, G. P., & Schacter, D. L. (1991). *Awareness of deficit after brain injury*. New York: Oxford University Press.

Sarno, M. T. (1981). *Acquired aphasia*. New York: Academic Press.

Sohlberg, M. M., & Mateer, C. A. (2001). *Cognitive rehabilitation: An integrative neuropsychological approach*. New York: Guilford Press.

Squire, L. R., & Schachter, D. L. (Eds.). (2003). *The neuropsychology of memory*. New York: Guilford Press.

Wertz, R. T., LaPointe, L. L., & Rosenbek, J. C. (1991). *Apraxia of speech in adults: The disorder and its management*. San Diego: Singular Publishing Group.

Zemlin, W. R. (1988.) *Speech and hearing science: Anatomy and physiology*. Englewood Cliffs, NJ: Prentice-Hall.

Zuckerman, E. L. (2005). *Clinician's thesaurus*. New York: Guilford Press.

CHAPTER 12

Sexuality and Disability

Catherine Moore
Donald D. Kautz
Michelle Cournan

LEARNING OBJECTIVES

At the end of this chapter the reader will be able to

- Outline the role of the nurse in addressing intimacy and sexual concerns of those with chronic illness and disability and their partners.
- Describe the stages of sexual development of children and adults.
- Describe the changes in the sexual response due to aging, chronic illness, and disability, and common responses to these changes.
- Discuss strategies to overcome vaginal dryness and erectile dysfunction.
- Identify practical advice and sexual resources for couples.
- Implement appropriate strategies that promote intimacy in community, long-term care, and inpatient rehabilitation settings.
- List strategies to extinguish sexually inappropriate behavior.

KEY CONCEPTS AND TERMS

Desire	Inorgasmia	Premature ejaculation
Excitement	Intimacy	Sexuality
Erectile dysfunction	Orgasm	Vaginal dryness
Human sexual response	PLISSIT model	Viagra

SEXUALITY AND DISABILITY

All disabilities and chronic illnesses have the potential to impact **sexuality** and **intimacy**. This chapter outlines some of the common problems men and women with disabilities and their sexual partners need to overcome and adapt to in order to have fulfilling intimate relationships.

A basic human need of people of all ages is intimacy with others. This chapter is designed to assist the rehabilitation nurse in promoting appropriate sexual development in children with disabilities and enhanced romantic intimacy and sexual function in adults with chronic illness and disability. People with chronic illness and disability are a diverse group, and romantic intimacy and sexual expression among the disabled vary greatly.

Despite decades of research showing that people with disabilities want to discuss intimacy and sexual concerns (Bauer, McAuliffe, & Nay, 2007; Higgins, Barker, & Begley, 2006; Magnan, Reynolds, & Galvin, 2005), these needs continue to be ignored by healthcare professionals, for several reasons. Addressing sexuality or sexual function is not seen as a priority for either the patient or the provider, and sexual concerns often are not addressed in healthcare encounters. Members of the rehabilitation team do not see any consequences to not addressing sexual concerns. Sexuality is seen as separate from healthcare concerns rather than integral to quality of life. Anxiety and fear of embarrassment prevent patients, families, nurses, and other rehabilitation team members from bringing up sexual concerns. Further, team members may fear they may not have the resources to assist patients to overcome sexual problems.

Most sexual problems that result from chronic health illnesses, aging, and disability are within the realm of nursing practice (Kautz, 2007; McAuliffe, Bauer, & Nay, 2007; Mick, 2007; Steinke, 2008). Yet instead of helping, nurses may contribute to sexual dysfunction by ignoring the underlying health problems that lead to sexual problems. For example, sending a patient home with an indwelling Foley catheter will certainly interfere with sexual intercourse. Teach a woman to tape the catheter up onto her abdomen and wear some type of t-shirt to prevent the catheter from rubbing during intercourse or to wear a crotchless teddy or crotchless panties to keep the catheter out of the way. A man with an indwelling catheter can fold the catheter back over an erect penis and then put on a condom. Partners report not being able to feel the catheter during intercourse, and ejaculation will occur unimpeded around the catheter. Both techniques have been recommended for decades, and they are not thought to increase the chances of urinary tract infection (Anderson, Kautz, Bryant, & Clanin, in press). Yet again, nurses regularly fail to teach clients who are discharged with catheters these effective and safe techniques.

> *A basic human need of people of all ages is intimacy with others.*

We also miss many opportunities to assist our clients in overcoming problems. Most health-promotion strategies have the potential to make a positive impact on sexual relationships and sexual function. Smoking cessation, limiting fat in the diet, losing weight, regular aerobic exercise, and drinking only moderate amounts of alcohol all may reverse the sexual changes that occur with chronic illnesses, obesity, and aging (Kautz, Van Horn, & Moore, 2009). If patients realize that heightened intimacy and regained sexual function may result from these lifestyle changes, they may be more motivated to make the changes.

The most widely cited model for practitioners to use when addressing sexual concerns of patients and their partners is the **PLISSIT model**, developed by Annon (1976). The PLISSIT acronym stands for the levels of intervention by members of the rehab team, which include permission (encouraging patients and their partners to voice sexual concerns), limited information (providing information for overcoming sexual problems by giving patients and their partners pamphlets, video resources, and information about helpful websites), specific suggestions (treatments for **vaginal dryness**, erectile dys-

function, and/or vaginal dryness, adopting comfortable positions for intercourse, methods of managing spasticity during intercourse), and intensive therapy (marital or sex therapy, which requires special training). All members of the healthcare team should be able to bring up sexual issues and provide limited information and then refer patients and their partners for more intensive therapy to specially trained sex therapists or relationship counselors. All rehabilitation facilities need a list of qualified counselors and sex therapists to refer clients to if they request these services.

Kautz, Van Horn, and Moore's (2009) integrative review of research on sexuality after stroke revealed that sexual issues with any chronic illness or disability could be addressed by all members of the rehabilitation healthcare team. Perhaps physicians would be best in addressing the effects of medications and problems with chronic illness. Physical therapists could focus on bed and wheelchair mobility during sexual activities. Occupational therapists, with their expertise in activities of daily living and cognitive impairment, may focus on managing the fine motor skills and cognitive aspects of sex and intimacy. For example, one quadriplegic said he believed he had truly been "rehabilitated" when he learned to unhook a bra with his teeth. Speech and language pathologists may focus on communication issues involving sex. For example, one aphasic stroke survivor and his partner had a special sign they shared to say "I love you." Each would point to the other, then make a fist and tap his or her own chests. The message was "you are in my heart."

Anecdotal reports and some literature show that indeed physical therapists, occupational therapists, and speech and language pathologists are asked by patients about sexual issues. Social workers and psychologists can provide counseling on intimacy and how to maintain relationships with chronic illnesses and disability. Recreational therapists can assist couples to adapt their leisure activities, especially those that have been coupled with intimacy. Kautz (1995) found that couples with chronic illnesses who continued to share leisure activities were more likely to be satisfied with both intimacy and sex.

Rehabilitation nurses can address bowel and bladder issues related to sex as well as many of the issues mentioned previously. Case managers and team coordinators can support the interventions that are implemented and address any remaining or unresolved issues. However, the type of holistic team care requires that all team members are adequately prepared and willing to address sexual concerns, which is not currently the case. For this reason, nurses can address all these sexual concerns.

ADDRESSING SEXUAL CONCERNS FROM AN EVIDENCE-BASED PRACTICE PERSPECTIVE

Reviewing research literature led Steinke (2008) and Wilmoth (2007) to determine that those with disabilities and chronic illnesses want information to help them cope with and overcome sex and intimacy problems. When sexual issues are addressed, one option practitioners have is to refer couples to websites and written materials related to the couple's specific areas of concern. This is the approach taken in this chapter. Unfortunately, there are several problems in documenting the effectiveness of this approach. First, those producing sex and intimacy resources rarely indicate how the information in their resources was obtained. The following questions should be asked: Did those with the disabilities report what helped them? Did the authors come up with these recommendations themselves? Second, the evidence for the information provided to assist in overcoming sexual problems is likely not to have been tested through research. Because the disabled person and his or her sexual partner may not be able to have sex in the days after receipt of the information, nurses likely do not know whether or not the interventions were effective. Finally, sex and intimacy issues are so complicated that it may be impossible to tell what is causing a couple's specific problems. Additionally, those who have overcome problems may not be able to specifically identify what helped them.

SEXUAL DEVELOPMENT IN CHILDREN: NURSING INTERVENTIONS

Nurses who work with children with disabilities may not believe that this chapter has any relevance for them. Yet, sexual development starts at a very early age, and some children with disabilities and chronic illnesses will have questions about sexuality and intimacy. Nurses working with children need to be sure to include parents in these discussions. Some topics may include the following: Do children who are disabled grow up to be lovers? How can children protect themselves against sexual abuse? What do disabled children need to know about dating and contraception? Can people with disabilities be good parents?

Sexual development begins at birth. Babies are raised as girls or boys and observe how girls and boys interact with each other. From birth, boys have erections, and girls experience vaginal lubrication. Toddlers may want to compare genitalia and learn the difference between boys and girls. Elementary school-aged children learn about sexual development of boys and girls, proper behavior for boys and girls, how adults who are in love interact, and the social norms for sex and intimacy.

Teens experience puberty and all the social norms that accompany the transition from being a child to being a teen who becomes like an adult in appearance. Yet all research shows that teens who wait until they are adults to become sexually active with others enjoy sex more and avoid the problems of pregnancy, sexual abuse, and sexually transmitted diseases—all of which are common in teens.

Young adults begin lifelong patterns of intimate relationships. Sexual development does not end there. Young adults may begin childbearing and raising children. Middle-aged adults learn how to balance intimacy, passion, lifelong commitments, work, and raising families. Older adults learn to maintain intimacy as the body ages and may experience a maturing of sexual intimacy. Table 12.1 provides resources for each of these stages. For resources specific to sexuality and children with disabilities, visit http://www.med.umich.edu/yourchild//topics/disabsex.htm

At all stages of sexual development, nurses can assist children, adults, and parents to anticipate developmental changes in intimacy. Children need to learn about safe sex, delaying sex until adulthood, and how to prevent the spread of sexually transmitted diseases. (For information on specific sexually transmitted diseases, visit http://www.cdc.gov/std/default.htm.) Finally, children and adults need to learn how to protect themselves from physical, mental, and sexual abuse. (For information on preventing child abuse, visit the following websites: http://www.childwelfare.gov/preventing/ or http://www.cdc.gov/ViolencePrevention/childmaltreatment/. For information on the prevention of adult abuse and violence, visit http://www.cdc.gov/ViolencePrevention/index.html/.)

Although all children and adults need to protect themselves against diseases and abuse, there are heightened concerns for those with disabilities. In 2007, of the reported cases of child abuse, 7.6% were classified as sexual abuse. Of these cases, 35.3% were children between the ages of 12 and 15, 23.8% were between 8 and 11 years old, and 23.3% were between 4 and 7 years of age (U.S. Department of Health and Human Services, 2007). In a 2010 report to Congress, it was stated that 1.4

TABLE 12.1	Resources for Various Levels of Sexual Development	
Developmental Level	**Common Behaviors**	**Resources**
Preschool (<4 years)	Exploring and touching genital areas (in public or private)	http://nctsn.org/nctsn_assets/pdfs/caring/sexualdevelopmentandbehavior.pdf
	Showing genitals to others	http://www.cfchildren.org/issues/abuse/touchsaferules/
	Taking clothes off	http://www.cfchildren.org/issues/abuse/touchsafety/
	Attempting to see others naked	http://www.familiesaretalking.org
	Asking questions about their bodies	
	Talking with other children about bodily functions	
Young child (4–6 years)	Purposely masturbating (sometimes in public)	
	Attempting to see others naked	
	Mimicking behaviors such as kissing or holding hands	
	Talking about private parts	
	Exploring genitals with other children of similar age	
School-aged child (7–12 years)	Purposely masturbating (in private predominantly)	
	Playing games involving sexual behavior with other children of similar ages	
	Attempting to see others naked	
	Interest in pictures/other media that show nudity and sexual content	
	Wanting more privacy	
	Sexual attraction to peers	
Teen	Participating in sexual conversations with peers	http://www.focusas.com/SexualBehavior-Range.html
	Flirting and courtship with peers	
	Interest in pornography	
	Individual masturbation	
	Hugging, kissing, holding hands	
	Foreplay and masturbation with peers	
	Intercourse with one sexual partner at a time	
Young adult	Participate in sexual and emotional relationships	http://www.themediaproject.com/facts/development/18_over.htm
	Have defined their sexual orientation	
	Understand the connection between sexuality and commitment	

disabled children per 1,000 were at risk of being sexually abused (U.S. Department of Health and Human Services, 2010).

SEXUAL DEVELOPMENT IN OLDER ADULTS

Contrary to what some believe, adults continue to develop sexually throughout their lives. Chronic illnesses have the potential to affect sexual function, and the older adult who continues to have sex may need to adapt to many changes. Most adults over 65 were raised not to talk about sex, and they may not talk with their partners about their sexual desires or preferences. They may see this silence as a way of protecting their partner, even though the silence results in loss of intimacy (Kautz, 1995).

A misconception that may be held by younger nurses is that because older adults do not talk about sex, they know very little about sex. However, the oldest among us have lived through several sexual revolutions and are much more informed than many believe. The first sexual revolution was in the roaring 20s, when women earned the right to vote and gained a great deal of sexual freedom. The second came shortly after World War II, when Kinsey published *Sexuality in the Human Male* in 1948 and *Sexuality in the Human Female* in 1952. The third was in the 1960s and early 1970s with the advent of the birth control pill and legalization of abortion. A fourth revolution occurred with the discovery of HIV, which led to the promotion of safe sex and the use of condoms. Some might argue that another sexual revolution is occurring now due to the advent of better treatments for erectile dysfunction and vaginal dryness and the constant barrage of television, newspaper, magazine, and website ads for products to treat these problems.

TRIPHASIC SEXUAL RESPONSE

Kaplan (1990), building on early work by Masters and Johnson, identified a triphasic model of **human sexual response**. The three phases are **desire**, **excitement**, and **orgasm**. The desire phase includes the sensations that move one to seek sexual pleasure. Sexual desire is probably stimulated by endorphins, and pleasure centers are stimulated by sex, whereas pain inhibits sexual desire. Love is a powerful stimulus to sexual desire. The excitement phase primarily occurs due to myotonia, or increased muscle tone and vasodilation of the genital blood vessels. In men the penis becomes erect. In women the vagina becomes lubricated, the clitoris and vagina become longer and wider, and the labia minora extend outward. Sexual excitement is controlled by the sympathetic nervous system, and fear inhibits sexual excitement. The orgasm phase is a climactic release of the genital vasodilation and myotonia of the excitement phase. Orgasm is an automatic spinal reflex response. Typically, sexual problems can be classified as either desire, excitement, or orgasm phase disorders, or combinations of the three.

Desire, excitement, and orgasm phase problems are common in adults at all ages. The most common problem is a lack of desire, due to fatigue, work, and family pressures. All adults who wish to maintain intimate relationships need to remember that love is a verb and requires daily action to ensure that love stays alive. Harry

Kautz told his son, Don, on his wedding day, "the key to any relationship is to show your love every day, whether or not you are feeling that love." Love has been shown to increase sexual desire, and, conversely, sex increases love. The most common sexual excitement problems are vaginal dryness and erectile dysfunction, which are discussed later in the chapter. The most common orgasm phase problems in adults are **inorgasmia** (the lack of orgasm) in women and **premature ejaculation** in men. Inorgasmia in women may be caused by premature ejaculation in men. Table 12.2 provides resources for information and comfortable positions for intercourse, and Table 12.3 contains a list of reputable sex education websites where resources can be obtained to overcome all these problems.

Changes in Sexual Response due to Neurological Disabilities

Spinal cord injury, stroke, head injury, cancers of the brain and spinal cord, and degenerative neurological disorders (e.g., multiple sclerosis, Parkinson's disease, dementias) change the neurological component of the sexual response. Paralysis and loss of sensation, whether bilateral in spinal cord injury, unilateral in stroke, and/or some variation of the two, which may occur with head injury, or due to peripheral neurological damage, frequently impairs either the excitement phase (erections and vaginal lubrication) or orgasm. (See Chapter 15 on stroke, Chapter 16 on brain injury, and Chapter 17 on spinal cord injury for more information on the specific types of impairments.)

TABLE 12.2   Resources for Information and Comfortable Positions for Intercourse

Being close. COPD and intimacy. Available from http://lungline.njc.org

Chronic low back pain and how it may affect sexuality. Available from http://ukhealthcare.uky.edu/patiented/booklets.htm

Sex and arthritis. Available from http://www.orthop.washington.edu

Sex after stroke. Available from http://www.strokeassociation.org

Sex and cancer (several Web articles by American Cancer Society). Available from http://www.cancer.org

Intimacy and diabetes. Available from http://www.netdoctor.co.uk

TABLE 12.3 Sex Education Websites
The following are a few professional websites that are highly recommended by the authors for people with disabilities and elders to obtain sex education materials. Reassure patients and their partners that these are legitimate sex education websites and are not "porno sites."
http://www.goodvibes.com
http://www.hivwisdom.org (HIV wisdom for older women)
http://www.womenshealth.org
http://www.erectile-dysfunction-impotence.org
http://marriage.about.com
http://www.sexualhealth.com (Sexual Health Network)
www.4woman.gov (Sexuality and disability for women)
Sex after stroke
http://www.aphasia.ca
http://www.stroke.org
http://stroke.about.com
Sex and chronic illness
http://www.arthritis.org
http://www.diabetes.org
http://www.tiny.cc/sexafterMI

Changes in Sexual Response due to Aging

Changes in sexual response have for decades been considered normal consequences of aging. Desire may or may not change with aging; levels of desire may remain the same throughout life. However, both men and women experience changes in excitement with age. Achieving an erection may require more direct stimulation and take longer, and the erection may be softer. Ejaculation may not be as forceful, and it may not occur with every sexual encounter. Vaginal lubrication is often decreased, and women find the need for more direct stimulation. Orgasms for women include uterine contractions, and changes in the uterus may change the way an orgasm feels.

Responses to Changes in Sexual Response in the Elderly and in Those with Disabilities

Those with chronic illnesses, disabilities, and advanced age differ greatly in their response to physiological changes in sexual response. Some couples adapt by increased genital fondling and caressing, taking more time, and paying more attention to each other's needs. Sex may be better than before the changes. This is a key piece of information: Research has shown many couples report that sex is actually better after a disability or as they age. For example, rehab practitioners who began their careers in the 1980s were told that men with spinal cord injury were sterile, yet some men with spinal cord injuries who are sexually persistent have been able to reach orgasm and father children. One man with a spinal cord injury who initially was unable to achieve an erection but was able to later perform and father children jokingly referred to sex as "physical therapy for my penis."

Other couples may welcome an end to sex. Still others may transcend the need for sex and actually become closer (Kautz, 1995). If an elder abstains from sex for months to years when in a sexless relationship or due to loss of a sexual partner, desire will eventually decrease. This loss of sexual desire has been thought to be permanent; however, there are anecdotal reports that when a person who has not been involved in a sexual relationship for many years meets a new partner, desire will return. When those who have stopped having sex for many years start with a new partner, some regain erectile function and vaginal lubrication after several weeks of manual or oral genital stimulation. Still others may seek help from their healthcare provider, which has led to what some call the **Viagra** revolution, or what MacDougall (2006) described as a remaking of the "real man." According to the Viagra website, 20 million men have had "the Viagra conversation" (www.viagra.com).

VAGINAL DRYNESS AND ERECTILE DYSFUNCTION

The decreased ability of a man to achieve and maintain an erection and decreased ability of a woman to achieve vaginal lubrication have, for decades, been considered normal consequences of aging (Ebersole, Hess, Touhy, Jett, & Luggen 2007). As with most changes associated with aging, changes in sexual function may begin as early as age 40, and they occur in almost every adult by age 80. One study of a diverse sample of 3,005 adults aged 57 to 85 identified several problems (Lindau et al., 2007). Among women, 43% complained of low desire, 39% complained of vaginal dryness, and 34% had problems with orgasm. Erectile dysfunction (37%) was the most common problem among men, and estimates vary as to the percentage of men who seek treatment. One expert estimated that less than 50% of men (Steggall, 2007) and women seek treatment (Malatesta, 2007), either because of embarrassment or because they are not bothered by the problems. Some may not discuss the issue with their partners.

Current recommendations for the therapeutic management of **erectile dysfunction** and vaginal dryness include stopping smoking, drinking only a moderate amount of alcohol, exercising more, and reducing obesity, especially belly fat. The physiological rationale for this is that smoking, obesity, and a sedentary lifestyle increase atherosclerosis in genital blood vessels, and there is excellent evidence that smoking cessation, losing weight, and doing aerobic exercises reverse this process. Vaginal dryness in women is the physiological correlate of erectile dysfunction in men, and thus it is possible that the same illnesses and lifestyle habits are correlated with vaginal dryness in women.

The introduction of sildenafil (Viagra) in 1998 and more recently vardenafil (Levitra) and tadalafil (Cialis) have changed the norms for sexual dysfunction. (For more information on these medications, see Cranwell-Bruce, 2010.) The constant barrage of ads in print media and junk mail, on television, and through Internet providers imply that erectile dysfunction is common, almost expected, and it is the norm is to seek treatment. Twenty years ago erectile dysfunction and vaginal dryness may have been a private matter for a couple. However, it is now literally impossible for couples to escape these media blitzes. Ads put pressure on men and women who otherwise might not have considered treatment or not thought the problem was important to seek treatment (Hanash, 2008). In addition, a woman may not want sex anymore, but she may go along when the man seeks treatment because she believes that whether or not they have sex is the man's decision (Kautz, 1995). Traditionally, vaginal dryness has been treated with lubricants or the oral or cream form of estrogen. Although there are no medications for women that are direct corollaries of Viagra, Levitra, and Cialis, women are bombarded with ads to relieve vaginal dryness and increase sexual desire with hormonal medications and nutritional/natural supplements. There are also constant ads for nutritional supplements and natural remedies for erectile dysfunction.

Clinical literature has long recommended that maintaining a healthy lifestyle leads to more satisfying sexual relationships. Many reputable websites, maintained by healthcare organizations including the Mayo Clinic and Dr. Orinsh, and self-help groups such as the Diabetes and Heart Associations advocate healthy behaviors as a first step in overcoming problems with erections and vaginal dryness. Nurses can focus patient education on the adoption of healthy behaviors as one step in overcoming sexual dysfunction. Because both erectile dysfunction and vaginal dryness may be early signs of hypertension, heart disease, dementia, or diabetes and in fact are predictive of heart disease and stroke (O'Sullivan & Savage, 2009), all patients should be told to see their physician for problems with erectile dysfunction or vaginal dryness to ensure there are not underlying problems and to explore all treatment options.

Belly fat, especially a waist of over 40 inches in either men or women, has been associated with both erectile dysfunction and vaginal dryness. Loss of belly fat, when combined with exercise, is an effective treatment for erectile dysfunction (McCoid, 2007) in men and vaginal dryness in women (Malatesta, 2007). Loss of belly fat is recommended in the clinical literature, on reputable websites, and in books (Edgson & Marber, 2004; Kleiner & O'Connell, 2006) as a way to increase erectile ability in men and vaginal lubrication in women. Similarly, adopting the Mediterranean diet, which also decreases belly fat, has been shown to increase erectile ability (Giugliano, Giugliano, & Esposito, 2006).

Although studies have examined the effectiveness of Viagra in improving both erectile function and quality of life in men, little is known about couples' experiences with these medications. Men receive the prescription for Viagra, but it is possible that women may be the ones taking the medication. Researchers are now beginning to study the effectiveness of Viagra in women (Basson, McInnes, Smith, Hodgson, & Koppiker, 2002). Dr. Irwin Goldstein, director of the Institute of Sexual Medicine at Boston University School of Medicine, has suggested that women use Viagra for vaginal dryness (Kautz & Upadhyaya, 2010). It is also unclear whether couples use lubricants during intercourse to help the man achieve an erection through stimulation or to assist the woman to overcome vaginal dryness.

Finally, the differences in views and experiences of men and women are unknown. Most studies of Viagra have only examined the men taking it, not their partners. One study noted a dearth of information on the perspectives and experiences of women whose partners take Viagra and found several detrimental effects for women when their partners took Viagra (Potts, Gavey, Grace, & Vares, 2003). Rehabilitation nurses should be reminded of the side effects of Viagra, especially cardiovascular effects, so that users can be informed about adverse reactions or potential drug–drug interactions that could worsen existing conditions or put a person at risk for additional health problems. Table 12.4 provides a list of medication that could affect sexual function.

TABLE 12.4 Medications and Sexual Functioning
The following groups of medications have been shown to contribute to sexual dysfunction by decreasing sexual desire in men and women, promoting vaginal dryness in women or erectile dysfunction in men, or causing delayed or absent orgasm in men or women. These sexual side effects may lessen 6 to 8 weeks after starting the medication. If the sexual dysfunction persists, a general recommendation for those experiencing sexual dysfunction is to contact the healthcare provider who prescribed the medication and ask if a different medication from the same class or another class can be prescribed. Sometimes, despite changing medications the side effects persist, and the person taking the medication will need to seek treatment for the sexual dysfunction.
Antidepressants: including tricyclics, monoamine oxidase inhibitors, and selective serotonin reuptake inhibitors; especially decreasing sexual desire in women and delayed or absent orgasm in both men and women
Antihypertensives: especially thiazide diuretics and beta-blockers. Centrally acting alpha receptor blockers and peripherally acting antiadrenergics may also cause problems
Anticholinergics: probanthine and atropine
Anticonvulsants: phenytoin, phenobarbital, carbamazepine
H_2 blocking agents: cimetidine, ranitidine
Lipid-lowering agents: niacin, clofibrate
Digoxin
Opioids

Sources: Bostwick, J. M. (2010). A generalist's guide to treating patients with depression with an emphasis on using side effects to tailor antidepressant therapy. *Mayo Clinic Proceedings, 85,* 538–550; Ginsberg, T. B. (2010). Male sexuality. *Clinics in Geriatric Medicine, 26,* 185–195; Krychman, M. L., & Kellogg-Spadt, S. (2009). Female sexual dysfunction: Working toward new understanding. *Women's Health Care: A Practical Journal for Nurse Practitioners, 8*(5), 37–48; Mintzer, S. (2010). Metabolic consequences of antiepileptic drugs. *Current Opinion in Neurology, 23,* 164–169.

PROMOTING SEXUAL PLEASURE IN THOSE WITH DISABILITIES RESIDING IN THE COMMUNITY

Nurses can have a tremendous impact in assisting those who reside in the community and wish to maintain sexual function in spite of myriad health problems and physical limitations. Those who wish to maintain an active sex life need to learn to overcome and compensate for the changes. Articles have been written by nurses to assist clients to overcome sexual problems due to stroke (Kautz, 2007), heart and lung disease (Steinke, 2005) (see Box 12.1), and the sexual problems of psychotropic medications taken to treat depression (Kennedy & Rizvi,

2009). Whatever the underlying cause(s), major obstacles to sexual intimacy that need to be overcome include fatigue, pain, mobility difficulties, finding comfortable positions for giving and receiving of pleasure, and memory and attention problems. These obstacles may occur for either men or women and for either one partner or both. However, there are practical ways to help overcome these problems. Tell couples that what works for one couple may or may not work for another. Encourage them to try different activities until they find one that both works and is acceptable to them. Trying something new may increase intimacy and sexual excitement!

BOX 12.1 Web Exploration 12.1
Visit http://www.tiny.cc/sexafterMI to find the common sexual and intimacy recommendations for people who have had a myocardial infarction.

Overcoming Fatigue and Pain

Overcoming fatigue and pain is essential to feeling desire and having the stamina to give and receive pleasure. Common ways to overcome fatigue are to plan for sex when rested, which is often in the morning. Another key factor is to plan one's activities to save some time and energy for pleasure.

Pain is a hallmark of a disability. Back and neck injuries, spinal cord injuries, head injuries, arthritis, and other chronic illnesses may have a chronic pain component that lasts until one dies. Most pain management strategies leave some residual pain, which may interfere with sexual desire and sexual excitement. The irritability, fatigue, and depression that accompany chronic pain can also have an impact on a couple's sexual relationship. Recommendations include planning for sex at a time when the pain is at its lowest level, often mid-morning for those with rheumatoid arthritis or when pain medications have their peak action (Newman, 2007). Incorporating massage, a hot bath for chronic arthritic pain, or cold packs for acute inflammation or using an electric massager or vibrator may relax sore muscles, relieve stiffened joints, and, when done with a partner, stimulate sexual excitement. Women may focus the water jets from a hot tub on their clitoris, and both men and women may use the vibrator for sexual stimulation. Anecdotal reports from those with arthritis suggest that the relaxing effects of these pain relief strategies and orgasm actually relieve chronic pain for many hours. This effect is thought to be due to endorphin release during the relaxing treatment and sexual stimulation.

Overcoming Mobility Difficulties (Paralysis, Spasticity, and Dyskinesias)

Those with spinal cord injuries, head injuries, stroke, multiple sclerosis, cerebral palsy, Parkinson's disease, and other musculoskeletal disorders may have the inability to move body parts to a specific sexual position or respond to a partner in a physically desired manner. Muscles spasms may also inhibit attempts at specific desired sexual positions. Several authors have addressed these issues (Kautz, Van Horn, & Moore, 2009; Moore, 2007; Parkinson's Disease Foundation, 2007, 2009). For some, exercising and stretching and taking medication for pain and muscle spasms approximately 20 minutes before planned sexual activities may be helpful. Arm and leg weights may be used to assist with the control of spasms. Alternate sexual positions, including side-lying, may be helpful. Many report that although sexual intercourse is no longer pleasurable, holding hands, cuddling, and sharing intimate moments are very satisfying.

Adopting New Positions and Learning New Techniques for Lovemaking

Because of limitations from disease and disability, some with chronic illnesses and disabilities need to adopt new positions for lovemaking. Table 12.5 lists resources that give suggestions for comfortable positions as well as additional information about sex and intimacy for specific chronic illnesses. The illustrations in Figure 12.1 provide examples of positions for intercourse when adapting to chronic illness or disability. For example, individuals with shortness of breath may have decreased stamina for sex and a decrease in sexual desire. Recommendations to overcome these problems include communicating with one's sexual partner about endurance and trying alternative sexual positions that reduce the amount of physical exertion necessary for sexual activity. These positions also facilitate the use of oxygen during sex. Note that shortness of breath is common with cardiac and lung disease as well as neurological diseases that impact breathing, including myasthenia gravis or quadriplegia after spinal cord injury. Thus, adopting these alternative positions is a recommendation that can be made to those with a wide variety of chronic illnesses and disabilities.

Overcoming Poor Attention Span, Memory Loss, and Loss of Initiative

Those with multiple sclerosis, head injury, stroke, or Parkinson's disease may miss subtle verbal and nonverbal sex and intimacy clues between partners or may be unable to focus on sexual activities. On the other hand, those who have memory loss or a poor attention span may pressure a partner for frequent sex. Some may lack the cognitive ability to take an active role in creating the mood for sexual or intimate activities. Anderson et al. (in press), the Patient Resource Center (2009), and the Parkinson's Disease Foundation (2007, 2009) recommend decreasing distractions during sexual activity, such as turning television and music off, using low lighting, and choosing a calm time of the day for intimacy and sexual activity. For those who request frequent sex, keeping a log or diary of sexual activities may help. Couples may find a sexual log a wonderful reminder of nice times they have shared. For those with a loss of initiative, the unaffected partner may need to be the primary initiator and provide a romantic environment. Couples may find creating an intimate setting to be a highlight of sexual activity.

TABLE 12.5 Books and Video Resources on Sexuality and Disability
For a comprehensive list of materials, go to the Association of Rehabilitation Nurses website (www.rehabnurse.org) and find the resource list "ARN 2009: Hope for Love: Practical Advice for Intimacy and Sex" compiled by Catherine Moore.
Books
Kaufman, M., Silverber, C., & Odette, F. (2007). *The ultimate guide to sex and disability: For all of us who live with disabilities, chronic pain & illness.* San Francisco: Cleis Press.
Kroll, K., & Klein, E. L. (2001). *Enabling romance: A guide to love sex, and relationships for people with disabilities (and those who care about them).* Bethesada, MD: No Limits Communications.
Schweir, K. M., & Hingsburger, D. (2000). *Sexuality: Your sons and daughters with intellectual disabilities.* Baltimore, MD: Brookes Publishing Company.
Videos & Webcasts
National Multiple Sclerosis Society: *Sex and Intimacy.* See resources at http://www.nationalmssociety.org/living-with-multiple-sclerosis/relationships/intimacy/index.aspx
University of Alabama at Birmingham (2005). *Sexuality and Sexual Function with SCI.* Go to http://www.spinalcord.uab.edu/show.asp?durki=97417 for information on ordering the video series.
Kessler Medical Rehabilitation Research and Education Corporation (1992). *Sexuality Reborn.* Available from Kessler Medical Rehabilitation Research and Education Corp.

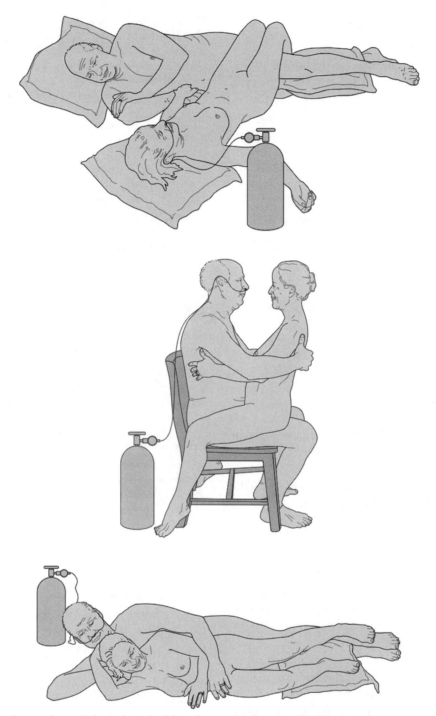

FIGURE 12.1   Positions that may be used when either or both have decreased endurance, COPD, hip or knee replacement, or stroke. Those with GERD may find sitting in the chair will not exacerbate their symptoms.

Source: Mauk, K. L. (2010). Gerontological Nursing: Competencies for Care. Sudbury, MA: Jones and Bartlett.

Communication Problems

Those with aphasia from a stroke or with impaired communication or speech as a result of a head injury or degenerative diseases, including multiple sclerosis and Parkinson's disease, may need to find ways to express intimate feelings and communicate sexual desire to their partners. Lemieurx, Cohen-Schneider, & Holzapfel (2001) developed and tested tools to help couples when the stroke survivor has aphasia to communicate about sex. Box 12.2 provides a website with further information on assessing sexual health in those with aphasia.

BOX 12.2   Web Exploration

Visit http://www.aphasia.ca to find the tools developed for a nurse to use in assessing sexual health in a person who is aphasic.

Bowel and Bladder Dysfunction

Those with urinary incontinence or bladder dysfunction should empty their bladder before sexual intercourse and then drink a glass of fluids after intercourse to reduce the occurrence of urinary tract infection (Anderson et al., in press; Parkinson's Disease Foundation, 2007). The management of indwelling catheters was addressed previously in the first section, Sexuality and Intimacy.

For those with bowel dysfunction due to a disability, maintaining a bowel elimination routine avoids discomfort from bowel distension and accidental leakage during sexual activities. Persons should consider their bowel routine when planning sexual activities and plan these activities for a time when the bowel is empty.

RESOURCES FOR COUPLES WHO WANT MORE INFORMATION

Table 12.5 contains a list of books, videos, and webcasts that may be of assistance for nurses who wish to address sexual concerns as well as patients and their partners. Some rehabilitation facilities have regularly scheduled sex and intimacy classes for patients and their partners. Some show sex education videos developed to assist the disabled and their partners. If therapists and nurses or couples are uncomfortable viewing the videos at rehabilitation centers, then the videos should be available for couples to view at home.

PROMOTING ROMANTIC AND SEXUAL RELATIONSHIPS IN REHABILITATION FACILITIES

Another issue that is rarely addressed in the literature is intimacy and sex among adults residing in long-term care facilities and rehabilitation centers. Barriers exist in virtually all facilities, including lack of privacy and door locks, lack of queen size beds, and literally lack of opportunities for romance. Inability to leave a facility overnight without "losing the bed" prevents couples who have had long-term relationships from getting away for even one night. Although it is important for staff to protect patients from sexual abuse and ensure safety, policies and environmental design go overboard to prevent intimacy. Studies confirm that staff members continue to be uncomfortable with sexual behavior of those in long-term care facilities (Bouman, Arcelus & Benbow, 2006; Roach, 2004). A timeless story of love in a nursing home, *The Notebook* by Nicolas Sparks (1999), shows us what is possible if nursing staff respect the rights and privacy of those who have entrusted us with the last years of their lives.

Some staff may actually promote romance and sex in long-term care, but they may not reveal these efforts for fear of reprisal. The American Medical Directors Association of long-term care facilities have developed policies that are available on their website, *Caring for the ages*, at www.amda.com/caring/february2002/sex.htm. Messinger-Rapport, Sandhu and Hujer (2003) provide guidelines for sex in the nursing home, taking into account the issues of what to do if a resident is cognitively impaired, what are the health needs of the residents, and how to keep the staff informed so that the privacy of the couple can be maintained. These materials can be adapted for use in other rehabilitation facilities. The authors recommend the video, *Freedom of sexual expression: Dementia and resident rights in long term care facilities*, developed by the Hebrew Home for the Aged, a facility that is nationally known for its policies of promoting intimacy between residents. (Their current policies and information about the video can be obtained at http://www.hebrewhome.org). This film and many others on a wide range of topics on aging, including intimacy and sexuality, are available through Terra Nova Films (www.terranova.org). Evidence-based practice guidelines are needed that balance safety with the lifelong need for intimacy. The need to be touched and held by someone who loves us and the need to feel loved, not just cared for, does not diminish with age or with physical or cognitive impairment (Edwards, 2004).

EXTINGUISHING SEXUALLY INAPPROPRIATE BEHAVIOR

Unfortunately, nursing staff may sometimes be confronted with either a man or a woman who displays sexually inappropriate behavior. Most incidents reported involve men, but women may display these behaviors as well. Sexually inappropriate behaviors include inappropriate language ("won't you get in the bed with me?"), inappropriate requests for personal care ("make sure and wash my penis really good"), inappropriate gestures ("sticking the tongue out and wiggling it at staff"), exposing one's self or masturbating in public places, and inappropriate touching (grabbing a breast or buttock when in close proximity). All these behaviors constitute sexual harassment and are not to be tolerated. These behaviors may reflect a power issue, a loss of inhibition due to cognitive impairment, or a combination of these. The behaviors make it difficult or impossible to care for the patient exhibiting them. The goal is to extinguish the behavior while maintaining the dignity of the patient.

Nursing staff need to confront the patient calmly and firmly, saying "This behavior is inappropriate, interferes with me doing my job, and will not be tolerated." Laughing it off, reacting violently, or showing anger all are likely to encourage the behavior. Saying, "Oh Mr. _____ you wouldn't know what to do even if you could," although meant lightheartedly, is demeaning and may encourage the patient to try the behavior with someone else. Ask other staff if the behavior is a pattern and be sure to inform others so they will not be caught off guard. One quadriplegic client told a nurse that he had rubbed the breasts of every nursing staff member on the unit with his upper arm when they were leaning over him to assist in dressing. He had gotten away with this behavior for weeks because the staff had not talked with each other about this behavior. The nurse informed the other staff, and two nursing staff firmly and compassionately confronted him together, and the behavior ended. Confronting him led several staff members to talk with him about his fears of dating and being seen as attractive, which was the underlying need behind this behavior.

Although extinguishing sexually inappropriate behavior is necessary to care for older adults, there is some good news about this behavior. It is an indicator of recovery in a client who has been too ill to think or worry about his or her sexuality. It may be an expression of power or anger, both of which are expressions of independence. Interest in sexuality can aid in the rehabilitation process. After confronting a patient and ensuring he or she is not going to act out again, the nurse can initiate discussions about recovery and how to take an active role in that process.

Confronting cognitively impaired clients who act out may be effective in extinguishing the behavior. If this strategy does not work, other strategies may extinguish the behavior. If a client has a habit of inappropriately touching staff during a bath or bed-to-chair transfer, put a washrag in the client's hand during the bath or place the patient's hand on the armrest to assist in the transfer.

Approach a client from the weaker side, which will both protect the staff member and discourage the client from acting out. Another strategy is to encourage appropriate behaviors and ignore inappropriate behaviors. In rehabilitative settings, rewarding appropriate behaviors can be included as a part of a behavioral modification program. If possible, get family involved in extinguishing the behavior. Do not assume that the behavior is a premorbid or lifelong behavior and try not to feed into perceptions of the client as a "dirty old man."

Another strategy is to avoid using language the client may misinterpret as sexual. Nurses typically say, "I am your nurse today," or "I am going to take care of you," both of which may be misinterpreted as flirting. Instead say, "I am going to work with you" or "I am going to assist you," which sound much more business-like. Lesser, Hughes, Jemelka, and Griffith (2005) outline pharmacological therapies that may be necessary when sexually inappropriate behaviors continue despite the interventions already outlined above.

DEALING WITH MASTURBATION IN PUBLIC PLACES IN HOSPITALS OR LONG-TERM CARE

Masturbation is self-limiting and has no known harmful effects. It does not spread sexually transmitted diseases, and it can be performed with minimal cognitive and hand function. However, masturbation is only appropriate in private. Public masturbation is best extinguished using the strategies previously described for sexually inappropriate behaviors. The goal is to allow privacy yet not draw undue attention. If "privacy" signs are necessary, keep them innocuous. Try to provide privacy even if clients' rooms are only semiprivate by giving the client some private time. Schover and Jenson (1988), who worked extensively with head injury survivors, noted that some clients benefited from an inflatable doll for which to have intercourse. Clients using sex toys or explicit materials should do so in private and store them in their own private space, away from public view.

PATIENTS DISPLAYING SEXUALLY EXPLICIT MATERIALS ON THE UNIT OR IN THE HOME

Display of sexually explicit materials is a problem that is ignored in the nursing literature. Nursing staff may need to set some ground rules with patients in regard to posters, jokes, magazines, or cards on display on the patient's room wall or on dressers or over-bed tables. Staff members need to recognize that although having these materials is the patient's choice, openly displaying them is a form of sexual harassment. A good rule is that materials with a PG-13 rating, such as the *Sports Illustrated* swimsuit issue, are acceptable, but those with naked bodies are not. Rules apply equally to men and women and apply regardless of the patient's sexual orientation. Rules also apply to staff areas; the inside of a staff members locker may be his or her private space, but when the door is open in a public lounge and others have to view the pictures, that is a form of sexual harassment. Pictures are not the only problem; get-well cards that overtly encourage sexual relationships with patients and nursing staff are also inappropriate. If a patient has displayed these materials, calmly tell the patient why they are inappropriate and encourage the patient or family to remove them. Use respect when approaching a patient about offensive material. It is the patient's home too, especially for a long rehabilitation stay. Try a compassionate approach first, focusing on your feelings. Keep the confrontation one on one if possible.

Occasionally, nursing staff who visit patients in their homes may encounter sexually explicit materials on display. Tell patients you cannot work with them in the rooms in which the materials are displayed. Negotiate with the patient for one room of the house where treatment can occur where there are no explicit materials.

SUMMARY

Each person has the right to be a sexual being. This is no less true for persons with chronic illness or disability. Sexuality is a part of the human makeup and needs to be addressed in holistic care. Rehabilitation nurses can play an important role in educating patients and families, directing them to medically correct information and resources and answering questions as needed. All rehabilitation nurses can participate in sexuality education through the first phase of the PLISSIT model by giving each patient permission to be a sexual being.

CRITICAL THINKING

1. Go to "Google" or another Internet search engine. Choose a chronic illness or disability that you wish to know more about. Search "sex and . . . (the chronic illness or disability you chose)." Find a patient education resource to help a patient and his or her partner

adapt to the changes they will experience. Share this resource with another nurse.
2. Talk with a person you know who has a chronic illness or disability about sexuality or intimacy issues. Did a healthcare provider talk with them? Have they found information from a website or self-help group? What information would they like?
3. Visit a local bookstore and go to the "sexuality" section. What books do they have available? Also go to the "self-help" or "disease management" section. Look for books on how to live with a chronic illness (e.g., cancer, heart disease, etc.) or a disability (e.g., spinal cord injury, multiple sclerosis, Parkinson's disease, etc.) What information does the book contain about sexuality and intimacy and relationships?

Personal Reflection

- Do you have any friends or relatives with disabilities or chronic illnesses? Have you ever talked with them about sex and intimacy issues? Would you be willing to share information in this chapter with them?
- What chronic illness(es) do you believe you might have later in your life? What do you believe your family history and current health conditions will make you susceptible to developing? How will your life change with this illness? How will the clinical manifestations of this illness change your relationship with others, especially an intimate partner? Would you be willing to make some of the adaptations recommended in this chapter?
- How might your own personal values facilitate or interfere in talking about sex or intimacy in those who are single? Married? Straight? Gay? Someone who is HIV positive?

REFERENCES

Anderson, C. D., Kautz, D. D., Bryant, S., & Clanin, N. (in press). Physical healthcare patterns and nursing interventions. In C. Jacelon (Ed.), *The specialty practice of rehabilitation nursing: A core curriculum* (6th ed.). Glenview, IL: Association of Rehabilitation Nurses.

Annon J. S. (1976). The PLISSIT model: A proposed conceptual scheme for the behavioral treatment of sexual problems. *Journal of Sex Education and Therapy, 2*(2), 1–15.

Basson, R., McInnes, R., Smith, M. D., Hodgson, G., & Koppiker, N. (2002). Efficacy and safety of sildenafil citrate in women with sexual dysfunction associated with female sexual arousal disorder. *Journal of Women's Health & Gender Based Medicine, 11*(4), 367–377.

Bauer, M., McAuliffe, L., & Nay, R. (2007). Sexuality, health care and the older person: An overview of the literature. *International Journal of Older People Nursing, 2*(1), 63–68.

Bouman, W. P., Arcelus, J., & Benbow, S. M. (2006). Nottingham Study of Sexuality & Ageing (NoSSA I). Attitudes regarding sexuality and older people: A review of the literature. *Sexuality and Relationship Therapy, 21*, 149–161.

Cranwell-Bruce, L. A. (2010). Drugs for erectile dysfunction. *MEDSURG Nursing, 19*, 185–191.

Ebersole, P., Hess, P., Touhy, T., Jett, K., & Luggen, A. S. (2007). *Towards healthy aging: Human needs and nursing response* (7th ed.). Philadelphia: Elsevier.

Edgson, V., & Marber, I. (2004). *The food doctor—fully revised and updated: Healing foods for the mind and body.* New York: Collins & Brown.

Edwards, D. J. (2004). Sex and intimacy in the nursing home. *Nursing Homes, 52*(2), 18–23.

Giugliano, D., Giugliano, F., & Esposito, K. (2006). Sexual dysfunction and the Mediterranean diet. *Public Health Nutrition, 9*, 1118–1120.

Hanash, K. A. (2008). *New frontiers in men's sexual health: Understanding erectile dysfunction and the revolutionary new treatments.* Westport, CT: Praegar Publishers.

Hardin, S. (2007). Cardiac disease and sexuality: Implications for research and practice. *Nursing Clinics of North America, 42*, 593–603.

Higgins, A., Barker, P., & Begley, C. M. (2006). Sexuality: The challenge to espoused holistic care. *International Journal of Nursing Practice, 12*, 345–351.

Kaplan, H. S. (1990). Sex, intimacy, and the aging process. *Journal of the American Academy of Psychoanalysis, 18*, 185–205.

Kautz, D. D. (1995). The maturing of sexual intimacy in chronically ill, older adult couples. Dissertation Abstracts International. Doctoral dissertation, University of Kentucky.

Kautz, D. D. (2007). Hope for love: Practical advice for intimacy and sex after stroke. *Rehabilitation Nursing, 32*, 95–103.

Kautz, D. D., Van Horn, E. R., & Moore, C. (2009). Sex after stroke: An integrative review and recommendations for clinical practice. *Critical Reviews in Physical and Rehabilitation Medicine, 21*(1), 25–41.

Kautz, D. D. & Upadhyaya, R. C. (2010). Appreciating diversity and enhancing intimacy. In K. L. Mauk (Ed.), *Gerontological Nursing: Competencies for Care* (pp. 602–627). Sudbury, MA: Jones and Bartlett.

Kennedy, S. H., & Rizvi, S. (2009). Sexual dysfunction, depression, and the impact of antidepressants. *Journal of Clinical Pharmacology, 29*, 157–164.

Kleiner, S. (2007). *The good mood diet: Feel great while you lose weight.* New York: Warner Books.

Kleiner, S., & O'Connell, J. (2006). *The powerfood nutrition plan: The guy's guide to getting stronger, leaner, smarter, healthier, better looking, better sex good!* Emmaus, PA: Rodale Press.

Lemieux, L., Cohen-Schneider, R., & Holzapfel, S. (2001). Aphasia and sexuality. *Sexuality and Disability, 19*(4), 253–266.

Lesser, J. M., Hughes, S. V., Jemelka, J. R., & Griffith, J. (2005). Sexually inappropriate behaviors: Assessment necessitates careful medical and psychological evaluation and sensitivity. *Geriatrics, 60*, 34–37.

Lindau, S. T., Schumm, L. P., Laumann, E. O., Levinson, W., O'Muircheataigh, C. A., & Waite, L. J. (2007). A study of sexuality and health among older adults in the United States. *New England Journal of Medicine, 357*, 762–774.

MacDougall, R. (2006). Remaking the real man: Erectile dysfunction palliatives and the social re-construction of the male heterosexual life cycle. *Sexuality and Culture, 10*(3), 59–90.

Magnan, M. A., Reynolds, K. E., & Galvin, E. A. (2005). Barriers to addressing patient sexuality in nursing practice. *Dermatology Nursing, 18*, 448–454.

Malatesta, V. J. (2007). Sexual problems, women and aging: An overview. *Mental Health Issues of Older Women: A Comprehensive Review for Health Care Professionals, 19*, 139–154.

McAuliffe, L., Bauer, M., & Nay, R. (2007). Barriers to the expression of sexuality in the older person. *International Journal of Older People Nursing, 2*, 69–75.

McCoid, J. D. (2007). Therapeutic management of erectile dysfunction. *Nurse Prescribing, 5*, 143–147.

Messinger-Rapport, B. J., Sandhu, S. K., & Hujer, M. E. (2003). Sex and sexuality: Is it over after 60? *Clinical Geriatrics, 11*(10), 45–53.

Mick, J. M. (2007). Sexuality assessment: 10 strategies for improvement. *Clinical Journal of Oncology Nursing, 11*, 671–675.

Moore, L. A. (2007). Intimacy and multiple sclerosis. *Nursing Clinics of North America, 42*, 606–619.

Newman, A. M. (2007). Arthritis and sexuality. *Nursing Clinics of North America, 42*, 621–630.

O'Sullivan, B., & Savage, E. (2009). Erectile dysfunction and CHD: Related risk factors and implications for nursing practice. *British Journal of Cardiovascular Nursing, 4*, 170–176.

Parkinson's Disease Foundation. (2007). Parkinson's disease Q & A (5th ed.). Retrieved July 1, 2010, from http://www.pdf.org/pdf/PDF_QA_07_Final.pdf

Parkinson's Disease Foundation. (2009). Medications. Retrieved July 1, 2010, from http://www.pdf.org/en/meds_treatments

Patient Resource Center. (2009). *Patient resource cancer guide: A treatment and facilities guide for patients and their families.* Retrieved November 9, 2009, from http://patientresource.net/Cognitive_Dysfunction.aspx

Potts, A., Gavey, N., Grace, V. M., & Vares, T. (2003). The downside of Viagra, women's experiences and concerns. *Sociology of Health & Illness, 25*, 697–719.

Roach, S. M. (2004). Sexual behaviour of nursing home residents: Staff perceptions and responses. *Journal of Advanced Nursing, 48*, 317–379.

Schover, I. R., & Jenson, S. B. (1988). *Sexuality and chronic illness: A comprehensive approach.* New York: Guilford Press.

Sexuality Information and Education Council of the United States. (n.d.). Retrieved July 1, 2010, from http://www.familiesaretalking.org.

Sparks, N. (1999). *The Notebook*. New York: Warner Books.

Steggall, M. J. (2007). Erectile dysfunction: Physiology, causes and patient management. *Nursing Standard, 21*(43), 49–56.

Steinke, E. E. (2008). Evidence-based guideline: Sexual counseling. In B. Ackley, G. Ladwig, B. A. Swan, & S. Tucker (Eds.), *Evidence-based nursing care guidelines: Medical-surgical interventions* (pp. 744–750). St. Louis, MO: Mosby.

Steinke, E. E. (2005). Intimacy needs and chronic illness: Strategies for sexual-counseling and self-management. *Journal of Gerontological Nursing, 31*(5), 40–50.

U.S. Department of Health and Human Resources. (2007). Child maltreatment 2007. Retrieved July 1, 2010, from http://www.acf.hhs.gov/programs/cb/pubs/cm07/cm07.pdf

U.S. Department of Health and Human Resources. (2010). Fourth national incidence study of child abuse and neglect (NIS-4): Report to Congress. Retrieved July 1, 2010, from http://www.acf.hhs.gov/programs/opre/abuse_neglect/natl_incid/nis4_report_exec_summ_pdf_jan2010.pdf

Wilmoth, M. C. (Ed.). (2007). Sexuality and chronic illness: Assessment and interventions. *Nursing Clinics of North America, 42*, 507–514.

CHAPTER 13

Educating Clients and Families

Pam Farrell
Robin Raptosh

LEARNING OBJECTIVES

At the end of this chapter, the reader will be able to

- Define the impact of health literacy and sociocultural beliefs on client/caregiver education and adherence.
- Explain the role of education in preventive health care and health maintenance.
- Describe how learning occurs and how new memories are laid down and retrieved.
- List strategies for determining learning needs and learner readiness.
- State guidelines for developing outcome-oriented learning goals with clients/caregivers.
- Discuss nursing diagnoses and interventions related to client/caregiver education.
- Identify strategies for evaluating effectiveness of teaching.

KEY CONCEPTS AND TERMS

Activation of prior knowledge	Encoding	Intrinsic load
Adult learning theory	Expertise reversal effect	Locus of control
Andragogy	Extraneous load	Motivational interviewing
Attention	Extrinsic load	Retrieval
Cognitive dissonance	Geragogy	Schema
Cognitive load theory	Health belief model	Self-efficacy
Elaboration and rehearsal	Health literacy	Working memory

They never told us anything! Regardless of the time spent educating and the resources used, all too often this is the response of clients and caregivers in the months after receipt of care by the rehabilitation team. Why?

A small study of clients with brain injury and their family caregivers is just one of many to investigate this issue. Interviews with the clients and family caregivers between ten months and two years after injury were compared with interviews of rehabilitation staff and their documentation (Paterson, Kieloch, & Gmiterek, 2001). Providers indicated that education was extensive. Written material explaining traumatic brain injury and listing resources was provided and discussed with the family during rehabilitation care and sent to the home after discharge. Yet, only *one* family member could recall receiving information about resources and services, and most families remained uncertain about

the patient's condition and health implications. Is this simply a case of poor adherence? Differences in client perception point to barriers associated with educating clients during extremely stressful situations. This study (Paterson, Kieloch, & Gmiterek, 2001), like others, identified the emotional state of the learner as a barrier to learning and inconsistency, poor timing, and a lack of relevance to the *learner's* perceived needs as additional factors contributing to the learner's inability to retrieve and use information (Bastable, 2006; Paterson, Kieloch, & Gmiterek, 2001).

Reductions in length of stay, increases in acuity, movement of the patient across the continuum of care, and decreased access to resources have changed the face of care delivery and created barriers to patient and caregiver education, in spite of the expansion of information via a wide variety of media. When clients and caregivers indicate they have no memory of being taught, in spite of extensive effort by the healthcare team, providers become frustrated, wondering why they were so ineffective. Unfortunately, many members of the team are ill-prepared for client and caregiver teaching in the current healthcare environment (Hoeman, 2008). Hoving, Visser, Mullen, and van den Borne (2010) analyzed the delivery of healthcare education over the last 50 years, observing a shift from authority to shared decision-making models. But, they point out that the most significant challenge of the future is that both clients and healthcare providers need to develop skills to optimize the process of client education. Not only are healthcare providers poorly prepared in how to best teach clients, clients do not know how to learn.

Healthcare education is a requirement of every setting in the continuum of care. No single entity in the continuum has the time or resources to do it all. This variety of care providers can add additional barriers when educational messaging is inconsistent between team members and between the different care settings. Education is more effective when all healthcare providers within the continuum coordinate educational efforts and recognize that each contact with the client or caregiver is a teachable moment in which role modeling, knowledge-sharing, and skill development can occur.

The rehabilitation team considers a person's learning styles, needs, strengths, and preferences before teaching begins. The Commission on Accreditation of Rehabilitation Facilities (CARF) standards also requires the team to assess the effectiveness of education and to focus on improvement of educational efforts if learning outcomes are not achieved. Education is targeted at an identified need that can include, but is not limited to, prevention of recurrence and complications, primary healthcare needs, utilization of health resources, health promotion, and needed skills for discharge. To meet accreditation standards, a mechanism is required for each client to demonstrate skills achieved before discharge. Simply teaching and documenting that the activity of educating has occurred is not sufficient.

The effective healthcare professional participating in client and caregiver education is aware that *teaching occurs to support a change in behavior*. Evaluation must then assess whether that change in behavior has occurred and whether the client/caregiver has the resources to sustain the identified behaviors. This requires awareness of available resources, knowledge of how learning occurs, the ability to exploit learning strategies to facilitate the learner's retrieval of learned skills and knowledge, and the ability to prioritize learning goals for each step in the continuum of care. Coordination and consistency in messaging across the team and across the continuum is critical to high-quality outcomes. When the behavior of the learner does not change to reflect the knowledge, skills, or attitudes addressed in learning activities, there is a barrier to learning that needs to be addressed.

NEED FOR EDUCATION

Achievement of maximal functional gain for rehabilitation clients requires learning about new ways to manage daily routines and health, to prevent problems, to adapt to new lifestyles, to conquer new social mores, to address new financial and legal issues, and to cope with life changes. The entire rehabilitation team is invested in client and caregiver education and has a duty to teach skills and knowledge to those in their care. A successful rehabilitation outcome is evidence of the ability of the client and/or caregiver to incorporate learned skills and knowledge into daily life, enabling them to live as independently as possible in the environment of their choice.

> *The effective healthcare professional participating in client and caregiver education is aware that teaching occurs to support a change in behavior.*

The ability of the client and/or caregiver to learn is limited by the stress of the situation, which includes more than simply emotional stress. Sleep deprivation, physical discomfort, and worry about abilities and performance are among the factors that impair even the most motivated learner's ability to learn. Poor health literacy often steepens the learning curve, creating great disparity between the common knowledge of healthcare providers and those they are teaching (Bastable, 2003).

The movement of the patient across the continuum of care, reductions in the length of time during which care is provided throughout the continuum, shortages of professional personnel, reductions in budgets, technology, and changes in care processes can negatively impact client education (Hoeman, 2008). These changes in care processes have supported paradigm shifts that emphasize increased consumer involvement in self-management of chronic disease and disability, increased participation of an informed consumer in healthcare decisions, and increased demand for coordinated and contiguous care across healthcare systems. Consider the client who has sustained a spinal cord injury and is discharged from acute rehabilitation care to outpatient care within four weeks of injury. This client has reentered the community while still recovering from the acute injury, likely restricted in movement or activity to support continued healing of a spinal fracture while experiencing changes in function and the development of new problems such as spasticity. The handoff across the continuum of care, the level of preparation and support provided to the client and caregiver, and the responsiveness of the healthcare system in addressing the client's changing needs all impact outcomes and costs of care.

Outcomes are better and costs are reduced when clients and caregivers partner to holistically address needs and manage resources. This requires that the healthcare professional value the client and caregiver's participation, knowledge, and role in maintaining health and preventing complications. Levine (2000) directly confronts this view of the caregiver as an informed and vested participant in care planning and evaluation, commenting that they often know more about the patient than the professionals do and that their perspective must be valued. She emphasizes the need for emotional support and true understanding of the workload and stress placed on the family caregiver who has "no extra hands to help out in a crisis and no experienced colleagues to ask for advice" (p. 78).

HEALTH LITERACY

Health literacy is defined in Healthy People 2010 as "the degree to which individuals have the capacity to obtain, process, and understand basic health information and services needed to make appropriate health decisions." (U.S. Department of Health and Human Services., 2000, p. 112). Differing from general literacy, health literacy encompasses "the individual's ability to act on the information received and to effectively access and navigate the healthcare system at the appropriate time, place, and level of service" (Rudd, 2007, p. S8). Health literacy is influenced by educational, social, and cultural factors that, in turn, influence an individual's beliefs, perceptions, preferences, fears, and expectations.

The Partnership for Clear Health Communication (2008) at the National Patient Safety Foundation remarks that research shows that most consumers need assistance to understand healthcare information (Box 13.1). In their evaluation they also find that literacy skills are so important they are stronger predictors of health status than are age, income, employment status, educational level, or racial/ethnic group. They impact personal and community health in many ways. Low literacy can increase the likelihood that clients will experience shame or con-

fusion, which can lead to behaviors such as making false excuses for nonadherence, late or missed appointments, or life-threatening mistakes (Chang & Kelly, 2007).

BOX 13.1   Implications of Poor Health Literacy for Healthcare Providers

- Poorer health outcomes, adherence, and self-management skills; only about 50% of all patients take medications correctly
- Increased costs of care—up to four times higher for those with low health literacy
- Lack of skills needed to negotiate healthcare system
- Higher risk for hospitalization
- Higher risk for medication or treatment errors
- Higher utilization of services
- Increased health disparity

Source: Modified from Partnership for Clear Health Communication (2008).

Accreditation agencies consider poor health literacy a patient safety issue, noting that as healthcare and health literacy collide across the continuum of care, the risk of patient harm increases. Additionally, as previously noted, the stress, fatigue, pain, effects of medications, and vulnerability that occur when a person is in need of health care limits the abilities of even the most literate person to understand healthcare information received in an often brief interaction with providers. Therefore, accrediting agencies expect that providers not only provide education but also ensure the education is understood and the receiver of the education is able to follow instructions (Joint Commission, 2007).

Health literacy is not the sole responsibility of the provider. It requires conscious effort on the part of the healthcare consumer; insurance companies; providers of services, products, and care; and health policymakers (Joint Commission, 2007). Providers of services and care, insurance companies, and health policymakers must be competent in communicating health information effectively and in creating systems that are accessible to the individuals they serve if they want to decrease barriers to healthcare literacy (Institute of Medicine, 2004). Rehabilitation nurses can directly influence the health literacy of their clients by teaching

- Self-management of disease.
- How to locate and evaluate the relevance and credibility of healthcare resources
- How to analyze the risks and benefits of treatment options.

Educating clients and caregivers provides the resources to support shared decision making, creates active involvement, and reduces risk (Joint Commission, 2007). Decision-support aids, such as those found at http://decisionaid.ohri.ca/index.html, provide interactive tools that guide decision making based on knowledge, values, and goals (Wittmann-Price & Fisher, 2009).

PREVENTION

Preventive care empowers clients with knowledge that helps them to influence long-term outcomes. Chronic diseases are costly and often preventable. In 2005 almost half of the adult population, or 133 million Americans, suffered from chronic illness (Centers for Disease Control and Prevention {CDC}, 2010). According to the CDC (2004), lifestyle behaviors related to physical exercise, alcohol abuse, poor nutrition, and tobacco use are directly linked to the illness, suffering, and early death associated with chronic disease. Healthcare providers must approach clients in a manner that encourages them to embrace preventive care efforts through the recognition that chronic conditions are not curable and that self-care strategies significantly impact the course of the condition and quality of life (Table 13.1).

Rehabilitation nurses teach preventive care throughout the continuum and at the community and individual level. A proactive approach of integrating prevention and health promotion in the caregiving process is a significant factor in the achievement of optimum outcomes and the prevention of further complications. Quality of life is improved and costs of care diminished when preventive approaches are included in care (Hoeman, 2008).

LEARNING

Instructional scientists have done an incredible amount of work over the past several decades to provide us with evidence-based strategies for teaching. These strategies facilitate learning by avoiding information overload and leveraging learning processes to help manage the barriers created by current healthcare environments.

How Does Learning Occur?

Learning is a physiological and psychological process. Simply put, it is a step-by-step procedure for encoding new information. The components of learning are attention, activation of prior knowledge, elaboration and rehearsal, encoding, and retrieval (Figure 13.1).

For learning to occur, the learner must first focus **attention** on relevant information. This requires that the learner have the capacity to screen out irrelevant data to avoid overloading **working memory**. The more attention directed at a situation, the more it will be remembered and more easily retrieved (Medina, 2008). **Activation of prior knowledge** occurs as the brain searches for hooks on which to hang new information. Stored information is moved into working memory for comparison

TABLE 13.1	Levels of Prevention in Health Care		
Level of Prevention	**Description**		**Examples**
Primary	Targeted at preventing the occurrence of a disease or injury. Precedes the disease or injury and is concerned with those who have not yet developed it. Includes health promotion, education, and specific interventions, including those targeted at limiting exposure to risk.		Risk assessment, health education, immunization, and other preventive care behaviors such as exercise and diet management.
Secondary	Encourages early detection and treatment of illness to limit its severity or impact. The illness or disease has occurred, but it has not yet been noticed or detected.		Health maintenance activities, screenings for cancer, diabetes, hypertension, etc., prevention of complications by administering medications, initiating dietary changes to improve bowel function.
Tertiary	Facilitates care, recovery, or rehabilitation after the occurrence of an injury or illness. Prevents further damage or slows down the disease process, prevents the development of complications, and supports a return to optimum health and function.		Rehabilitation activities associated with recovery from stroke or other injury (relearning self-care, mobility, etc., self-management of diabetes, pressure ulcer preventive care through the use of pressure reliefs).

Source: Modified from the Centers for Disease Control and Prevention (2004) and U.S. Department of Health and Human Services (2003).

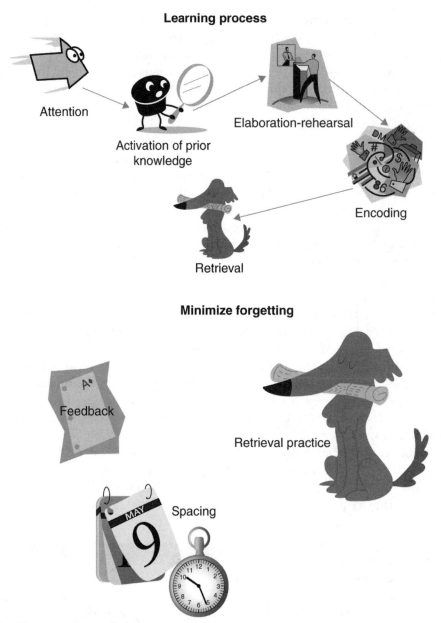

FIGURE 13.1   Principles of learning and remembering.

(*Source:* Modified from Clark, R., Nguyen, F. & Sweller, J. (2006). Efficiency in Learning: Evidence-Based Guidelines to Manage Cognitive Load. San Francisco, CA: John Wiley & Sons, Inc.)

and analysis. **Elaboration and rehearsal** occur as the working memory integrates old and new information, transforming it into new and expanded schemas. Chunks, or **schema**, are the meaningful relationships and patterns found in conceptual and factual knowledge. **Encoding** into long-term memory places the information into permanent storage. When the information is needed again, **retrieval** from long-term memory places the schema back into working memory for utilization and further learning. Frequently-repeated tasks become a large schema that

is mostly automated so that it requires less effort from working memory (Clark, Nguyen, & Sweller, 2006).

Learning can be supported or hindered by a breakdown in any step of this process. It is important to note that attention can easily be interrupted and that working memory can quickly become overloaded. We truly cannot multitask without a loss of information or reduction in speed of processing. Additionally, encoding requires physiological support, including adequate sleep, for completion to occur (Medina, 2008).

George Miller identified the limits of working memory in 1956, publishing the magical number of 7 ± 2 as the maximum number of chunks of information that can be held in working memory. Unless new information is kept alive in working memory through repetition, even small amounts of information disappear from consciousness in a few seconds (Clark et al., 2006). Evidence of the effort of working memory is readily seen by the actions taken to remember an unfamiliar phone number long enough to dial it. An interruption in this thought process quickly leads to loss of the number. Continuing research has reinforced the concept of working memory as a limited and easily-distracted resource but has also expanded our understanding of how the brain maximizes its capacity in spite of this limitation by the variation in the size of the information chunks it uses and its parallel processing of visual and auditory information.

The manner in which a person chunks information depends on the person's previous exposure to that information. Smaller chunks of information are required when the subject is unfamiliar. Familiar subjects are quickly incorporated into information already stored in the brain and can be processed by working memory in larger chunks (Clark et al., 2006). This concept supports the educational principle of determining what the patient or caregiver already knows before embarking on an educational journey. Our mental models and schemas of information define how new information is received and processed.

Cognitive Load Theory

Cognitive load theory is defined as "a universal set of learning principles that are proven to result in efficient instructional environments as a consequence of leveraging human cognitive learning processes" (Clark et al., 2006). This theory is universal and applies to all types of learning. Cognitive load refers to the intrinsic, extrinsic, and extraneous load on cognitive processes during learning activities (Figure 13.2).

- **Intrinsic load** refers to the amount of mental work required on the part of the learner by the complexity of the content to be learned. This is directly related to the expected outcomes or behaviors that should occur following education.
- **Extrinsic** or germane **load** is the relevant load imposed by the teaching strategies used to improve learning outcomes.
- **Extraneous load** is mental work that is irrelevant to the learning task at hand. It wastes mental resources.

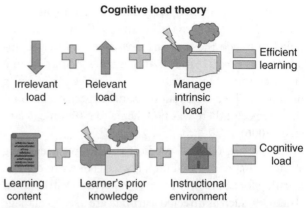

FIGURE 13.2   Dynamics of Cognitive Load Theory.

(*Source:* From Clark, R., Nguyen, F. & Sweller, J. (2006). Efficiency in Learning: Evidence-Based Guidelines to Manage Cognitive Load. San Francisco, CA: John Wiley & Sons, Inc.)

This is often under the control of the educator (Clark et al., 2006).

Cognitive load theory guides education efforts, requiring that educators minimize extraneous load when learning tasks are complex and learners are novices. It also requires that the educator recognize that complexity is highly individualized, because it depends on the learner's previous knowledge and experience (Clark et al., 2006). The strategies used to manage extrinsic load can help to increase retention of new knowledge and skills. Repetition, associating new information with old information, placing new information into context, focusing on retrieval practice, and spacing it out across time reduces the speed of forgetting (Thalheimer, 2009).

It should be noted that forgetting also has a purpose that supports the brain's overall function. Forgetting allows us to prioritize events. Some things are forgotten so that others can be remembered, and prioritization occurs during this process (Medina, 2008). Additionally, high-quality sleep is important to remembering and the storage of new information into long-term memory (Medina, 2008).

Another component of learning that influences remembering is the **expertise reversal effect**. The classic example of this effect is shown in repeatable studies with expert and novice chess players. When both groups are shown a chessboard in mid-play and asked to reconstruct it, the experts did so with few look-backs at the original board for confirmation, whereas the novices required many more look-backs. When that test is repeated with a random chess board, the novices perform better than the experts. Why? The random board disrupted the schema the experts had in their brains, requiring much more cognitive work to resolve the conflicting view that failed to match the patterns that were expected to appear on the board (patterns are parts of schema allowing larger chunks of information to be managed in working memory). The novice had the same experience in both situations and there was no schema to overcome (Clark et al., 2006).

Expertise reversal predicts that a given teaching strategy that works well for a novice is likely to depress learning for a person with more expertise. Instructional strategies, such as directed learning, are used to manage cognitive load for novices, helping the working memory to organize information. Experienced learners do not need this support. It burdens the working memory and depresses learning. Guided discovery is more helpful for experts who can use inductive learning strategies (Clark et al., 2006). Thus, training plans across the continuum should support learners as they grow from novices to higher proficiency in any given task (Box 13.2).

BOX 13.2 Example of Teaching Trajectory as Novice Gains Experience

Consider the teaching trajectory for a novice caregiver learning about preventing falls:

- New information is provided in structured manner with support of written materials, how to identify risk, and demonstration of how to use strategies to prevent falls
- As awareness of risk increases, teacher asks questions about application of strategies in different situations
- As skills increase and as part of mental rehearsal, teacher provides opportunities to solve problems that have not yet occurred
- Teacher provides feedback, praises efforts, and encourages independent problem solving in a variety of situations

---

Teaching strategies need to change as proficiency increases. Educators can gradually move from fully working through a skill with the learner to coaching and supporting as the learner completes more and more of the activity, until the learner fully completes the activity independently. Move at the learner's speed and plan for transfer of skills to other settings by rehearsing in similar settings (Clark et al., 2006).

Psychosocial Models and Theories

There is no single cookbook approach to client and family education. The multitude of factors that influence teaching and learning require that the healthcare provider expand skills and use resources from the social sciences, as well as the healthcare fields, to develop expertise in client and family education.

Health Belief Model

The **health belief model** has been shown to predict a wide variety of health improvement or preventive behaviors for many groups with chronic diseases (Turner, Kivlahan, Sloan, & Haselkorn, 2007). It is useful in assessing readiness to learn and can be used to guide the customization of learning activities. The health belief model states that learners are more receptive to changes in behavior if there is belief that the risk is real and personal, that it will negatively affect them, that benefits of action outweigh barriers to action, and if they are confident they can take that action to improve the situation (Figure 13.3).

Varying components of the health belief model have been found to be helpful in predicting adherence to healthcare regimens. In a study with a small group of patients with multiple sclerosis, perceived benefit was found to be the most important factor in predicting adherence to disease-modifying therapies (Turner et al., 2007). In another study regarding antibiotic use in young adults, a higher perception of perceived risk combined with lower perceived barriers was correlated with compliance to antibiotic therapy (Sangasubana, Yang, Bentley, Thumula, & Mendonca, 2009).

The rehabilitation team often needs to influence a client or caregiver's beliefs to prevent complications and promote optimal function. A mother who wants to believe her son is going to be safe and able to make appropriate judgments in the community after a brain injury, despite the fact that he gets lost and cannot find his way around the rehabilitation setting after three weeks in that setting, needs more evidence to believe the risk is real and significant. Until she believes this, she will likely not act to keep her son safe after discharge. Nor will the client with spinal cord injury follow skin care guidelines unless he believes the negative consequences are a significant and real possibility, that the skin care regimen is worth doing, and that he can be successful in preventing this complication.

Self-Efficacy

Confidence in the ability to perform required actions refers to **self-efficacy**. The self-efficacy theory (Bandura, 1977) is a social learning theory. If one's perceptions of self-efficacy levels are low, the person is less likely to attempt a change in behavior. Several programs have supported the impact of self-efficacy in the long-term

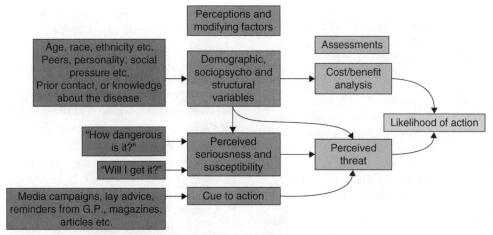

FIGURE 13.3   Factors impacting the likelihood of action in the Health Belief Model.

(*Source:* Adapted from Banyard, P. (2002). *Psychology in Practice: Health*. London: Hodder & Stoughton, page 137.)

management of chronic illness and disability. The Arthritis Self-Management Program and the Group Visit program designed by Dr. John Scott of the Kaiser Health System in Denver demonstrated behavioral changes that improved coping and reduced costs for care with higher correlations to perceptions of self-efficacy than to type of strategy learned for disease management. This may be the most important outcome of learning activities (Holman & Lorig, 2004).

The rehabilitation team that actively supports the development of competence in self-care and problem-solving encourages the development of self-efficacy. Many family caregivers are learning a new role. The team supports the development of knowledge and provides the opportunity to practice, with feedback, to build confidence in providing care and solving problems, thereby increasing self-efficacy.

Locus of Control

Locus of control is a social psychology theory describing personal beliefs regarding the amount of control one has over one's own health and the ultimate outcomes from injury or illness. Persons with an internal locus of control believe their actions influence outcomes. Persons with an external locus of control believe that outcomes are up to fate, God, or other authority (Wallston, Wallston, & DeVellis, 1978). These self-perceptions are heavily influenced by culture. Cultural values and traditions may become especially important during the stress of illness and life-changing situations that limit influence and control. If the culture strongly supports an external locus of control, it is unlikely that a change in behavior

will occur. When care providers assess for and identify a person's locus of control, they can adjust teaching plans accordingly. Persons with an internal locus of control more easily participate as partners in learning and in self-care. The client who actively participates in goal setting and takes responsibility to pursue activities that facilitate return to the community demonstrates an internal locus of control. The team can actively engage this patient in the caregiving process.

In those with an external locus of control, providers likely need to reduce focus on personal responsibility when teaching, finding alternative approaches that are acceptable and reasonable for each client (Hoeman, 2008). The team may need to more actively drive the plan of care in this population.

Cognitive Dissonance

Cognitive dissonance (Festinger, 1957) is a social theory that addresses the level of discomfort felt when what one does differs from what one believes. A person experiencing cognitive dissonance usually puts forth effort to reduce the levels of discomfort. This discomfort can be a significant motivating factor, increasing the need to know and making a person more receptive to teaching. By creating dissonance, the provider can influence readiness to learn. The rehabilitation nurse can determine a caregiver's belief regarding her husband's need to control carbohydrate intake and compare that with the frequency with which she brings him sweets to help him feel better. Addressing this dissonance, the rehabilitation nurse can help the caregiver learn alternative methods of helping her husband feel better.

Adult Learning Theory

Knowles' **adult learning theory** (1990) emphasizes prior knowledge and partnerships in learning. He coined the term "**andragogy**" to compare and contrast this approach with that of pedagogy. **Geragogy** is an alternative approach that emphasizes learning strategies that accommodate the functional changes that occur with aging (John, 1988). Each of these approaches has its place, based on the skills and needs of the learner (Box 13.3). An understanding of the differences in these approaches to teaching is helpful in designing teaching strategies for learners. They are not truly age-bound but rather are best applied according to prior experience and knowledge of the learner. Those with little experience to fall back on are likely to benefit from a pedagogical approach, whereas those with more experience to draw on and who are more self-directed in acquiring new skills and information will benefit more from an andragogical approach (Box 13.4).

Research continues to be prolific in the evaluation of these approaches to education. A recent, small study by Kimball et al. (2010) found that a geragogy teaching method did not significantly improve knowledge when compared with a standard method of education regarding medication administration. This emphasizes the need for continued research to identify those strategies that are most influential in improving outcomes.

Change Theory

If teaching occurs to effect a change in behavior, an understanding of change theory is relevant. Change theories reflect on the motivation to change, the contemplation involved in determining which action to take, and the energy required to solidify and maintain a change in behavior (Table 13.2).

In Lewin's change theory, change occurs when driving forces exceed restraining forces. The transformational model of change describes the process of change as a series of stages that one progresses through on a journey to a new behavior set. The journey may not be straightforward. A person may slide backward and move forward again

TABLE 13.2 Change Theories	
Theory	**Summary**
Change theory (Lewin, 1951)	Dynamic balance of opposing forces. Driving forces facilitate change. Restraining forces hinder change. Unfreezing starts the process of moving from the status quo. Movement results in change and refreezing solidifies that change into a new status quo.
Transformational model of change (Prochaska & Velicer, 1997)	A series of stages describing the process of change: precontemplation, contemplation, preparation, action, and maintenance.
Theory of reasoned action (Ajzen & Fishbein, 1980)	Behaviors are determined by beliefs, attitudes, and intentions and motivation is heavily influenced by beliefs regarding what an individual believes others think he or she should or should not do (subjective norms). An individual's intent to behave in a certain manner can be predicted by the relative weights of attitudes and subjective norm.

multiple times based on experiences and the energy available for the change process. The theory of reasoned action introduces the influence of peer pressure and attitudes as subjective norms that heavily influence the actions a person will take. It is used to predict the likelihood that a person will follow through with intended behaviors.

BOX 13.5   RULE Principle of Motivational Interviewing

- **R**esist the righting reflex: The healthcare provider acknowledges challenges and works to reframe resistance. By decreasing defensiveness, the risk of the client becoming entrenched in defending current behaviors is decreased. The more the client defends the current state, the more committed he or she is to it.
- **U**nderstand client's motivations: The healthcare provider uses therapeutic communication to understand the client's perspective regarding the change to be made. Ask why the client would want to change and how that might be accomplished.
- **L**isten with empathy: The healthcare provider uses active listening to fully understand the client. Answers lie within the client, and the healthcare provider must listen to identify them.
- **E**mpower the client: The healthcare provider supports healthy choices and uses a strong knowledge base to assist the client in the process of change, encouraging hope and optimism. The client's resources and ideas are key; he or she must be an active participant in planning and changing behavior.

Source: Adapted from Rollnick, William, & Butler (2008).

Motivational interviewing is one strategy that facilitates self-efficacy and self-responsibility by focusing on the client's readiness to change (Box 13.5). Motivational interviewing reflects the transformational model of change by recognizing that change is not a discrete behavioral activity but rather a process that occurs over time. The interaction with the client shifts from providing information to guiding the client to the next stage of the change process. This supports the client in focusing on the next stage in the process of change, a more manageable activity than focusing on completely altering a behavioral pattern. Effective motivational interviewing, by virtue of the collaborative process, facilitates the transition from the client simply receiving instruction to the patient being in charge of the changes in daily self-care management. The nurse provides the information and expertise and then supports the patient's efforts to achieve personal empowerment. Instead of using terms such as "patient compliance," the focus then shifts to the transition or change process, using terms such as "self-care choices" and "self-management."

Process of Client and Family Education

Teaching clients and facilitating changes in behavior are complex processes, as this review of learning theories indicates. Expertise in teaching develops through study, practice, and experience. The reality of chronic disease and disability is that success depends on active participation in self-management by clients and their caregivers and on effective coordination and communication throughout the continuum of care. Through this coordination and communication, providers can continue and reinforce teaching, ensure consistency of messages, support learning and practice efforts, and effectively change behavior over time. Rarely does a single teaching interaction address a learning need.

CASE STUDY 13.1

You are caring for a 70-year-old man, Jesse Gomez, who has suffered a right middle cerebral artery stroke. He received emergent care and is making progress in recovery from his hemiplegia. He has been taking oral medications to manage his type II diabetes for 16 years. His history also includes hypertension and atherosclerotic cardiovascular disease. During his initial assessment he and his wife note they have completed diabetic education classes at three different times over the years. He seldom checks his blood sugar at home because he understands from his family practice physician that the medication he is taking will take care of the diabetes. His medical record indicates an A_{1C} of 10%. The team observes that family members often bring high-carbohydrate snacks to Jesse, who has been placed on an insulin regimen during his inpatient stay. Jesse is now asking why he is getting so much insulin, indicating that he would "rather just take his pill and forget about it."

Questions

1. What response is best in this situation?
2. How will you learn what Jesse and his wife already know and believe regarding diabetes, its relation to his stroke, and its impact on his general health?
3. How will you identify what is preventing the practice of effective diabetic management?
4. What method will likely work best to establish learning goals?
5. What strategies need to be included to support learning and retrieval practice?
6. How should learning be evaluated?

There are many impacts on daily life and community living when a disability is present. Emotional responses to the situation also influence behavioral choices. Healthcare providers planning teaching activities need to recognize that clients and their caregivers are often new to the role of being active partners in care, needing to learn how to participate effectively in this role at the same time they are learning about living with a newly acquired disability. Teaching activities do not stand alone as tasks to be completed. These activities often force clients and caregivers to address losses and methods for accommodating them. Providers must listen to the needs of the learner and blend psychosocial support and encouragement into teaching activities.

Assessment

Assessment of learning needs and abilities starts with the first interactions with clients and family members. Many of them are unfamiliar with rehabilitation care. Education often begins with admission to rehabilitation services when the program and its processes are explained. This is a necessary and required step of care and can be used to evaluate how the client and family process information.

Develop Rapport

The team has much to learn about the needs of those new to their care. Rapport development is critical to building trust and enhancing communication. Team members must actively listen to the perceptions and beliefs of clients and their caregivers, recognizing that a few members of the team may develop a better rapport with them than others. This rapport is a tool that can be used to facilitate learning

Identify Prior Knowledge and Beliefs

While assessing the situation for a new client, the team can get to know the learner, paying careful attention to the knowledge, skills, attitudes, culture, and beliefs that the learner brings to the situation. Assessment of the developmental stage and cognitive functioning of the learner allows the team to teach in a manner that accommodates the learner's abilities.

Cultural sensitivity, which is defined as an "awareness and utilization of knowledge related to ethnicity, culture, gender, or sexual orientation in explaining and understanding situations and responses of individuals in their environments," (Chang & Kelly, 2007, p. 412). facilitates understanding of client and caregiver behaviors. A culturally sensitive nursing assessment addresses the client's perception of the illness, including

its cause and treatments, the perceived role of the sick person and family, expressions of pain, communication behaviors, folk healthcare beliefs, past healthcare experiences, and language. Using younger or opposite-gender family members to translate may impede the care process and compromise patient dignity. Utilization of professional translation services, when possible, reduces this risk.

It would not be surprising to learn that clients and their families are uninformed about bodily functions or naive of the amount and type of care that may be required now that they are in need of rehabilitation. Theories of change and the health belief model emphasize the importance of understanding the learner's perception of the situation and beliefs surrounding any topic of education. Be respectful of their prior knowledge and experiences. Family members often know a great deal about how a client responds to interventions and can identify strategies to facilitate success. Appreciate their expertise and learn from them. However, be alert. Ask questions and listen to conversations to fully understand their views. Research with patients with obstructive pulmonary disease has shown that patients significantly underestimate the severity of their disease and overestimate how well controlled their disease is (Carlson, Ivnik, Dierkhising, O-Byrne, & Vickers, 2006). Perceptions between clients and their caregivers may vary as well, with clients being less anxious and depressed regarding their situations than caregivers are (Levine, 2000).

Identification of the client's and caregiver's prior knowledge is also an essential part of a learning needs assessment (Box 13.6). We know enough about how a person learns to recognize that the strategy for teaching should be changed according to the prior knowledge and beliefs regarding the topic for learning. Asking questions to identify what the learner already knows also helps to bring schema into working memory to practice retrieval of old information and to prepare mentally to learn new information.

BOX 13.6   Client Education Tip

Assessment

Learn what the learner already knows and believes.

Learning styles have received a great deal of attention and are indeed interesting. However, there has not been valid, replicated evidence that teaching to popular learning styles facilitates better learning. Rather, the research shows that the one individual difference that requires a change in instructional technique is prior knowledge.

This is easier to assess and more reliably determined than learning styles (Bastable, 2003; Clark et al., 2006).

Determine Learner Readiness

Learner readiness refers to whether the learner is ready, willing, and able to participate in the learning process (Box 13.7). Teachable moments often occur during conversations when a client or caregiver asks a question, indicating readiness to learn. Timing is important, and flexibility in addressing learning needs in these moments of opportunity is both effective and efficient.

BOX 13.7   Using PEEK to Determine Readiness to Learn

- **P**hysical: ability, complexity, environment, health
- **E**motional: anxiety, support system, motivation, risk-taking behavior, attitude, developmental stage
- **E**xperiential: level of aspiration, past coping strategies, culture, locus of control, self-efficacy
- **K**nowledge: present knowledge, cognitive ability

Source: Adapted from Bastable (2003, p. 85).

One strategy that is helpful in assessing readiness to learn is to understand previous adherence and history in management of functional and healthcare needs. If a mother comments that her son walked on his cast when he was not supposed to after he broke his leg last summer, further discussion is warranted to understand his behavioral choices and how they may relate to willingness to learn and apply self-care skills in the current situation.

The rehabilitation team often has to look for ways to create a need-to-know. When they understand what the learner is ready to learn, they can adjust learning activities to match the current interest and level of readiness. A patient who indicates that she does not need to know how to catheterize herself will not learn how to do so, even if forced through the motions, until she changes her perspective and becomes ready to learn.

Identify Needs

Research has shown that several patterns to need identification in client education (Box 13.8). One of the most important points for providers to understand is that clients and their caregivers have very different concepts of what is most important to learn (Carlson et al., 2006). Providers often fail to address needs that are of most concern to the client/caregiver at the time they are of concern. This failure leads learners to tune out other information that is shared, even though it too may be important (Paterson et al., 2001).

BOX 13.8   Client Education Tip

- Identify needs
- Identify what the learner wants to know (perceived learning needs)

Clients and their families place a high priority on the information and skills they will need for survival (Box 13.9). They may organize this information differently from the way healthcare providers do (Carlson et al., 2006). Much of their focus will likely be on how to cope with the physical, mental, social, and financial impacts of the current situation. A family caregiver who is now the sole provider for the family will have a very difficult time learning medication management when he is frightfully concerned about paying for basic needs if he is forced to leave his job to care for his spouse.

Address first what the learner wants and needs to know to reduce stress and clear the brain for learning other information. Several studies of those with chronic illness have found that when they are encouraged to ask questions or to select topics to address, they eventually work through all relevant and needed topics, though not necessarily in the order providers would have selected (Holman & Lorig, 2004). Study after study reinforces the need for healthcare providers to ask clients what their concerns are and what they want to learn to individualize teaching and actively engage clients in the learning process (Lewis, Stabler, & Welch, 2010; White, Bissell, & Anderson, 2010).

BOX 13.9   What Clients and Families Want

- Access to information (diagnosis, course of disease and its impacts, available treatments with pros and cons, impact on the future)
- Coordination of care between services and specialists
- Continuity of care and ready access to it
- Advice, instruction, and support regarding ways to cope with all the changes they are facing (symptoms, pain, fatigue, disability, changes in roles, loss of independence, uncertainty, fear, depression, anger, loneliness, sleep disorders, memory loss, exercise needs, nocturia, sexual dysfunction, stress, care of the caregiver)
- Advice on access to resources and assistance for home care
- What to look for that indicates things are going wrong and what to do about it

Source: Adapted from Holman & Lorig (2004), Boughton & Halliday (2009), and Levine (2000).

Problem Identification

Clinicians spend a great deal of effort and energy in determining what the client and family need to know in order to progress to the next level of care or to be successful in the community. Unfortunately, many of them have not been in the role of continuous caregiver, and this alters their perception when developing a prioritized problem list (Box 13.10). Clearly stated, problem lists can be generated with clients and their caregivers, helping to invest them in the plan, to prioritize their needs, and to prepare them for the future. The more specifically the problem is described, the better it is understood by all team members addressing it. Consider the differences when identifying a problem as caregiver role strain versus describing it as caregiver role strain related to loss of family income and insurance due to husband's injury and lack of family support system to provide assistance following discharge.

BOX 13.10   Nursing Diagnoses

- Caregiver role strain
- Ineffective health maintenance
- Deficient knowledge
- Ineffective therapeutic regimen management

Source: From NANDA International (2007).

Goals and Objectives

Goals are important tools for focusing learning efforts. It follows naturally that if clients and caregivers are active participants in problem identification, they can be active in goal setting as well (Box 13.11). Setting targets focuses energy and helps to create a need-to-know. Goals should purposely focus on the skills and knowledge needed to safely move to the next level of care.

BOX 13.11   Client Education Tip

- Mutual goal setting
- Set goals with learners to meet needs, develop a need-to-know, and create investment in the plan.

There is a difference between goals and objectives (Box 13.12). In many care-planning situations objectives may be likened to short-term goals. Goals and objectives combined provide a map to guide the education plan (Bastable, 2003).

Goals are more global than objectives. An example goal is as follows: *The client will maintain intact skin.* Objectives address specific tasks that need to be accom-

---

BOX 13.12   Objectives (Short-Term Goals)

- Who
- Does what
- Under what circumstances
- Meeting what performance criteria
- By when

Examples

- Wife administers medications using medication guide at scheduled times, by Monday.
- Client performs self-catheterization at scheduled times with no more than two verbal cues, by Friday.
- Client uses chin tuck consistently at each meal with no more than one verbal cue per meal, by Wednesday.

---

plished to achieve the goal. They answer the question of what the learner needs to do and in what situation it needs to be done. An example objective is this: *The client will direct pressure relief every 30 minutes while in the wheelchair.* Mager (1997) provides many examples and a quick template for developing high-quality objectives by clearly defining the performance expected, the conditions in which a learner is expected to perform, and criteria for success. In our previous example the performance is *directing pressure relief*, the conditions are *while up in the wheelchair*, and the criteria is *every 30 minutes*.

Objectives or short-term goals written in this manner make it easier to document progress toward overall goals. Documentation for our example situation quickly indicates progress toward goals with something like this: *Remembered to direct pressure relief in a timely manner while up in wheelchair during the evening until visitors arrived. While visitors were present, required 100% cuing to direct pressure relief at the appropriate time.* The next logical step in care for this situation is a discussion about why it was hard to remember this activity when distracted by the visitors and the development and communication of a plan of approach to improve success in the future. Documentation of this conversation and plan demonstrate the dynamic response of the team to the patient's performance.

The most common mistakes made by the rehabilitation team when developing goals are (Bastable, 2003)

- Failure to develop them with the learner
- Describing the work of the teacher rather than the work of the learner
- Using vague terminology
- Developing goals that are unattainable in the amount of time available

It may be helpful to look at objectives in relationship to the learning domains involved to enhance adherence. The learning domains, cognitive, psychomotor, and affective, holistically address learning tasks (Bloom, 1956). Reviewing medication self-management from this perspective reminds the healthcare provider of the need to address affective issues such as the client's attitudes toward self-management, the costs of the drugs, side effects, and so on. This may need to precede the psychomotor practice of self-administration (such as drawing up insulin), which may need to be preceded with knowledge of what the medications are and why they should be taken. Learning during the assessment that a client wants to take as few medications as possible would guide the team in developing a teaching strategy that provides sufficient information to the client to support decision making around the value of each medication prescribed.

Teaching Interventions

As problems are identified and interventions are planned to meet goals, the team should carefully consider the resources, abilities, and settings the client will move on to after their care. Teaching should be focused on achieving the outcomes desired. Teaching strategies should move beyond talking at clients and families toward providing ample opportunity to practice and build self-confidence. This type of learner-centered technique has been well documented as a method of increasing involvement, improving performance, and increasing retention. Learning is an intentional process that requires focused attention. Attention drifts easily for passive participants in the learning process.

To those involved in rehabilitation care, it seems that almost every moment of contact with the client and family has the potential to be a teaching moment. The team is often teaching with role modeling when unaware of doing so. This reinforces the fact that the rehabilitation milieu should be a meaningful, supportive, and safe learning environment. Indeed, teachable moments are common and should be fully embraced by the team (London, 2009). When effective communication is used across the team, these moments build throughout the care process, increasing the team's efficiency.

There are many reasons a healthcare provider experiences teachable moments with clients and caregivers. When there is trust and rapport, there is confidence in getting questions answered. Fear, curiosity, and a need-to-know promote the asking of questions. The art of listening to the question, body language, and even anticipating the unasked question is a skill healthcare providers must develop in the hurry-along, task-driven environment of

care. Listening allows ongoing assessment of attitudes, fears, and interpretations of what has been learned from others. A few questions can change the entire focus of a teachable moment: "So, how long have you had diabetes?" "How does diabetes affect your life?" "What kinds of things do you do to take care of yourself and manage it?" "Why do you think you need to do those things?" "Are there other things you think you could be doing?" "Why are you not doing them?" "What worries you about the fact that you have diabetes and have to do these things?" "How can I help you feel more confident in managing your diabetes?" (London, 2009).

Teaching strategies selected by the team influence the efficiency and effectiveness of learning (Box 13.13). Learning should be intentional and in context. It should involve meaningful repetitions with retrieval practice and feedback. Skill development should be done in a step-by-step approach to avoid overloading the working memory. Attention to the details of the learning activities and learning environment enable management of extraneous load that can limit learning in a learner already stressed by the situation and its demands (Clark et al., 2006; Thalheimer, 2009).

Learning is faster and performance is more accurate when learning context is similar to performance context. Context helps to make learning both relevant and focused on solving real-world problems (Clark et al., 2006). During practice sessions, focus on using real-life resources that will be available when the learner needs to perform or solve a problem independently so that access to these resources becomes part of the schema the learner develops.

BOX 13.13   Client Education Tip

Teaching Strategies

- Actively support the connection of new information with information the learner already knows.

- Teach in context. Situation-based learning is more effective.

- Use meaningful repetitions and space them over time. Support the organization of new learning into meaningful activities that can be applied to currently-needed life skills.

- Provide opportunities for retrieval practice and problem solving.

- Provide feedback and reinforcement to groom performance.

- Consistency in messaging reduces extraneous load and avoids confusion.

The team recognizes that the success of the client depends on the ability to generalize learning from one situation to another in which it applies. This process of carryover is a component of practice that supports the need for clients to practice what is learned with one member of the team when the same situation is faced with another member of the team. An example of this type of repetition and retrieval practice to support the learning process for transfers is practicing the same technique at the bedside as is learned on the mat in physical therapy. This type of meaningful repetition, when consistently applied, supports encoding and rehearsal, facilitating long-term memory storage and retrieval. During these practice sessions, the focus is on guiding the learner in self-cueing for retrieval of necessary knowledge and skills.

Spacing repetition strengthens retrieval skills, and feedback keeps the learner on track. Shortly after being exposed to new information, retrieval of that information is fairly specific and detailed. When memories are retrieved later, the brain fills in missing gaps to complete the details of a memory that is fragmented and incomplete. Memory is truly reconstructive and readily includes misinformation or false information to make a coherent story (Medina, 2008). This reinforces the importance of consistency in messaging, of providing corrective feedback, and of retrieval practice to strengthen the details of the memory and improve the accuracy of performance. Combined with context, these activities increase the likelihood that environmental cues will trigger spontaneous remembering of the correct information and skills when they are needed (Thalheimer, 2009).

A consistent theme in studies of clients and their caregivers has been the need to increase their confidence in their ability to provide the care that is needed with the resources they have in the community. Education plans that include ample opportunity for coached practice also build confidence and improve perceptions of self-efficacy (Boughton & Halliday, 2009). Helpful teaching principles for improving confidence include breaking tasks into smaller, more easily achievable steps to support the building of new chunks of information and using feedback to groom and encourage success. This requires the educator to change strategies according to the learner's readiness to learn and participate in the learning process, to provide clear directions, to create an opportunity for practice, and to model the desired behavior, while guiding and praising the learner's efforts (Table 13.3).

The concept of a personal coach has been found to be helpful in achieving behavioral change in patients receiving diabetic and cardiac rehabilitation education. This approach emphasizes empowerment of the client and caregiver and reinforces their involvement as active participants in achieving a goal. When clients developed rapport with the coach, reporting and analyzing progress became important drivers toward goal achievement (Koenigsberg, Bartlett, & Cramer, 2004; Williams, 2004). The rehabilitation team can use such an approach by selecting an individual team member to coach the client and caregiver in much the same way through learning activities, using fellow team members as resources toward goal achievement.

Group learning can provide both support and avenues for problem solving and sharing of experiences. Some clients find this type of learning to be highly rewarding as members help each other out (Holman & Lorig, 2004). However, it should be recognized that group learning can have limitations when barriers such as anxiety, low literacy, and embarrassment exist (Hoeman, 2008).

Use of Technology

Technology is becoming more and more common in everyday life. It can provide the team with additional avenues for teaching. Empowerment of clients and their caregivers supports the use of technological resources, providing convenient opportunities for at-will education, encouraging independence, facilitating informed decision making, and promoting lifelong learning.

Benefits to using the Internet include 24-hour access to a wide range of current information, presented in a variety of teaching formats, that allow consumers to connect with resources and other people who share common issues and concerns. Patients who are disabled or isolated glean psychosocial benefits as well. Patients, families, and caregivers can use online resources to find information, formulate questions, understand symptoms, and explore alternative treatments (Anderson & Klemm, 2008).

A study by Matter et al. (2009) from the Center for Technology and Disability Studies at the University of Washington, Seattle, reports that respondents using the Internet prefer "Physician: SCI Expert/Rehab Specialist" interaction for gaining information about spinal cord injury but use the "Web pages/Internet" more frequently. This shift from a paternalistic provider–client relationship to shared decision making encourages Internet use for easy access to health information, often before clients have consulted with a provider. The potential for effective patient education or the dissemination of errant facts abounds with consumer Internet use, especially if the consumer is not informed regarding how to evaluate Internet resources. As clients and caregivers continue to

TABLE 13.3   Rehabilitation Learning Readiness Assessment Guide (RLRAG) as a One-Page Information Guide

Stage	Dependent	Involvement	Engagement	Self-Initiation	Self-Direction
Learning readiness process	Need for direction and support of the nurses in maintaining basic self-care functions	Process of assimilating new knowledge and skills	Responses and behaviors of patients (both positive and negative) to the learning of self-care regimens	Use of positive energy to master self-care competencies	Ability to thoughtfully plan, implement, and evaluate care with/without a partner/guide
Examples of learning readiness and obstacles	Physical and psychosocial complications	Denial of need to learn Procrastination Delays Lack of availability of caregivers to teach	Information overload Energy demands Grief responses Resistive forms of learning behavior	Over/underconfident Discouragement Insecurity Setbacks	Maintaining autonomy/independence Continuing education Availability of consultation as needed
Teaching role	Authority	Guide	Motivator	Mentor	Consultant/Partner
Teaching goals	Providing direction and care	Organizing involvement	Facilitating optimal participation	Supporting self-initiated behavior	Promoting autonomy and self-direction of care
Teaching activities	Monitoring of physical/emotional status Intervening for clients Directing care Providing comfort	Assessing self-care Monitoring status Encouraging Instructing Guiding Discussing Explaining Role model Reviewing Reteaching	Monitoring progress Encouraging participation Clarifying Cueing Reemphasizing Reminding Coaching Confronting Reinforcing	Delegating Encouraging practice Reinforcing Evaluating Mutual problem solving Challenging Correcting Negotiating Overseeing Supervising	Advising Suggesting Consulting

Source: From Olinzock (2008).

use the Internet to search out information, it becomes important for all healthcare providers to promote safe use of these resources. The sheer volume of information available can be overwhelming, difficult to navigate, or impossible to understand if clients and caregivers are unable to access the accurate and easy-to-use material that facilitates their learning. Barriers and drawbacks of Internet use as a primary tool for client education can also include lack of access and privacy issues (Anderson & Klemm, 2008).

Online resources for healthcare information vary in accuracy and reliability. Rehabilitation nurses have an opportunity to improve the way patients use the Internet by teaching them how to determine site validity and by providing a list of appropriate online resources (Box 13.14). Resources for guiding Internet use are provided by agencies such as Health on the Net, the Food and Drug Administration, and the National Institutes of Health. The Medical Library Association has a special section on their website dedicated to consumer health information, older adult populations, and Spanish-speaking clients. Older clients can experience frustration with technology, and even younger clients can experience difficulty understanding content that is often designed at the high-school-age reading level (Anderson & Klemm, 2008). Clients should be instructed about assessing sites for security and cautioned about the potential pitfalls of making online purchases or listing personal information.

BOX 13.14   Checklist for Internet Use

Use the following checklist to ensure health information you are reading online can be trusted.

- Can you easily see who sponsors the website?
- Is the sponsor a government agency, a medical school, or a reliable health-related organization, or is it related to one of these?
- Is there contact information?
- Can you tell when the information was written?
- Is your privacy protected?
- Does the website make claims that seem too good to be true? Are quick, miraculous cures promised?

Source: From National Institute on Aging *(2009).*

The information nurses retrieve from Internet sites can be shared with patients to reinforce the benefit of Internet utilization. Patients who are intimidated by technology and reluctant to risk failure can be encouraged by healthcare providers who break learning into manageable increments. Volunteers with computer savvy can further assist patients who wish to explore resources on clinic computers (Anderson & Klemm, 2008). In addition to the health information resources listed in this chapter, *U.S. News and World Report* (2010) provides a list of the top rehabilitation hospitals in the United States, with direct links to each website. Information can be found on these sites related to disease/disabilities, treatments, patient education, and relevant trials and studies. Healthcare providers may also access online educational opportunities and download patient handouts on some of these sites. A list of Internet resources is included in Resources and Readings at the end of this chapter.

Technology will continue to develop. Northeastern University has developed a virtual discharge advocate named Louise, an animated character on a touch-screen display mounted on an articulated arm of a mobile cart. Functioning as a virtual nurse, Louise uses synthetic speech and animation to interact with clients according to the selections they make by touching the screen. Louise displays a copy of the discharge instructions identical to the paper copy provided to the client. The comments made by Louise are dynamically generated from the client's individual medical data and the questions asked. Louise also tests the client's understanding of key facts

and produces a report of the client's issues and questions for human professional caregiver follow-up that could not be answered. Clients indicate they like Louise better than her human counterparts because she takes more time to answer questions, discusses each point in more detail, is more patient in repeating unclear information, and evaluates understanding! (Jack et al., 2009)

Documentation of Learning Activities

A learning plan helps to target the most urgent skills that need to be developed at each level of care. All team members should be actively involved in identifying resources and designing documentation systems that support efficient planning, implementation, and evaluation of progress in achieving learning goals. Tools and processes should be designed to support consistent messaging and continuity of care. The sample in Box 13.15 demonstrates a documentation guide and form that reflects the development of client/caregiver competence and confidence in self-care while making it easy for caregivers to hand off teaching activities to each other. Tools such as this can easily be adapted to electronic documentation systems, altered to address individual topics, or organized to holistically reflect the self-care needs.

Whatever tool is used, it should demonstrate application of data collected during assessment to target learning needs, learning strategies used, who was taught, the response to learning activities, and the ability to demonstrate needed skills. The tool should readily show progress toward the learning goal and should make it easy for each caregiver to know what has been taught and the learner's response to it so that efficiency can be gained by consistent forward momentum in the learning process. Including a job aid, as noted in the heart failure example presented in Box 13.15, provides a way to support clinicians in remembering to address key issues and to orient new staff to the resources, tools, and learning activities available.

Documentation of learning activities and their effectiveness supports continuity of care across the continuum. Documentation tools can be incorporated into care maps, care plans, and/or the discharge plan. An effective documentation tools tracks progress, helps providers to avoid duplication, and focuses on necessary repetition, retrieval practice, and feedback. There should be obvious documentation of the work of the team to identify barriers to learning and the methods used to manage them.

Barriers to learning can occur at any step of the learning process. Constant evaluation, reevaluation, and attentiveness to the responses of the learner are required to address these barriers as they develop. Creativity and active support are often required to individualize interventions to remove barriers and allow achievement of the learning goal. Motivational interviewing can be used to address attitudinal barriers that are often difficult to overcome and that significantly limit changes in behavior.

Healthcare providers must remember that documentation tools support reimbursement, and they also are legal records (Hoeman, 2008). Healthcare providers often fail to document adequately and should be aware that this documentation can be the evidence or lack of evidence that determines the outcome of litigation (Bastable, 2003).

Evaluation of Learning

It is common to see documentation that a client or family caregiver has stated understanding of information provided. Although at times this is the only option the provider has due to the nature of the information being taught or the time available for practice and demonstration of understanding, this is very weak evidence that the learner has indeed learned something and is able to use this information. The evidence of the learner's ability to use new learning is in the *performance* of activities that require application of that learning. As noted previously, Commission on Accreditation of Rehabilitation Facilities standards of care require the team to assess the effectiveness of education and to focus on improvement of educational efforts if learning outcomes are not achieved.

There are many strategies for assessing application of learning. The client or caregiver can assume various parts of care as skill sets develop. The team can challenge them with questions and role playing regarding responses to anticipated problems. A written or computerized tool can be used to determine what has been learned and what still needs more practice or reinforcement. Simulation training is a form of role playing and is very valuable in providing context and retrieval practice. Healthcare providers must be aware of the amount of cuing and support provided when evaluating what has been learned. It is very easy to fail to recognize the level of cueing still needed, which can lead to failure when the support of the team is less available.

Peer Education

The rehabilitation nurse educates peers, new hires, and fellow caregivers across the continuum. The role of the rehabilitation nurse educator is defined by the Association of Rehabilitation Nurses at http://www.rehabnurse.

BOX 13.15   Heart Failure Education Documentation

Resource List and Key Teaching Points

Topics on the checklist are required learning for safe management of this problem. A patient/caregiver is considered competent when able to answer the questions without cues from staff. Midpoint on the competence scale is defined as being able to answer the questions or perform self-care with 50% or less prompting.

Tools Available

- Video: *Heart Failure* reviews physiology and importance of proactive management. The video is on the patient education computer in Video folder on desktop.
- Interactive Workbook: *Living Well with Heart Failure* focuses on self-care and self-management. This booklet is generally provided to patients in acute care to start the education process. Continue teaching from it. If it is not found with the patient, issue a new copy from the Krames folder in the patient education filing cabinet.
- Fast Guide: *Understanding Heart Failure* provides a quick guide to lifestyle changes and medical tests. Available from the Krames folder in the patient education filing cabinet.
- Tools: *Daily Weight Record*, *Pocket Medication List*, *Pocket Dietary Guide*, and *Appointment Reminders* are available for patient use in implementation. Print from our intranet under key word: HF/PtEd. Link for public use is printed on the bottom of each tool. Copies are available in the patient education filing cabinet.
- Internet Interactive Tool: Medline Plus tool that can be provided as an ongoing reference at: http://www.nlm.nih.gov/medlineplus/tutorials/congestiveheartfailure/htm/index.htm.

Other supportive tools or steps may include:

- Making sure there is a scale at home the patient is able to use
- Medication tracking sheet
- Referral to appropriate sources if competency or adherence is not at least 75% on discharge evaluation

Continues

BOX 13.15   Heart Failure Education Documentation   *(Continued)*

Heart Failure Education Documentation Form (page 1)

Persons taught: Pts wife Sarah and pt

Teaching resources used (record date initiated):

⊙ *Heart Failure* video _____5/9/09_____   ⊙ *Living Well with Heart Failure* _____5/9/09_____

⊙ *Understanding Heart Failure* _____   ⊙ *Daily Weight Record* _____5/12/09_____

⊙ *Pocket Medication List* _____   ⊙ *Pocket Dietary Guide* _____5/12/09_____

⊙ Medline Plus Reference: http://www.nlm.nih.gov/medlineplus/tutorialslcongestiveheartfailurefhtmlindex.
htm _____5/11/09_____

⊙ Other: _____
_____
_____
_____
_____
_____
_____
_____

Record dates in which the persons taught are able to do the following:

⊙ **Persons taught able to state simple explanation of HF.** (HF is a condition in which the heart does not pump blood
efficiently, causing fluids to collect in the lungs and other tissues.) _____5/11/09_____

Persons taught able to list symptoms of heart failure problems requiring contact with healthcare provider (may
reference resources provided to them) _____5/22/09_____

⊙ Sudden weight gain of 2lbs in one day or 5lbs in 5 days   ⊙ Worsening shortness of breath

⊙ Increased swelling in feet, legs, or abdomen   ⊙ Needing more pillows to sleep or using recliner

⊙ Waking from sleep to catch breath   ⊙ New or worsening dizziness

⊙ Cough that does not go away   ⊙ New or increasing irregularity in heart rate

⊙ Any problems with heart failure medicines

Persons taught able to identify when to go to the emergency department or call 911. _____5/22/09_____

⊙ Severe shortness of breath   ⊙ Coughing up pink, frothy sputum

⊙ Chest discomfort, pain, or pressure that is not relieved by rest or nitroglycerine

Persons taught able to self-manage treatment plan (may reference resources provided to them). _____5/23/09_____

⊙ Identifies medications that are for HF by name/reason for taking

⊙ Lists side effects to watch for from medications

⊙ Manages medication schedule (self-med program or calls for medications at correct time)

⊙ Manages daily weights (completes and records independently or directs others)

⊙ Follows dietary recommendations for salt restriction and weight management

⊙ Describes plan for compliance to salt restrictions and weight management that will be used at home

⊙ Demonstrates balance of rest and activity

Persons taught will plan for participation in follow-up care for HF (after issuing follow-up appointment
cards). _____5/26/09_____

⊙ Describes reason for MD visits (medication and symptom monitoring that may include blood tests)

⊙ Describes reason for nutrition consultation (dietary management and support)

⊙ Identifies what should be brought to each appointment (refers to follow-up appt card which lists this information)

Continues

BOX 13.15   Heart Failure Education Documentation   *(Continued)*

Heart Failure Education Documentation Form (page 2)

Comments (barriers identified, problems encountered, strategies to support self-management, etc.):

5/9/09: Pt and wife very concerned, as did not know pt had heart failure till admission for the stroke. Wife able to show in the workbook the progress made in learning about it. Wife has many questions about reducing salt intake—dietician will meet with her on the 12th. Pt unhappy about salt restriction but notes is able to breathe more easily already. Will be working on pages 12–16 in workbook next few days. NN

5/11/09: Still complains about salt restriction, but is following guidelines consistently. Investigating salt-free snacks, but wants to try to wean into this. Discussed consequences of a slow weaning process on overall health. Reviewed reasons to call the doctor or the emergency room. Symptoms frightened wife. She is leading plans for "healthy living" and studying workbook. KB

5/12/09: Progressing well through workbook. Provided self-tracking tools and helped to start completing them. Discussing strategies for daily weights at home, considering pt's mobility limitations. Sister has a scale that is more stable for standing, so they will likely trade scales hoping that pt will be able to stand quietly for short periods of time for weights. Will bring it in closer to discharge for practice. PM

5/15/09: Wife participating in self-med management and will be administering meds at home. Provided medication resource sheets for all HF medications today. Highlighted most important points. She will study them and be ready for our questions to test her understanding as we review with her over the next few days. KB

5/22/09: Wife able to answer all questions on medications and problems to watch out for. Did not remember that pt needed to weigh before eating breakfast. Still concerned about meeting dietary restrictions. Went to hospital cafeteria for lunch and had difficulty selecting foods that met dietary restrictions for pt. Reminded to use dietary pocket guide. Will try again tomorrow. NN

5/23/09: Wife more confident today. Many questions re: medications, diet, and when pt should rest. Practiced observation of respiratory pattern. Actively participated in checking weight, edema, and diet selection in cafeteria using dietary pocket guide. Pt does much less complaining about lack of salt. Brought in scale from home and compared results to zero it. Pt able to stand on it for weight if uses walker to get on it and then can let go for a moment to read weight. NN

5/25/09: Issued discharge instructions and reviewed HF follow-up recommendations and their purpose. Wife was mildly anxious and wanted to review again when to call the doctor. Reminded of resources and she quickly accessed information. Role play of problems she thought she might encounter and how to respond seemed to ease anxiety. Reminded her we would HF information with the rest of her materials tomorrow before discharge on 5/27. KB

5/26/09: Wife directed care re: HF today (weight, diet, meds, edema check, rest periods). Able to answer all questions on meds and when to seek help. States confident in being able to manage at home and plans to keep follow-up appts. PM

Evaluation of competence in self-management (mark with date/initials):

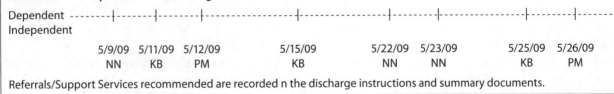

| Dependent -------- | -------- | -------- | ---------------- | ---------------- | -------- | ---------------- | -------- | ------- |
| Independent |

| 5/9/09 | 5/11/09 | 5/12/09 | 5/15/09 | 5/22/09 | 5/23/09 | 5/25/09 | 5/26/09 |
| NN | KB | PM | KB | NN | NN | KB | PM |

Referrals/Support Services recommended are recorded n the discharge instructions and summary documents.

Sample documentation sheet. Reprinted with permission from *See One, Do One: Patient & Family Education in Rehabilitation*, (2010) Salt Lake City, UT: Rehab ClassWorks, LLC.

org/pubs/role/educator.html. All strategies presented for client and caregiver education can be applied to the education of professionals and their associates as well. Again, a focus on context, retrieval practice, and feedback is extremely valuable to improving performance, as is noted in the high level of success achieved with simulation training. Simulation, a powerful teaching tool that supports context of learning, rehearsal, and retrieval practice, can be as simple as putting a glob of peanut butter in a specimen cup to simulate a stool sample to as complex as a simulation lab with a computerized mannequin that provides symptoms and records responses of care providers.

Community Education and Prevention

Participation in community-level education to reduce the risk of injury from accidents through the use of seat belts, child safety seats, helmets, and other safety gear is a role of the rehabilitation nurse. An act as simple as role modeling safe behavior and discussing it with family and friends demonstrates application of this principle of prevention. Rehabilitation nurses can also chose to participate in community-level education through involvement with community groups, local healthcare systems, and other forms of volunteerism.

Additional Information on Learning Domains and Memory

Learning Domains (Cognitive, Psychomotor, Affective)

Bloom (1956) focused much of his research on the study of educational objectives and, ultimately, proposed that any given task favors one of three psychological domains: cognitive, affective, or psychomotor. The cognitive domain deals with a person's ability to process and use (as a measure) information in a meaningful way. The affective domain relates to the attitudes and feelings that result from the learning process. Finally, the psychomotor domain involves manipulative or physical skills.

Working Memory

Working memory (previously referred to as short-term memory) is the part of the brain that provides temporary storage and manipulation of information during complex cognitive tasks. Working memory involves simultaneous storage and processing of information. It contains three subcomponents: (1) the central executive, the attentional-controlling system, and two slave systems; (2) the visuospatial sketch pad, which manipulates visual images; and (3) the phonological loop, which stores and rehearses speech-based information. Working memory has a limited capacity and is active in the selection, initiation, and termination of information-processing functions such as encoding, storing, and retrieving data.

CRITICAL THINKING

1. Explore the expectations of the role of the rehabilitation nursing educator at the Association of Rehabilitation Nursing website at http://www.rehabnurse.org/pubs/role/educator.html. Discuss your findings with a peer.
2. What would you do to create *teachable moments* when caring for a patient with a language barrier when the interpreter is not available?
3. What does resiliency have to do with coping and learning after the occurrence of an injury or illness resulting in disability?

PERSONAL REFLECTION

- Identify the most common barrier you face during client and caregiver education and reflect on how the principles of motivational interviewing may help to remove the barrier.
- What strategies can or do you use to *educate* rather than *inform* clients and their caregivers?
- What are your personal biases regarding involvement of clients/caregivers as active participants in the learning process?
- How often do you assess what your clients/caregivers *want* to know? How might you incorporate this important component of client education into your care in the future?
- What strategies of client/caregiver education do you believe work best to create a change in behavior in your learners and why? When was the last time you tried a new approach? What are your strengths? How can you reduce your weaknesses?
- What strategies can you use to determine what your learners already know?
- How can you reduce extraneous load when you are teaching? How do you support working memory?
- What are some techniques you can use to reduce the amount of last-minute discharge teaching for clients/caregivers?
- Are there strategies that should be used to improve documentation and hand off communication re-

garding client education for those in your care? Are learning goals clearly documented?

RESOURCES AND READINGS

General

Health Care Education Association at www.hcea-info.org

London, F. (2009). No time to teach: The essence of patient and family education for health care providers (pocket guide). Atlanta, GA: Pritchett & Hull Associates.

Partnership for Clear Health Communication and the National Patient Safety Foundation at http://www.npsf.org/pchc/index.php

Ostwald, S. K., Davis, S., Hersch, G., Kelley, C., & Godwin, K. M. (2008). Evidence-based educational guidelines for stroke survivors after discharge home. *Journal of Neuroscience Nursing, 40*(3), 173–179, 191.

Evaluating Internet Resources

Medical Library Association: *A user's guide to finding and evaluating health information on the web* at http://www.mlanet.org/resources/userguide.html

Medline Plus: *Evaluating health information* at http://www.nlm.nih.gov/medlineplus/evaluatinghealthinformation.html

Medline Plus: *Guide to healthy web surfing* at www.nlm.nih.gov/medlineplus/healthywebsurfing.html

National Cancer Institute: *Evaluating health information on the internet* at http://www.cancer.gov/cancertopics/factsheet/Information/internet

National Institute on Aging: *Online health information: Can you trust it?* at http://www.nia.nih.gov/healthinformation/publications/onlinehealth.htm.

National Library of Medicine: *FAQ: National Library of Medicine guide to finding health information* at http://www.nlm.nih.gov/services/guide.html.

Office of Dietary Supplements: *How to evaluate information on the internet: Questions and answers* at http://ods.od.nih.gov/Health_Information/How_To_Evaluate_Health_Information_on_the_Internet_Questions_and_Answers.aspx

Resources for Clients and Caregivers

American Heart Association at http://www.heart.org

American Spinal Injury Association at http://www.asia-spinalinjury.org

American Stroke Association at http://www.strokeassociation.org/presenter.jhtml?identifier=1200037

Brain Attack Coalition at http://www.stroke-site.org/disclaimer/disclaimer.html

Brain Injury Association at www.biausa.org

Centers for Disease Control and Prevention at http://www.cdc.gov/doc.do/id/0900f3ec80093c90

Centers for Medicare & Medicaid Services: *Caregiver information* at http://www.medicare.gov/caregivers

Internet Stroke Center at http://www.strokecenter.org

Mayo Clinic at http://www.mayoclinic.com

Medical Library Association at http://www.mlanet.org/resources/consumr_index.html

MedlinePlus at http://medlineplus.gov

Multiple Sclerosis Association of America at http://www.msaa.com

National Aphasia Association at http://www.aphasia.org

National Institute of Child Health and Human Development at http://www.nichd.nih.gov/health

National Institute of Neurological Disorders and Stroke at www.ninds.nih.gov

National Spinal Cord Injury Association at www.spinalcord.org

National Stroke Association at http://www.stroke.org/site/PageNavigator/HOME?cvridirect=true

Paralyzed Veterans of America at www.pva.org

U.S. Department of Health and Human Services: *Quick guide to healthy living* at http://www.healthfinder.gov

U.S. National Institutes of Health at http://clinicaltrials.gov

RECOMMENDED READINGS

Clark, R., Nguyen, F., & Sweller, J. (2006). *Efficiency in learning: Evidence-based guidelines to manage cognitive load.* San Francisco: John Wiley & Sons.

Johnson, J., & Pearson, V. (2000). The effects of a structured education course on stroke survivors living in the community. *Rehabilitation Nursing, 25*(2), 59–65.

Levine, C. (2000). *Always on call: When illness turns families into caregivers.* New York: United Hospital Fund.

Manchusco, J. M. (2008). Health literacy: A concept/dimensional analysis. *Nursing and Health Sciences, 10,* 248–255.

Paterson, B., Kieloch, B., & Gmiterek, J. (2001). "They never told us anything": Postdischarge instructions for families of persons with brain injuries. *Rehabilitation Nursing, 26*(2), 48–53.

Rollnick, S., William, R., & Butler, C. C. (2008). *Motivational interviewing in health care: Helping patients change behavior.* New York: Guilford Publications.

Suter, P. M., & Suter, W. N. (2008). Timeless principles of learning: A solid foundation for enhancing chronic disease self-management. *Home Health Nurse, 26*(2), 82–88.

REFERENCES

Ajzen, I., & Fishbein, M. (1980). *Understanding attitudes and predicting social behavior.* Englewood Cliffs, NJ: Prentice-Hall.

Anderson, A. S., & Klemm, P (2008). The Internet: Friend or foe when providing patient education? *Clinical Journal of Oncology Nursing, 12*(1), 55–63.

Bandura, A. (1977). Self-efficacy: Toward a unifying theory of behavioral change. *Psychological Review, 84*(2), 191–215.

Banyard, P. (2002). *Psychology in practice: Health*. London: Hodder & Stoughton.

Bastable, S. B. (2006). *Nurse as educator: Principles of teaching and learning for nursing practice*. Sudbury, MA: Jones & Bartlett.

Billings, D. M., & Halstead, J. A. (2009). *Teaching in nursing* (3rd ed.). St. Louis, MO: Saunders Elsevier.

Bloom, B. S. (1956). *Taxonomy of educational objectives, handbook 1: Cognitive domain*. New York: Longman.

Boughton, M., & Halliday, L. (2009). Home alone: Patient and care uncertainty surrounding discharge with continuing care needs. *Contemporary Nurse, 33*(1), 30–40.

Bradshaw, B. G., Richardson, G. E., & Kulkarmi, K. (2007). Thriving with diabetes: An introduction to the resiliency approach for diabetes. *The Diabetes Educator, 33*, 643–649.

Brunner, L. S. & Suddarth, D. S. (2004). Medical surgical nursing (10th ed.). Philadelphia: Lippincott Williams & Wilkins.

Carlson, M. L., Ivnik, M. A., Dierkhising, R. A., O-Byrne, M. M., & Vickers, K. S. (2006). A learning needs assessment of patients with COPD. *MEDSURG Nursing, 15*(4), 204–212.

Centers for Disease Control and Prevention. (2010). Chronic diseases and health promotion. Retrieved December 1, 2009, from http://www.cdc.gov/chronicdisease/overview/index.htm

Centers for Disease Control and Prevention. (2004). Levels of disease prevention. Retrieved July 1, 2010, from http://www.cdc.gov/excite/skincancer/mod13.htm#levels

Chang, M., & Kelly, A. E. (2007). Patient education: Addressing cultural diversity and health literacy issues. *Urologic Nursing, 27*(5), 411–417. Retrieved from http://www.medscape.com/viewarticle/564667

Clark, R., Nguyen, F., & Sweller, J. (2006). *Efficiency in learning: Evidence-based guidelines to manage cognitive load*. San Francisco: John Wiley & Sons.

Festinger, L. (1957). *A theory of cognitive dissonance*. Stanford, CA: Stanford University Press.

Hoeman, S. P. (2008). *Rehabilitation nursing prevention, intervention, & outcomes* (4th ed.). St Louis, MO: Mosby Elsevier.

Holman, H., & Lorig, K. (2004). Patient self-management: A key to effectiveness and efficiency in care of chronic disease (Viewpoint). *Public Health Reports*, May 1, 2004.

Hoving, C., Visser, A., Mullen, P. D., & van den Borne, B. (2010). A history of patient education by health professionals in Europe and North America: from authority to shared decision making in education. *Patient Education Counsel, 78*(3), 275–281.

Institute of Medicine. (2004). Crossing the Quality Chasm. Washington, DC: National Academy Press.

Jack, J. B., Chetty, B. K., Anthony, D., et al. (2009). A reengineered hospital discharge program to decrease re-hospitalization: A randomized trial. *Annuals of Internal Medicine, 150*(3), 178–187.

John, M. (1988). *Geragogy: A theory for teaching the elderly*. New York: Hearth Press.

Joint Commission. (2007). *What did the doctor say? Improving health literacy to protect patient safety*. Oakbrook Terrace, IL: Author.

Kimball, S. Buck, G. Goldstein, D, Largaespada, E., Logan, L. Stebbins, D. Halvorsen, L., & Kalman-Yearout, K. (2010). Testing a teaching appointment and geragogy-based approach to medication knowledge at discharge. *Rehabilitation Nursing, 35*(1), 31–40.

Koenigsberg, M. R., Bartlett, D., & Cramer, J. S. (2004). Facilitating treatment adherence with lifestyle changes in diabetes. *American Family Physician, 69*(2), 309.

Knowles, M. (1990). Andragogy: Theory into practice. Retrieved July 1, 2010, from http://tip.psychology.org/knowles.html

Levine, C. (2000). *Always on call: When illness turns families into caregivers*. New York: United Hospital Fund.

Lewin, K. (1951). *Field theory in social science*. New York: Harper.

Lewis, A. L., Stabler, K. A., & Welch, J. L. (2010). Perceived informational needs, problems, or concerns among patients with stage 4 chronic kidney disease. *Nephrology Nursing Journal, 37*(2), 143–148, 149.

London, F. (2009). *No time to teach: The essence of patient and family education for healthcare providers*. Atlanta, GA: Pritchett & Hull Associates.

Mager, R. F. (1997). *Preparing instructional objectives* (3rd ed.). Atlanta, GA: Center for Effective Performance.

Matter, B, Feinberg, M., Schomer, K. Harniss, M, Brown, P, & Johnson, K. (2009). Information needs of people with spinal cord injuries. *Journal of Spinal Cord Medicine, 32*(5) 545–554.

Medina, J. J. (2008). The biology of recognition memory. *Psychiatric Times*. Retrieved October 15, 2010, from http://www.brainrules.net/pdf/JohnMedina_PsychTimes_June08.pdf

Miller, G. A. (1956). The magical number seven, plus or minus two: Some limits on our capacity for processing information. *Psychological Review, 63*(2), 81–97.

NANDA International. (2007) *Nursing diagnoses: Definitions & classification 2007–2008*. Philadelphia: NANDA International.

National Institute on Aging. (2009, August 19). On line health information: Can you trust it? Retrieved October 15, 2010, from http://www.nia.nih.gov/healthinformation/publications/onlinehealth.htm

National Library of Medicine. (2009). FAQ: National Library of Medicine guide to finding health information. Retrieved July 1, 2010, from http://www.nlm.nih.gov/services/guide.html

Olinzock, B. J. (2008). Enhancing learning for patients with SCI: A patient education tool. *SCI Nursing, 25*, 10–19. Retrieved October 15, 2010, from http://www.aascin.org/pdf/scinursing-spring08.pdf

Partnership for Clear Health Communication. (2008). Health literacy stats at a glance. Retrieved September 15, 2010, from http://www.npsf.org/askme3/pdfs/STATS_GLANCE_EN.pdf

Paterson, B., Kieloch, B., & Gmiterek, J. (2001). "They never told us anything": Postdischarge instructions for families of persons with brain injuries. *Rehabilitation Nursing, 26*(2), 48–53.

Prochaska, J. O., & Velicer, W. F. (1997). The transtheoretical model of health behavior change. *American Journal of Health Promotion, 12,* 38–48.

Rollnick, S., William, R., & Butler, C. C. (2008). *Motivational interviewing in health care: Helping patients change behavior.* New York: Guilford Publications.

Rudd, R. E. (2007). Health Literacy Skills of U.S. Adults. *American Journal of Health Behavior 31* (Suppl 1), S8–18.

Sangasubana, N., Yang, Y., Bentley, S. I., Thumula, V., & Mendonca, C. M. (2009). Applying the health belief model to predict intention to comply with antibiotic regimen in young adults. Paper presented at the annual meeting of the American Association of Colleges of Pharmacy. Retrieved April 3, 2009, from http://www.allacademic.com/meta/p260787_index.html

Suter, P. M., & Suter, W. N. (2008). Timeless principles of learning: A solid foundation for enhancing chronic disease self-management. *Home Health Nurse, 26*(2), 82–88.

Thalheimer, W. (2009, January). Aligning the learning and performance context: Creating spontaneous remembering. Retrieved July 1, 2010, from http://www.work-learning.com/catalog.

Turner, A. P., Kivlahan, D. R., Sloan, A. P., & Haselkorn, J. K. (2007). Predicting ongoing adherence to disease modifying therapies in multiple sclerosis: Utility of the health belief model. *Multiple Sclerosis, 13,* 1146–1152

U.S. Department of Health and Human Services. Healthy People 2010 (2000). Understanding and Improving Health. 2nd ed. Washington, DC: U.S. Government Printing Office.

U.S. Department of Health and Human Services. (2003). A comprehensive approach to cancer prevention and control: A vision for the future. Retrieved July 1, 2010, from http://health.usnews.com/best-hospitals/rankings/rehabilitation

U.S. News and World Report. (2010). U.S. News Best Hospitals: Rehabilitation. Retrieved July 1, 2010, from http://www.huffingtonpost.com/2009/07/16/best-hospitals-in-the-us_n_235718.html

Wallston, K. A., Wallston, B. S., & DeVellis, R. (1978). Development of the multidimensional health locus of control (MHLC) scales. *Health Education Monographs, 6,* 160–170.

White, S., Bissell, P., & Anderson, C. (2010). Patients' perspectives on cardiac rehabilitation, lifestyle change and taking medicines: Implications for service development. *Journal of Health Services Research and Policy, 15*(Suppl 2), 47–53.

Wittmann-Price, R. A., & Fisher, K. M. (2009). Patient decision aids: Tools for patients and professionals. *American Journal of Nursing, 109*(12), 60–63.

CHAPTER 14

The Art of Caring: Addressing Psychosocial and Spiritual Issues

Spirituality, Coping, Depression, Grieving, Adjustment, and Adaptation

Gail L Sims

LEARNING OBJECTIVES

At the end of this chapter, the reader will be able to

- Describe how at least two nursing theorists have advocated for the spiritual support of rehabilitation patients.
- State three coping strategies for adjustment to disability.
- Synthesize techniques of assessment, implementation, and referral to obtain spiritual resources.
- Define the role of the professional rehabilitation nurse in providing spiritual care.
- Appreciate the importance of making meaning of patients' experiences, listening, and being present.

KEY CONCEPTS AND TERMS

Acceptance and Action Questionnaire	Emotion-focused behavior	Problem-focused behavior
Adolescent Coping Scale	Existential spirituality	Religious spirituality
Anxiety	Family Crisis Oriented Personal Evaluation Scale	Roy's Adaptation Model
Beck Depression Inventory	Five stages of death and dying	Spinal Cord Lesion Coping Strategies Questionnaire
Caritas consciousness relationship	Health-related quality of life	Spinal Cord Lesion Emotional Wellbeing Questionnaire
Catastrophizing	Inner strength	Spirituality
Coping	Intercessory prayer	Spiritual care
Daily Spiritual Experiences	Lewin's Change Theory	Spiritual distress
Depression	Optimism	Therapeutic use of self
Dispositional optimism	Perceived Support from God Scale	

The stories of team members in case study 14.1 are not unique, as they are shared among professional rehabilitation nurses across the world and over the ages. Making meaning of these experiences is the spirit, the very essence, and the heart of rehabilitation nursing practice. For some of us it is a calling, for some it is a ministry, for everyone it is, and forever will be, a mystery. Many have been called into this specialty of rehabilitation nursing to be healers, mentors, advocates, and teachers. In offering ourselves, we open our hearts and our minds to this sacred work. Exploring our own spiritual and philosophical views, we find meaning and inner strength to serve in this noble profession. Listening to our own hearts and sharing our stories with others is truly what sustains

Seven nurses sat in the beautiful, sun-filled conference room during the first Caring Council with the flicker of an artificial candle and the fragrance of lavender around the circle. We shared the deepest emotions surrounding one of our most challenging experiences. Authentic presence was at the heart of our sharing the memory of our first encounters with a middle-aged gentleman and his partner who came to our facility 3 weeks ago after sustaining a C4–5 complete spinal cord injury. The director of rehab operations shared her experience of opening her heart with compassion for this man. Sharing from the deepest place, she gave a testimony of her own personal journey about a family member with a similar level of injury. The first clinical rehabilitation nurse who cared for this patient at our hospital expressed the fear she felt. Could she meet the needs, demands, and expectations of the new arrivals? Did she have the energy and expertise within her being to cope with the physical, emotional, and spiritual pain they were experiencing? Could she sustain focused energy because she knew this would be an extremely long and challenging case? The next nurse who cared for this individual and his family added her own concerns about having the fortitude to sustain her own self while instilling hope and maintaining the bond of trust initially established. As we shared our emotions surrounding this encounter, we were profoundly touched and our lives were changed.

us. These encounters enrich our own lives as we give of ourselves. As we perform our daily tasks, we may be privileged to see into the heart and soul of others. Having the courage to search for these opportunities, peer into these open doors, and be fully present is a spiritual gift we have also received.

Simple attention allows us to be fully present to connect with another person. Often, we discover the greatest healing can lie within the smallest gestures of a loving touch, a caring word. The gift of a compassionate heart allows us to extend ourselves beyond the boundaries of our own personal worlds. Attention is a way to connect us inwardly with our thoughts, feelings, and desires. Listening without judgment or resistance is to begin to know and understand ourselves and is the source of wisdom.

DEFINITIONS OF SPIRITUALITY

Definitions of **spirituality** are complex and ambiguous. One conceptualization of spirituality stems form the theoretical work of Reed (1992), who described spirituality as a sense of making meaning through connectedness to a power greater than oneself, to others and the environment, and within oneself. This transcendence or connectedness is viewed as critical in driving values and derives meaning from daily experiences and the expressions of connectedness to others and to self.

Spirituality has evolved dramatically over the past few years in health care. This essential component of our work is now known to be an essential, required objective according to the *Joint Commission Journal on Quality and Safety* (Clark, Drain, & Malone, 2003). Standard RI.1.3.5 refers to the provision of pastoral care and other spiritual services, although meeting the spiritual needs of persons served is not a role delegated to one particular discipline. It is the responsibility of each individual to address the emotional and spiritual needs of patients and families we meet on our lives' journey.

Spirituality is often defined as religious or existential. **Religious spirituality** can be defined as a relationship with God or a higher power and typically is seen among individuals who attend organized services within a community (Colon, 1996). **Existential spirituality** is not directly related to a specific place of worship or an agreed on set of ideals. It refers to a worldview or perspective in which persons seek purpose in their life and come to understand their life as having meaning and value (Brady, Peterman, Fitchett, Mo, & Cella, 1999). It is suggested that studies include both religious and existential spirituality, because persons who have survived a catastrophic illness or injury may have mobility challenges that limit their ability to attend religious services in a community setting.

The concept of spirituality in nursing is deeply rooted in the history of our profession. Jenkins, Wikoff, Amankwaa, and Trent (2009) remind us that this concept is often overlooked in nursing practice, although it as an essential component in the holistic care of clients. Findings from their study revealed that nurse leaders' perception of **spiritual care** was of a religious nature, involving pastoral care visits as a primary intervention. The leaders interviewed stated the provision of spiritual care as a comfort measure was the primary benefit to patients, but most of them were not aware of holistic or spiritual care policies in their departments of nursing. Most had no influence from their supervisor or a job description to guide their role in providing spiritual care. Many of these leaders were not familiar with The Joint Commission guidelines related to spiritual care. They saw holistic care as a trend that might influence their role in the future. Many nurse leaders in this study reported being uncomfortable providing spiritual care for patients but perceived their staff was comfortable providing this care. Therefore, they were unable to advocate for spiritual care if they lacked understanding and direction. They had no prior education on spiritual care. A clear definition of spiritual care was lacking, and interventions were not expected of them or their nursing. This study suggested that the role of the nurse leader in the provision of spiritual care for patients was inadequate at the time of this study. Further training, encouraging staff, and advocating for a spiritual assessment tool was suggested.

NURSING MODELS FOR SPIRITUAL CARE AND ADAPTATION

Jenkins et al. (2009) explain the concept of spirituality in nursing as being deeply rooted in the history of our profession. Jean Watson's original work (1979) offered a conceptual framework for nursing and provided the foundation for the science and art of human caring. Her contributions describe 10 carative factors that are the original and evolved core for professional nursing practice. She explains that "when we include caring and love in our science, we discover our caring; healing professions and disciplines are much more than a detached scientific endeavor, but a life-giving and life-receiving endeavor for humanity" (Watson, 2005, p. 3).

> *Rehabilitation nurses are in key positions to foster the spiritual growth for themselves and others.*

The origin of what Jean Watson calls **caritas consciousness relationship** is actually found in Florence Nightingale's work. *Caritas* is the Latin word closely related to the original term "carative" but conveying a deep form of transpersonal caring and love. Jean Watson's theoretical framework explains the caring relationship as transpersonal in nature, meaning it involves both a giving and receiving interaction between the nurse and the patient. The nurse must be consciously aware of the need to exercise care and compassion in the relationship with others. This component of mindful presence expressed in a truly caring manner is an essential component of spiritual care.

Jean Watson's theory is based on authentic, intentional caring as a way to honor and respect the dignity of all humanity. The transpersonal caring relationship occurs when the caregiver enters into the life space of another person and detects that individual's condition of being on a spiritual or soul level. The caregiver must feel this condition within his or her being and respond in a way that allows the other person to release feelings, thoughts, and tension according to Watson's theory (George, 2002).

Roy's Adaptation Model provides a framework for modeling the integration of spiritual care. Roy's model proposes that all of life has purpose and meaning. Care of patients and family members is based on a multidimensional, holistic, and human experience. Provision of spiritual care to instill hope is critical to integration of the spiritual dimension into the plan of care and to achieve patient centered goals. Weiland (2010) integrates the spiritual domain into the nursing plan of care to positively influence health and wellness. The application of Roy's model into clinical practice emphasizes the role of the professional nurse to integrate spiritual care into the care environment. She states this role is not curative but healing in a way that assists the patient to reconstruct life plans and realize meaning from his or her extreme adversity.

MODELS FOR ADAPTATION TO DISABILITY

There are several models we refer to in rehabilitation nursing to describe ways in which patients cope with changes. **Lewin's Change Theory** (1947) covers unfreezing, movement, refreezing, and the forces and processes that can facilitate of impede change. Variables that influence **coping** efforts include age, severity of impairment, visibility of the impairment, sense of control, prior coping abilities, values (spiritual, cultural, philosophical, and religious), and perceived social support.

Livneh (1991) describes five stages of adaptation in his work that are applicable to adjustment to disability. Initial impact of shock and **anxiety**, defense mobilization, the initial realization of great turmoil, retaliation, and reintegration occur as the individual and his or her support system attempt to make meaning of the catastrophic events of their lives.

The classic model of adaptation to loss and grief is found in the famous work of Elizabeth Kubler-Ross (1982). The **five stages of death and dying** are applicable to the phases individuals experience in coping with disability and disease. Shock, denial, anger, depression, and finally acceptance and adjustment occur for most in the transformation of healing and rebuilding the narrative story of life purpose.

COPING STRATEGIES AND SCALES

Adaptation to illness and injury demands reliance of various coping strategies, especially in cases were permanent changes in functioning are present. Lazarus and Folkman (1984) suggested two categories of coping behaviors. **Emotion-focused behavior** uses avoidance efforts to divert away from thoughts and feelings caused by stress. These behaviors are maladaptive and result in poor outcomes. The other is **problem-focused behavior**, which utilizes adaptation and results in improved outcomes.

Kortte, Veiel, Batten, and Wegener (2009) studied the use of the **Acceptance and Action Questionnaire** as a tool to detect avoidance coping characterized by both active and passive attempts to avoid thoughts, feeling, memories, and bodily sensations the individual considers negative. Because these forms of ineffective coping can be extremely destructive and are related to increased levels of depression, detection of this maladaptive behavior is critical for prevention of complications in selected rehabilitation outcomes. Intervention to prevent avoidance is likely to produce positive outcomes. Promotion of acceptance and encouraging a strong commitment to engage in 3 hours of inpatient therapy as well as outpatient sessions and physician appointments is essential for long-term success. Wellness clinics are also important links in the continuum of care.

Jones and colleagues (2008) studied racial differences in coping with chronic osteoarthritis pain. Conclusions were drawn using the Coping Strategies Questionnaire, which revealed in a large sample size that African Americans' perception of prayer's helpfulness, as well as hoping and praying coping strategies, scored significantly higher than Whites. Another study by Hodge and Roby (2010) involving African women living with HIV/AIDS explored general and spiritual coping strategies. Using open-ended questions, a survey based on Koenig et al.'s (1992) three-item coping index was used. Questions were asked such as "How do you cope?", "How do you keep from getting depressed?", and "Do your spiritual or religious beliefs or activities help you cope?" It was determined that services that provided material assistance for food, medications, and counseling were helpful in coping. Spirituality in the form of prayer, singing, worship, and music was the second most popular means of coping. Social support was listed third most important for these women.

There is great need for reliable standardized, condition-specific instruments to assess the coping efforts made by persons with spinal cord injury. An article published in *Spinal Cord* (Migliorini, Elfstrom, & Tonge, 2008) used the **Spinal Cord Lesion Coping Strategies Questionnaire** to provide specific coping mechanisms of acceptance, fighting spirit, and social reliance used by respondents. The **Spinal Cord Lesion Emotional Wellbeing Questionnaire** indicated emotional consequences to the spinal cord injury and evaluated the positive emotional outcomes of personal growth and the negative outcomes of helplessness and intrusion. This study provided strong predictors of mental health outcomes and supported the usefulness of scales such as these for improved results. Using questions from these instruments enhances the assessment of coping strategies and emotional well being by the rehabilitation team.

Analysis of cognitive dysfunction, coping, and depression in multiple sclerosis was conducted by Rabinowitz and Arnett (2009). This study evaluated the hypothesis that coping mediates the relationship between cognitive dysfunction and depression in patients with multiple sclerosis. Negative coping styles were present with cognitive dysfunction. Maladaptive coping was shown to increase likelihood of depression. Cognitive deficits were believed to impair an individual's ability to use adaptive coping strategies and contributed to greater likelihood of using maladaptive coping strategies. Implications may be relevant in persons with other diagnoses that involve cognitive decline such as traumatic and nontraumatic brain injuries.

Coping with disabilities has been well researched. Physical, emotional, mental, and spiritual disabilities of all ages and a multitude of diseases and disorders have been discussed in the literature. Although instruments for the assessment of degrees of coping are used extensively by psychologists and neuropsychologists, it is valuable for rehabilitation nurses to be aware of these tools. Examples include the **Family Crisis Oriented Personal Evaluation Scale**, which shows the degree of faith and religious belief in relation to medical care, and the Coping Health Inventory for Parents, which determines parent's belief and faith related to their child's health. The implications of using instruments such as these are to determine degrees of coping and the role spirituality plays in this mechanism (Allen & Marshall, 2010).

Coping styles and strategies in students with and without learning disabilities should be considered when developing educational materials and designing methods of instructing persons with physical disabilities. The **Adolescent Coping Scale** was used by Firth, Greaves, and Frydenberg (2010) and revealed a need to provide adolescents with resources and strategies that addressed the risks of passive coping styles. Maladaptive coping may contribute to complications after spinal cord injuries, strokes, and brain injuries. Therefore, the rehabilitation nurse needs to use resources from school records and other diagnostic tools such as this instrument to determine the degree of coping strategies in the adolescent population. Teaching materials should be designed to encourage productive coping strategies such as problem-solving, focusing on the positive, and recreation and relaxation. Nonproductive coping strategies should be identified and addressed to prevent adverse outcomes. Some potentially destructive strategies include self-blame, isolation, worry, and wishful thinking.

Although age is an indicator of coping, the astute nurse can work with all age groups effectively, with these important needs taken into account. It is clear that persons with learning disabilities may be at risk for using passive coping strategies. With increased research and emphasis on hidden disabilities such as autism spectrum disorders, the rehabilitation nurse must adjust teaching styles and methods to promote positive outcomes.

RELATIONSHIP BETWEEN SPIRITUALITY AND OUTCOMES

Randolph Byrd's (1988) research study on **intercessory prayer** showed positive therapeutic effects of intercessory prayer in coronary care unit populations. Ten years later, McCaffrey, Eisenberg, Legedza, Davis, and Phillips (2004) concluded an estimated one-third of adults (n = 2,055, 60% weighted response rate) used prayer for health concerns in 1998. The current statistics on the frequency of using prayer may have changed since that time, although prayers can take many forms from a variety of faith traditions. A more recent study was conducted on the effects of intercessory prayer as an intervention for individuals with health challenges (Roberts, Ahmed, Hall, & Davison, 2009). This review brought together the relevant research evidence and sought to resolve uncertainties about the effects of intercessory prayer. Various forms of complementary and alternative medicine, including prayer and meditation, were used among 62% of all adults in the United States according to the 2002 National Health Interview Survey, conducted by the Centers for Disease Control and Prevention's National Center for Health Statistic (2002).

It is believed that prayer can be used effectively in conjunction with medical care (Dossey, 1993). The clinical issues and implications of prayer were described as holistic in nature by Taylor (2007). DiJoseph and Cavendish (2005) expanded further on the relevance of prayer

to holistic care. Spiritual practices may help one cope by facilitating acceptance of illness or disability and may counteract the feelings of isolation that may accompany illness or debilitating injuries.

Nurses must address psychosocial and spiritual issues in relationship to the person with an acute or chronic condition. Physicians are now taught to consider the role of spirituality in health care, which bodes well for the future according to Dr. Fuentes-Afflick (2009). As a resident, Dr. Fuentes-Afflick was not instructed on how to address religious or spiritual issues with patients and families. Although she assumed the mother of one of her disabled patients was Catholic, she had not discussed with her beliefs about the role of God in her life. She had not explored the mother's perception of a divine explanation for her child's developmental delay and seizure disorder. As a physician, Dr. Fuentes-Afflick was stunned by a question asked by this concerned parent during a routine clinic visit one day. The mother asked, "Do you believe that God answers our prayers?" The reason for her inquiry was more important to explore than the physician's response. The open door to communication was what really mattered most in this moment of authentic presence. The doctor's only response was "Si." She sat with the mother who was then encouraged to share the real reason for her asking. The doctor simply reached across the desk to hold her hand, sat in silence, and the mother relaxed and stopped crying. She then explained her concern centered around her own prayer that God would take her child before she and her husband died. She did not want her daughter to be left with no one to care for her. The acceptance the mother felt from her encounter with the physician eased the grief as several years later her child died after a seizure in the home.

Although training can help to prepare healthcare workers for the moment just described, the real question is not what we do but how we do it that really matters. Being authentically present and listening are critical. Validating this mother's beliefs and honoring her was the most important component of that encounter.

A review of literature offers several extensive studies on quality of life measurement. Quality of life and the concept of connectedness are described by Register and Herman (2010) as a universally recognized and highly desirable outcome in postmodern society. Spirituality, social networks, supportive communities, and a variety of health-promoting activities were associated with improved quality of life, whereas loneliness, depression, fear, and isolation were associated with decreased quality of life.

Spiritual care in rehabilitation nursing is about making meaning of life's experiences, catastrophic as they may be. When disability occurs, whether sudden or gradual, the narrative of that person's life is broken. The struggle is to create a new narrative, or mend the broken one. Alison Bonds-Shapiro survived two brainstem hemorrhagic strokes to discover the power of this amazing transformation (Shapiro, 2009). She described her profound experience of having "a little bit of blood in the wrong place" that caused her to suddenly lose her ability to speak, swallow, and control her emotions, her bowel, and her bladder. She stated it is virtually impossible to imagine the depth of this type of injury and the overwhelming struggle necessary to rebuild a life that has been broken.

The concept of spirituality is frequently associated with health outcomes as well as quality of life. The relationship between religiousness, spirituality, and health outcomes in the rehabilitation population was studied by Johnstone and Yoon (2009). They concluded that positive spiritual experiences and willingness to forgive are related to better physical health, whereas negative spiritual experiences are related to poor physical and mental health to persons with disabilities. The study also concluded that spiritual experiences are related to health outcomes, although religious practices and congregationally based social support are not. It was further determined in this study that positive emotions associated with a loving higher power are associated with better health, and negative emotions associated with an abandoning, punishing higher power are associated with worse health, consistent with previous research findings (Rippentrop, Altmaier, Chen, Fomd, & Keffela, 2005).

FINDING MEANING, PURPOSE, AND SIGNIFICANCE

Victor Frankl (1959), survivor of a concentration camp and also a psychiatrist, developed a theory of why some people survived and others died. He observed that life has purpose and meaning in all types of situations and that psychological problems may occur when person's search for meaning is impeded. Frankl stated that one's purpose in life is not solely dependent on physical health or external circumstances. He said people could find meaning and purpose in any situation and that survival was due to having a life purpose in any surroundings and circumstances. Life purpose is an important thread in health and critical care nursing according to Hodges (2009). The philosophical nature of life purpose, its attributes, definitions, and theoretical frameworks, as well as differences in theories and empirical support are explored in this work. Purpose in life affects the capacity to respond to opportunities and to manage life problems and challenges.

The gentleman described in the case study 14.1 was desperately trying to find meaning and purpose in his life after a traumatic spinal cord injury. Everything about his surroundings, his livelihood, and his relationships to others had suddenly changed, in the blink of an eye, as one fall put a halt to his dreams and hopes for the future. As rehabilitation nurses search for ways to create meaning, they find comfort in a variety of resources. Prayers such as the one stated below can provide comfort and purpose. Nurses may share with each other or with patients and families words of hope and encouragement when appropriate (Hake & Boone, 2004, p. 201):

> "Broken bodies, broken hearts. I look around me and see those whose lives have been shattered … . The progress is slow, unpredictable, and hard won. Help us to see each step as a victory, even the smallest skill as a triumph. Remind me this isn't just a time to master the body; it is a time to rebuild the spirit."

In times of extreme challenge, Christian African Americans' faith in a higher power provided strength and hope, liberating them from the cruelties of slavery (Cone, 2002). Their religious thought gave them inspiration and hope for survival. Christian African Americans depended on their personal relationship and connection to a higher power called God through prayer, trust, and support.

Mendes, Roux, and Ridosh (2010) explored the development of inner strength in women and found improvement in health outcomes and quality of life. This study supported previous works that described the outcome of inner strength is living a new normal. Four themes associated with the theory of inner strength emerged: anguish and searching, connectedness, engagement, and movement. A definition of **inner strength** evolved as having the capacity to build self through a developmental process that positively moves an individual through challenging life events. The outcome of this process is living a new normal as defined by Roux, Dingley, and Bush (2002).

Hamilton, Crandell, Carter, and Lynn (2010) evaluated the reliability and validity an instrument known as the **Perceived Support from God Scale**. This scale was used to assess components of spirituality in health care not found in other instruments. The instrument measured support derived from a dynamic, communicative exchange between individuals and God. The positive influence of spirituality on health outcomes can aid healthcare practitioners in meeting the spiritual needs of persons recovering from injury and illness.

Quality of life has been studied from a generative context. The concept of spiritual and social connectedness has emerged in the literature. Burkhardt (1994) studied elements of belonging in women, and Hill (2004) examined this concept in Native American. The quality of life and life purpose is described in a variety of ways by different groups. Psychological well-being, religiosity, and spirituality are used to describe the positive aspects of life purpose. Krause (2004) asserted that believing one's actions have a place in the larger order of things and one's behavior fits into the larger whole of society. Having a sense of direction, order, and a reason for living, personal identity and a greater social consciousness helps one define life purpose. On the contrary, lack of life purpose is stated by Lyons and Younger (2001) as a frustration when life purpose is lacking or absent in cases of severe conditions such as those living with HIV. Life purpose can be discovered by suffering as well as by experiencing love and by doing good deeds. Coping, inner strength, and courage are often associated with life purpose after recovery from neurological impairments such as stroke and spinal cord injury. Facing one's mortality, letting go of fear and turmoil, identifying and making lifestyle changes, and seeking higher purpose and meaning in life are ways in which spirituality influenced recovery after acute myocardial infarction (Walton, 2002).

Optimism was significantly correlated with spirituality in a recent study by Mazanec, Daly, Douglas, and Lipson (2010). Spirituality was a significant predictor of overall **health-related quality of life** and social, emotional, and functional well being. Mofidi, DeVellis, Devellis, Blazer, Panter, and Jordan (2007) studied the relationship between spirituality and depressive symptoms and postulated there was a relationship between spirituality and optimism that is bidirectional in that spirituality may foster optimism and optimism may support spirituality. Matheis, Tulsky, and Matheis (2006) explored the relationship between spirituality and quality of life among individuals with spinal cord injury; 98.7% of respondents reported using some form of spiritual-based coping. Quality of life was highest among those participants who used existential spiritual as opposed to religious spiritual coping. It was suggested that spiritual-based coping should be used as a strategy for improving life quality and that clinicians should be aware of spiritual practices

of persons with spinal cord injuries. Honoring these practices and supporting their expression may be a powerful tool to assist the healing or restoration of another human being.

ROLE OF THE INTERDISCIPLINARY TEAM MEMBER IN SPIRITUAL ASSESSMENT

Spiritual inquiry in health care is viewed as controversial, although spirituality and religiosity have been correlated with reduced morbidity and mortality, improved physical and emotional well being, reduced stress and illness prevention, and improved coping skills (McCord et al., 2004). Although many professionals, including physicians, lack spirituality training, there has been a movement toward development of a more holistic, patient-centered assessment of spiritual and religious beliefs.

The Office of Research of the Northeastern Ohio Universities College of Medicine designed a questionnaire to assess spirituality. One of their findings included that respondents' reasons for wanting their physician to know about their spiritual beliefs centered on understanding them better as people and understanding their decision making. Providing compassion, encouraging realistic hope, and referral to a spiritual counselor were endorsed by over 50% of participants. Providing understanding, compassion, and hope are hallmarks of good healthcare providers.

A strictly scientific approach to medicine does not consider the importance of meaning of life and hope to patients' well being, according to Ellis (2002). Referral to a spiritual advisor has been identified as an acceptable course of action to bridge the gap between medicine and spirituality. Healthcare providers must identify, coordinate, and use referral sources for patient requests. Koenig (2000) stated that for many patients spirituality is an important part of wholeness and that ignoring the spiritual dimension of a person leaves one with a feeling of incompleteness and may interfere with healing.

Several spiritual assessment tools are found in the literature and should be used to assess the unique needs of all patients. Based on the spiritual assessment concepts discussed in the literature, assessment tools using mnemonics devices should be incorporated into the rehabilitation nurse's dialogue, such as HOPE. (Ananderajah & Hight, 2001). *H* represents sources of hope, meaning, comfort, strength, peace, love, and connection; *O* means organized religion; *P* stands for personal spirituality and practices; and *E* represents effects on medical care, disability, and possibly end-of-life decisions. Use of mnemonics was recommended by Rieg, Mason, and Preston (2006) to prompt nurses to inquire about sources of support, important affiliations, consequences related to current illness, and treatment concerns. Dialogue initiated by the nurse was suggested to form connectedness with patients and families to meet the holistic and spiritual needs of patients. When we embrace the need for spiritual care and share our values with others, it generates a set of behaviors that encourages others by role modeling the art of caring.

Mazanec and colleagues (2010) demonstrated the relationship between what they called **dispositional optimism** and quality of life as a critical step in developing effective screening tools and targeting interventions for psychological care. Dispositional optimism is the belief in positive outcomes in the future. Although this study was not conclusive of a direct correlation, it is suggested that persons with poor functional status, young age, low levels of spirituality, and high levels of depression may be vulnerable for negative outcomes.

NURSING INTERVENTIONS

Interventions must be of a nonjudgmental nature, as definitions of spirituality differ, based on a variety of worldviews and opinions. Because spirituality is a broad concept, it transcends religious boundaries. Spiritual care must be delivered in a manner that is culturally sensitive and based on the patient's, not the caregiver's, beliefs. Nurses must develop their own style of intervention in a manner in which they are comfortable. Religious affiliation is not the same as a person's spirituality. Persons receiving rehabilitation services often struggle to integrate their old self into a new self. Rieg et al. (2006) emphasized the importance of formulating one's own worldview, appreciating the attributes that foster one's spiritual sense such as love, understanding, wisdom, and faith. Discovering one's own spiritual foundation can prepare the nurse to distinguish the actual needs of patients from the nurse's own spiritual perspectives.

The essence of delivering spiritual care is **therapeutic use of self**. Engaging oneself in the interaction, the nurse needs to be aware that spiritual care must be patient led, not nurse directed. Skills of listening, observing, and presence are essential in nursing and support spiritual care. When the nurse is fully present and sensitive to a patient's cues, spiritual care often occurs spontaneously and purposefully during their stay. It is important for the nurse to become comfortable asking questions that produce valuable spiritual assessment data. This nurs-

TABLE 14.1   Questions to Ask Patients Related to Providing Spiritual Care
Where are you in your spiritual journey?
Would you like to speak with the hospital chaplain on call?
Would you like me to pray with you?
How are your spirits today?
What role has faith played in your life in the past?
Is there a spiritual leader, pastor, priest, rabbi, or other person who can be called for you?
What items from home would be helpful in practicing your faith or religion?

ing process can be implemented by asking a few, simple, open-ended questions (Table 14.1). Focusing on feeling, concerns, needs, or hurts provide situational assessment questions. Diagnosis and plan of care starts with analyzing the assessment. Determination of spiritual well being leads to a nursing diagnosis, and the plan is established from this information.

Determining the best person on the team to provide interventions of spiritual care may occur at the first team conference. Some rehabilitation nurses refer to psychologists, chaplains, and social workers to provide spiritual and psychological support to patients and families. Regardless of which discipline provides this service, open communication facilitates the rehabilitation process for both patients and family members (Duhamel & Talbot, 2004). Ways to inspire hope in the rehabilitation setting and generic prayers that can be used by nurses for persons of various faiths to open the door to spiritual conversations are described by Kautz (2008). A Web link to world prayers can be found in Box 14.1.

BOX 14.1   Web Exploration
Go to http://www.worldprayers.org to view a collection of many prayers from all different faiths. Consider how you might use any of these prayers in your practice as a rehabilitation nurse.

The Institute of Medicine recently shared the importance of psychosocial services and interventions to optimize the health-related quality of life of patients and families with cancer (Mazanec et al., 2010). The benefit of implementing these services includes the development of a tailored plan of care to address individual needs and address follow-up care. The need for more effective screening tools and interventions was highlighted as a research priority to assist clinicians to meet the standards for psychosocial care. Screening and interventions for rehabilitation patients is noteworthy. Nursing diagnoses and interventions must encompass a spiritual rather than a religious-based identification. The role of the rehabilitation nurse is to support and facilitate the person's own unique values and promote spiritual health.

IMPLEMENTING TOOLS FOR THE PREVENTION AND DETECTION OF DEPRESSION, ANXIETY, ANGER, AND WITHDRAWAL IN THE REHABILITATION SETTING

Depression, anxiety, and various forms of mental distress and disorder are discussed by Loewenthal (2007) in relation to religious beliefs and practices. The relationship between religion, spirituality, and mental distress, though controversial, must be examined to demonstrate the positive, and rarely negative, effects that spirituality and religion may have on well-being. Faith and interpersonal processes influence coping and resilience. Blumenthal et al (2007) examined the relationship between spiritual experiences and health in a sample of persons who survived an acute myocardial infarction with depression or low social support. Using the **Beck Depression Inventory** and the **Daily Spiritual Experiences** questionnaire, respondents shared about spirituality variables of worship attendance, prayer, or meditation. Although religion and religious practices provide psychological comfort, support, and reassurance to persons with serious medical conditions, the physical health benefits of spirituality, religion, and prayer remain controversial. Further study is suggested in the future.

Anger, depression, or withdrawal in the rehabilitation setting is not uncommon during any phase of recovery. Depression is also a major health issue in the elderly. Depression severity is associated with decreased quality of life, functional decline, and disability (Lenze et al., 2005). Mann and colleagues (2008) examined changes in impairment level, functional status, and the use of assistive devices by older persons with depression. Because the rehabilitation team prescribes and trains any individual to use assistive devices, it is important to assess for their ability to use the equipment safely and appropriately to maintain functional ability. Consideration of emotional factors can help to determine whether there are additional barriers to learning and carryover. With this information being taken into consideration, therapists and nurses may determine that additional time is needed for reinforcement or that neuropsychology, social services, or chaplaincy personnel need to become involved to ensure optimal outcomes.

A recent study published by Molton and colleagues (2009) described the relative importance of psychosocial factors in pain experienced by persons with spinal cord injury. Simplification of pain appraisal and coping responses were used. It was found that passive coping and **catastrophizing** were significant independent predictors of the degree of pain interference. Catastrophizing is characterized by unrealistic and excessively negative self-statements in response to pain. Examples of catastrophizing chronic pain are labeling pain sensations as awful, horrible, and unbearable (Gracely et al., 2004). Negative beliefs and coping variables such as disability and catastrophizing have stronger relationships with pain interference and mental health outcomes in this study than did the positive beliefs and coping variables such as control or task persistence. Implications for nursing practice include the importance of decreasing suffering and managing pain in not only persons recovering from spinal cord injury, but for all diagnostic groups. Consideration of psychosocial factors needs to be made along with pain intensity. Negative or maladaptive coping strategies and beliefs need to be addressed to improve outcomes. Negative beliefs such as the perception of poor pain control, ineffective or maladaptive coping, and catastrophizing pain appear to interfere with positive outcomes. It is the rehabilitation nurse's role to advocate for proper pain management. This is done through collaboration and problem solving with the patient and the entire clinical rehabilitation team during team and family conferences. Advocacy is critical for the successful promotion of patients to achieve functional gains and healthy coping strategies.

Feelings of depression, anxiety, anger, and withdrawal may be a person's own unique way of searching for meaning in the experience. Learning to listen for questions with "why" in them is an important skill. Open-ended questions may allow for more in-depth inquiry. Listening, reflection, and touch, when used together, provide the support to explore and find meaning. Interactions can flow out of this encounter. Journaling, imagery, reminiscence, and life review also may help. Presence or mindfulness can be the most profound quality, enabling the nurse to center and focus on the patient. Kornfield (1993) explains there is no formula for practicing presence or mindfulness. Being compassionate and available to others requires that we listen and attend, understand our own motivation, and ask ourselves what action can be helpful.

The essence of providing spiritual care is the therapeutic involvement of the nurse's full presence or self into the interaction. Spiritual care must be patient focused and not directed by the nurse. Questions that can assess the spiritual needs of patients in rehabilitation may include "How are your spirits today?", "Has faith been important to you at other times in your life?", and "Is faith or spirituality important to you at this time?" The rehabilitation nurse must discover which type of inquiry yields results that enable them to support the patient and family through recovery. Recognizing that expression of feelings is normal and natural, it is important for the nurse to know when these feelings interfere with progress and halt rehabilitation efforts. The rehabilitation team may consult with neuropsychology or psychiatry for management of these behaviors.

Various methods can be used in addition to those previously mentioned. Humor is often used to relieve stress, increase the ability to cope, and maintain hope (Kylma & Juvakka, 2006). Chinery (2007) found that humor promotes relaxation, wellness, and hopefulness. Rehabilitation nurses who exercise the gift of humor in their interactions with others help themselves, their coworkers, patients, and families to cope. Incorporating laughter into the day to day routine can lift spirits and promote healing (Box 14.2). As the nurse develops rapport with patients and families over the course of the inpatient stay, there can be further assessment of which techniques are most effective. The nurse must monitor the patient's mood and determine when and how to apply these interventions.

BOX 14.2   Web Exploration
Check out Brian Regan's comic monologue called "The Emergency Room" on YouTube at www.youtube.com. Share it with a nurse friend.

RESOURCES FOR THE PROVISION OF SPIRITUAL CARE

Resources for the provision of emotional and spiritual support include books, music, multimedia such as a television channel dedicated to both visual and auditory sensory stimulation, meditation, prayer facilities and environment, and support groups that include community- and hospital-based programs, recovery, and specific diseases to provide the resources and common ground for sharing unique experiences (Table 14.2). Many facilities have migrated away from traditional chapels to honor all faiths and belief systems. Quiet rooms that offer silence and a tranquil atmosphere may appeal to some, although

TABLE 14.2   Additional Rehabilitation Unit Strategies for Promoting Spiritual Health
• Books
• Music
• Multimedia such as a television channel dedicated to both visual and auditory sensory stimulation
• Meditation
• Prayer facilities and environment
• A facility chapel
• A dedicated prayer or quiet room for meditation on each unit
• Support groups, which include community- and hospital-based programs, recovery, and disease specific
• Resources on faith, spiritual comfort, forgiveness, etc. provided on the unit in a binder
• Groups to share unique experiences, such as healing circles
• Labyrinths and gardens to promote wellness and peace
• Chaplain or spiritual support person available or on call 24 hours per day
• Programming that include both denominational and nondenominational
• Create a caring environment (healing touchstones, blessing baskets, nursing lounges)

outdoor environments have emerged into the modern architecture of hospitals to include labyrinths and gardens to promote wellness and peace. Administrative support must be present to promote these modalities to more forward with this caring model.

Some organizations have created quality improvement teams dedicated to the research and implementation of emotionally and spiritually supportive individualized interventions. Resource guides have been developed to assist healthcare workers in the provision of culturally competent care. One example of such a resource is "A Provider's Handbook on Culturally Competent Care" designed to meet the needs of individuals with disabilities (Sandel et al., 2004). Some facilities use resources through the chaplaincy department to ensure resources are available to meet spiritual and emotional needs of persons served.

EVALUATION OF EFFECTIVENESS

The effectiveness of providing emotional and spiritual care can take many forms. Subjective data from both staff and supervisor nursing rounds can provide valuable feedback. Satisfaction surveys can provide data from which to benchmark progress in this area. Objectively, the utilization of resources provided in the patient and family education binder may imply that spiritual needs are being addressed and at least partially met. The expression of interest and participation in activities to promote spiritual wellness, such as a healing circle, religious services, or programs in the inpatient setting, can be an indication of the effectiveness of needs being met. Affiliation of the chaplaincy or pastoral care team is a valuable method of keeping abreast of how well the rehabilitation team is meeting the spiritual needs of the disabled population. Encouraging programs that are both denominational and nondenominational provide avenues for meeting the needs of the persons served, and evaluation of these programs is critical for continuous improvement.

> *Spiritual sensitivity is a way to support patients in their own search for spiritual meaning and solace without injecting one's own opinions or values (Lackey, 2009).*

Spiritual sensitivity in nursing care is defined by Sarah Lackey (2009) as a way to support patients in their own search for spiritual meaning and solace without injecting one's own opinions or values. Listening carefully is the key to opening the door to the deepest level of nursing practice. She offers a simple method to sorting out the cues of religious activity from spiritual searching in our assessment. Contacting clergy or chaplain as a resource to meet the patient's needs is one step in allowing the patient to practice his or her own beliefs. Being supportive and nonjudgmental in your approach helps the patient find his or her own answers to make meaning of the experience. Identification of **spiritual distress** is accomplished by using several basic tools of observation, active listening, reflection, and touch. Clues indicating spiritual distress may include anger, depression, or withdrawal. Spiritual distress can be a sign that a person is searching for the meaning or purpose behind the events of life. Noting the patient's connections, the nurse begins to recognize, respect, and support the individual's process of spiritual searching. Providing emotional support and maintaining a nonjudgmental approach during the patient's search for meaning helps the individuals find his or her own answers. Acceptance is the key to support the process of spiritual searching. Simply being present with the patient, even when the nurse truly cannot find words to share, is the best intervention. Though silence can be awkward, being silently present can support the patient's spiritual process in unknown ways.

Lisa Copen (2009) shared her views as a patient when she stated open communication is the key to the success of the nurse–patient relationship. The nurse's presence can determine how well the patient copes with situations and how well one is able to emotionally process the outcome. From a patient's perspective, nurses who contributed the greatest degree of improvements in the quality of care were advocates when no one else would listen or those who simply held a hand of a patient experiencing pain or feeling lonely. Rehabilitation nurses and their patients and families who improve understanding of one another and each other's needs often sustain a long-standing relationship. The celebration of the smallest successes can be the highlight of a patient's day. Nurses must realize how powerful their words are, when giving compliments such as "You have a great attitude," or "I admire how well you are coping." Making eye contact, touching a shoulder, or holding someone's hand can make all the difference.

ETHICAL CONSIDERATIONS

The American Nurses Association code of ethics mandates the inclusion of spiritual care for all patients. Provision 1.3 states that "the measures nurses take to care for the patient enable that patient to live with as much physical, emotional, social, and spiritual well-being as possible" (American Nurses Association, 2001, p. 7). Spiritual support scales often focus on support from a religious community, clergy, or healthcare providers. Spirituality has been associated with quality of life (Tarakeshwar et al., 2006). Spiritual preferences have a profound effect on the rehabilitation process. Belief systems can influence patient's outcomes in positive or negative ways. The provision of nonjudgmental spiritual support inspires hope for recovery.

CULTURE OF CARING EMERGING

Creating a culture of caring is essential to a healthy workplace. It is imperative that we examine closely the culture we are creating for patients, families, and healthcare providers. Green, McArdle, and Robichaux (2009) examined the creation of a caring culture that addressed the needs of patients and families while valuing the contribution of healthcare practitioners. Attention to physical comfort and promotion of teamwork, healing, and support are cornerstones of a culture of caring. Attributes of a caring culture must be present in the provision of patient care as well as the provision of caring for each other as colleagues.

Finfgeld-Connett (2008) defined caring in nursing as being derived from a metasynthesis of the concept of "an interpersonal process that is characterized by expert nursing, interpersonal sensitivity and intimate relationships" (p. 198). There must be a need for and an openness to caring. The environment must value caring over simple task completion. Caring is the focus of the nursing profession. The role of caring must be fully understood. Caring must work in both directions, with both patients and nurses involved in the process. Although technology has advanced, the delivery of care may change, but the true work of nursing must always be centered on caring. Teamwork, support, and connecting supports a culture of caring.

> *Healing touchstones, blessing baskets, nursing lounges, and waiting rooms are evolving into symbols of caring environments.*

Jean Watson's theory of human caring includes basic beliefs that we are human beings caring for others. We are all caregivers who are giving care through kindness and compassion. We provide patient-centered care in a holistic approach to meeting others' needs. Families, friends, and loved ones are essential in the healing process. Jean Watson used Lewin's Change Theory (1947) to help create a culture of care. Her theory honors the caring practices of nurses, defining how caring practice is valued and developing nursing knowledge within a caring framework.

The cultural climate of the organization frames and shapes the behaviors of employees. As we share the importance of spiritual care, we create the type of climate that fosters holistic patient care in a nurturing and healing environment. Leaders in rehabilitation nursing have a profound influence on the transdisciplinary team as well as on other healthcare providers that can transform an organization, improve service scores and retention in all departments, and provide exceptional care. Sharing caring theories and giving permission to create healing environments have been known to permeate not only the patient's immediate circle, but these concepts have begun to shape the interactions in team conferences, nursing huddles, and cut across to other departments in the organization. Inclusion of spiritual care education in nursing orientation and the provision of in-services

train nurses in the use of this model and incorporating Jean Watson's Caring Theory into nursing practice is a way to promote this important component into our daily routines.

Care councils, committees, or groups known as caring advocates have formed as examples of the implementation of Watson's caring environment. Exploring the carative factors with the goal of sharing the theory in everyday practice is becoming part of the change in nursing practice. Several practices are immerging in the hospital settings to create an environment of caring, healing, and peace. Healing touchstones, blessing baskets, nursing lounges, and waiting rooms are evolving into symbols of caring environments. Care channels are becoming an available source for patients, families, and healthcare workers. Setting the tone and intention of a calm atmosphere has reduced the sense of institutional darkness. As we implement other practices that honor our own humanity, our coworkers, and other staff we interact with, we are taking ownership of our professional nursing practice. We are making meaning of our experiences and transforming healing and spirituality in an extraordinary and interdisciplinary way. Staff meetings are held in circular fashion with a candle in the center to remind us that we are the light in our institutional darkness. Patients and their families are the focus of our family conferences rather than the traditional reading of functional levels. We are now taking ownership of rehabilitation nursing practice through the utilization of the caring theory.

SUMMARY

Spiritual care is no longer reserved for one discipline. Chaplains, social workers, hospital administrators, physicians, therapists, and nurses are responsible for discovering their own worldview and for creating an environment that supports and encourages communication, authentic presence, and making meaning of life events. Rehabilitation nurses are in key positions to foster the spiritual growth for themselves and others. Assessing, implementing, and referring our patients and families to resources promote adaptation and healthy coping strategies. With advances in medical technology, spirit is calling us back to our roots to be the healers, mentors, and teachers of the ancient art of caring in its purest form. With our spiritual toolbox stored deep in our soul, we make meaning of our own spiritual journey and support the experiences of others.

CRITICAL THINKING

1. Consider meeting with other nurse colleagues and inviting a hospital chaplain to explore ways in which the nursing staff in your facility can further integrate spiritual care into rehabilitation care.

2. Visit or contact another rehabilitation center to gather additional information regarding spiritual assessment instruments and share ideas about creating or expanding a culture of caring in your setting.

3. Access Internet sites such as the Medical Home Portal at http://www.medicalhomeportal.org to explore resources and spiritual support sites for persons with disabilities.

4. Access Jean Watson's Internet website at www.watsoncaringscience.org to obtain more information and resources to aid in creating or expanding your own culture of caring environment.

PERSONAL REFLECTION

- As we aspire to create a compassionate, healing environment, centered around caring for the rehabilitation patient and family, how do you plan to personally deliver this care in your professional role?

- Describe an example of a caring moment you have personally experienced and journal your answer in your private diary.

- How do you motivate others to focus less on the tasks of nursing and more on the whole patient? What would you personally commit to changing in your behaviors and interactions with others to role model this?

- Imagine providing rehabilitation nursing care to a 22-year-old woman who is ventilator dependent after sustaining a spinal cord injury. You have an excellent rapport and trust established. She has just returned from an outing to the beach where she attempted to drive her power wheelchair off the peer to end her life. What would you do to support her? How would you handle this situation, and what resources would you obtain? What would you do for yourself and your colleagues after this incident?

Questions

1. What is the benefit of team members sharing feelings and emotions in this way?

2. What resources discussed in this chapter could be used to assess the spirituality of the patient in this case?

3. How could the nurses in this situation use therapeutic use of self to provide spiritual care to this patient?

REFERENCES

Allen, D., & Marshall, E. (2010). Spirituality as a coping resource for African American parents of chronically ill children. *American Journal of Maternal/Child Nursing, 35*(4), 232–237.

American Nurses Association. (2001). *Code of ethics for nurses with interpretive statements.* Silver Springs, MD: American Nurses Association.

Anandarajah, G., & Hight, E. (2001). Spirituality and Medical Practice: Using the HOPE Questions as a Practical Tool for Spiritual Assessment. *American Family Physician, 63*(1), 81–89.

Blumenthal, J., Babyak, M., Ironstone, G., et al. (2007). Spirituality, religion, and clinical outcomes in patients recovering from an acute myocardial infarction. *Psychosomatic Medicine, 69*, 501–508.

Blumenthal, J. A., Babyak, I. G., Thoresen, C., Powell, L., Czajkowski, S., Catellier, P., et al. (2007). Spirituality, religion, and clinical outcomes in patients recovering from an acute myocardial infarction. *Psychosomatic Medicine, 69*, 501–508.

Brady, M. J., Peterman, A. H., Fitchett, G., Mo, M., & Cella, D. (1999). A case for including spirituality in quality of life measurement in oncology. *Psycho-Oncology, 8*, 417–428.

Burkhardt, M. A. (1994). Becoming and connecting: elements of spirituality for women. *Holistic Nursing Practice, 8*(4), 12–21.

Byrd, R. (1988). Positive therapeutic effects of intercessory prayer in a coronary care unit population. *Scientific Medicine Journal, 81*(7), 826–829.

Chinery, W. (2007). Alleviating stress with humor: A literature review. *Journal of Perioperative Practice, 17*, 172–182.

Clark, P., Drain, M., & Malone, M. (2003). Addressing patient's emotional and spiritual needs. *Joint Commission Journal on Quality and Safety, 29*(12), 659–670.

Colon, K. (1996). The healing power of spirituality. *Minnesota Medicine, 79*, 12–18.

Cone, J. H. (2002). *God of the oppressed.* Maryknoll, NY: Orbitz Books.

Copen, L. (2009). Nurses and chronically ill patients: Open communication is key. Retrieved October 15, 2010, from http://www.copingwithdisability.com.

DiJoseph, J., & Cavendish, R. (2005). Expanding the dialogue on prayer relevant to holistic care. *Holistic Nursing Practice, 19*, 147–154.

Dossey, L. (1993). *Healing words: The power of prayer and the practice of medicine.* San Francisco: Harper.

Duhamel, F., & Talbot, L. R. (2004). A constructive evaluation of family systems nursing interventions with families experiencing cardiovascular and cerebrovascular illness. *Journal of Family Nursing, 10*, 12–32.

Ellis, M.R. (2002). Challenges posed by a scientific approach to spiritual issues. *Journal of Family Practice, 51*, 259–260.

Fawcett, T. N., & Noble, A. (2004). The challenge of spiritual care in a multi-faith society experienced as a Christian nurse. *Journal of Clinical Nursing, 13*(2), 136–142.

Finfgeld-Connett, D. (2008). Meta-synthesis of caring in nursing. *Journal of Clinical Nursing, 17*, 196–204.

Firth, N., Greaves, D., & Frydenberg, E. (2010). Coping styles and strategies: A comparison of adolescent students with and without learning disabilities. *Journal of Learning Disabilities, 43*(1), 77–85.

Frankl, V. (1959). *Man's search for meaning.* New York: Pocket Books.

Fuentes-Afflick, E. (2009). A mother's prayer. *Academic Pediatrics, 9*(1), 15–17.

George, J. B. (2002). *Nursing theories: The base for professional nursing practice.* Upper Saddle River, NJ: Prentice Hall.

Gracely, R. H., Geisser, M. E., Giesecke,T., Grant, M.A., Petzke, F., Williams, D. A., et al. (2004). Pain catastrophizing and neural responses to pain among persons with fibromyalgia. *Brain, 127*(4), 835–843.

Green, M., McArdle, D., & Robichaux, C. (2009). Creating a culture of caring to foster a healthy workplace. *Critical Care Nursing Quarterly, 32*(4), 296–304.

Hake, C., & Boone, D. (2004). *Light unto my path for nurses.* Uhrichsville, OH: Barbour Publishing.

Hamilton, J., Crandell, J., Carter, J., & Lynn, M. (2010). Reliability and validity of the perspectives of support from God scale. *Nursing Research, 59*(2), 102–109.

Hill, D. L. (2006). Sense of belonging as connectedness: American Indian worldview and mental health. *Archives of Psychiatric Nursing, 20*(5), 210–216.

Hodge, D., & Roby, J. (2010). Sub-Saharan African women living with HIV/AIDS: An exploration of general and spiritual coping strategies. *Social Work, 55*(1), 27–37.

Hodges, P. (2009). The essence of life purpose. *Critical Care Nursing Quarterly, 32*(2), 163–170.

Jenkins, M., Wikoff, K., Amankwaa, L., & Trent, B. (2009). Nursing the spirit. *Nursing Management, 40*(8), 29–36.

Johnstone, B., & Yoon, D. (2009). Relationships between the brief multidimensional measure of religiousness/spirituality and health outcomes for heterogeneous rehabilitation population. *Rehabilitation Psychology, 54*(4), 42–431.

Jones, A. C., Kwoh, C. K., Groeneveld, P. W., Mor, M., Geng, M., & Ibrahim, S. (2008). Investigating racial differences in coping with chronic osteoarthritis pain. *Journal of Cross Cultural Gerontology, 23*, 339–347.

Kautz, D. (2008). Inspiring hope in our patients, their families, and ourselves. *Rehabilitation Nursing, 33*, 148–153.

Kautz, D., & Horn, E. (2009). Promoting family integrity to inspire hope in rehabilitation patients: Strategies to provide evidence-based care. *Rehabilitation Nursing, 34*(4), 168–173.

Kemp, B. (2010) Coping with disability. A challenge at all ages. Retrieved from http://codi.buffalo.edu/graph_based/.aging/.conf/.coping.htm

Koenig, H. G. (2000). Religion, spirituality and medicine: application to clinical practice. *Journal of the American Medical Association, 284*(13), 1708.

Koenig, H. G., Cohen, H. J., Blazer, D. G., et al (1992). Religious coping and depression among elderly hospitalized medically ill men. *American Journal of Psychiatry, 149*, 1693–1700.

Kornfield, J. (1993). *A path with heart.* New York: Bantam.

Kortte, K., Veiel, L., Batten, S., & Wegener, S. (2009). Measuring avoidance in medical rehabilitation. *Rehabilitation Psychology, 54*(1), 91–98.

Kubler-Ross, E. (1982). *Living with death and dying.* New York: MacMillan.

Krause, N. (2004) Stressors arising in highly valued roles, meaning in life and the physical status of older adults. *Journal of Gerontology and Behavioral Psychological Science and Social Science, 59*, 5287–5297.

Kylma, J., & Juvakka, T. (2006). Hope in parents of adolescents with cancer: Factors endangering and engendering parental hope. *European Journal of Oncology Nursing, 11*, 262–271.

Lackey, S. (2009). Opening the door to spiritually sensitive nursing care. *Nursing, 39*(4), 46–48.

Lazarus, R. S., & Folkman. S. (1984). *Stress, appraisal, and coping.* New York: Springer.

Lenze, E., Schulz, R., Matire, L., et al. (2005). The course of functional decline in older people with persistently elevated depressive symptoms: Longitudinal findings from cardiovascular health status. *Journal of the American Geriatric Society, 53*, 569–575.

Lewin, K. (1947). Frontiers in group dynamics: Concepts, methods and reality in social science. *Human Relations, 5*(1), 5–42.

Livneh, H. (1991). Unified approach to existing models of adaptation to disability: A model of adaptation. In H. Livneh (Ed.), *The psychology and social impact of disability* (pp. 111–138). New York: Springer.

Loewenthal, K. (2007). *Religion, culture, and mental health.* Cambridge, MA: Cambridge University Press.

Lyons, D., & Younger, B. (2001). Purpose in life and depressive symptoms in persons living with HIV disease. *Journal of Nursing Scholarship, 33*(2), 129–133.

Mann, W., Johnson, I., Lynch, L., et al. (2008). Changes in impairment level, functional status, and use of assistive devices by older people with depressive symptoms. *Journal of Occupational Therapy, 62*, 9–17.

Matheis, E. Tulsky, D., & Matheis, R. (2006). The relationship between spirituality and quality of life among individuals with spinal cord injuries. *Rehabilitation Psychology, 51*(3), 265–271.

Mazanec, S., Daly, B., Douglas, S. & Lipson, A. (2010). The relationship between optimism and quality of life in newly diagnosed cancer patients. *Cancer Nursing, 33*(3), 235–243.

McCaffery, A., Eisenberg, D. Legedza, A., Davis, R., & Phillips, R. (2004). Prayer for health concerns. *Archives of Internal Medicine, 164*, 858–862.

McCord, G., Gilcrest,V. Grossman, S., et al. (2004). Discussing spirituality with patients: A rational and ethical approach. *Annuals of Family Medicine, 2*, 256–361.

Mendez, B. Roux, G., & Ridosh, M. (2010). Phenomenon of inner strength in women post-myocardial infarction. *Critical Care Nursing Quarterly, 33*(3), 248–258.

Migliorini, C. E., Elfstrom, M. L., & Tonge, B. J. (2008). Translation and Australian validation of the spinal cord lesion related coping strategies and emotional wellbeing questionnaires. *Spinal Cord, 46*, 690–695.

Mofidi, M., DeVellis, R., Devellis, B., Blazer, D., Panter, A., & Jordan, J. (2007). The relationship between spirituality and depression symptoms: Testing psychosocial mechanisms. *Journal of Nervous Mental Disorders, 195*(8), 681–688.

Molton, I., Stoelb, B. Jensen, M., Ehde, D., Raichle, K., & Cardenas, D. (2009). Psychosocial factors and adjustment to chronic pain in spinal cord injury: Replication and cross-validation. *Journal of Rehabilitation Research and Development, 46*(1), 31–43.

National Center for Health Statistics. (2002). National Health Interview Survey. Public use data release. NHIS Survey Description. Retrieved October 15, 2010, from ftp://ftp.cdc.gov/pub/Health_Statistics/NCHS/Dataset_Dpci,emtatopm/MHIS/2002/srvydesc.pdf

Rabinowitz, A., & Arnett, P. (2009). A longitudinal analysis of cognitive dysfunction, coping, and depression in multiple sclerosis. *Neuropsychology, 23*(5), 581–591.

Reed, P. G. (1992) An emerging paradigm for the investigation of spirituality in nursing. *Research in Nursing and Health, 15*(5), 349–357.

Register, M., & Herman, J. (2010). Quality of life revisited: The concept of connectedness in older adults. *Advances in Nursing Science, 33*(1), 53–63.

Rieg, L. S., Mason, C. H., & Preston, K. (2006). Spiritual care: Practical guidelines for rehabilitation nurses. *Rehabilitation Nursing, 31*(6), 249–256.

Rippentrop, A. E., Altmaier, E. M., Chen, J. J., Fomd, E. M., & Keffela, V. J. (2005). The relationship between religion, spirituality and physical health, mental health, and pain in the chronic mental health and pain population. *Pain, 114*, 311–321.

Roberts, L., Ahmed, I., Hall, S., & Davison, A. (2009). Intercessory prayer for the alleviation of ill health. *Cochrane Database of Systematic Reviews, 3*, 1–42.

Roux, G., Dingley, C., & Bush, H. (2002). Inner strength in women: metasynthesis of qualitative findings in theory development. *Journal of Theory Construct Test, 4*(2), 36–39.

Sandel, E. Delmonico, R., Giap, B., Josten, T., Kaplan, D., Kinavey, et al. (2004). *Provider's handbook on culturally competent care designed to meet the needs of individuals with disabilities.* Vallejo, CA: Kaiser Permanente.

Shapiro, A. (2009). *Healing into possibilities.* Novato, CA.: H.J. Kramer and New World Library.

Tarakeshwar, N., Vanderwerker, L. C., Paulk, E., Pearce, M. J., Kasl, S. V., & Prigerson, H. G. (2006). Religious coping is associated with the quality of life of patients with advanced cancer. *Journal of Palliative Medicine, 9*(3), 646–657.

Taylor, E., J. (2007). Prayer's clinical issues and implications. *Holistic Nursing Practice, 17*, 179–188.

Walton, J. (2002). Discovering meaning and purpose during recovery from an acute myocardial infarction. *Dimensions of Critical Care Nursing, 21*(1), 36–43.

Watson, J. (1979). *Nursing: The philosophy and science of caring.* Boston: Little, Brown.

Watson, J. (1988). *Nursing: Human science and human care.* Norwalk, CT: Appleton-Century-Crofts.

Watson, J. (2005). *Caring science as sacred science*, Philadelphia: F.A. Davis.

Weiland, S. (2010). Integrating spirituality into critical care: An APN perspective using Roy's Adaptation Model. *Critical Care Nursing Quarterly, 33*(3), 282–291.

CHAPTER 15

Stroke

Sylvia A. Duraski
Florence A. Denby
Linda V. Danzy
Susan Sullivan

LEARNING OBJECTIVES

At the end of this chapter, the reader will be able to

- Define stroke.
- Name two common types of stroke.
- Identify two modifiable and nonmodifiable risk factors.
- List three ways in which brain tissue is injured during stroke.
- Discuss two areas on which to focus patient education regarding secondary stroke prevention.
- Describe two areas of nursing assessment and two nursing interventions for each of the following poststroke complications: deep vein thrombosis, pneumonia, seizures, pain, bowel and bladder elimination, skin integrity, motor deficits, safety, vision deficits, sensory complications, perceptual complications, communication deficits, cognitive deficits, depression, sexuality, sleep, education, and community reintegration.

KEY CONCEPTS AND TERMS

Agnosia
Aneurysm
Aphasia
Apraxia
Apraxia of speech
Arteriovenous malformation
Aspiration pneumonia
Ataxia
Atrial fibrillation (AF)
Attention process training
Bobath
Brain attack
Central poststroke pain
   syndrome (CPSP)
Central sleep apnea
Cerebrovascular accident
Constraint-induced movement
   therapy
Deep vein thrombosis (DVT)
Dysphagia
Dysarthria

Emboli
Embolic stroke
Emotional lability
Hemiparesis
Hemiplegia
Hemorrhagic stroke
Homonymous hemianopsia
Hypersomnia
International Normalized Ratio
Ischemic stroke
Intracerebral hemorrhage (ICH)
Intracranial pressure
Intraparenchymal
Intraventricular
Lacunar infarction
Modified Ashworth Scale
Neglect syndrome
Neuroplasticity
Percutaneous endoscopic
   gastrostomy (PEG) tube

Poststroke depression (PSD)
Proprioceptive neuromuscular
   facilitation
Pulmonary embolism (PE)
Shoulder subluxation
Sleep disordered breathing
   (SDB)
Sleep–wake disorders (SWDs)
Spasticity
Speech-language pathologist
   (SLP)
Stroke
Stroke syndromes
Subarachnoid hemorrhage
Thrombotic stroke
Thrombus
Transient ischemic attack
Videofluoroscopic swallow
   study

Stroke, also known as **cerebrovascular accident** or **brain attack**, is a nontraumatic brain injury caused by disruption in blood flow to part of the brain from either occlusion of a blood vessel (ischemic stroke) or rupture of a blood vessel (hemorrhagic stroke). When blood flow is interrupted, the brain is deprived of nutrients and oxygen, resulting in cell death.

IMPACT OF STROKE

Each year about 795,000 people experience a stroke. About 600,000 of these are first strokes, and 185,000 are recurrent strokes. On average, someone in the United States has a stroke every 40 seconds. As many as 55,000 more women than men have a stroke each year. Blacks have almost twice the risk of first stroke as Whites (Kleindorfer et al., 2005), and a higher incidence of stroke has also been found among Mexican Americans as compared with non-Hispanic Whites (Morgenstern et al., 2004).

Mortality

Stroke is the leading cause of disability and the third leading cause of death in the United States. On average, someone dies of a stroke every 4 minutes (National Center for Health Statistics, 2008; U.S Department of Health and Human Services, 2004). Among persons 45 to 64 years of age, 8% to 12% of ischemic strokes and 37% to 38% of hemorrhagic strokes result in death within 30 days (Rosamond et al., 1999). Because women live longer than men, more women than men die of stroke each year. Women accounted for 60.6% of U.S. stroke deaths in 2005 (American Heart Association [AHA], 2009).

Cost

The estimated direct and indirect cost of stroke for 2010 was $73.7 billion. Severe strokes cost twice as much as mild strokes, and the presence of comorbidities such as ischemic heart disease and atrial fibrillation predict higher costs (Diringer, et al., 1999; Metz, 2003).

TYPES OF STROKE

Strokes are classified as ischemic or hemorrhagic. The clinical presentations of stroke vary because of the complex anatomy and vasculature of the human brain. Thus, no two strokes are exactly the same, and all require individualized medical and nursing care and management (Harvey, Roth, & Yu, 2007).

No matter what type of stroke occurs, the result is compromised cerebral blood flow and brain injury lead-ing to neurological deficits. These deficits may include paralysis, loss of motor control, altered sensation, cognitive changes, language impairment, disequilibrium, or coma (Summers et al., 2009).

Ischemic Stroke

Eight-seven percent of all strokes are ischemic. In ischemic brain injury the blood vessel becomes occluded, interrupting blood flow to the brain and depriving neurons and other cells of essential nutrients, including oxygen. This results in cerebral ischemia that can quickly lead to brain cell death. Irreversible ischemic injury, or infarct, occurs with prolonged interruption of blood flow (Caruso & Silliman, 2010), but brain cell death can likely be avoided if blood flow is restored within a few minutes. Without blood flow, death of brain tissue occurs within 4 to 10 minutes (Smith, English, & Johnston, 2010). **Ischemic stroke** is further classified as thrombotic or embolic, depending on the origin of the occluding factor.

Thrombotic Stroke

A **thrombus** is a blood clot that forms in an area previously damaged by atherosclerosis. Fatty deposits, or plaques, can also clog and gradually block blood flow to the brain, resulting in a **thrombotic stroke**. Two types of thrombosis cause stroke, large vessel thrombosis and small vessel disease (**lacunar infarction**).

Large vessel thrombosis is the most frequent type of thrombotic stroke. The most common cause of large vessel thrombosis is a combination of long-term atherosclerosis and rapid clot formation. The damage that results depends on how long the vessel is occluded, the flow rate remaining after the thrombosis, and the effectiveness of collateral circulation (Smith et al., 2010).

Small vessel thrombosis or lacunar infarction is the result of blood flow blockage to very small arterial vessels. Lacunar infarcts are small lesions that occur with complete occlusion of small branches of the major cerebral arteries (Roth & Harvey, 2000). The word "lacune" means lake and describes the small cavity remaining after the products of deep infarct have been removed by the body. Lacunar infarcts are caused by either atherosclerosis or degenerative changes in the arterial walls that are related to chronic hypertension. In addition to hypertension, diabetes mellitus is associated with lacunar stroke as a result of chronic microvascular changes (Caruso & Silliman, 2010; Harvey et al., 2007). Twenty-five percent of ischemic strokes are due to small vessel disease that causes lacunar or subcortical strokes (Summers et al., 2009).

Embolic Stroke

Emboli are clots that can travel from the heart or extracranial arteries to the brain. Once in the brain the clot travels to and blocks a small blood vessel, causing a stroke. **Embolic strokes** cause a sudden onset of neurological deficits with no prior symptoms, and most embolic strokes have a cardiac source of emboli, such as from atrial fibrillation (National Stroke Association, 2003).

Other cardiac origins of emboli may include emboli formation after myocardial infarction or cardiac surgery; emboli secondary to cardiomyopathy, and a thrombus within the left ventricle. Mechanical heart valves can also cause cerebral emboli if anticoagulation is insufficient, and infectious endocarditis can lead to septic emboli (Harvey et al., 2007).

Hemorrhagic Stroke

Hemorrhagic stroke refers to a process by which weakened cerebral blood vessels rupture and spill blood into nearby intracranial spaces or brain tissue. Cerebral hemorrhage is the third most common cause of stroke and is associated with a 50% mortality rate. Types of hemorrhagic stroke include **intracerebral hemorrhage (ICH)** and **subarachnoid hemorrhage**.

Bleeding in the brain may be labeled **intraventricular** (into the ventricular spaces where cerebrospinal fluid is produced and stored) or **intraparenchymal** (into the tissues). Intraparenchymal hemorrhages usually occur from the rupture of small penetrating arteries and occur in the basal ganglia, thalamus, pons, and cerebellum. The onset of symptoms is rapid, developing over 30 to 90 minutes, and almost one-half of the patients die. In substance abuse of cocaine and amphetamines, there is a rapid increase in blood pressure, leading to vessel rupture, whereas bleeding associated with anticoagulation therapy develops slowly over 24 to 48 hours.

ICH accounts for 10% of all strokes (Rosamond et al., 2008). Small vessels deep in the brain burst and bleed into brain tissue, putting pressure on tissue and causing vessel tearing, brain shifting, and herniation. The result can be immediate stupor and coma with death within hours (Smith et al., 2010). Free blood in the brain tissue also irritates adjacent vessels and causes vasospasms. Risk factors for ICH include hypertension, bleeding disorders, African American ethnicity, aging, vascular malformations, bleeding into a tumor, excessive use of alcohol, and liver dysfunction. Phenylpropanolamine use has also been linked with ICH, as has cocaine.

Subarachnoid hemorrhage refers to bleeding into the subarachnoid space caused by rupture of a vessel in the protective lining of the brain. Subarachnoid hemorrhage can be the result of an **aneurysm** within the brain vasculature or an **arteriovenous malformation** on the surface of the brain. Blood in the spaces surrounding the brain causes pressure on the brain itself, increasing intracranial pressure, affecting brain function, and causing ischemic damage.

Hemorrhagic stroke can cause ischemia and elevated **intracranial pressure**. Symptoms of severe headache, nausea, and vomiting appear suddenly. In acute hemorrhage the blood pushes against and squeezes the bordering tissue, leading to more ischemic injury. The affected tissue becomes swollen and necrotic. Cellular changes occur, and macrophages phagocytize the blood and dead tissue. The area is liquefied, and a cavity forms as part of the inflammatory response (Frizzel, 2005).

Less Common Causes of Stroke

Hypercoagulable disorders can cause increased risk of venous thrombosis. This may occur as a complication of oral contraceptive use, may occur during pregnancy and the postpartum period, or may be due to conditions such as inflammatory bowel disease, meningitis, or dehydration. Patients with thrombophilia are also at higher risk for stroke, as are women who take oral contraceptives and have the prothrombin G20210 mutation. Moyamoya disease is an occlusive disease involving large intracranial arteries that can cause stroke (Rosamond et al., 2008).

Other uncommon causes of stroke include disorders such as protein C deficiency, protein S deficiency, antithrombin III deficiency, antiphospholipid syndrome, sickle cell anemia, beta-thalassemia, polycythemia vera, systemic lupus erythematosus, homocysteinemia, thrombotic thrombocytopenic purpura, and vasculitis. Drugs, amphetamines, and cocaine use can cause stroke due to acute hypertension or drug-induced vasculitis (Rosamond et al., 2008).

RISK FACTORS FOR STROKE

Eighty percent of strokes are preventable. Risk factors for stroke are classified as modifiable (can be changed) and nonmodifiable (cannot be changed) (Table 15.1). For more information about risk factors for stroke, refer to

TABLE 15.1   Risk Factors for Stroke

Modifiable	Nonmodifiable	Other
Hypertension	Age	Socioeconomic factors
Coronary heart disease	Gender	Geographic location
Peripheral artery disease	Ethnicity	
	Family history	Alcohol abuse
Diabetes		Substance use and abuse
Obesity		
Smoking		
Atrial fibrillation		

the American Stroke Association website at http://www.americanheart.org, the National Stroke Association website at http://www.stroke.org, or the National Institute of Neurological Disorders and Stroke website at http://www.ninds.nih.gov.

WARNING SIGNS OF STROKE

The five warning signs of stroke are

- Sudden weakness on one side of the body involving the face, arm, or leg
- Dizziness, loss of balance or coordination
- Sudden severe unexplained headaches
- Sudden confusion and difficulty understanding or speaking
- Visual impairment of one or both eyes.

Rapid recognition of stroke symptoms is important to prevent a delay in treatment and to optimize chances for survival. The AHA has developed several programs designed to assist facilities with early recognition and management of stroke: recommendations for development of Primary Stroke Centers accredited by the AHA, Acute Stroke Treatment Program, and Get with the Guidelines. Further information on these topics can be found at http://www.strokeassociation.org/presenter.jhtml?identifier=1200037

It is not within the scope of this chapter to review acute care of the stroke patient in detail. Therefore, the provided AHA website is an excellent resource for more information on that topic.

STROKE SYNDROMES RELATED TO BLOOD SUPPLY

A syndrome is a collection of symptoms that, when found together, are characteristic of a disease. **Stroke syndromes** can be predicted if the arteries affected by stroke are known, but the extent of impairment will vary depending on the specific arteries affected and the size of the infarction. Table 15.2 describes predictable stroke syndromes typical of major cerebral arterial and branch occlusions (Harvey, 2009). Table 15.3 describes less predictable stroke syndromes such as those associated with lacunar strokes and ICH. Stroke syndromes are important because they predict potential deficits and can thus assist in the planning and implementation of care. By being familiar with these stroke syndromes,

TABLE 15.2   Cerebral Stroke Syndromes

Cerebral Artery	Area of Brain Supplied	Deficits After Stroke
Anterior cerebral artery	Anterior three quarters of the interhemispheric cortical surface of the frontal and parietal lobes.	Contralateral hemiplegia, lower limb worse distally
		Foot drop
		Left limb disconnection apraxia
		Head and eyes deviated toward side of lesion
		Forced hand grasping
		Contralateral hemianesthesia, lower limb worse distally
		Flat affect
		Impulsivity
		Abulia: reduction in speech or movement
		Amnesia
		Dominant: transcortical motor aphasia, decreased auditory comprehension

Continues

TABLE 15.2   Cerebral Stroke Syndromes *(Continued)*

Cerebral Artery	Area of Brain Supplied	Deficits After Stroke

Middle cerebral artery	The frontal lobe and the lateral surface of the temporal and parietal lobes.	Main stem
		 Contralateral hemiplegia
		 Contralateral hemianesthesia
		 Contralateral hemianopia
		 Head or eyes turning toward the lesion
		 Dysphagia
		 Uninhibited neurogenic bladder
		 Dominant: global aphasia, apraxia
		 Nondominant: hemineglect, aprosody: absence of pitch in speech, affective agnosia, dressing apraxia, anosognosia
		Upper division
		 Contralateral hemiplegia not as severe in face and hand and worse in leg
		  Language comprehension deficits not as severe
		  Dominant: Broca's aphasia, apraxia
		  Nondominant: aprosody, hemineglect, visuospatial deficits
		Lower division
		  Impaired language
		  Impaired vision
		  Poor awareness of deficits
		  Homonymous hemianopsia
		   Dominant: Wernicke's aphasia
		   Nondominant: Affective agnosia

Posterior cerebral circulation	The temporal and occipital lobes	Hemisensory deficits Homonymous hemianopsia Cortical blindness Color agnosia Alexia without agraphia

rehabilitation nurses can anticipate potential safety issues or education needs.

> *Stroke syndromes are important because they predict potential deficits and can thus assist in the planning and implementation of care.*

SECONDARY STROKE PREVENTION

One of five stroke survivors will have a second stroke within 5 years. Secondary strokes are often more severe and have a higher rate of death and disability because of the trauma and injury the brain has already sustained from the first stroke; the brain is no longer as resilient. Thirty-five percent of people who have experienced **transient ischemic attacks** will have a stroke as well

(National Stroke Association, 2006). Most modalities used to prevent first strokes are also crucial in preventing secondary strokes as well. Risk factors contributing to a second stroke include hypertension, obesity, poorly managed diabetes, hyperlipidemia, smoking, and physical inactivity.

NEUROPLASTICITY

Neuroplasticity is the ability of the brain to rearrange the connections between its neurons and alter its behavior in response to new information, sensory stimulation, development, damage, or dysfunction. Plasticity consists of laying out preferred pathways within the brain for circulating important information. If we regularly perform a very skilled motor task, the cortical representation for

TABLE 15.3	Brainstem/Lacunar Stroke Syndromes	
Syndrome	**Location**	**Deficits**
Weber syndrome	Medial basal midbrain	Ipsilateral third nerve palsy
		Contralateral hemiplegia
Wallenberg syndrome	Lateral medulla	Ipsilateral hemiataxia
		Ipsilateral loss of facial pain and temperature sensation
		Nystagmus: involuntary movements of the eyes
		Ipsilateral Horner's syndrome: myosis, ptosis, anhydrosis
		Dysphagia
		Dysphonia: difficulty in speaking loudly
Locked-in	Bilateral basal pons	Quadriplegia
		Bilateral cranial nerve palsy
		Laryngeal weakness
		Upward gaze is spared
Benedikt syndrome	Tegmentum of midbrain	Ipsilateral third nerve palsy
		Contralateral loss of pain and temperature sensation
		Contralateral loss of joint position sense
		Contralateral ataxia and chorea
Pure motor stroke	Posterior limb of internal capsule	Contralateral hemiplegia of face, arm, hand, leg and foot
	Corona radiata	
	Ventral pons	
Dysarthria-clumsy hand stroke	Anterior limb of internal capsule	Dysarthria
		Unilateral facial weakness
	Base of pons	Mild upper limb paresis
Pure sensory stroke	Lateral thalamus	Hemisensory deficits of the extremities, face and trunk

the muscles involved remains large (Johansson, 2000). Neuroplasticity is the foundation of memory formation and learning processes and can also be important in compensating for brain damage by allowing the brain to create new networks of neurons.

Basic science and clinical research strongly suggest that any new intervention for promoting motor recovery after stroke must be coupled with appropriate behavioral interventions (e.g., rehabilitation therapy) aimed at facilitating neuroplastic processes (Harvey et al., 2007). This information points to the importance of comprehensive interdisciplinary rehabilitation after stroke.

OUTCOME PREDICTORS

It is very difficult to predict how much recovery a person will experience after stroke. Potentially important factors that influence specific individual outcomes include type,

distribution, pattern, and severity of physical impairment; cognitive, language, communication, and learning ability; number, types, and severity of comorbid medical conditions; ongoing health functions, coping ability, and coping style; nature and degree of family and other social supports; and type and quality of specific rehabilitation programs (Harvey et al., 2007). The severity of the initial deficits after stroke is inversely proportional to the prognosis for recovery.

> *Most recovery occurs during the first 3 to 6 months after the stroke and decelerates over time.*

Most functional recovery occurs within the first two months after stroke. Rehabilitation during this early poststroke period is considered to be most beneficial and effective. Most recovery occurs during the first three to six months after the stroke and decelerates over time (Teasell, Foley, & Salter, 2009). This does not mean recovery cannot occur after the six-month period, but the rate at which recovery is experienced when compared with the first six months is less.

EFFECTS OF STROKE

Musculoskeletal and Motor Deficits

Synergy

Muscle weakness has clinically been recognized as one of the limiting factors in the rehabilitation of patients after stroke (Bourbonnais & Vanden Noven, 1989; Duncan & Badke, 1987). A well-documented factor limiting the motor rehabilitation of patients after stroke is the presence of abnormal muscle activation patterns or loss of control over select muscle groups, resulting in paired joint movements that are often inappropriate to complete the desired task (Brunnstrom, 1970; Waters, Frazier, Garland, Jordan, & Perry, 1982). These coupled or paired joint movements are known as synergy patterns of movement. For the leg, these movements have been grouped into extension synergy (internal rotation, adduction, and extension of the hip; extension of the knee; and extension and inversion of the ankle) and flexion synergy (external rotation, abduction, and flexion of the hip; flexion of the knee; and flexion and eversion of the ankle) (Brunnstrom, 1956; Michels, 1982; Sawner & LaVigne, 1992; Waters et al., 1982). In synergy patterns, movement in each muscle group cannot be isolated or separated but rather occurs together.

Rehabilitation nurses should be aware of these patterns of movement, because over time these patterns can cause the individual pain and discomfort. These patterned movements can lead to contractures and loss of function. The affected extremities should always be placed in neutral positions. Positioning devices should be applied as ordered by the therapy team, and the need to perform range of motion and stretching exercises on a daily basis should be reinforced with families. Rehabilitation nurses should recognize patients whose discomfort is interfering with function so the medical or therapy team can be notified immediately for proper intervention.

Paralysis

Hemiplegia or **hemiparesis** causes decreased motor control of voluntary activities. Stroke survivors' decreased abilities to perform their hygiene, dressing, toileting, and eating, along with their decline in mobility, including impaired balance and gait, lead to decreased function

and require a coordinated rehabilitation plan. A primary objective in rehabilitation is to help the stroke survivor maximize mobility and self-care skills so they can return to the community.

Research generally supports early mobilization of the person with an acute stroke to prevent deep vein thrombosis, skin breakdown, contracture formation, constipation, and pneumonia. The AHA/American Stroke Association Stroke Clinical Practice Guidelines recommend that rehabilitation therapy start as early as possible and that survivors receive as much therapy as needed to adapt, recover, and/or reestablish their premorbid or optimum level of functional independence (Duncan et al., 2005).

Ataxia

Ataxia is the inability of muscles to perform synchronized movements, a disorder of coordination and rhythm. Ataxia occurs after lacunar stroke and is found in 3% of the stroke population. The diagnosis of ataxic hemiparesis predicts small deep infarcts, usually in the internal capsule or base of the pons. With rehabilitation therapy, survivors with ataxia have good recovery (O'Dwyer, Ada, & Neilson, 1996).

Balance

Balance is a complex process that requires coordination between the vestibular, visual, proprioceptive, musculoskeletal, and cognitive systems. It is the ability to maintain equilibrium in a gravitational field by keeping or returning the center of body mass over its base of support. Balance allows the body to react to destabilizing forces to regain stability through postural adjustments and requires the organized activities of ankle, knee, hip, and trunk muscles to resume equilibrium and maintain balance (Karatas, Cetin, Bayramoglu, & Dilek, 2004). Stroke may disrupt both sitting and standing balance, both of which are necessary to perform activities of daily living (ADLs), self-care, and mobility. Balance in stroke survivors is also influenced by other factors such as spasticity. During stroke recovery, balance usually improves with physical therapy and gait training.

Contracture

One of the most painful complications after stroke is contracture. Contracture is a condition of fixed, high resistance to passive stretching that results from fibrosis and shortening of tissues that support muscles or joints. In stroke, the muscle and supporting tendons contract, resulting in reduced flexibility and a reduction in compliance that is due to remodeling of muscle connective tissue. Thus, the range of motion is reduced both by shortening of the muscle fibers and by loss of muscle compliance. The focus of rehabilitation therapy to prevent contractures and treatment needs to be initiated early in stroke recovery. Supporting the affected limb in an anatomically correct position that opposes the pattern of spasticity and regularly ranging the limb are both traditional measures of prevention.

Contractures of the affected limb or joint can be painful and may compromise rehabilitation and limit recovery. Once a contracture occurs, corrective measures include splinting and/or serial casting that may progress the joint into improved anatomical and comfortable positions. Sometime a contracture requires serial casting, providing a prolonged slow stretch of the affected joint and muscle (Agency for Health Care Policy and Research, 1995). Also, specially made splints with a gauge that can be dialed and set at a specific degree of angle stretch can be used in the upper limb for elbows and wrists.

Spasticity

Spasticity is a velocity-dependent increase in tonic stretch reflexes (muscle tone) in resistance to muscle stretch that develops after an upper motor neuron injury within the central nervous system (O'Dwyer et al., 1996; Roth & Harvey, 2000). Increased stretch reflexes cause hypertonia and increased resistance to passive movement. Symptoms of spasticity are hypertonia (increased muscle tone), clonus (a series of involuntary rapid muscle contractions), exaggerated deep tendon reflexes, and scissor gait, and over time spasticity leads to shortened tendons and fixed joints (contractures). The degree and location of spasticity is individual and depends on the severity of the stroke.

Spasticity interferes with ADLs, mobility, and function and is adversely affected by cold weather, fatigue, and stress. After stroke, spasticity is more common in the affected arm than the leg. Upper extremity spasticity can push the hand and wrist into flexion with the elbow with the arm also moved in flexion contraction against the chest.

The **Modified Ashworth Scale** is a quick and easy way to evaluate spasticity. The Modified Ashworth Scale is best done when the patient is supine. The test is done a maximum of three times for each joint. If it is done more than three times, the short-term effect of a stretch influences the score. The joints usually assessed are elbow, wrist, fingers, thumb, hamstrings, quadriceps, gastroc-

nemius, and soleus (Bohannon & Smith, 1987). Box 15.1 shows the Modified Ashworth Scale.

Physical and occupational therapies are extremely important in spasticity management. The therapist's assessment includes identifying which muscles or muscle groups are affected by spasticity and how the stroke survivor's life and function are affected by the spasticity. As a part of the treatment team, the rehabilitation nurse evaluates and recommends treatment for any skin breakdown or irritations that may be the result of spasticity. The nurse assists in positioning the affected limb, correctly applying splints. Pain is also a complication of spasticity, which the rehabilitation nurse assesses and manages appropriately.

BOX 15.1   Modified Ashworth Scale

0 = No increase in tone or normal tone

1 = Slight increase in muscle tone, manifested by catch and release or minimal resistance at the end of ROM when the affected body part is moved in flexion or extension

2 = Marked increase in muscle tone through most of the ROM but affected part(s) are easily moved

3 = Considerable increase in muscle tone; passive movement is difficult

4 = Affected part is rigid in flexion or extension

ROM, range of motion.

Botox, also known as botulinum toxin type A, injections are used as an effective treatment of spasticity. Botox therapy for the treatment of spasticity is off-label because it has not been approved by the U.S. Food and Drug Administration for this use. Many controlled clinical trials of Botox injections for focal muscle spasticity have shown prolonged improvement in spasticity with few adverse side effects. The effect of Botox usually only lasts three to four months, but during that time the stroke survivor often gets improved results while participating in complementary therapies such as physical and occupational therapies (Vanek & Menkes, 2007).

Oral medications can also effectively treat spasticity. Baclofen or lioresil is a gamma-aminobutyric acid agonist and acts on the central nervous system to relax muscles. Studies show that oral baclofen improves clonus, flexor spasm frequency, and joint range of motion, resulting in better functional skills and improved self-care. Patients with renal insufficiency need to be monitored because baclofen is cleared in the kidneys. Tolerance to baclofen can develop, and it must be tapered slowly to prevent withdrawal effects.

Dantrium or dantrolene acts directly on the muscle, blocking the signals that cause muscles to contract so it can lessen muscle tone, clonus, and muscle spasm. Because Dantrium acts at the level of the muscle fiber, it is less likely to cause drowsiness or cognitive changes. It can cause generalized weakness, fatigue, and diarrhea.

Zanaflex or tizanidine is an effective therapeutic option that temporarily reduces spasticity by blocking nerve impulses. It has been shown to decrease spasticity without reducing muscle strength. Zanaflex is sometimes used in combination with baclofen or benzodiazepines to maximize therapeutic results, but there are increased potential side effects such as addiction, sedation, or liver toxicity (Vanek & Menkes, 2007).

Other treatments for spasticity include an implanted pump and nerve block. Intrathecal baclofen therapy delivers baclofen in liquid form directly into the spinal fluid. A programmable pump is surgically implanted just below the skin in the lower abdomen and delivers continual small doses of baclofen as programmed. There are fewer side effects with intrathecal baclofen than with oral baclofen because of the drug delivery technique. Nerve blocks consist of a bolus injection of phenol, either a perineural injection of a motor nerve or intramuscular nerve blocking (Gould & Barnes, 2009; Vanek & Menkes, 2007). Phenol causes chemical denervation by denaturing protein, and it has a short-term anesthetic effect through a longer duration nerve block. The improvement may last a few weeks to years.

Nonpharmacological therapies discussed earlier include anatomical positioning away from the spasticity, daily scheduled range of motion, and serial casting with possible splinting. Slow, prolonged stretching is the gold standard of effective nonpharmacological spasticity management. The rehabilitation nurse plays a critical role in the positioning and mobility of the person with spasticity.

Shoulder Subluxation

Shoulder subluxation is a frequent complication in stroke survivors with hemiplegia that can impair functional recovery and mobility by limiting range of motion. Subluxation is a partial or incomplete dislocation due to changes in the anatomy of the shoulder joint. It occurs early in the course of recovery as a result of the flaccidity of supporting shoulder musculature. It appears to be the result of the weight of the flaccid arm applying direct mechanical stretch to the joint capsule and pulling on the unsupportive shoulder muscles (Gould & Barnes, 2009). Trained clinicians can diagnose subluxation by palpating and measuring anatomical landmarks (fingerbreadths and calipers) during exam. Performing shoulder palpation to diagnose subluxation can be reliably graded as well as verified by radiographic measures.

After a stroke the body goes through stages of flaccidity, spasticity, and synergy. In the United States shoulder pathology with resulting pain is common in hemiplegic patients, with 85% of hemiplegic survivors experiencing spastic symptoms and 18% of survivors, flaccid symptoms. Eighty-one percent of survivors develop subluxation.

The correlation between shoulder subluxation and shoulder pain remains controversial. Numerous cases of subluxation without pain have been documented as have cases of a painful shoulder without subluxation (Gould & Barnes, 2009). Treatment of subluxation is also controversial. Slings, arm boards, troughs, and lap trays have not proven to be effective and sometimes may provide overcorrection. Sling use may cause lateral subluxation, impede proprioception, promote synergy, and interfere with functional activities. Even though sling use and other supportive devices are not considered beneficial in the treatment of subluxation, they continue to be used because painful shoulder subluxation can improve with joint reduction. Early prevention of subluxation is necessary because shoulder pain is often refractory to treatment. Neuromuscular electrical stimulation has been shown to be successful in the prevention and treatment of shoulder subluxation and, with that, improve motor recovery.

Falls

Falls are one of the most frequent complications in stroke rehabilitation. The reported percentages of stroke patients who fall during their hospitalization include 14% in acute care, 24% in acute rehabilitation, and 39% in geriatric rehabilitation (Batchelor, Hill, Mackintosh & Said, 2010; Nyberg & Gustafson, 1995). Falls in community-dwelling stroke survivors have been documented to be as high as 73% (Batchelor et al., 2010; Yates, Lai, Duncan & Studenski, 2002). Falls in the stroke population may result in serious injury, with fracture rates up to four times higher than the general population (Batchelor et al., 2010). Injuries and other consequences of falls lead to restricted activity due to fear of falling and are likely to have a negative effect on rehabilitation (Batchelor et al., 2010).

Early identification of fall-prone stroke survivors is of great importance. A number of risk factors have been identified by various research studies, including

TABLE 15.4 Fall Prevention Tools
Timed Up and Go: Identifies gait and balance problems
Get Up and Go Test: Assesses risk of falling and identifies balance problems
Berg Balance Scale: Rates ability to maintain balance while performing ADLs
Dynamic Gait Index: Assesses ability to modify gait in response to changing task demands
Tinetti Performance Oriented Mobility Assessment: Rates ability to maintain balance during ADLs
Activities-specific Balance Confidence: Rates confidence in maintaining balance during ADLs
Falls Efficacy Scale: Assesses confidence in performing ADLs without falling
Morse Fall Scale: Risk assessment tool for inpatients.
Hendrich Fall Risk Assessment: Risk assessment tool used in long-term care
St. Thomas Risk Assessment Tool: Identifies risk factors and creates a risk profile

TABLE 15.5 Hospital Safety Interventions
Wheelchair or bed exit alarms
Call light within reach
Bedside commode or regular toileting program
24-hour supervision
Frequent staff safety checks
Signs or visual cues in the environment
Bed enclosures
Low to floor beds
Nonskid shoes
Plenty of lighting
Use or hearing devices and glasses

behavioral impulsivity (Rapport et al., 1993), a history of falls, impaired decision-making ability, restlessness, generalized weakness, abnormal hematocrit level (Byers, Arrington, & Finstuen, 1990), postural sway or the body motion during stance, increased motor response time to visual stimuli, perceptual deficits, visual impairments, confusion, disorientation, problems with communication, acute illnesses, depression, and medication side effects (Forster & Young, 1995; Webster et al., 1995). Greater stroke severity (Schmid, Kapoor, Dallas, & Bravata, 2010), Barthel score of less than 15 less than or equal to 12 weeks from stroke onset, visuospatial neglect, age greater than 65 years (Czernuszenko, & Czlonkowska, 2009), and depressive symptoms (Jorgensen, Engstad, & Jacobsen, 2002) have also been associated with an increased risk of falls in stroke patients.

The entire interdisciplinary treatment team must work on preventing falls and injuries among stroke survivors. Fall risk should be assessed with an evidence-based, reliable, and valid assessment tool so the appropriate interventions can be implemented. Table 15.4 provides a list of fall prevention tools. The least restrictive safety measures should then be implemented so that mobility is maintained while still injury is prevented. Table 15.5 provides hospital safety interventions. Families should also be educated regarding the need for continued safety measures in the home environment. Table 15.6 lists home safety interventions.

Sensory Perception

For some stroke survivors, visual-spatial perceptual deficits are the most troublesome deficits experienced (Harvey et al., 2007). Stroke survivors with visual-spatial perceptual deficits tend to do poorly in rehabilitation and have a poorer prognosis for recovery. There are several types of sensory perceptual deficits.

Vision

Between 30% and 85% of stroke survivors experience some type of visual dysfunction. The visual changes associated with stroke can be divided into three categories: sensory deficits, which involve visual acuity and visual field; motor deficits, which involve impaired extraocular muscle movement; and perceptual deficits (Khan, Leung, & Jay, 2008). In those stroke survivors who have a preexisting visual acuity problem, the problems remain and

TABLE 15.6 Home Safety Interventions
Remove loose rugs, electrical cords, or other items that could lead to tripping, slipping, and falling
Ensure adequate lighting in all areas inside and around the home (including stairwells and entrance ways)
Avoid ice, wet or polished floors, or other potentially slippery surfaces, and avoid walking in unfamiliar areas outside
Ensure properly fitted, nonslip footwear
Do not leave unattended
Bedside commode or routine toileting program
Grab bars or raised toilet seat in bathroom
Medication review

may worsen due to the stroke. Previous forms of compensation may not be as effective as before the stroke.

Visual field defects after stroke differ based on the location of the lesion along the optic chiasm. One commonly seen visual field deficit that causes bilateral visual field loss is **homonymous hemianopsia**. Hemianopsia refers to one half of the visual field of each eye. Homonymous indicates the loss is on the same side of each eye (Khan et al., 2008). Cranial nerve damage after stroke can cause paralysis of the eye muscles responsible for movement. Double vision is a common complaint that can result when the eyes are unable to move together. Unilateral neglect is the most common visual perception problem seen after stroke. Known also as hemispatial neglect, hemineglect, spatial neglect, or **neglect syndrome**, it is defined as a deficit in awareness of one side of space or one side of the body opposite to the lesion.

Those with visual sensory, visual motor, or visual perceptual deficits are often assessed by an occupational therapist for potential problems before being referred to a neuro-optometrist or neuro-ophthalmologist for further evaluation. Patients may admit to problems seeing or complain of blurred vision when attempting to read. Patients may also be seen constantly closing one eye, which could signal blurred vision. Patients may make errors when filling out menus, complain of dizziness, run into objects on the unit, or miss objects on one side of their meal tray, bedside table, or in their room.

Stroke survivors with visual acuity problems often respond best to magnification. Nurses should make sure the survivor has his or her glasses from home. Further magnification can be achieved by using a magnifying glass or sheet (Khan et al., 2008). Good lighting and color contrast can help improve visual acuity. Large-print reading material can also help decrease errors and problems with visual acuity.

Visual field deficits can be compensated for by relocating objects from the nonseeing to the seeing area. This is done by using mirrors or prisms on eyeglasses (Khan et al., 2008). Prism glasses are prescribed by a neuro-optometrist should be worn routinely.

Extraocular muscle paralysis or weakness may spontaneously resolve after a period of time. Often, patients independently correct blurred or double vision by keeping one eyelid closed. Another way to resolve blurred vision is to provide a small patch over the affected eye. If a full field patch is used, it should be alternated from eye to eye to avoid depriving one eye of sensory stimulation (Khan et al., 2008). Visual rehabilitation professionals may provide the stroke survivor with diplopia eyeglasses with strips of tape over the affected eye lens. This allows for peripheral information to be perceived by allowing light and color through the tape. As the vision improves, strips of tape can be removed.

For those with unilateral neglect, prisms can be used to shift objects into the neglected side (Khan et al., 2008). The therapy team will spend a great deal of time and effort training the survivor to scan into the visual field of the neglected side or use cues to bring their vision to midline. Rehabilitation nurses should be aware of compensatory techniques being used by the treatment team to assist the stroke survivor with neglect to scan to the affected side. Safety of the stroke survivor is very important. Clutter should be limited to prevent injury. Objects should be placed in the survivor's visual field when left alone, and when supervised, the objects can be moved to midline or to the affected side to cue the survivor to turn their head. Family should be educated regarding any deficits and potential safety issues.

Sensation

Sensory loss after stroke is very common. Over half of survivors suffer some sensory impairment (Cambier, DeCorte, Danneels, & Witvrouw, 2003). Sensory loss occurs in conjunction with motor deficits because the motor and sensory strips in the brain are so close in proximity (Figure 15.1). Sensory impairments may affect light touch, pain, temperature, vibration, and position sense. The loss may be complete or partial. Sensory loss is considered to be a precursor to the recovery of movement and functional activity and is an important part of widely used physiotherapy approaches such as Bobath and Brunnstrom (Tyson, Hanley, Chillala, Selley, & Tallis, 2008).

Usually, the medical staff or occupational therapist will formally test for sensory loss after stroke, but rehabilitation nurses may become aware of these losses when performing care or by simply observing the patient during activities on the unit. These patients are at higher risk for injuries due to the slow reaction time to sensory input or lack of awareness of what is being held.

Little has been written about the treatment of sensory impairments after stroke. Therapists may treat those survivors with sensory loss by providing different levels of sensory stimulation. The objective is to provide information similar to that which would be experienced during movement or performance of a task. Using objects of varying textures and temperatures is part of the therapy. Although rehabilitation nurses do not provide the sensory stimulation therapy, they should ensure survivor safety

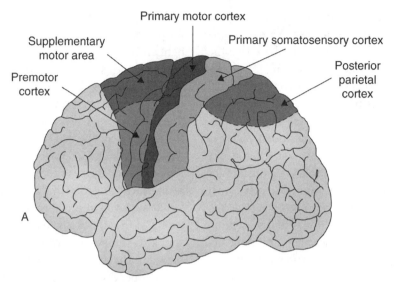

FIGURE 15.1 Primary motor cortex and primary somatosensory cortex.

Source: From *Motor Control: Theory and Practical Applications* [p.78] by A.Shumway-Cook & M.H. Woollacott, 2001, Philadelphia:Lippincott Williams &Wilkins. Copyright 1995 by Lippincott Williams & Wilkins. Reprinted by permission.

and education. Survivors and families should be taught about safety for the affected extremities.

Apraxia

Apraxia is defined as the lack of ability to perform previously learned motor skills either on command or by imitation (Baggerly, 1991). This occurs after a right hemisphere stroke and is a problem conceptualizing, planning, and executing skilled or purposeful motor patterns not related to paralysis or comprehension problems (Baggerly, 1991). There are several main types of apraxia that affect the extremities (Wheaton & Hallett, 2007). Table 15.7 provides a more thorough description of apraxia. Stroke survivors with apraxia are often more impaired in other

areas such as language and motor skills. They tend to have larger lesions than do stroke patients without apraxia, and the lesions are frequently found in the right parietal and frontal areas of the brain (Buxbaum et al., 2008).

Numerous tests can be used to assess for apraxia. The two most common are the Test of Oral and Limb Apraxia and the Florida Apraxia Battery. Rehabilitation nurses commonly observe apraxia during ADLs on the unit. The stroke survivor with apraxia often appears to be unmotivated or unable to start actions due to the inability to get the steps of the activity in the correct order.

The goal of treatment for any apraxia is to compensate for the lack of the skill. Rehabilitation nurses should provide supervision or hand over hand assistance with all activities. Just as with other visual perceptual deficits, potential for injury is a huge problem. Distractions should be limited so the patient can focus on the task at hand, and steps to a task should be minimized to decrease the frequency of errors.

Agnosia

Agnosia is defined as a series of perceptual deficits that describe a marked indifference to or lack of awareness of the paralyzed side of the body and disregard to the environment on the affected side. Unlike hemianopsia, which refers to a visual field cut, an agnosia may be tactile or auditory in nature (Baggerly, 1991). Table 15.8 provides more information on the types of agnosia.

Much like the other visual perceptual deficits, formalized testing can be performed by an occupational

TABLE 15.7	Types of Apraxia
Type	**Definition**
Limb kinetic	The inability to make precise movements with an affected arm or leg
Ideomotor	The inability to make the proper use of familiar tools or items
Ideational	The inability to coordinate activities with multiple sequential movements such as dressing, eating, or grooming
Verbal	The inability to coordinate mouth and speech movements.
Constructional	The inability to copy, draw, or construct simple figures

TABLE 15.8	Types of Agnosia
Type	**Definition**
Alexia	Inability to recognize text
Receptive agnosia	Inability to recognize musical notes or rhythms
Anosognosia	Denial of disability
Auditory agnosia	Inability to distinguish nonverbal and auditory cues
Color agnosia	Inability to recognize color
Prosopagnosia	Inability to recognize familiar faces
Asterognosia	Inability to recognize objected by touch
Somatognosia	Inability to recognize body structure and the relationship of body part to each other
Visual agnosia	Inability to recognize objects visually

therapist. Rehabilitation nurses may see these behaviors during ADLs on the unit. When approached by the affected side, stroke survivors seem confused or paranoid because they are not aware that part of their body or environment exists. When approached about their disability, they may become argumentative because the stroke survivor may not be aware of their deficits and how that impacts returning home. During ADLs, the stroke survivor with agnosia may ignore the affected side of the body for bathing, shaving, applying makeup, and combing hair (Baggerly, 1991).

Because the individual with apraxia has had their stroke in the right hemisphere, this means the left hemisphere and verbal skills are generally intact, and the survivor may appear more cognitively aware. Rehabilitation nurses should approach the stroke survivor from the center or midline position to get the person's attention and then cue them to turn to both the left and right side (Baggerly, 1991). The affected extremity should be used in ADLs as a passive assist in midline so that it is not off to the side where it can be ignored.

Cognition

Cognitive disorders can contribute to disability in everyday life after stroke. The consequences of cognitive disorders after stroke are critical in that they exert considerable influence on recovery and have been found to predict poorer functional outcomes (Lesniak, Bak, Czpiel, Seniow, & Czlonkowska, 2008). A number of studies have demonstrated that the incidence of impaired cognitive

functions can reach 40% to 60% in elderly patients during the first 6 months after transient ischemic attacks, minor strokes, and strokes with minimal neurological deficit (Vakhnina, Nikitina, Parefenow, & Yakhno, 2009).

Cognitive deficits can be categorized as mild, moderate, or severe. Severe deficits include dementia, resulting in significant difficulties in a stroke survivor's ability to perform daily activities. Moderate cognitive impairments have no influence on daily life but can have adverse effects on the more complex types of activities. Mild cognitive impairments are recognized subjectively but do not interfere with a patient's routine professional or social adaptation (Vakhnina et al., 2009). Most studies of cognitive disorders after stroke report vascular dementia as the main outcome. Eight percent to 26% of stroke survivors develop a dementia within 12 months (Rasquin et al., 2004).

Attention

Impaired attention is the "most prominent" stroke-related neuropsychological change, with rates of up to 46% to 92% reported in acute stroke survivors. Impaired attention can reduce cognitive productivity. Distractibility and attention are also associated with physical and social functional impairments. Attention deficits are linked to greater functional impairment and falls in community-dwelling stroke survivors (Barker-Collo et al., 2009).

There are several different levels of attention. Focused attention is the ability to concentrate on one specific stimulus and ignore all surrounding stimuli. Sustained attention is the ability to maintain focus on a prolonged stimulus. Selective attention is the ability to concentrate on one stimulus while another distracting or competitive stimulus is in the area. Alternating attention is the ability to shift focus between two different stimuli. Divided attention is the highest level of attention and requires the person to focus on two stimuli that are occurring simultaneously.

Memory

Between 20% and 50% of patients who survive a stroke demonstrate memory difficulties. There may be numerous reasons for memory difficulties related to the stroke: depression, medication side effects, and sleep disorders. Some researchers believe the location of the brain injury may be the cause of the memory difficulties, such as the hippocampus or amygdale. Short-term memory or working memory is defined as lasting less than a minute before the memory is dismissed or moved into long-term memory. Long-term memory lasts more than several minutes and is for permanent storage (Lim & Alexander, 2009).

Executive Functioning

The area of executive functioning includes several integrative cognitive processes by which an individual can monitor, manage, and regulate the orderly "execution" of goal-directed activities (Cicerone et al., 2005). Executive functioning components include planning, organization, problem solving, execution, thought flexibility, time management, and self-monitoring. These components are also known as initiation, cognitive persistence, flexibility, self-monitoring, and abstract thinking (Ownsworth & Shum, 2008). Most studies have suggested that cognitive decline has been related to stroke severity, but other studies have suggested that executive function decline may begin before stroke (Zinn, Bosworth, Hoenig, &

Swartzwelder, 2007). It is reasonable to consider that there may be a gradual loss of executive function processing in cerebrovascular disease before stroke that becomes worse with a lesion (Zinn et al., 2007).

Cognitive Assessment

A simple bedside cognitive assessment for attention that can be performed is to ask the stroke survivor to spell the word "world" backward or say the days of the week or the months of the year backward. The first is less difficult than the second. Those patients with impaired attention demonstrate difficulty in focusing long enough to complete the task.

Other tests used to assess for attention deficits include a letter cancellation test, the Stroop color word test, and the Mini Mental State Examination (Table 15.9). The Mini Mental State Examination contains a variety of brief

TABLE 15.9   Folstein's Mini Mental State Examination

Examination	Maximum Score
Orientation	1 point for each correct answer
Ask for the year	Maximum score of 10
Ask for the season	
Ask for the date	
Ask for the month	
Ask for day of the week	
Ask for the state	
Ask of the county	
Ask for the town	
Ask for the name of hospital	
Ask for the floor/department	
Registration	1 point for each correct answer
Name three objects: "ball, shoe, window"	Maximum score of 3
Ask to repeat all three objects	
Attention and calculation	1 point for each correct answer
Ask to spell the word "world" backward	Maximum score of 5
Recall	1 point for each correct answer
Ask to repeat three object said in registration section	Maximum score of 3
Language	1 point for each correct answer
Ask to name pencil	(1 point for each command followed)
Ask to name watch	Maximum score of 9
Ask to repeat the phrase "No, ifs, ands, or buts"	
Ask to follow a three-step command such as "Take a piece of paper, fold it in half, and put it on the floor"	
Read and obey the following command: "Close your eyes"	
Write a sentence	
Copy a design of two intersecting shapes	

tasks that assess a wide spectrum of cognitive domains and has proven to be a valid means of detecting cognitive dysfunction in acute stroke patients (Lee et al., 2008). A full neuropsychological assessment is the best way to assess for cognitive function, but it is time-consuming and requires special expertise to administer and interpret (Nokleby et al., 2008).

A simple bedside cognitive assessment for memory that can be performed by the rehabilitation nurse is to ask the stroke survivor first to repeat three random words, such as "ball," "shoe," and "window." This tests for immediate memory. The stroke survivor should then be asked to repeat the same three words after several minutes have passed. This tests for short-term memory. To test for long-term memory, the stroke survivor can be asked the name of the current president or vice president or important dates or events. Other more complex tests used to test for memory deficits include the Auditory Verbal Learning Test, which is used to measure episodic memory; the Wechsler Memory Scale, used to measure verbal memory and visual memory; the Digit Span from the Wechsler Adult Intelligence Scale, used to measure working memory; and the California Verbal Learning test (Lesniak et al., 2008).

A simple bedside cognitive assessment for executive function that can be done by a rehabilitation nurse is to have the stroke survivor participate in the "Go, no go" test. This has the stroke survivor begin a simple motor response and then inhibit that response. This tests the person's ability to control motor behavior. The Verbal Similarities test has the stroke survivor identify similarities and differences between two common objects such as an apple and orange. The Trail Making test is a visual attention task. Many of the trails are prefabricated and the stroke survivor connects the dots between numbers or letters (Figure 15.2).

The Verbal Fluency test asks the stroke survivor to list as many words as possible from a given category in 60 seconds. An example is to list all the animals seen in a zoo or all the animals seen on a farm (Sachedev, Brodaty, Valenzuela, Lorentz, & Koschera, 2004).

Neuropsychological testing is also the best measure for executive function deficits. For executive functioning, several tests need to be performed to best capture the area of deficit. For example, Picture Completion tests for abstract reasoning deficits and the Color Form Sorting Text tests for mental flexibility. The Delis-Kaplan Executive Function Systems is a relatively new test battery comprising nine new or existing tests of executive function from which an examiner can select specifics tests according

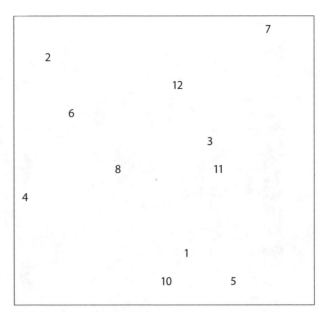

FIGURE 15.2   Trail Making TestF.

to the needs of the stroke survivor and the assessment context (Ownsworth & Shum, 2008).

Language and Communication Deficits

One of the biggest challenges facing stroke survivors is the loss of communication and language skills. Approximately one-third to one-half of stroke survivors experience speech and language disorders (Harvey et al., 2007). Aphasia, apraxia of speech, and dysarthria are the three most common types of speech and language disorders encountered by the stroke survivor. Language is an organized set of symbols used for communication that allows us to speak, to listen, and to understand meaning, ask questions, read and understand, and write. The extent to which areas of language and communication are impacted depends on the severity and location of the stroke. Much of our ability to use language and communicate is located in the left hemisphere of the brain.

Aphasia

Aphasia is the general term used to describe the reduction of language production and comprehension following a stroke. Aphasia can affect all modes of communication, including expression and comprehension. Aphasia can impact communication profoundly on a daily basis and contribute to feelings of isolation and depression (American Stroke Association, 2009). Aphasias are classified base on fluency of speech production, auditory comprehension, and repetition. There are multiple types of aphasia, shown in Table 15.10.

TABLE 15.10 Types of Aphasia

Type	Brain Injury	Fluency	Auditory Comprehension	Repetition	Reading	Writing	Naming
Broca's	Lesion in the posterior portion of the dominant frontal lobe	Nonfluent Phrase length is less than 4 words Automatic speech is intact	Intact	Impaired	Impaired	Reflects verbal output	Impaired
Wernicke's	Lesion in the posterior, superior temporal lobe	Fluent Hyperfluent speech Empty speech that is well articulated	Impaired	Impaired	Impaired	Comparable with speech	Impaired
Global	Lesion in the frontal temporal lobe	Nonfluent May speak a few words No consistent language skills	Impaired	Impaired	Impaired	Impaired	Impaired
Conduction	Arcuate fasiculus Neural pathway connection between Broca's and Wernicke's areas	Fluent Paraphasic errors	Impaired	Impaired	Impaired	Comparable with speech	Impaired
Anomic	Lesion in the angular gyrus	Fluent Difficulty with word retrieval	Intact	Intact	Intact	Intact	Impaired
Transcortical motor	Lesion in the anterior superior frontal lobe	Nonfluent	Intact	Intact	Intact	Impaired	Intact
Transcortical sensory	Lesion in the temporal occipital parietal junction	Fluent	Impaired	Intact	Impaired	Worse than speech	Impaired

Apraxia

Apraxia of speech is a neurological disorder characterized by loss of the ability to execute or carry out learned purposeful movements, despite having the desire and the physical ability to perform the movements. Apraxia of speech is the inability to sequence syllables into sounds and words and can be mild or severe. With apraxia of speech the person knows what they want to say but is unable to form sounds into meaningful words. Communication can be incredibly frustrating. Their rate of speech is slow; however, automatic speech, such as a "hi, how are you?" may be spared. Apraxia of speech is diagnosed by a **speech-language pathologist (SLP)**. The SLP can work with the individual to retrain and strengthen the muscles needed to shape sounds into words (American Speech Language Association, 2010).

Dysarthria

Dysarthria is a motor speech disorder due to damage in the central nervous system. The stroke survivor will have imprecise articulation, which will make him or her difficult to understand. Aspects of speech production affected in dysarthria include respiration, phonation, articulation, and prosody, the stress and intonation in language. Comprehension, reading, and writing are usually intact. Table 15.11 provide the characteristics of dysarthria.

Assessment

Although a language and communication assessment is normally performed by an SLP, rehabilitation nurses are often the first individuals to interact with the stroke survivors and in some locations may need to communicate with them for several days without input from an SLP. Rehabilitation nurses should be able to assess various areas of communication to identify potential ways to interact with the stroke survivor with aphasia until a more thorough assessment can be performed by the SLP. Knowing the survivor's primary language and level of education helps to rule out any issues with language barriers and difficulties with reading or writing that may not be associated with the stroke. The rehabilitation nurse should assess the survivor's ability to express him- or herself verbally, including the rhythm and fluency of speech, the use of words and ability to repeat, the level of frustration with his or her communication ability, automatic speech, auditory comprehension, the ability to name objects correctly, as well as the ability to read or

TABLE 15.11 Characteristics of Dysarthria			
Type	**Brain Injury**	**Characteristics**	**Diagnoses**
Flaccid dysarthria	Damage to cranial nerve X	Hypernasality Reduced tone Slurred speech	Brainstem stroke Traumatic brain injury
Spastic dysarthria	Damage to the pyramidal tract	Harsh, strained or strangled voice quality Low pitch Hypernasality Bursts of loudness	Bilateral strokes Traumatic brain injury Multiple sclerosis Cerebral palsy
Ataxic dysarthria	Lesion in the cerebellum	Harsh vocal quality Increased loudness Explosive speech	Stroke Multiple sclerosis Brain tumors
Hypokinetic dysarthria	Lesion in the substantia nigra	Hoarseness Low volume Muffled pitch Hypernasality	Parkinson's disease
Hyperkinetic dysarthria	Lesion in the basal ganglia	Voice quality is harsh, strained or strangled Hypernasality Fluctuating loudness	Stroke Encephalitis Traumatic brain injury

write as a potential method of communication if verbal output is poor.

Genitourinary and Gastrointestinal Complications After Stroke

Urinary Incontinence

Urinary incontinence is a common problem after stroke. Approximately 50% of stroke survivors have incontinence during their acute admission for stroke. However, that number decreases to 20% by 6 months after stroke. Increased age, increased stroke severity, the presence of diabetes, and the occurrence of other disabling diseases increases the risk of urinary incontinence in stroke (Duncan et al., 2005). Most survivors with moderate-to-severe stroke are incontinent at presentation, and many are discharged incontinent. Urinary incontinence is a major burden on caregivers once the patient is discharged home.

Management of bladder problems should be seen as an essential part of the survivor's rehabilitation, because it can seriously hamper progress in other areas. Although the acute use of an indwelling catheter may facilitate care, the use of an indwelling catheter for more than 48 hours after stroke increases the risk of urinary tract infection (Duncan et al., 2005; Nakayama, Jorgensen, Peterson, Raaschou, & Olsen, 1997). The indwelling catheter should be removed within 48 hours to avoid urinary tract infections, and urinary retention should then be assessed through the use of a bladder scanner or postvoid catheterization. An individualized training program should then be implemented for those who are incontinent of urine (Duncan et al., 2005). The stroke survivor with urinary incontinence often experiences urge incontinence. This is due to a loss of cortical inhibition of the voiding reflex. The symptoms are usually exacerbated by the loss of mobility, cognition, or communication that often occurs with a stroke, because more time may be required to get to the toilet.

Simple measures (use of a bedside commode, timed/prompted voiding, and avoidance of bladder irritants such as caffeine) may be used for management of incontinence after stroke. Other more advanced therapies require a level of motivation and muscle control that may not be present in all patients but may be quite effective in properly chosen survivors (Duraski, Denby, & Clemons, 2009).

A toileting program should be initiated by the rehabilitation nurse. The use of a voiding diary helps to identify patterns of voiding so that nursing staff can anticipate voiding needs. Until a pattern can be established, timed voiding can be used to anticipate voiding needs. Rehabilitation nurses can also educate survivors and families regarding fluids and equipment that will help improve continence. In some cases rehabilitation nurses need to work with medical staff to prescribe medication

---

CASE STUDY 15.1

Dr. N. is a 39-year-old physician who suffered a pontine stroke. He was readmitted to the rehabilitation unit 18 months after his original stroke. His wife was returning to work and he needed more therapy so he could stay home alone while she was away. His goal was to be able to toilet himself independently while she was away. He does not want a caregiver. Currently, the patient is 80% continent. He relies on his wife toileting him during the day and at night. If he does not get to the bathroom immediately, he is incontinent.

Questions

1. What nursing diagnosis would the rehabilitation nurse use for this patient?
2. What other information does the rehabilitation nurse need to obtain to identify goals and nursing interventions?
3. What nursing interventions are appropriate to help the patient achieve his identified goal?

Answers

1. Alteration in bladder elimination secondary to altered mobility
2. What fluids does the patient normally drink during the day?
   How much fluid does the patient drink at a time?
   How quickly after the urge to void does the patient have to get to the bathroom?
   Can the patient tell when he has to have a bowel movement?
   Is he continent of bowel?
3. Toileting schedule to anticipate need
   Education about fluid schedule
   Avoid fluids that cause urinary urgency and frequency
   Work with physical therapy regarding transfers so they can be practiced on the unit
   Work with occupational therapy on clothing management so it can be practiced on the unit

management. The management of urinary incontinence is a team effort. Rehabilitation nurses should work with other team members on timing, transfers, clothing management, and communication to be successful. Chapter 9 provides additional information on establishing bowel and bladder patterns.

Fecal Incontinence

Fecal incontinence occurs in a substantial proportion of patients after a stroke but clears within two weeks in most survivors if the stroke survivor's recovery includes improved cognitive awareness and mobility (Brockelhurst, Andrews, Richards, & Laycock, 1985). Continued fecal incontinence signals a poor prognosis. Constipation and fecal impaction are more common after stroke than incontinence. Immobility and inactivity, inadequate fluid or food intake, depression or anxiety, the inability to perceive bowel signals, lack of transfer ability, and cognitive deficits may each contribute to this problem after stroke.

The management of fecal incontinence after stroke is often easier to address than urinary incontinence. Depending upon the problem, stool may need to be softened for easier passage or bulked up to increase sensory input (Duraski et al., 2009). Treatment should be cause specific (Duncan et al., 2005). Goals of management are to ensure adequate intake of fluid, bulk, and fiber; improved exercise and activity; and a regular toileting schedule. Bowel training is more effective if the schedule is consistent with the patient's previous bowel habits. Stool softeners and the judicious use of laxatives may be helpful (Duraski et al., 2009; Venn, Taft, Carpentier, & Applebaugh, 1992).

Rehabilitation nurses should take the lead role in the management of fecal incontinence. Identification of the problems leading to incontinence will help the nurse decide whether fluids, fiber, exercise, or toileting is needed. Encouraging stroke survivors to use the toilet after meals uses the gastrocolic reflex to the patient's advantage. Just as with the management of urinary incontinence, the management of fecal incontinence is a team effort. All team members should be recruited to assist with transfers, clothing management, communication, and medication management.

Nutrition

Dysphagia, or impaired swallowing, occurs in approximately one-third to one-half of all stroke survivors and places the stroke survivor at risk for aspiration and pneumonia, malnutrition, and dehydration. Malnutrition is common, being present in about 15% of all survivors admitted to the hospital and increasing to about 30% over the first week after stroke. Malnutrition is associated with a worse outcome and a slower rate of recovery (Intercollegiate Stroke Working Party, 2004).

About 83% of survivors receiving a **videofluoroscopic swallow study** receive referrals to other specialists, swallowing therapy, prescribed compensatory strategies to improve swallowing, changes in mode of nutritional intake, and/or diet modifications (Hormer, Massey, Riski, Lathrop, & Chase, 1988; Martin-Harris, Logemann, McMahon, Schleicher, & Sandidge, 2000). All survivors should receive evaluation of nutrition and hydration as soon as possible after admission.

The best treatment for malnutrition after stroke is prevention. Calorie counts and intake and output should be monitored for all those survivors who are at risk for malnutrition. Weekly weights should be performed to monitor for weight loss. Oral mucosa should be assessed for moisture and skin turgor assessed for moisture and elasticity. Urine color can also identify dehydration as can increased heart rate or complaints of fatigue. In some cases altered mental status and confusion can be very serious effects of dehydration and malnutrition.

Focus should be placed on specific problems that interfere with intake. For those survivors with very poor attention, difficulty self-feeding, or fatigue after a period of time, providing assistance in feeding may help improve oral intake. For those who complain of feeling full or who are overwhelmed by the amount of fluid or food they must consume, offering small frequent meals or consistently offering fluid by mouth is an effective intervention. Having the survivor carry a water bottle filled with fluid may also help serve as a reminder to drink. Catering to food preferences or asking family or friend to bring in foods from home may also improve intake (Duncan et al., 2005). Oral supplements can increase caloric or fluid intake.

Psychosocial Issues

Poststroke Depression

According to the AHA 2005 guidelines, **poststroke depression (PSD)** is common and under-diagnosed. Assessment of emotional disorders is challenging in the stroke survivor because of aphasia, flat affect, aprosodic speech, and lack of standardized testing. With this knowledge the rehabilitation nurse and team need to observe the stroke survivor's behaviors and speak with family to gain insight into the psychosocial history to aid in determining if these are new neuropsychological disorders or preexisting conditions. As rehabilitation team members, psychologists or psychiatrists with experience working in stroke rehabilitation can be valuable resources in the development of the stroke recovery plan (Bates et al., 2005).

PSD is described as the most frequent and important neuropsychiatric consequence of stroke, as approximately one-third of stroke survivors experience depression both early and late after stroke. The etiology of PSD is controversial, but PSD has been found to be associated with diminished recovery after stroke (Gianotti & Marra, 2002; Williams et al., 2007). Factors associated with increased risk for PSD include female gender, past history of depression or psychiatric illness, social isolation, functional impairment, and cognitive impairment (Salter, Bhogal, Teasell, Foley, & Speechley, 2009).

Assessment

Clinical depression is a sense of hopelessness that disrupts a person's ability to function and appears to be the emotional disorder most commonly experienced by stroke survivors. Some of the signs of clinical depression include sleep disturbances, a radical change in eating patterns that lead to weight loss or gain, lethargy, social withdrawal, irritability, fatigue, self-loathing, and suicidal thoughts (Office of Communications and Public Liaison, 2008).

Treatment

The initiation of pharmacological treatment soon after stroke may help prevent PSD. There is strong evidence that early initiation of antidepressant therapy in nondepressed stroke survivors is effective in preventing PSD impairment (Salter et al., 2009). Table 15.12 provides more information on antidepressant medications.

Motivated depression is a reactive depression, and symptoms are common in survivors with both major and minor PSD impairment (Salter et al., 2009). Symptoms of motivational disturbances include loss of interest, psychomotor change, less energy, and difficulty with thinking or concentration. Stroke survivors with apathy often have a frontal lobe disturbance. Apathy has been described as a lack of motivation and a decrease in behavioral, cognitive, and emotional responses to goal directed behavior (Marin, Firinciogullari, & Biedrzycki, 1994).

In the first 6 months after stroke, poststroke emotionalism affects approximately 25% of stroke survivors' impairment (Salter et al., 2009). **Emotional lability**, or uncontrollable episodes of laughter, crying, or both, is often seen in stroke survivors. Emotional outbursts can occur without a clear relationship to the event or may be triggered by an insignificant or nonspecific stimulus. In response, the stroke survivor may not experience any subsequent change in feeling. Lability causes embarrassment and social isolation and can interfere with rehabilitation (Tang et al., 2009). Antidepressants can reduce the frequency and severity of crying or laughing episodes, but the effect does not seem specific to one drug or class of drugs (House, Hackett, Anderson, & Horrocks, 2009). Table 15.13 describes nonpharmacological interventions.

Caregiver Issues

Caregivers of stroke survivors assume their role suddenly and with little preparation (King et al., 2007). Numerous studies highlight the problems and emotions experienced by these caregivers. Understanding stroke-related problems reported by family caregivers is important because they are risk factors for caregiver depression, which also is a known risk factor for a negative impact on the stroke

---

CASE STUDY 15.2

FX is a 43-year-old woman with a past medical history of migraines who suffered a left medullary stroke confirmed by brain magnetic resonance image in March 2010 resulting in left facial droop, vertigo, left hand clumsiness, hypophonia, dysphagia, and diplopia. Videofluoroscopic swallow study on March 8 revealed severe pharyngeal dysphagia. A PEG was tube placed on March 9. Initially, FX was transferred for acute rehabilitation on March 10. At the time of her transfer she presented with a persistent cough and pain at her PEG tube site. FW developed an elevated white count and drainage coming from her PEG tube with continued pain.

Questions

1. What precautions should nursing be the least concerned with?
2. Which precautions should be initially implemented?
3. Would you say FX has an infection?
4. What would be the most likely source of her infection?
5. What comfort measures could nursing provide for her abdominal wound pain?

TABLE 15.12   Antidepressant Medications

Class of Drugs	Names	Action	Benefits	Side Effects/Risks
Heterocyclic antidepressants (HCA)	Amitriptyline Desipramine Imipramine Nortriptyline	Block the reuptake of serotonin & norepinephrine, thus increasing level of neurotransmitters	Improves anxiety symptoms and recovery of ADLs as measured by FIM	Confusion, drowsiness, agitation, especially in elderly Do not use in patients with cardiac arrhythmia, heart block, glaucoma Has been linked to adverse cardiovascular, anticholinergic & antihistamine effects
Selective serotonin reuptake inhibitors (SSRIs)	Citalopram Fluoxetine Sertraline	Selectively block serotonin reuptake rather than blocking both serotonin & norepinephrine reuptake	Improves anxiety, hostility, restlessness Shown to be faster acting than HCA Side effects are mild & transient	Weight loss in the elderly
Selective noradrenaline reuptake inhibitors (NRI)	Reboxetine	Inhibit noradrenaline reuptake for treatment of patients with lethargy, poor initiation	Effective treatment of depression with poor initiation, lethargy	Constipation, headache hyperperspiration, drowsiness, decreased libido
Serontonin and noradrenaline reuptake inhibitors (SNRIs)	Venlafaxine	Inhibits reuptake of serotonin, norepinephrine, and to lesser extent dopamine	Has been used safely with the geriatric population	Increase blood pressure There is little evidence that SNRIs are a safe and effective treatment for PSD
Gamma-aminobutyric acid (GABA) compounds	Nefiracetam	Affects neurotransmission, regional blood flow & glucose utilization	Has not been proven to be beneficial	Has not been shown to be more effective than placebo in the treatment for PSD
Psychostimulants	Methylphenidate	Heighten mood affecting neurotransmitter systems, blocks the reuptake of serotonin & norepinephrine & has dopaminergic activity May correct the depletion of biogenic amines caused by stroke	Early onset Treats apathy Affects the cortical & subcortical areas of the brain Heightens mood by affecting several neurotransmitter systems, especially noradrenergic system	Can be addictive; Nervousness, insomnia, decreased appetite, diarrhea, heartburn, dry mouth, headache, restlessness, muscle tightness, decreased libido

Note: FIM, Functional Independence Measure

survivor, and because they increase risk of nursing home placement (Haley et al., 2009).

Several problems are commonly identified by caregivers: stroke survivors not being independent enough to do things for themselves or to be left alone; difficulty dealing with emotions of stroke survivor such as anger or depression; problems managing comorbid conditions such as fluctuations in blood sugar; onset of flu symptoms; weight gain; problems balancing roles, commitments, and activities required in addition to caring for the stroke survivor; problems getting stroke survivor to do home exercise program; and sleep issues (Pierce, Steiner, Hicks, & Holzaepfel, 2006). One study noted that caregivers reported dealing with patient anxiety, needing help with transportation, trouble remembering recent events, difficulty walking or climbing stairs, and problems with

TABLE 15.13   Nonpharmacological Intervention in the Treatment of PSD

Intervention	Technique/Response	Benefit
Electroconvulsive therapy (ECT)	Electroshock therapy seizures are electrically induced in an anesthetized patient. Reported risk of relapse after treatment. Transient memory loss, muscle soreness.	Relatively safe & effective treatment but unsure of long-term effect on cognition.
Repetitive transcranial magnetic stimulation (rTMS)	Uses focused magnetic impulses to stimulate the brain in the prefrontal cortex. Excites neurons in the brain through weak electrical currents induced in the tissue by electromagnetic induction.	Noninvasive treatment used in patients who have failed other treatments. Moderate evidence that shows it is well tolerated in PSD with mild adverse side effects and has longer effects than TMS.
Cognitive behavioral therapy	Problem-solving approach through goal-oriented, systematic procedure.	Has not been shown to be beneficial in the treatment of PSD.
Combined therapy	Combining psychosocial, problem-solving intervention with antidepressant medication.	Moderate evidence that shows psychosocial intervention in addition to antidepressant medication is more effective that medication alone.
Music therapy	Provides stimulation, motivation, and enhances social interactions.	Music therapy is noninvasive and may improve PSD.

vision or hearing (Haley et al., 2009). Another study identified caregiver problems in the first month after discharge from the hospital as safety, ADLs, and managing cognitive, behavioral, and emotional changes exhibited by the stroke survivor (Grant, Glandon, Elliot, Giger, & Weaver, et al., 2004).

Sexuality

In the months after a stroke, lingering sequelae result in changes in sexual intimacy for both the stroke survivor and their partner. These changes can be devastating to the relationship (Forsberg-Warleby, Moller, & Blomstrand, 2002; Korpelainen, Nieminen, & Myllyla, 1999; Murray & Harrison, 2004). Common sexual problems after stroke include loss of desire, feelings of being less attractive, fatigue, chronic aches and pain, depression, persistent vaginal dryness, erectile dysfunction, inability to find a comfortable position for intercourse, lack of satisfaction or pleasure in sex, concern about masturbation, speech difficulties, incontinence, memory problems, and difficulty expressing emotions (Forsberg-Warleby et al., 2002; Korpelainen et al., 1999; Murray & Harrison, 2004).

Treatment

Unfortunately, sexual issues are not always addressed by the rehabilitation team. It has been recommended that sexual issues are discussed during rehabilitation and addressed again after transition to the community when the poststroke survivor and partner are ready (Duncan et al., 2005). The stroke survivor and partner must first understand that sexual activity is not contraindicated. Couples

should be encouraged to take their time, communicate, share concerns, and just be together before sexual intercourse. For those without partners, stroke survivors may need to be encouraged to take care in their appearance and learn where and how to meet potential new partners. Younger stroke survivors should be educated about birth control methods and prevention of pregnancy. Certain birth control methods may need to be avoided because they increase the risk of blood clotting.

Letting the stroke survivor know that sexuality concerns are common is the beginning of treatment. Giving general information about sexuality after stroke helps to dispel myths. Management of depression, timing of pain medication, use of vaginal creams or lubricants, timing of antispasticity medication, and positioning can help address commonly identified sexuality issues after stroke.

MEDICAL COMPLICATIONS POSTSTROKE

Medical complications are unfortunately not uncommon after a stroke. Risk factors that lead to stroke can lead to other medical conditions, and immobility and treatments for stroke can cause complications.

Cardiovascular Complications

Venous Thromboembolism

Stroke survivors who have suffered an acute thromboembolic stroke are at increased risk for further venous thromboembolism events (VTE). These events include both **deep vein thrombosis (DVT)** and **pulmonary embolism (PE)**.

The incidence of DVT in the first two weeks after stroke is between 27% and 75% in untreated survivors. An untreated DVT can break loose from the venous wall and travel, potentially causing another stroke, PE, or myocardial infarction. The most common signs of a DVT are calf swelling, pain, altered temperature, and fever. Homan's sign, pain associated with forced dorsiflexion of the ankle, is often part of the physical assessment of the person with a suspected DVT. Numerous studies have documented the unreliability of Homan's sign. Estimates of the accuracy of Homan's sign range from it being positive in 8% to 56% of cases of proven DVT and positive in greater than 50% of symptomatic patients without DVT (Urbano, 2001). The diagnosis of DVT is confirmed by a venous ultrasound (Teasell, Foley & Bhogal, 2006). Other diagnostic tests include a venography or a D-dimer blood test.

PE is responsible for approximately 25% of early deaths after stroke. PE is the third leading cause of death in stroke survivors after the stroke itself (Hara, 2008; Sherman, 2006). The most common signs of a PE are tachycardia, tachypnea, pleuritic chest pain, and fever. The diagnosis of a PE is confirmed by a ventilation/perfusion lung scan or spiral computed tomography.

Survivors of thromboembolic stroke should receive either low-dose unfractionated heparin or low-molecular-weight heparin, or heparinoids (danaparoid) (Sherman, 2006). Intermittent pneumatic compression boots are used continuously in the acute care setting and can be used at bedtime in the rehabilitation setting. When possible, the stroke survivor should weight-bear or ambulate. Graduated compression stockings can be used as an adjunct to anticoagulation medications or as an alternative to anticoagulation for survivors who have had a hemorrhagic stroke and cannot take anticoagulants (Duncan et al., 2005).

Rehabilitation nurses play a vital role in early identification of a stroke survivor with a DVT as well as early mobilization and prevention of DVT. Rehabilitation nurses should also educate the survivor and family on thromboprophylactic measures.

Atrial Fibrillation

Atrial fibrillation (AF) is the most common type of heart rhythm abnormality after stroke. AF, often paroxysmal, is often detected only after it has caused a cardioembolic stroke. When cardiac output is compromised, arrhythmias may further aggravate an already damaged cerebral blood flow.

Some people with AF may not have symptoms. Others may experience light-headedness, fainting, anxiety, fatigue, shortness of breath, or the feeling of an increased or irregular heart rate. Electrocardiogram is the gold standard in diagnosing AF. AF may be intermittent, requiring a 24-hour Holter monitor to diagnose if AF is suspected but not seen on routine electrocardiogram (Stein, Silver, & Frates, 2006).

AF can be treated by either restoring the heart to a normal rhythm through cardioversion or controlling the heart rate with medication. If cardioversion is not the best treatment or fails, then rate-controlling medications are used. In some cases medications cannot control AF and a pacemaker is implanted or a Cox-Maze procedure performed, which involves cutting into the atria to stop the abnormal electrical impulses. Stroke survivors with a history of AF are often prescribed Coumadin. Using Coumadin is challenging because of the complex pharmacokinetics and narrow therapeutic window. The adjusted dosing of Coumadin maintaining a target **International Normalized Ratio** between two and three prevents ischemic stroke with an acceptable hemorrhagic risk but requires frequent blood draws and dietary adjustment.

Pulmonary Complications

Aspiration Pneumonia

With one-third to one-half of all stroke survivors experiencing some level of dysphagia, or impaired ability to swallow, the risk of **aspiration pneumonia** is high. Pneumonia impedes blood oxygenation and slow recovery. The stroke survivor must be evaluated to determine the risk of aspiration.

Signs of aspiration pneumonia can include coughing or choking on food, water, or even saliva. In the case of silent aspiration, no signs are apparent. Aspiration pneumonia is generally seen more frequently in the right lung, whereas regular viral or bacterial pneumonia is often seen equally in either lung or bilaterally.

All stroke patients should have their swallowing function screened before initiating oral intake of fluids or foods. A bedside screening can be completed by an SLP or nurses trained to look for signs of dysphagia. If the swallow screening is abnormal, an examination should be performed by the SLP who will define swallow physiology and make recommendations about management and treatment (Duncan et al., 2005). A videofluoroscopic swallow may be ordered in which the therapist can visually observe how, where, and to what extent the person's swallow is impaired.

In 1984, Frazier Rehabilitation in Louisville Kentucky, implemented a water protocol. It is based on the assumptions that aspiration of water poses little risk to the patient if oral bacteria associated with the development of aspiration pneumonia can be minimized; allowing free water decreases the risk of dehydration, increases patient compliance with swallowing precaution, and improves quality of life. Water intake is unrestricted before meals and is allowed 30 minutes after a meal. Aggressive oral care is provided with twice-daily brushing, suctioning oral secretions as needed, and oral rinse with 1.5% hydrogen peroxide three times a day. The only published research is by Garon, Engle, and Ormiston (1997). One group of dysphagia patients received thickened liquids, whereas another group received thickened liquids and water between meals. No patients in either group developed aspiration pneumonia or dehydration during the study or during a 30-day follow-up period (Garon et al., 1997).

Rehabilitation nursing interventions are key to preventing pneumonia in stroke survivors. For instance, in the case of severe dysphagia, a feeding tube should be placed to provide nutrition, fluids, and medication. To prevent aspiration of feedings, nasogastric tube placement verification must be done by chest x-ray each time a tube is inserted and before any feedings being initiated. After that, the nasogastric tube length should be measured before each feeding. If the measurement is more than 10 cm different from the previous measurement, a chest x-ray should be repeated to verify placement. A gastric tube or **percutaneous endogastric gastrostomy (PEG) tube** may also be placed into the stomach, but again the risk of aspiration remains. Feedings should be administered only when the patient is in an upright position to prevent emesis or aspiration. Nurses should ensure patients are not scheduled to have therapy that requires lying down close after the time of a tube feeding to prevent the potential for aspiration.

In those who are transitioning from enteral to oral feedings, rehabilitation nurses should monitor stroke survivors very closely during meals. SLPs often make recommendations on compensatory techniques to improve swallow (e.g., chin tuck, head turns, small bites/sips). It will fall to the rehabilitation nurse to cue survivors on these techniques to decrease the risk of aspiration. Rehabilitation nurses also need to ensure the survivor is using these same techniques when medications are administered. During this period, auscultation of lung fields and moni-

---

CASE STUDY 15.3

Mrs. P. is a 76-year-old White woman with a history of atrial fibrillation and a left-sided stroke. The residual effects from the stroke were bilateral hemianopsia. While visiting her daughter in Poland, Mrs. P. noted transient blurred vision in her right eye that spontaneously resolved. Two days later she was admitted with continued visual problems and was found to have a right posterior cerebral artery infarct. While in the hospital she developed slurred speech, left facial droop, and left hemiplegia. She was found to have a right middle cerebral artery occlusion and a partial thrombectomy was performed.

Questions

1. Was Mrs. P. at greater risk for a recurrent stroke and, if so, why?
2. On what areas of education should the rehabilitation nurse focus?

Answers

1. Yes, she has a previous history of stroke and atrial fibrillation.

2. Education should focus on risk factors of stroke, signs and symptoms of stroke, and methods to prevent future or recurrent stroke.

After an inpatient rehabilitation stay, Mrs. P. was transferred to day rehabilitation. She received continued physical, occupational, and speech-language therapies and nursing services for medication education and blood draws to monitor her Coumadin levels. Mrs. P. was discharged with contact guard assistance for ambulation and supervision for her ADLs.

Questions

1. What nursing diagnosis would best describe any issues this patient may have once discharged from day rehabilitation?
2. What nursing interventions would best address the identified issue?

Answers

1. Potential for injury
2. Education regarding Coumadin and safety measures in the home environment to prevent falls and injuries

toring for any elevations in temperature may cue the nurse to possible aspiration signs. Changes in lung sounds, shortness of breath, or an elevated temperature should be pointed out to the medical team immediately.

Nosocomial Pneumonia

Nosocomial pneumonia is prevalent in poststroke survivors who cannot manage their respiratory secretions. One study puts the incidence as high as 21% in the intensive care unit. Poststroke survivors with pneumonia have a higher mortality rate and poorer functional outcome than survivors who remain pneumonia free (Hilker et al., 2003).

Preventing nosocomial pneumonia includes basic rehabilitation nursing interventions such as frequent repositioning, postural drainage, and use of incentive spirometer. A tracheostomy tube may be needed for survivors requiring long-term mechanical ventilation, patients who are unable to cough effectively to clear secretions, and survivors with an obstructed airway. The increase in activity, strength, and endurance related to rehabilitation may mean that the survivor is more able to cough up secretions independently or rely less frequently on tracheal suctioning. Once suctioning is no longer required, a weaning program may be initiated.

The patient may be discharged home with the tracheostomy tube still in place if they are not able to consistently clear secretions independently, if they have ongoing active respiratory issues, or if they have an upcoming surgical procedure. If that is the case, the family or a caregiver will need to learn suctioning and tracheostomy management. If the survivor is able, they too should be taught to direct family members in suctioning and tracheostomy management. If a survivor goes home with a tracheostomy tube that is capped continuously, family should still learn how to suction and manage the tracheostomy for emergency purposes.

Sleep Disordered Breathing

Sleep disordered breathing (SDB) and **sleep–wake disorders (SWDs)** are frequent after stroke. The brain injury from the stroke itself can impair the regulation of sleep and wake breathing control mechanisms. Other causes include immobilization, pain, hypoxia, and depression that may affect the same mechanisms. SDB and SWDs can arise from similar predisposing or risk factors (Bassetti, 2005).

The most common form of SDB in stroke survivors is obstructive sleep apnea. In the first few days after stroke, **central sleep apnea** and/or Cheyne Stokes breathing

may be present and in fact even predominate in up to 30% to 40% of survivors (Bassetti, 2005). Symptoms of SDB include difficulty falling asleep, respiratory noises, irregular or periodic respiration, apneas, agitated sleep with increased motor activity and frequent awakenings, sudden awakenings with or without choking sensations, shortness of breath, palpitations and fear, orthopnea and increased sweating (Bassetti, 2005).

SWDs are found in at least 20% to 40% of survivors who most commonly present with increased sleep needs (hypersomnia), excessive daytime sleepiness, or insomnia. Often SWDs are mild and/or transient (Hermann, Siccoli, & Bassetti, 2003). **Hypersomnia** is defined by an increased sleep propensity with excessive daytime sleepiness and/or increased sleep needs. Increased sleep needs may correspond to an increase of physiological sleep or of sleeplike behavior with normal or altered posturing and breathing patterns. Insomnia is defined by difficulty initiating or maintaining sleep, early awakenings, insufficient sleep quality, and corresponding poor daytime functioning (lack of energy, fatigue, concentration problems, mood swings, irritability). Insomnia may be accompanied by an inversion of the sleep–wake cycle with insomnia and agitation during the night and hypersomnia during the day (Bassetti, 2005).

SWDs are often multifactorial in origin. In addition to the brain injury, environmental factors may contribute to the development of SWD. Cardiorespiratory disorders, seizures, infections, fever, and drugs may aggravate sleep fragmentation and result in further sleep disturbances. Anxiety, depression, and psychological stress frequently accompany and complicate stroke and may further contribute to SWD (Bassetti, 2005).

SDB is best diagnosed by respiratory polygraphy in which nasal airflow and thoracic and abdominal respiratory movements in addition to oximetry are monitored. Conventional polysomnography offers additional information (Bassetti, 2005). Polysomnography provides a comprehensive recording of the physiological changes that occur during sleep. The polysomnography monitors many body functions through electroencephalogram, electrooculogram, electromyogram, and electrocardiogram during sleep. Due to the complexity of the machinery required, polysomnography is costly, labor intensive, and inconvenient to the study subject.

The recognition of poststroke SWDs is primarily clinical. In survivors with poststroke hypersomnia sleep, for example, electroencephalogram may reveal both a reduction, less commonly an increase, of non–rapid eye movement and/or rapid eye movement sleep.

Actigraphy may be helpful to estimate changes in sleep–wake rhythms and sleep/rest needs after stroke (Bassetti, 2005). An actigraph is a small portable tool that can be attached to the wearer's arm, leg, or waist to monitor activity or movement by miniaturized acceleration sensors that translate physical motion to a numeric representation (Sadeh, Hauri, Kripke, & Lavie, 1995).

Treatment of SDB should always include prevention and early treatment of secondary complications and cautious use or avoidance of alcohol and sedative hypnotic drugs, which may all negatively affect breathing control during sleep. For rehabilitation nurses, proper patient positioning is important to maintain oxygen saturation. Teaching weight loss and use of lateral sleeping positions can also improve SDB.

Continuous positive airway pressure, or CPAP, is the treatment of choice for obstructive sleep apnea. CPAP treatment prevents the collapse of the upper airway, acting as a pneumatic splint (Hermann et al., 2003). Compliance with use of CPAP is between 50% and 70%. Rehabilitation nurses can prove to be important in educating survivors regarding the need to use the machine and identify reasons for poor compliance (Bassetti, 2005). Improvement of Cheyne Stokes breathing can be obtained in stroke survivors with oxygen (Hermann et al., 2003).

Treatment of poststroke SWDs is also multifactorial. Various medication categories can be used to manage poststroke hypersomnia. For instance, modafinil is approved by the U.S. Food and Drug Administration for the management of narcolepsy. Other drug categories used to manage poststroke hypersomnia include dopaminergic agents, stimulating antidepressants, and stimulants. Treatment of an associated depression with sedative antidepressants may also improve poststroke insomnia (Bassetti, 2005). Treatment of postacute stroke insomnia should include environmental factors. Placement in a private room, protection against noise and light at night, increased activity with exposure to light during the day, avoidance of caffeine, avoidance of fluids immediately before sleep, avoiding heavy meals 3 hours before bedtime, and no naps during the day are all environmental factors that can be considered.

Behavioral modifications can also help with SWDs. Management of pain issues, medication timing, and treatment of urinary issues can impact sleep–wake cycles. Although some medications are used to improve wakefulness, timing of these medications should be closely examined. If taken too late in the day, these medications may contribute to insomnia. Short-term use of sedative hypnotics or herbal treatments can help those with insomnia. Herbal medicines should always be reviewed with the stroke's healthcare practitioner to ensure no drug interactions with prescription medications. Table 15.14 provides information on sleep medications.

TABLE 15.14	Sleep Medications	
Drug Class	**Medications**	**Adverse Effects**
Over the counter	dimenhydrinate (Dramamine)	Do not use in those with glaucoma, BPH, GI obstruction, asthma or pulmonary patients, CV disease or hypertension, PUD
	diphenhydramine (Benadryl, Excedrin PM, Tylenol PM)	
	doxylamine (Unisom)	
Benzodiazepines	triazolam (Halcion)	Rapid onset, daytime sleepiness, dizziness, headache, lightheadedness, constipation, decreased memory, uncoordination
	temazepam (Restoril)	
	estazolam (ProSom)	
	flurazepman (Dalmane)	
	alprazolam (Xanax)	
	clonazepam (Klonopin)	
Hypnotics (nonbenzodiazepines)	zolpidem (Ambien)	Unpleasant taste, hallucinations, worsening depression, headache, dizziness, altered color perception, vertigo malaise
	zaleplon (Sonata)	
	eszopiclone (Lunesta)	
Antidepressants	amitriptyline (Elavil)	Anticholinergic side effects, daytime somnolence, dyspepsia, hypotension, blurred vision, cardiac toxicity, sexual dysfunction
	trazodone (Desyrel)	
Melatonin receptor agonist	ramelteon (Rozerem)	Caution with hepatic or renal disease

CV, cardiovascular; BPH, benign prostatic hypertension; GI, gastrointestinal; PUD, Peptic ulcer disease

Neurological Complications

Poststroke Seizure Disorder

Seizures occur in about 10% of all stroke survivors. Five percent of poststroke seizures occur within 24 to 48 hours after stroke. The other 5% are late-onset seizures, weeks to months after stroke. Those stroke survivors who have early seizures are less likely to have chronic seizures. Those with late seizures are more likely to require seizure management on a longer term. Those who suffer larger strokes are more likely to have late seizures. Recurrent seizures develop in 3% to 4% of stroke patients. Among older adults, stroke is the most common cause of a new-onset seizure disorder. The use of antiseizure medication as a preventative measure immediately after a stroke is not uncommon. The use of seizure medication for late seizures is a medical decision based on the occurrence of seizure, type and location of the stroke, and information from other diagnostic tests such as the electroencephalogram (Pathak, 2006).

Rehabilitation nurses play a very important role in identifying stroke survivors who may be having seizures. Seizures can occur quickly and may not be witnessed by staff, but changes in a survivor's behavior or cognition may be observed instead. Medical staff should be notified of any unexplained behavior and cognitive or functional changes in the stroke patient. The family should be educated on how to manage potential seizure activity at home. Survivors and families need to be taught about the proper administration of medication, the need to avoid missing or skipping doses, and whether monitoring of blood levels is required. Table 15.15 provides more information on antiepileptic medications.

Pain

Central Pain Syndrome

Central poststroke pain syndrome (CPSP) or thalamic pain is a neuropathic pain disorder caused by damage to the central nervous system. It is especially common in left brain hemispheric strokes and can affect up to 18% or more of stroke survivors who have sensory deficits. CPSP generally develops 3 to 6 months after the stroke, but this can vary from immediately after stroke to years poststroke. The exact etiology of CPSP remains unknown. CPSP is described by patients as burning and/or tingling, often in the hands and feet; shooting pains; or pain like an electrical current on the affected side. A definitive diagnosis of CPSP is difficult because of the variety of pain symptoms that can be present and because other types of pain may be present simultaneously, which clouds the picture. There are no clear diagnostic criteria for evaluating CPSP. Pain scales, such as the numeric pain intensity score or the visual analog scale, are helpful in determining the pain intensity, but there are no scales developed specifically to measure CPSP (Klit, Finnerup & Jensen, 2009).

CPSP does not respond to analgesic pain medication (Klit et al., 2009). The goal of treatment is not to completely eradicate the pain but to calm the pain to a point where the person can continue to participate in daily activities and maintain an acceptable quality of life. Treatment often involves the use of antidepressants such as tricyclics or selective serotonin-norepinephrine reuptake inhibitors. Another class of medications that seems to be effective is anticonvulsants or antiepileptics, such as gabapentin and Lyrica. Opioids have limited effects for

TABLE 15.15 **Antiepileptic Medications Used After Stroke**			
Agent	**Dose**	**Lab Monitoring**	**Adverse Effects**
Gabapentin (Neurontin)	Min: 300 mg TID Max: 3,600 mg/day	Yes	Weight gain, edema
Levetiracetam (Keppra)	Min: 500 mg BID Max: 1,500 mg BID	No	Irritability, sedation, diarrhea
Carbamazepine (Tegretol)	Min: 200 mg BID Max: 1,200 mg/day	Yes	Nystagmus, blurred vision, dizziness, dry mouth, rash, granulocytopenia
Phenytoin (Dilantin)	15–20 mg/kg	Yes	Gingival hypertrophy, peripheral neuropathy, osteomalacia, folic acid deficiency
Valproic acid (Depakene, Depakote)	Min: 15 mg/kg/day Max: 60 mg/kg/day	Yes	Somnolence, dizziness, alopecia, nausea, vomiting, diarrhea, thrombocytopenia

neuropathic pain, and the adverse effects are such that they need to be closely monitored and used sparingly. Often, an antidepressant may be combined with gabapentin and the dosages adjusted until the patient reports a decrease in pain or that the pain has become tolerable. This is a random trial and error method of treatment that varies from individual to individual. Table 15.16 further describes medications used to treat CPSP.

Nonpharmacological forms of treatment are also important in treatment of CPSP (Kumar, Selim, & Caplan, 2010). These include transcutaneous nerve stimulation, desensitization techniques such as rubbing the affected area with materials of different textures, joint contracture prevention, and psychological interventions. Surgery is the last intervention when all forms of medical and rehabilitative treatments have failed.

CPSP can be exacerbated by physical movement, emotional stress, loud noises, changes in weather, and cold or light touch (Teasell et al., 2006). Caution should be used when handling the affected extremity, and family and staff should be educated in methods of preventing exacerbation of the pain.

Hemiplegic Shoulder Pain Syndrome.

Another common type of poststroke pain is hemiplegic shoulder pain syndrome. The incidence of hemiplegic shoulder pain is between 5% and 84%. Symptoms can be apparent in the first few weeks or surface much later.

TABLE 15.16   Medications Used to Treat Central Poststroke Pain

Drug Class	Medications
Antidepressants	Amitriptyline
	Fluvoxamine
Anticonvulsants	Carbamazepine
	Lamotrigine
	Gabapentin
N-methyl-D-aspartate antagonist	Ketamine
	Dextromethorphan
Opioids	Morphine
	Naloxone
	Levorphanol
	Tramadol
Anesthetics	Lidocaine
	Propofol
	Pentothal

Hemiplegic shoulder pain can be a deterrent to upper extremity movement and motor skill restoration, limiting the stroke survivor's recovery. Hemiplegic shoulder pain needs to be effectively treated and managed to facilitate rehabilitation and recovery (Domerick, Edwards, & Kuma, 2008).

Risk factors for hemiplegic shoulder pain include glenohumeral subluxation, neglect of the affected side, poor muscle tone, spasticity, or any premorbid shoulder injury. The causes of shoulder pain range from rotator cuff injury, bursitis, tendonitis, and brachial plexis neuralgias to referred pain originating from another source (Dromerick et al., 2008).

Treatment of hemiplegic shoulder pain depends on the etiology of the pain. The pain can be difficult to diagnose because it may be due to multiple factors such as mild subluxation, inflammation, rotator cuff tears, and central stroke pain. The treatment for hemiplegic shoulder pain may include splinting, slinging, strapping or taping, soft tissue massage, range of motion exercises, icing, heat, intraarticular injections, and anti-inflammatory medications (Duncan et al., 2005). Proper positioning of the upper extremities is an important preventive factor, and the limb should never be pulled or tugged. Range of motion exercises are an important factor in treatment, and slings and splints must be applied properly to prevent further pain or injury to the affected shoulder. The patient should also be evaluated for pain on the nonaffected side because it will be subjected to increased movement and stress to compensate for the affected limb. The nonaffected side can become overused as those muscle groups take on more and more of the work. In time, the nonaffected arm can become inflamed, tender, and sore.

The management of pain in the poststroke survivor, whether it is central poststroke pain, hemiplegic shoulder pain, or just plain musculoskeletal pain is important to allow the person to maintain quality of life, limit depression, and allow for maximal rehabilitation and return to function.

Integumentary Complications

The National Survey of Stroke found that 14.5% of stroke survivors develop pressure sores. Those stroke survivors who are comatose, more severely paralyzed, obese, incontinent of urine or stool, or have spasticity are at greatest risk of skin breakdown (Agency for Health Care Policy and Research, 1995). Chapter 8 provides additional information on maintaining skin integrity in rehabilitation patients.

REHABILITATION

Musculoskeletal Rehabilitation

Multiple approaches are used by the therapist in the treatment of stroke. Based on a review of the literature's best practice, there is no evidence available for the superiority of any approach. It is believed that evidence-based guidelines rather than therapist preference should serve as the basis from which to derive the most effective treatment (Kollen et al., 2009).

The **Bobath** approach is an exercise therapy used in the care of survivors with brain injuries. Also referred to as neurodevelopmental treatment, Bobath therapy is for survivors with injuries to the central nervous system, adults with stroke, and hemiplegia. Developed by a physiotherapist and her husband, the Bobath concept is based on the brain's ability to reorganize and recover after neurological insult (neuroplasticity). This is one of the most popular treatment approaches used in stroke rehabilitation but it remains controversial on its effectiveness. A systematic literature search was conducted regarding the evidence on the Bobath concept in stroke rehabilitation and the review confirmed that Bobath is not superior to other approaches (Kollen et al., 2009).

Another therapy approach is **proprioceptive neuromuscular facilitation**, a technique originally developed in the 1940s for polio patients. It is based on neurophysiological mechanisms. When used in combination with Botox A, it often facilitates the physical activity and function after stroke. The effectiveness of proprioceptive neuromuscular facilitation for specific objectives such as increasing range of motion, improving voluntary movement, and improving gait training skills demonstrates that proprioceptive neuromuscular facilitation is beneficial within physical therapy sessions (Szymon, Banach, Longawa, & Windak, 2005).

A technique that is gaining more support in the literature and in clinical practice is **constraint-induced movement therapy**. This technique combines active training with the affected arm by constraining the unaffected arm. Constraint-induced movement therapy is based on using the paretic arm for functional activities while restraining the stronger limb through wearing a mitten for specific time every day. This type of relearning functional skills is associated with changes in cortical physiology by overcoming learned nonuse of the affected limb (Sawner & LaVigne, 1992). Constraint-induced movement therapy has demonstrated upper extremity functional improvements over a 5-year period. Constraint-induced move-

ment therapy has been shown to enhance recovery after stroke (Rowe, Blanton, & Wolf, 2009).

Body weight–supported treadmill training is a recent gait-training technique that supports a percentage of the stroke survivor's body weight while walking on a treadmill. Clinical studies have found that treadmill exercise improves gait training. One clinical study found that stroke subjects with body weight–supported treadmill training had better walking abilities than walking with no support (Vistin, Barbeau, Korner-Bitensky, & Mayo, 1998). It is interesting to note that in gait retraining and upper extremity retraining there are brain activity changes with improvements in function associated with cortical activation changes with some differences in the involved cortical area (Enzinger et al., 2009).

Stroke rehabilitation has inspired the development of equipment and devices to improve the quality of life of the stroke survivor. In Greek, the word *orthosis* means to make straight. In orthotics management, trained orthotists develop devices to help straighten affected limbs by preventing or modifying spasticity or contractures. The field of orthotics makes equipment with the goals of improving gait stability, increasing functional skills, and decreasing further complications from stroke. Because there are many various complications from stroke, there are as many devices to treat or to compensate for the stroke impairment. For orthoses to work for the stroke survivor, they need to be safe and there needs to be follow-up regarding fit and function. When a stroke survivor is issued an orthotic device, skin must be checked for irritation or breakdown and proper application and use of device needs to be done. Survivors and their families need to be trained regarding the safe use and care of the device (Fatone, 2009).

Language and Communication

Interventions

When working with stroke survivors who have communication or language deficits, the survivor should always be treated as an adult. Distractions should be limited to help the survivor focus. The speaker should face the survivor when speaking and supplement verbal messages with nonverbal cues. The use of gestures may help with communication. The survivor should be given plenty of time to communicate.

For those with Broca's or transcortical motor aphasia, the survivor should be asked yes or no questions or provided with the opportunity to complete a sentence with a one- or two-word response. For those with nonfluent aphasia an SLP may use "total communication," a treatment method using gestures, communication boards, or facial expressions to communicate. Oral reading for language uses printed sentences and paragraphs with the SLP pointing to each word as the patient and therapist read together. The complexity increases as the patient progresses. Melodic intonation therapy is another treatment that presents the nonfluent aphasic survivor with a hierarchy of sentences that are musically intoned. The most recent treatment technique is supported conversation for adults with aphasia. A therapist or trained communicator is given a black marker, unlined paper, and pictures. The communicator uses simple brief statements, asks yes or no questions or multiple-choice questions, and uses pictures, gestures, or facial expressions during communication. More information about supported conversation for adults with aphasia is available on the National Aphasia Institute website at www.aphasia.org (Aphasia Institute, 2009).

Nonverbal forms of communication are used with those with Wernicke's or transcortical sensory aphasia, and the survivor is asked questions to verify comprehension. For those with global aphasia, all forms of communication are attempted, including communication boards, picture boards, or pointing and gesturing. Total communication and oral reading for language are treatments used for those with fluent aphasia. Survivors with dysarthria should be cued to slow down and overemphasize their articulation (Harvey, Roth, & Yu, 2007).

The practice of oral motor exercises provided by the SLP should be emphasized. Rehabilitation nurses should also work closely with the treating SLP to find the best method of communication to identify the basic needs of the survivor. Once a form of communication is established, that method or technique should be continued and feedback on its effectiveness provided to the SLP.

Cognition

Interventions

Patients with multiple areas of cognitive impairment may benefit from a variety of cognitive remediation techniques. **Attention process training** is a method typically used by neuropsychologists, occupational therapists, SLPs, and other rehabilitation specialists, as is appropriate within their scope of practice (Barker-Collo et al., 2009). Although this intervention has been proven to be effective, rehabilitation nurses can easily apply simple nursing interventions to help those stroke survivors with atten-

tion deficits succeed in their environment. One simple environmental or behavioral change is maintaining eye contact with the survivor to ensure they are listening. Reducing attention demands in the environment helps keep the survivor focused on what is important and limits the possibility of distractions. Scheduled rest periods for the stroke survivor with attention problems can help to prevent attention deficits. Prioritizing activities and focusing on what is important helps to prevent overloading the patient. Breaking tasks into parts helps the stroke survivor be more successful with less chances of making errors.

Studies of the remediation of memory deficits have continued to focus on the use of compensatory strategies as well as the use of assistive technology. Internal compensatory strategies that rehabilitation nurses can encourage their stroke patients to use include mnemonics, acronyms visual imagery, rhymes, association, grouping, and repetition.

In this age of technology, numerous devices are available to use with memory deficits. These include portable pagers to improve independence in people with memory and planning problems, cellular phones, personal digital assistants, and electronic watches (Cicerone et al., 2005). Some less expensive compensatory external memory aids can be used for those who cannot afford the more expensive devices, including reminder notes, calendars, alarms, or planners for daily activities.

Executive function deficits remediation integrates several cognitive processes. Simple interventions that can be implemented by rehabilitation nurses include limiting stimuli that the stroke survivor with executive deficits can find overwhelming; underlining, circling, or highlighting important information; and using mnemonics, verbal rhymes, or other verbal mediation strategies.

The rehabilitation nurse can assist the stroke survivor with problem recognition, exploring solutions, implementing solutions, and evaluating the effectiveness of those solutions. The stroke survivor may need help with self-prediction and self-evaluation for those who may overestimate their abilities or fail to check their work. Although some of these areas may appear to be beyond a nurse's scope of practice, all these areas can impact those topics that rehabilitation nurses educate their patients (e.g., medication management, dressing changes, and safety).

Education

The amount of time allocated to inpatient education on prevention, stroke management, and safety in performing ADLs is scarce due to shorter stays, leaving survivors and their caregivers less opportunities to absorb and practice all the knowledge and skills needed to return home safely. In addition, stroke survivors often have multiple comorbidities and complications that need to be addressed for prevention of future strokes, such as understanding the necessity of their medications and encouraging adaptation of a healthy lifestyle (Ostwald, Davis, Hersch, Kelley, & Godwin, 2008). A stroke education plan needs to be flexible so it can be adapted to stroke survivors' and their caregivers' ages, educational and literacy levels, and lifestyles.

When developing an educational plan, age needs to be considered. Young and middle aged adults are usually working and may be responsible for raising children. Because of time constraints, stroke education needs to be presented simply so that it is understood and can be practiced and retained. The educational plan needs to be applicable to all ages, stroke deficits, home environments, and accessibility of local community resources that are available to stroke survivors and their families. Stroke survivors who are better educated and informed about their stroke and prognosis make better functional recoveries than poorly informed survivors (Ostwald et al., 2008). Stroke survivors may also more greatly benefit from teaching at certain times during the recovery and rehabilitation process (Mauk, 2006). Box 15.2 provides a web link on interacting with stroke survivors for readers to explore. Chapter 4 provides some theories and models that may be useful when planning teaching for stroke survivors. In addition, Chapter 13 gives many excellent suggestions for educating patients and families.

BOX 15.2   Web Exploration

Visit the American Stroke Foundation's website at http://www.americanstroke.org/index.php?option=com_content&task=view&id=91&Itemid=125 for *Ten Guidelines for Interacting with a Stroke Survivor*. Discuss with fellow nurses or students what you learned from this document.

Most of the 5.7 million living stroke survivors are cared for in the homes of family members (Singh & Cameron, 2005; Ski & O'Connell, 2005; Steiner et al., 2008). Most family caregivers feel unprepared for this role because stroke occurs suddenly, changing lives and future plans without warning. As the leading cause of disability, stroke requires care management across the continuum with the focus of care and the stroke survivor's needs changing over time. The days and weeks after the stroke event are stressful and uncertain for

families facing new and challenging experiences over the next year. Cameron and Gignac (2008) developed a "Timing It Right" framework outlining the changing support needs of stroke family caregivers from hospital to home. Designed into five phases, the framework outlines a general guide of stroke caregiver experiences that may be associated with changing needs over time. Phase one is the stroke event/diagnoses during acute hospitalization, whereas phase two is stabilization. Rehabilitation takes place during phase three, the preparation phase, covering the time before the patient goes home with the emphasis on maintaining safety in ADLs, teaching secondary stroke prevention, practicing family care, and addressing caregiver concerns about their ability to perform care. Caregivers want information on accessibility and availability of community resources, ordering supplies, and how to handle future caregiver problems. The last two phases are implementation and adaptation and follow the first few months after discharge and adjustment at home, respectively.

Families recognize the need for information on fall prevention, maintaining nutrition, keeping a healthy lifestyle, and dealing with emotional and mood changes. Emotional support is a recurring need of caregivers, and many find it informally. Complaints include a lack of information about stroke symptoms, medical terminology, treatment, and drugs. Nurses recommended four types of information: (1) understanding the disease process, (2) preventing pressure ulcers, (3) performing safe transfers, and (4) coping with impaired communication. A study of the self-care needs of stroke caregivers found safety issues accounting for three of the five self-care needs identified by therapists. Nurses use their leadership skills in coordinating care with the team in a smooth transition to home (Cook, Pierce, Hicks, & Steiner, 2006).

Rehabilitation nurses learn to identify specific stroke training goals and to make stroke survivors and their families' education a priority. Stroke caregivers have identified informational needs associated with clinical, practical problems and then learning to get additional help through resources such as in a stroke information database listing websites and phone numbers. Rehabilitation nurses are in the position to provide support and education by addressing the conditions and concerns of new stroke survivors and caregivers. Stroke survivors and caregivers often do not perceive involvement in goal setting and discharge planning, but this can improve continued care and compliance after discharge. Teaching sessions with short- and long-term goals need to be part of the daily plan. Stroke caregivers have to care for themselves and the stroke survivor. Peer visitor programs are often established within the hospital setting and provide stroke survivors with real examples of living with stroke. Nurses identify the benefit of a peer visitor and prepare the stroke survivor for the visit.

Stroke survivor and caregiver support can be accessed 24 hours through the Internet. The number of American adults seeking information online has increased as the availability of the Internet has exploded throughout the United States. Informal caregivers, over 73 million people, search the Internet for healthcare information and support (Fox & Rainie, 2002; Pierce, Steiner, & Smelser, 2009). Healthcare providers use the Internet and e-mail to educate and support their patients. Organizations, such as the ones listed in Table 15.17, provide information and support to both stroke survivors and caregivers through the Internet, phone, or e-mail.

Most stroke rehabilitation centers have established guidelines to ensure educational needs are addressed. Table 15.18 presents an outline of educational requirements for teaching and discussion before discharge and then reinforced while living in the community.

Community Reintegration

Medical Follow-up

In 1995 the risk of suffering a second stroke was 7% to 10% per year; today, one of every five stroke survivors (20%) is expected to have a second stroke within five years. All stroke patients should participate in a secondary prevention program. Postacute stroke survivors should be followed up by a primary care provider to address stroke risk factors and continue treatment of comorbidities. The survivor and family should be educated about pertinent risk factors for stroke (Duncan et al., 2005). Steps to control risk factors such as hypertension, tobacco use, diabetes mellitus, hyperlipidemia, and drug abuse should be pursued (Agency for Health Care Policy and Research, 1995).

For those stroke survivors who do not have a primary care physician, the rehabilitation nurse in conjunction with a case manager or social worker should assist the patient in locating one in their area. Survivors should follow up with their primary care physician within 2 weeks of discharge from inpatient rehabilitation. Those who have an active medical problem (e.g., uncontrolled hypertension, uncontrolled blood sugars, recent changes in medication) or require blood work should follow up with

their primary care physician within 1 week of discharge from inpatient rehabilitation. To ensure that a survivor does follow up with their primary care physician, an appointment with that physician should be made before discharge from rehabilitation. Those stroke survivors who are discharged to skilled nursing or extended care facilities will have a physician assigned to them who will follow their medical needs. The stroke survivor should also follow up with their rehabilitation practitioner within 1 month of discharge from inpatient rehabilitation.

Gaps in care may occur as responsibility shifts from the rehabilitation program to the primary care physician, other rehabilitation services, or community agencies. Physical regression may occur because of lack of stimulation, lack of confidence, or a physical environment that makes daily activities difficult to perform or if the family caregivers inadvertently suppress initiative by taking over rather than encouraging self-performance of activities (Agency for Health Care Policy and Research, 1995). The rehabilitation medical professional can make certain that the stroke survivor continues to make appropriate gains in the community. If the stroke survivor has other active medical conditions (e.g., congestive heart failure, uncontrolled diabetes, gastric ulcers), they should follow up with specialists such as a cardiologist, endocrinologist, or gastroenterologist.

Return to Work

The American Stroke Association (ASA) has stated that as more treatments for stroke are developed, more survivors will be facing the potential for reemployment (Agency for Health Care Policy and Research, 1995). It is recommended that stroke survivors who worked before their strokes should, if their condition permits, be encouraged to be evaluated for the potential to return to work (Agency for Health Care Policy and Research, 1995). This holds true for younger as well as older stroke survivors. All patients who were previously employed should be referred to vocational counseling for assistance with return to work (Agency for Health Care Policy and Research, 1995).

Vocational rehabilitation counseling has been around since the 1940s, but it was not until the availability of federal funding in 1954 that the profession began to grow. Many barriers to vocational reintegration must be addressed if the stroke patient is to return to work (Duncan et al., 2005). Referral to vocational rehabilitation services helps to overcome these barriers and helps stroke survivors identify the potential for return to work.

TABLE 15-17 Stroke Organizations

Organization	Purpose	Address	Phone	Website/E-mail
American Stroke Association (ASA)	Website contains information on stroke prevention, current news on stroke prevention & treatment, personal stories of survivors.	7272 Greenville Ave., Dallas, TX 75231	(888)-478-7653	www.strokeassociation.org
National Stroke Association (NSA)	Provides updates on stroke news on prevention & care. Publishes *Stroke Smart* magazine and books and pamphlets.	9707 East Easter Lane, Englewood, CO 80112-5112	(800) 787-6537	www.stroke.org
AHCPR Publication Consumer Guide Number 16 Publication No. 95-0664: May, 1995	Publishes a booklet about stroke rehabilitation, called "Recovering after a stroke: A patient and family guide."	AHCPR Publications Clearinghouse, PO Box 8547, Silver Spring, MD 20907	(800) 358-9295	www.ahrq.gov
National Aphasia Association	Information on general caregiving and listings of caregiver support sites by condition and region.	7 Dey St., Ste 600, New York NY 10007	(800) 922-4622	www.aphasia.org
Stroke Survivors Empowering Each Other (SSEEO)	Builds community, provides support, & shares information by connecting survivors, caregivers, health professionals. Sponsored by AHA/ASA.		(800) 677-5481	www.sseeo.org
Family Caregiver Alliance	Tips on caregiving, care, state resources and stats	180 Montgomery St., Ste 1110, San Francisco, CA 94104	(415) 434-8106 (800) 445-8106	www.caregiver.org e-mail: info@caregiver.org
Stroke Family Caregiving for African Americans	Site is a nonprofit web resource for information about stroke care and research, educational service of the Stroke Center at Barnes-Jewish Hospital & Washington University School of Medicine.	The Internet Stroke Center at Washington University School of Medicine		www.strokecenter.org
National Family Caregiver Assn (NFCA)/National Alliance for Caregiving (NAC)	Two organizations joined together to create a valuable resource that offers info from talking to insurance and hospital personnel to tips on caregiving problems.	NFCA, 9621 East Bexhill Drive, Kensington, MD 20895-3104 NAC,4720 Montgomery, Suite 642, Bethesda, MD 20814	(301) 942-6430	www.familycaregiving101.org

TABLE 15.18   Stroke Survivor and Family Education Guidelines

Stroke Recovery and Condition Info	Medical Care	Medications	Exercise/Mobility/Cognition/Speech	Discharge Plan and Follow-up	Caregiver and Equipment	Housing and Transportation	Education and Employment	Support and Wellness
Type of stroke	Bladder	Antiplatelet	ROM	Destination	Family training and participation	Accessibility	Vocational rehab	Intimacy
Etiology	Bowel	Anticoagulation	Stretching	SNF	Equipment	Ability to get to appointments		Sexuality
Risk factors	Cognition	Hypertension	Balance	Home	Mobility	Handicap Parking		Peer Support
Secondary prevention	Nutrition	CV	Fitness	Therapy	ADLs	Driver's Evaluation		Stroke Clubs
Stroke mgmt	Respiratory	Neurostimulants	Strengthening	Home	Bed			Volunteer
Understand deficits	Skin care	Sleep aids	Endurance	Outpatient				
	Positioning	Antidepressants	Compensatory techniques	Day				
	Safety	Antianxiety	Communication	Labs				
		Pulmonary	Swallowing	Scheduled				
		Bowel & bladder agents	Vision	Appts with appropriate care				

CV, cardiovascular; ROM, range of motion; SNF, skilled nursing facility.

Source: Adapted from Ostwald et al. (2008, p. 155) and from the Rehabilitation Institute of Chicago's *Patient and Family Resource Guide Stroke Program* (2009). Chicago, IL: Rehabilitation Institute of Chicago.

Vocational rehabilitation counselors assess the survivor, identify deficits resulting from the stroke, work with employers on modifications, assist survivors with resumes, fill out applications, set up interviews, and visit job sites. In some cases returning to school may be necessary for the stroke survivor to find a new line of work.

Return to Driving

For those survivors with moderate to severe strokes, many are left with persisting impairment after the rehabilitation period, yet up to 30% of stroke survivors return to driving (Marshall et al., 2007). Unfortunately for those unable to return to driving, this only further identifies the lack of independence that results from a stroke. It is recommended that the assessment of the ability of a disabled stroke survivor to drive a car should be based on neurological examination, behavioral observations, and evaluation by the state agency responsible for issuing drivers' licenses, including a standardized driving test (Agency for Health Care Policy and Research, 1995). In many cases stroke survivors do not lose their driver's license as a result of the stroke but may not be safe to return to driving. It is usually cognitive or perceptual deficits that prevent stroke survivors from returning to driving.

Most states have driver rehabilitation programs associated with rehabilitation facilities that provide assessments of motor, cognitive, perception, and reaction times. Most of these programs provide a therapy assessment as well as a behind the wheel assessment. The behind the wheel driving assessment is the typical gold standard for assessing fitness to drive for persons with disability. Despite its gold standard attributes, driver's evaluations can be costly for survivors. For this reason much effort has been directed at identifying and developing screening measures and protocols to assist in predicting which stroke survivors are able to return to driving (Marshall et al., 2007). Once the assessment is completed, recommendations are forwarded to the ordering practitioner who then decides whether the survivor is safe to return to driving or requires further interventions. For those survivors who have only motor deficits, there are adaptive devices such as mechanical or power hand controls that can help compensate for their disability.

Return to Leisure Interests

Another aspect of reintegrating back into the community after stroke is to resume leisure activities. Depending on the leisure activity, the person may be able to resume it without much adaptation or thought. For others, education

and awareness of potential new leisure activities should occur. The Agency for Health Care Policy and Research guidelines recommend that "leisure activities should be identified, encouraged and enabled" (1995, p. 156).

The stroke survivor may need assistance to consider ways to adapt leisure activities that they may have not thought of before their disability. Several things should be considered when deciding on a leisure activity after stroke. The stroke survivor should review valued activities against his or her current functional levels. They should develop strategies to overcome physical barriers in the home and community. They should identify new leisure activities to match their functional abilities and learn about available community resources (Agency for Health Care Policy and Research, 1995). Not only can leisure activities improve quality of life, but some have been documented to help promote recovery.

Animal assisted therapy has been studied specifically when working with aphasic patients. One study suggested that dogs serve as catalysts for human communication (LaFrance, Garcia, & Labreche, 2006). Other animals such as horses used in hippotherapy have also been documented to help with sensory input. Chapter 29 provides more detailed information on animal assisted therapy.

Art therapy was originally used to work with those with psychiatric disorders. Today, it has been documented to improve attention, memory, organization, motivation, and self-esteem and to decrease anger, anxiety, and depression (Kim, Kim, Lee, & Chun, 2008). Another form of art, specifically music therapy, has been found to enhance cognitive recovery and prevent negative mood (Sarkamo et al., 2008). Participation in adaptive sports programs is also available for those stroke survivors who prefer more active leisure activities. Sports such as golf, bowling, skiing, boating, kayaking, fishing, basketball, volleyball, biking, climbing, swimming, hockey, horseback riding, rowing, scuba diving, sailing, water skiing, tennis, rugby, archery, and soccer are all available for those with physical and cognitive disabilities. For those who are less athletic but want to remain physically active, personal trainers are being used to develop a fitness program designed to enhance the patient strength, range of motion, stability, balance, coordination, and functional strength (Burkow-Heikkinen, 2009).

SUMMARY

This chapter content discussed the physiology and effects of stroke. The residual effects of stroke vary according to the location and severity of the damage. While the effects of stroke for many people are long-lasting, there is hope for continued improvement through rehabilitation. The assistance of the interdisciplinary team and vocational rehabilitation counselors can promote reintegration into the community after stroke and foster increased quality of life.

CRITICAL THINKING

1. Look at the statistics presented in the beginning of the chapter. How large of a problem do you believe stroke is compared with other disorders such as breast cancer or diabetes? How does stroke differ from the pattern of chronic illness seen in neurological diseases such as multiple sclerosis or Parkinson's disease?

2. Find out if there is a stroke support group in your area. Ask if you can attend. Talk with survivors and their family members to see what their experience was like and how they coped with life after stroke.

3. Visit the American Stroke Association website at http://www.strokeassociation.org and browse the website for helpful educational information for both you and stroke survivors/families.

4. Of the stroke syndromes listed in Tables 15.2 and 15.3, which do you believe would be the most difficult for patient to have and why? Which of the problems would be the most difficult for a family member to deal with? Which pose the greatest challenge for the interdisciplinary rehabilitation team?

5. Read the book or watch the movie, *The Diving Bell and the Butterfly*. Discuss your feelings about this story with your classmates or colleagues.

PERSONAL REFLECTION

- Have you ever cared for a person with stroke or had a family member who experienced a stroke? If so, what type of stroke was it? Did the person receive inpatient rehabilitation? If so, in what setting? How would you describe that person's experience? And/or your experience as a caregiver of a stroke survivor?

- What did you learn in this chapter about how stroke affects the lives of survivors and their families?

- Imagine that you have had a severe stroke with expressive aphasia and hemiplegia. How would you communicate your needs to your family members and healthcare providers?

REFERENCES

Agency for Health Care Policy and Research. (1995). *Clinical practice guideline number 16: Post stroke rehabilitation.* Rockville, MD: U.S. Department of Health and Human Services.

American Heart Association (AHA). (2009). Heart disease and stroke statistics—2009 update. Retrieved July 1, 2010, from http://www.americanheart.org/presenter

American Speech Language Association. (2010). Apraxia of speech in adults. Retrieved September 1, 2010, from http://www.asha.org/public/speech/disorders/ApraxiaAdults.htm

American Stroke Association. (2009). *Aphasia.* Retrieved July 1, 2010, from http://www.strokeassociation.org/presenter.jhtml?identifier=4485

Aphasia Institute. (2009). Supported conversation for adults with aphasia. Retrieved September 1, 2010, from http://www.aphasia.ca/SCAtext.html

Baggerly, J. (1991). Sensory perceptual problems following stroke: The "invisible" deficits. *Nursing Clinics of North America, 26*(4), 997–1005.

Barker-Collo, S. L., Feigin, V. L., Lawes, C. M. M., Parag, V., Senior, H., & Rodgers, A. (2009). Reducing attention deficits after stroke using attention process training: A randomized controlled trial. *Stroke, 40,* 3293–3298.

Bassetti, C. L. (2005). Sleep and stroke. *Seminars in Neurology, 25*(1), 19–32.

Batchelor, F., Hill, K., Mackintosh, S., & Said, C. (2010). What works in fall prevention after stroke? A systematic review and meta-analysis. *Stroke, 14,* 1715–1722.

Bates, B., Choi, J. Y, Duncan, P. W., et al. (2005). AHA/ASA endorsed practice guidelines. Veterans Affairs/Department of Defense clinical practice guideline for the management of adult stroke rehabilitation care: Executive summary. *Stroke, 36,* 2049–2056.

Bohannon, R. W., & Smith, M. B. (1987). Interrater reliability of a modified Ashworth scale of muscle spasticity. *Physical Therapy, 67*(2), 206–207.

Bourbonnais, D., & Vanden Noven, S. (1989). Weakness in patients with hemiparesis. *American Journal of Occupational Therapy, 43*(5), 313–319.

Brocklehurst, J. C., Andrews, K., Richards, B., & Laycock, P. J. (1985). Incidence and correlates of incontinence in stroke patients. *Journal of the American Geriatric Society, 33,* 540–542.

Brunnstrom, S. (1956). Associated reactions to the upper extremity in adult patients with hemiplegia: An approach to training. *Physical Therapy Review, 36*(4), 225–236.

Brunnstrom, S. (1970). *Movement therapy in hemiplegia.* New York: Harper and Row.

Burkow-Heikkinen, L. (2009). The role of personal trainers for stroke rehabilitation. *Neurological Research, 31,* 841–847.

Buxbaum, L. J., Haal, K. Y., Hallet, M., Wheaton, L., Heilman, K. M., Rodrguez, A., et al. (2008). Treatment of limb apraxia:

Moving forward to improve action. *American Journal of Physical Medicine and Rehabilitation, 87,* 149–161.

Byers, V., Arrington, M. E., & Finstuen, K. (1990). Predictive risk factors associated with stroke patient falls in acute care settings. *Journal of Neuroscience Nursing, 22,* 147–154.

Cambier, D. C., DeCorte, E., Danneels, L. A., & Witvrouw, E. E. (2003). Treating sensory impairments in the post-stroke upper limb with intermittent pneumatic compression. Results of a preliminary trial. *Clinical Rehabilitation, 17,* 14–20.

Cameron, J. I., & Gignac, M. A. M. (2008). Timing it right: A conceptual framework for addressing the support needs of family caregivers to stroke survivors from the hospital to the home. *Patient Education and Counseling, 70,* 305–314.

Caruso, L. B & Silliman, R. A. (2010). Geriatric medicine. In A. S. Fauci, E. Brunwald, D. L. Kasper, S. L. Hauser, D. L. Longo, J. L. Jameson, et al. (Eds.), *Harrison's principles of internal medicine.* Retrieved September 1, 2010, from www.accessmedicine.com.ezproxy.galter.northwestern.edu

Cicerone, K. D., Dahlberg, C., Malec, J. F., et al. (2005). Evidence-based cognitive rehabilitation: Updated review of the literature from 1998 through 2002. *Archives of Physical Medicine and Rehabilitation, 86,* 1681–1692.

Cook, A. M., Pierce, L. L., Hicks, B., & Steiner, V., (2006). Self care needs of caregivers dealing with stroke. *Journal of Neuroscience Nursing, 38*(1), 31–36.

Czernuszenko, A., & Czlonkowska, A. (2009). Risk factors for falls in stroke patients during inpatient rehabilitation. *Clinical Rehabilitation, 23*(2), 176–188.

Diringer, M. N., Edwards, D. F., Mattson, D. T., Akins, P. T., Sheedy, C. W., Hsu, C. Y., et al. (1999). Predictors of acute hospital costs for treatment of ischemic stroke in an academic center. *Stroke, 30,* 724–728.

Dromerick, A. W., Edwards, D., & Kuma, A. (2008). Hemiplegic shoulder pain syndrome: Frequency and characteristics during inpatient stroke rehabilitation. *Archives of Physical Medicine and Rehabilitation, 89*(8), 1589–1593.

Duncan, P. W., & Badke, M. B. (1987). *Stroke rehabilitation: The recovery of motor control.* Chicago: YearBook Medical.

Duncan, P. W., Zorowitz, R., Bates, B., Choi, J. Y., Glasber, J. J., Graham, G. D., et al. (2005). Management of adult stroke rehabilitation care: A clinical practice guideline. *Stroke, 36,* e100–e143.

Duraski, S., Denby F., & Clemons, J. Q. (2009). Bladder and bowel management after stroke. In J. Stein, R. L. Harvey, R. F. Macko, C. J. Winstein, & R.D. Zorowitz (Eds.), *Stroke recovery and rehabilitation.* New York: Demos Publishing.

Enzinger, C., Dawes, H., Johansen-Berg, H., et al. (2009). Brain activity changes associated with treadmill training after stroke. *Stroke, 40,* 2460–2467.

Fatone, S. (2009). Orthotic management in stroke. In J. Stein, R.L. Harvey, R.F. Macko, C. J. Winstein, & R. D. Zorowitz (Eds.), *Stroke recovery & rehabilitation* (pp. 515–530). New York: Demos Medical.

Forsberg-Warleby, G., Moller, A., & Blomstrand, C. (2002). Spouses of first-ever stroke victims: Sense of coherence in the first phase after stroke. *Journal of Rehabilitation Medicine, 34*(3), 128–133.

Forster, A., & Young, J. (1995). Incidence and consequences of falls due to stroke: A systematic inquiry. *British Medical Journal, 311,* 83–86.

Fox, S., & Rainie, L. (2002). *Vital decisions.* Washington, DC: Pew Internet and American Life Project.

Frizzel, J. P. (2005). Acute stroke: Pathophysiology, diagnosis and treatment. *AACN Clinical Issues, 16*(4), 421–440.

Garon, B. R., Engle, M., & Ormiston, C. (1997). A randomized control study to determine the effects of unlimited oral intake of water in patients with identified aspiration. *Neurorehabilitation and Neural Repair, 11*(3),139–148.

Gianotti, G., & Marra, C. (2002). Determinants and consequences of post-stroke depression. *Current Opinion in Neurology, 15,* 85–89.

Gould, R., & Barnes, S. S. (2009). Shoulder and hemiplegia. Emedicine: Physical Medicine and Rehabilitation. Retrieved July 1, 2010, from http://emedicine.medscape.com/article/328793

Grant, J. S., Glandon, G. L., Elliott, T. R., Giger, J. N., & Weaver, M. (2004). Caregiving problems and feelings experienced by family caregivers of stroke survivors the first month after discharge. *International Journal of Rehabilitation Research, 27,* 105–111.

Haley, W. E., Allen, J. Y., Grant, J. S., Clay, O. J., Perkins, M., & Roth, D. L. (2009). Problems and benefits reported by stroke family caregivers: Results from a prospective epidemiological study. *Stroke, 40,* 2129–2133.

Hara, Y. (2008). Deep venous thrombosis in stroke patients during rehabilitation. *Keio Journal of Medicine, 57*(4), 196–204.

Harvey, R. L. (2009). Cerebral stroke syndromes. In J. Stein, R. L. Harvey, R. F. Macko, C. J. Winstein, & R. D. Zorowitz (Eds.), *Stroke recovery & rehabilitation* (pp. 83–94). New York: Demos Medical.

Harvey, R. L., Roth, E. J., & Yu, D. (2007). Rehabilitation in stroke syndromes. In R. L. Braddom (Ed.), *Physical medicine & rehabilitation* (3rd ed., pp. 1175–1212). Philadelphia: W. B. Saunders.

Hermann, D. M., Siccoli, M., & Bassetti, C. L. (2003). Sleep-wake disorders and stroke. *Schweizer Archives for Neurology and Psychiatry, 154,* 369–373.

Hilker, R., Poetter, C., Findeisen, N., Sobesky, J., Jacobs, A., Neveling, M., et al. (2003). Nosocomial pneumonia after acute stroke: Implications for neurological intensive care medicine. *Stroke, 34,* 975–981

Hormer, J., Massey, E. W., Riski, J. E., Lathrop, D. L., & Chase, K. N. (1988). Aspiration following stroke: Clinical correlates and outcome. *Neurology, 38,* 1359–1362.

House, A., Hackett, M. L., Anderson, C. S., & Horrocks, J. A. (2009). Pharmaceutical interventions for emotionalism after stroke (Review). Cochrane Library, issue 1. Retrieved September 1, 2010, from http://www.thecochranelibrary.com

Intercollegiate Stroke Working Party. (2004). *National clinical guidelines for stroke* (2nd ed.). London: Royal College of Physicians.

Johansson, B. (2000). Brain plasticity and stroke rehabilitation: The Willis lecture. *Stroke, 31*, 223–230.

Jorgensen, L., Engstad, T., & Jacobsen, B. K. (2002). Higher incidence of falls in long term stroke survivors than in population controls: Depressive symptoms predict falls after stroke. *Stroke, 33*(2), 542–547.

Karatas, M., Cetin, N., Bayramoglu, M., & Dilek, A. (2004). Trunk muscle strength in relation to balance and functional disability in unihemispheric stroke patients. *American Journal of Physical Medicine & Rehabilitation, 83*(2), 81–87.

Khan, S., Leung, E., & Jay, W. M. (2008). Stroke and visual rehabilitation. *Topics in Stroke Rehabilitation, 156*(1), 27–36.

Kim, S.-H., Kim, M.-Y., Lee, J.-H., & Chun, S.-I. (2008). Art therapy outcomes in the rehabilitation treatment of a stroke patient: A case report. *Art Therapy: Journal of the American Art Therapy Association, 25*(3), 129–133.

King, R. B., Hartke, R. J., & Denby F. (2007). Problem-solving early intervention: A pilot study of stroke caregivers. *Rehabilitation Nursing, 32*(2), 68–76.

Kleindorfer, D., Panagos, P. Pancioli, A., et al. (2005). Incidence and short-term prognosis of transient ischemic attack in a population based study. *Stroke, 36*, 720–723

Klit, H., Finnerup, N. B., & Jensen, T. S. (2009). Central post-stroke pain: Clinical characteristics, pathophysiology, and management. *The Lancet Neurology, 8*(9), 857–868.

Kollen, B. J., Lennon, S., Lyons, B., et al. (2009). The effectiveness of the Bobath concept in stroke rehabilitation: What is the evidence? *Stroke, 40*(4), e89–e97.

Korpelainen, J. T., Nieminen, P., & Myllyla, W. (1999). Sexual functioning among stroke patients and their spouses. *Stroke, 30*(4), 715–719.

Kumar, S., Selim, M. H., & Caplan, L. R. (2010). Medical complications after stroke. *The Lancet Neurology, 9*(10), 105–118.

LaFrance, C., Garcia, L. J., & Labreche, J. (2006). The effect of a therapy dog on the communication skills of an adult with aphasia. *Journal of Communication Disorders, 40*, 215–224.

Lee, B. H., Kim, E.-J., Ku, B. D., et al. (2008). Cognitive impairments in patients with hemispatial neglect from acute right hemisphere stroke. *Cognitive Behavioral Neurology, 21*(2), 73–76.

Lesniak, M., Bak, T., Czpiel, W., Seniow, J., & Czlonkowska, A. (2008). Frequency and prognostic value of cognitive disorders in stroke patients. *Dementia and Geriatric Cognitive Disorders, 26*, 356–363.

Lim, C., & Alexander, M. P. (2009). Stroke and episodic memory disorders. *Neuropsychologia, 47*, 3045–3058.

Marin, R., Firinciogullari, S., & Biedrzycki, R. C. (1994). Group differences in the relationship between apathy and depression. *Journal of Nervous and Mental Disease, 182*(4), 193–251.

Marshall, S. C., Molnar, F., Man-Son-Hing, M., et al. (2007). Predictors of driving ability following stroke: A systematic review. *Topics in Stroke Rehabilitation, 14*(1), 98–114.

Martin-Harris, B., Logemann, J. A., McMahon, S., Schleicher, M., & Sandidge, J. (2000). Clinical utility of the modified barium swallow. *Dysphagia, 15*, 136–141.

Mauk, K. L. (2006). Nursing interventions within the Mauk model for post-stroke recovery. *Rehabilitation Nursing, 31*(6), 259–267.

Metz, R. (2003). Cost-effective, risk-free, evidence-based medicine. *Archives of Internal Medicine, 163*, 2795.

Michels, E. (1982). Synergies in hemiplegia. *Clinical Management, 1*, 9–16.

Morgenstern, L. B., Smith, M. A., Lisabeth, L. D., et al. (2004). Excess stroke in Mexican Americans compared with non-Hispanic whites: The Brain Attack Surveillance in Corpus Christi (BASIC) Project. *American Journal Epidemiology, 160*, 376–383.

Murray, C. D., & Harrison, B. (2004). The meaning and experience of being a stroke survivor: An interpretative phenomenological analysis. *Disability and Rehabilitation, 26*(13), 808–816.

Nakayama H., Jorgensen H. S., Pedersen, P. M., Raaschou, H. O., & Olsen, T. S. (1997). Prevalence and risk factors of incontinence after stroke: The Copenhagen stroke study. *Stroke, 28*, 58–62.

National Center for Health Statistics, (2008). Compressed mortality file: Underlying cause of death 1979 to 2005. Atlanta, GA: Centers for Disease Control and Prevention.

National Stroke Association. (2003). What is a stroke/brain attack? Retrieved July 1, 2010, from http://www.stroke.org/site/DocServer/NSA_complete_guide.pdf?docID=341

National Stroke Association. (2006). Secondary (recurrent) risk. Retrieved July 1, 2010, from http://www.stroke.org

Nokleby, K. Boland, E., Bergersen, H., Schanke, A. K., Farner, L., Wagle, J., et al. (2008). Screening for cognitive deficits after stroke: A comparison of three screening tools. *Clinical Rehabilitation, 22*, 1095–1104.

Nyberg, L., & Gustafson, Y. (1995). Patient falls in stroke rehabilitation: A challenge to rehabilitation strategies. *Stroke, 26*, 838–842.

O'Dwyer, N. J., Ada, L., & Neilson, P. D. (1996). Spasticity and muscle contracture following stroke. *Brain, 119*, 1737–1749.

Ownsworth, T., & Shum, D. (2008). Relationship between executive functions and productivity outcomes following stroke. *Disability and Rehabilitation, 30*(7), 531–540.

Office of Communications and Public Liaison. (2008). NINDS, National Institutes of Health. Post-stroke rehabilitation fact sheet. Retrieved December 1, 2009, from http://www.ninds.nih.gov/disorders/stroke/poststrokerehab.htm

Ostwald, S. K., Davis, S., Hersch, G., Kelley, C., & Godwin, K. M. (2008). Evidence based educational guidelines for stroke survivors after discharge home. *Journal of Neuroscience Nursing, 40*(3), 173–179, 191.

Pathak, M. (2006). Stroke and seizures. Retrieved October 15, 2010, from http://www.strokesafe.org/resources/stroke_and_seizures.html

Pierce, L. L., Steiner, V., Hicks, B., & Holzaepfel, A. L. (2006). Problems of new caregivers of persons with stroke. *Rehabilitation Nursing, 31*(4), 166–152.

Pierce, L., Steiner, V., & Smelser, J. (2009). Stroke caregivers share ABC's of caring. *Rehabilitation Nursing, 34*, 5.

Rapport, L. J., Webster, J. S., Fleming, K. L., Lindberg, J. W., Godlewski, M. C., Brees, J. E., et al. (1993). Predictors of falls among right-hemisphere stroke patients in the rehabilitation setting. *Archives of Physical Medicine and Rehabilitation, 74*, 621–626.

Rasquin, S. M. C., Lodder, J., Ponds, R. W. H. M., Winkens, I., Jolles, J., & Verhey, F. R. J. (2004). Cognitive functioning after stroke: A one-year follow-up study. *Dementia and Geriatric Cognitive Disorders, 18*, 138–144.

Rosamond, W., Flegal, K., Furie, K., et al. (2008). Heart disease and stroke statistics: 2008 update: A report from the American Heart Association Statistics Committee and Stroke Statistics Subcommittee. *Circulation, 115*, e25–e146.

Rosamond, W. D., Folsom, A. R., Chambless, L. E., et al. (1999). Stroke incidence and survival among middle aged adults: Nine year follow up of the atherosclerotic risk in communities (ARIC) cohort. *Stroke, 30*, 736–743.

Roth, E. J., & Harvey, R. L. (2000). Rehabilitation in stroke syndromes. In R. L. Braddom (Ed.), *Physical medicine & rehabilitation* (2nd ed., pp. 1117–1163). Philadelphia, PA: W.B. Saunders.

Rowe, V. T., Blanton, S., & Wolf. S. L. (2009). Long term follow-up after constraint-induced therapy: A case report of a chronic stroke survivor. *American Journal of Occupational Therapy, 63*, 317–322.

Sachdev, P. S., Brodaty, H., Valenzuela, M. J., Lorentz, L., & Koschera, A. (2004). Progression of cognitive impairment in stroke patients. *Neurology, 63*, 1618–1623.

Sackley, C. M. (1991). Falls, sway and symmetry of weight-bearing after stroke. *International Disability Studies, 13*(1), 1–4.

Sadeh, A, Hauri, P. J., Kripke, D. F., & Lavie, P. (1995). The role of actigraphy in the evaluation of sleep disorders. *Sleep, 18*(4), 288–302.

Salter, K., Bhogal, S., Teasell, R., Foley, N., & Speechley, M. (2009). Post-stroke depression. Evidence-Based Review of Stroke Rehabilitation. (EBRSR) (12th ed., pp. 1–80). Retrieved September 1, 2010, from http://www.ebrsr.com

Sarkamo, T., Tervaniemi, M., Laitinen, S., et al. (2008). Music listening enhances cognitive recovery and mood after middle cerebral artery stroke. *Brain, 131*, 866–876.

Sawner, K., & LaVigne, J. (1992). *Brunnstrom's movement therapy in hemiplegia: A neurological approach* (2nd ed.). Philadelphia: J. B. Lippincott.

Schmid, A. A., Kapoor, J. R., Dallas, M., & Bravata, D. M. (2010). Association between stroke severity and fall risk among stroke patients. *Neuroepidemiology, 34*(3), 158–162.

Sherman, D. G. (2006). Prevention of venous thromboembolism, recurrent stroke and other vascular events after acute ischemic stroke: The role of low-molecular-weight heparin and antiplatelet therapy. *Journal of Stroke and Cerebrovascular Diseases, 15*(6), 250–259.

Singh, M., & Cameron, J. (2005). Psychosocial aspects of caregiving to stroke patients. *Axon, 27*(1), 18–24.

Ski, C., & O'Connell, B. (2005). Caring for carers: Stroke survivors in the community. *Australian Journal of Nursing, 13*(6), 31.

Smith, W. S., English, J. D., & Johnston, S. C. (2010). Cerebrovascular diseases. In A.S. Fauci, E. Brunwald, D. L. Kasper, S. L. Hauser, D. L. Longo, J. L. Jameson, et al. (Eds.), *Harrison's principles of internal medicine*. Retrieved September 1, 2010, from www.accessmedicine.com.ezproxy.galter.northwestern.edu

Stein, J., Silver, J., & Frates, E. P. (2006). *Life after stroke: Recovering your health and preventing another stroke*. Baltimore: John Hopkins University Press.

Steiner, V., Pierce L., Drahuschak, S., Norfiger, E., Buchman, D., & Szirony, T. (2008). Emotional support, physical help, and health of caregivers of stroke survivors. *Journal of Neuroscience Nursing, 40*(1), 48–54.

Summers, D., Leonard, A., Wentworth, D., et al. (2009). Comprehensive overview of nursing and interdisciplinary care of the acute ischemic stroke patient: A scientific statement from the American Heart Association. *Stroke, 40*, 2911–2944.

Szymon, P., Banach, M., Longawa, K., & Windak, F. (2005). Stroke rehabilitation conducted by PNF method, with and without the application of botulinum toxin—case reports. *Medical Rehabilitation, 9*, 5–24.

Tang, W. K., Chen, Y. K., Lu, J. Y., et al. (2009). Microbleeds and post stroke emotional lability. *Journal of Neurology Neurosurgery Psychiatry, 80*, 1082–1086

Teasell, R., Foley, N., & Bhogal, S. (2006). Evidence-based review of stroke rehabilitation: Medical complications post stroke (9th ed.). St. Louis, MO: Thomas Land Publishers.

Teasell, R. W., Foley, N., & Salter, K. (2009). Predictive factors for recovery. In J. Stein, R. L. Harvey, R. F. Macko, C. J. Winstein, & R. D. Zorowitz (Eds.), Stroke recovery and rehabilitation (pp. 587–597) New York: Demos Publishing.

Tutuarima, J. A., de Haan, R. J., & Limburg, M. (1993). Number of nursing staff and falls: A case-control study on falls by stroke patients in acute-care settings. *Journal of Advanced Nursing, 118*, 1101–1105.

Tyson, S. F., Hanley, M., Chillala, J., Selley, A. B., & Tallis, R. C. (2008). Sensory loss in hospital-admitted people with stroke: Characteristics, associated factors, and relationship with function. *Neurorehabilitation and Neural Repair, 22*(2), 166–152.

U.S. Department of Health and Human Services, National Institutes of Health, & National Heart, Lung and Blood Institute. (2004). The seventh report of the joint national committee on the prevention, detection, evaluation, and treatment of high blood pressure. NIH Publication No. 04-5230. Bethesda, MD: National Heart, Lung and Blood Institute.

Urbano, F. L. (2001). Homans' sign in the diagnosis of deep venous thrombosis. *Hospital Physician,119*, (1Suppl) 22–24.

Vakhnina, N. V., Nikitina, L. Y., Parefenow, V. A., & Yakhno, N. N. (2009). Post-stroke cognitive impairments. *Neuroscience and Behavioral Physiology, 39,* 719–724.

Vanek, Z. F., & Menkes, J. H. (2007). Spasticity. Retrieved December 1, 2009, from http://emedicine.medscape.com/article/1148826

Venn, M. R., Taft, L., Carpentier, B., & Applebaugh, G. (1992). The influence of timing and suppository use on efficiency and effectiveness of bowel training after a stroke. *Rehabilitation Nursing, 17,* 116–120.

Vistin, M., Barbeau, H., Korner-Bitensky, N., & Mayo, N. E. (1998). A new approach to retrain gait in stroke patients through body weight support and treadmill stimulation. *Stroke, 29*(6), 1122–1128.

Waters, R. L., Frazier, J., Garland, D. E., Jordan, C., & Perry, J. (1982). Electromyographic gait analysis before and after operative treatment for hemiplegic equinus and equinovarus deformity. *American Journal of Bone and Joint Surgery, 64*(2), 284–288.

Webster, J. S., Roades, L. A., Morrill, B., Rapport, L. J., Abadee, P. S., Sowa, M. V., et al. (1995). Rightward orienting bias, wheelchair maneuvering, and fall risk. *Archives of Physical Medicine and Rehabilitation, 76,* 924–928.

Wheaton, L., & Hallett, M. (2007). Ideomotor apraxia: A review. *Journal of the Neurological Sciences, 260*(1–2), 1–10.

Williams, L. S., Kroenke, K., Bakas, T., Plue, L. D., Brizendine, E., Wanzhu T., et al. (2007). Care management of poststroke depression: A randomized, controlled trial. *Stroke, 38,* 998–1003.

Yates, J. S., Lai, S. M., Duncan, P. W., & Studenski, S. (2002). Falls in community-dwelling stroke survivors: An accumulated impairments model. *Journal of Rehabilitation Research and Development, 39*(3), 385–394.

Zinn, S., Bosworth, H. B., Hoenig, H. M., & Swartzwelder, H. S. (2007). Executive function deficits in acute stroke. *Archives of Physical Medicine and Rehabilitation, 88,* 173–180.

CHAPTER 16

Traumatic Brain Injury

Paula M. Anton

LEARNING OBJECTIVES

At the end of this chapter, the reader will be able to

- Describe how brain injury affects the function of the brain.
- Discuss the major complications of traumatic brain injury.
- Recognize commonly used assessment tools, including appropriate interpretation of findings.
- Provide evidence-based cognitive interventions to assist the individual through the traumatic brain injury trajectory.

KEY CONCEPTS AND TERMS

Acquired brain injury
Behavior
Closed head injuries
Cognitive
Complex regional pain syndrome (CRPs)
Concussion
Contusion
Coup/contrecoup
Epidural hematoma
Focal injury
Functional assessment measures

Galveston orientation and amnesia test
Glasgow coma scale (GCS)
Headache
Hemorrhagic injuries
Intraparenchymal hemorrhage
Intraventricular hemorrhage
Loss of consciousness (LOC)
Mild brain injury
Moderate brain injury
Moment of impact injury
Neurological

Postconcussion syndrome
Posttraumatic amnesia
Primary injuries
Rancho Los Amigos levels of cognitive functioning scale
Secondary injuries
Severe brain injury
Subdural hematoma
Temporal lobe
Traumatic brain injury (TBI)

Traumatic brain injury (TBI), or **acquired brain injury**, is a complex injury with broad implications, occurring when there is disruption of brain tissue resulting from an impact to the head (Lovasik, Kerr, & Alexander, 2001) in which the head hits, is hit by, or is penetrated by an object. The severity and complexity of the injury depend on the amount of brain tissue that is disrupted and the extent of the damage. Brain injuries can be nonpenetrating (**closed head injuries**), such as those resulting from a blow to the head, or penetrating, in which a missile or other object pierces the scalp, skull, or brain.

EPIDEMIOLOGY

Prevalence and Incidence

Annually, some 1.7 million people sustain a TBI annually. Of these, 1,365,000 are seen in an emergency department. This means 1.4% of emergency room visits annually are the result of a head injury. Each year, 275,000 TBI victims are hospitalized and 52,000 die (2.1% of all deaths annually). Moreover, 80,000 people sustain permanent severe **neurological** disabilities as a result of brain injury. Of those whose injuries are less severe, 30% to 80% will experience some symptoms of postconcussion syndrome, another sequelae of brain injury that is rising in prevalence annually (Langlois et al., 2003; Corrigan, Selassie, & Orman, 2010).

Common causes of brain injury include falls, motor vehicle crashes, struck by or against an object, and assault. Langlois (2003) described at least 21% of brain injuries to be from "unknown or other" causes, including sports injuries, combat injuries (blast injury), and gunshot wounds.

Children younger than 14 years of age have the highest number of emergency department visits per year from TBI, and elderly adults have the highest prevalence of hospitalization and death from TBI annually. Males are more likely to suffer a head injury than females across all age groups, having a 1.4 times greater prevalence of TBI overall.

ANATOMY

Knowledge of brain anatomy and of the location of injury in the brain assists the healthcare professional to assess and understand deficits that result from injury to the brain. Figure 16.1 shows the anatomy of the brain.

The brain is made up of regions, or lobes, each of which contains centers for various functions to govern physiological processes. Table 16.1 summarizes the functions of the various parts.

PATHOPHYSIOLOGY

Brain injures are described based on when the damage occurs. For example, damage from **primary injuries** occurs from the initial insult. **Secondary injuries** result from the swelling and homeostatic responses to the initial brain injury.

Primary Injuries

These injuries occur at the moment of impact and result from the blow to the head and the movement of the brain within the skull. The **moment of impact injury** can be further described as **coup/contrecoup** injuries. These are the result of acceleration/deceleration of the brain within the skull at the moment of impact. The brain crashes into the skull by motion toward the impact area (**coup**) and then rebounds to the opposite side of the skull (**contrecoup**).

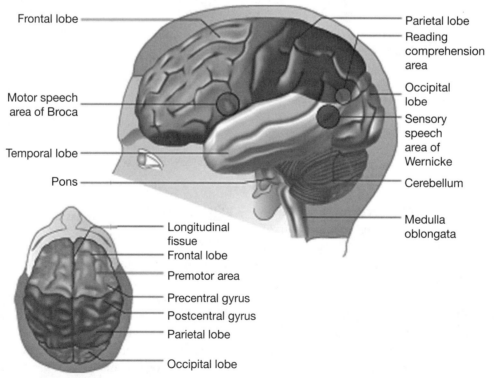

FIGURE 16.1   Anatomy of the brain.

Source: http://www.nlm.nih.gov/medlineplus/ency/imagepages/1074.htm

TABLE 16.1   Parts of the Brain and Their Functions

Part of the Brain	Function
Frontal lobe	Problem solving, planning, behavior, and emotion as well as primary motor cortex for movement of body parts and premotor cortex for eye and head movements and sense of orientation in space. Broca's area for language production is located in the frontal lobe as well.
Temporal lobe	Memory, emotion, hearing, and word understanding. Wernicke's area for language and speech resides generally in the temporal lobe.
Occipital lobe	Visual processing area of the brain, allowing for signals from the retina to be perceived.
Parietal lobe	Integrates sensory and motor information, allowing the subject to understand spatial relationships and position in space; assists with coordination of auditory visual, motor and sensory signals, and is the center for memory to identify objects.
Cerebellum	Controls movement, balance, equilibrium, posture, and muscle tone and is a center for some cognitive functions, including attention, language, and emotion.
Brainstem	Controls primitive function.
Pituitary gland	Master gland of the body, producing hormones.
Hypothalamus	Controls pituitary gland, eating and sexual behaviors, sleeping, and body temperature.
Pineal gland	Unclear function, possible light/dark response.
Thalamus	Pain sensation and alertness.
Spinal cord	Connects the brain to the rest of the body, for signal transmission.

Moment of impact injuries can be further described as **focal injuries**, which occur in a specific area of the brain. These include contusion of brain tissue, intracranial hemorrhage, or hematoma. Additional injuries include diffuse injury, in which the damage occurs in a widespread area, usually the result of shearing.

Diffuse axonal injury occurs at the moment of impact during which axons (long nerve fibers that traverse the white matter of the brain to connect nerve cells in the gray matter of the brain with distant nerve cells) become stretched, twisted, or damaged by the sudden twisting or torquing of the brain in acceleration/deceleration. This injury cannot be detected with current imaging options such as magnetic resonance imaging or computed tomography. Diffuse injuries are diagnosed by symptomatology of brain injury in the absence of hemorrhagic signs or contusions commonly seen on imaging studies.

Secondary Injuries

Brain swelling (edema) results from the inflammatory response to injury. Edema leads to crowding within the cranium, resulting in continued or worsening damage to brain tissue, and is mediated by several causes:

- Hypotension is a major determinant of outcome in patients with severe head injury, occurring in 34.6%

of these patients and associated with a 1.5 times increase in mortality. Furthermore, improvements in trauma care over time have not altered the adverse effects of hypotension on TBI outcomes (Chestnut et al., 1993).

- Hypoxia/hypoxemia is when brain tissue is deprived of oxygen due to states of decreased or absent cerebral blood flow, most commonly caused by cardiopulmonary arrest. Multiple mechanisms contribute to the injury on a microscopic level. The cell membrane is impaired, resulting in changes in inter- and intracellular ions and causing acidosis, further cell injury, and edema. There is secondary activation of destructive enzymes that break down neuronal tissue. With reestablishment of blood flow, edema and microhemorrhages result, causing further brain swelling (Greer, 2006).

- Electrolyte imbalance in severe TBI results in disturbed ionic and neurotransmitter homeostasis. This is thought to be an important mechanism contributing to cerebral edema after TBI. The injury leads to ion channel activation in which potassium moves out of the neuronal cell and sodium moves in, causing massive depolarization of the cells. The result is fluid imbalance and metabolic derangement (Katayama, Kawamata, & Tsubokawa, 1995; Reinert et al., 2000)

Types of Injuries

Injuries can be further broken down as follows:

- **Concussion** is a temporary loss of consciousness resulting from a blow to the head.
- **Contusion** is bruising of cerebral tissue.
- **Hemorrhagic injuries** are of several types:
  - **Subdural hematoma** is bleeding between the dura and arachnoid membranes, usually caused by tearing of vessels in the space from shearing injury. The blood collects outside the brain tissue (extraaxial).
  - **Epidural hematoma** is bleeding between the dura and the skull, usually caused by acceleration/deceleration injuries. This is also extraaxial bleeding.
  - Subarachnoid hemorrhage (SAH) is bleeding into the subarachnoid space between the arachnoid membrane and the pia mater, which is the brain covering. Subarachnoid hemorrhage usually results from a cerebral aneurism or head injury.
  - **Intraparenchymal and intraventricular hemorrhages** are intraaxial (within brain tissue) hemorrhages that usually result from trauma or hemorrhagic stroke.

Common signs and symptoms of TBI include overt signs seen at the time of or shortly after injury. These include **loss of consciousness (LOC)**, which can last from minutes to hours or days, and **posttraumatic amnesia** (PTA), which lasts for varied lengths of time. Some patients experience nausea and vomiting, seizure, focal neurological signs, **headache**, cerebrospinal fluid rhinorrhea or otorrhea, and skull fracture. These signs generally cause hospital admission for observation. Although TBI implies that just the brain in injured, nearly all body systems can be affected.

COMMON PROBLEMS EXPERIENCED BY PATIENTS AFTER TBI

Persons with brain injury may face a number of challenges associated with brain damage. These problems depend largely on the location and extent of brain injury as well as on the immediate care and rehabilitation received. Some common problems and complications associated with TBI are as follows:

- Affective disorders such as agitation, anxiety, depression, and posttraumatic stress disorder (PTSD).
- Autonomic system signs including hypertension, hypotension, tachycardia, temperature regulation abnormalities.
- Behavioral and psychological impairments, including aggression, dysinhibition, impaired awareness, sexual dysfunction, and substance abuse.
- Cardiovascular system problems such as cardiac ischemia or necrosis, arrhythmias, and deep vein thrombosis.
- **Cognitive** deficits such as arousal, attention abnormalities, loss of executive functioning, delay in initiation of tasks, language and communication deficits, and visuospatial perception disorders. (See Chapter 11 for more information on enhancing cognition, communication, and **behavior**.)
- Endocrine system abnormalities such as acne or rashes, appetite control problems, decreased cellular immune response, hyponatremia, hypernatremia, anterior pituitary disease, amenorrhea, and sleep irregularities.
- Gastrointestinal system problems, including constipation, diarrhea, bowel accidents, dysphagia, gastoesophageal reflux disease, gastritis, gastric ulcer, hepatic dysfunction, hiccups, hypermetabolism, decreased motility, and vomiting/nausea.
- Genitourinary system problems such as loss of cortical urinary control, bladder dyssynergia, urinary tract infections, and neurogenic bladder.
- Neurological system complications, including auditory, olfactory, and visual deficits and sensory disorders, neurogenic motor disturbances, neglect and lack of spatial awareness, peripheral nerve injuries, hydrocephalus, seizures, and sleep disturbances.
- Neuromuscular system problems such as contractures, rigidity, parkinsonism, tremors, akathisia, ataxia, athetosis, ballismus chorea, dystonia, cranial dystonia, oromandibular dystonia, cervical dystonia (torticollis), hemidystonia, palsies, stereotypy (tardive dyskinesia), tics, movement disorders, myoclonus, and spasticity.
- Orthopedic system complications such as fractures and heterotopic ossification.
- **Complex regional pain syndrome** (CRPs) complications include diffuse distal limb pain, loss of function, and autonomic dysfunction.
- Postconcussive syndromes include cervical acceleration/deceleration injuries, cervicogenic dizziness, and head pain/headache.
- Pulmonary system complications include airway

management problems, airway obstruction, tracheal granulomas due to prolonged tracheostomy tube placement, and hypooxemia/respiratory failure.

- Skin system problems such as skin breakdown and pressure ulcers and perioral redness due to drooling of oral secretions. (See Chapter 8 for more information on skin breakdown and pressure ulcers.)

CLASSIFICATION

Degree of brain injury is variable and depends on the mechanism of injury, length of time of LOC, and persistence of amnesia of the event. **Mild brain injury** can occur from direct contact injury or acceleration deceleration injury. There may be no LOC or brief LOC of 20 minutes or less, mild posttraumatic amnesia, and a **Glasgow coma scale (GCS)** score of more than 13. There usually is negative neuroimaging. This is the type of injury formerly called "concussion" but which is now called **postconcussion syndrome** (PCS). Symptoms can go unrecognized until they begin to interfere with activities of daily living (ADLs). Headache is the cardinal symptom. Other symptoms include dizziness, fatigue, irritability, anxiety, insomnia, concentration and memory disturbances, and noise sensitivity (Evans, 2006, 2010). Experts recommend patients who have mild head injury continue to undergo neuropsychological testing and continuing assessment (Ferullo & Green, 2010). It can take weeks to months of recovery without specific treatment.

Moderate brain injury can also occur from direct contact injury or acceleration/deceleration injury. The patient can have LOC longer than 20 minutes, posttraumatic amnesia, GCS score of 9–12, and cerebral edema and cerebral hemorrhages may be seen on neuroimaging tests. Symptoms include disturbed balance and coordination, agitation, seizures, dysphagia, and speech disturbances, depending on the areas of the brain affected. The patient usually requires rehabilitation and may experience long-term neurological deficits.

Severe brain injury involves LOC of greater than 6 hours, prolonged post traumatic amnesia and GCS of <8. There can be intracranial or subdural hemorrhage, tearing and shearing of brain tissue or penetration of brain tissue by an object or projectile, with deficits seen on neuroimaging tests. The patient requires intensive treatment in the acute phase to mitigate systemic complications and generally requires a long period of rehabilitation, even lifelong. Some patients with severe TBI remain in a vegetative state.

ASSESSMENT

Assessment of the patient with TBI includes the general systems assessment with additional specific assessments of neurological functioning. Widely used functional assessment measures administered by nurses and other allied health professionals include the GCS, the **Ranchos Los Amigos levels of cognitive functioning scale**, and the Galveston orientation and amnesia test.

The GCS, first described by Teasdale and Jennett (1974), comprises three tests, eye, verbal, and motor responses, to estimate consciousness (Table 16.2). This test is often administered at the scene of an injury by the first responders and is used over time to assess changes in consciousness. It is applicable in the intensive care unit through the acute phase and into the rehabilitative phase of care. The three values separately as well as their sum are considered. The lowest possible score (the sum) is 3 (deep coma or death) and the highest is 15 (fully awake) (Box 16.1).

TABLE 16.2 Glasgow Coma Scale

	1	2	3	4	5	6
Eyes	Does not open eyes	Opens eyes in response to painful stimuli	Opens eyes in response to voice	Opens eyes spontaneously	N/A	N/A
Verbal	Makes no sounds	Incomprehensible sounds	Utters inappropriate words	Confused, disoriented	Oriented, converses normally	N/A
Motor	Makes no movements	Extension to painful stimuli (decerebrate response)	Abnormal flexion to painful stimuli (decorticate response)	Flexion/withdrawal to painful stimuli	Localizes painful stimuli	Obeys commands

Source: From Teasdale and Jennett (1974).

BOX 16.1	Scoring the Glasgow Coma Scale

Eye-Opening Response

- Spontaneous, open with blinking at baseline (4 points)
- To verbal stimuli, command, speech (3 points)
- To pain only (not applied to face) (2 points)
- No response (1 point)

Verbal Response

- Oriented (5 points)
- Confused conversation but able to answer questions (4 points)
- Inappropriate words (3 points)

- Incomprehensible speech (2 points)
- No response (1 point)

Motor Response

- Obeys commands for movement (6 points)
- Purposeful movement to painful stimulus (5 points)
- Withdraws in response to pain (4 points)
- Flexion in response to pain (decorticate posturing) (3 points)
- Extension response in response to pain (decerebrate posturing) (2 points)
- No response (1 point)

Although Rowley and Fielding (1991) maintain that scoring of the GCS requires education to be done reliably and others question the reliability of the scales (Becker & Povlishock, 1988), it is widely used. Use of this scale involves assigning a score based on the best response elicited from the patient. Box 16.1 presents the scoring rubric for the three tests that comprise the scale.

The Rancho Los Amigos scale of cognitive functioning was originally developed in the 1970s at Rancho Los Amigos National Rehabilitation Center (Hagan, Malk-mus, & Durham, 1979). Over the years it has been modified to the current versions, resulting in the widely used 8-point scale and a newer expanded version, which is a 10-point scale proposed by the original author (Chris Hagan). For the purposes of this description, we use the eight-point scale, which has been validated and tested for reliability (Dowling, 1985; Hall & Johnston, 1994). Table 16.3 describes the Ranchos Los Amigos levels of cognitive functioning and describes patient characteristics at each level. This test can be administered by any member of

TABLE 16.3	Rancho Los Amigos Scale of Cognitive Functioning: Patient Characteristics
Cognitive Level	**The patient will**
I: no response	• not respond to sounds, sights, touch, or movement
II: generalized response	• begin to respond to sounds, sights, touch, or movement; • respond slowly, inconsistently, or after a delay; • respond in the same way to what he hears, sees, or feels. Responses may include chewing, sweating, breathing faster, moaning, moving, and/or increasing blood pressure.
III: localized response	• be awake on and off during the day; • make more movements than before; • react more specifically to what he sees, hears, or feels. For example, the patient may turn toward a sound, withdraw from pain, and attempt to watch a person move around the room; • react slowly and inconsistently; • begin to recognize family and friends; • follow some simple directions such as "look at me" or "squeeze my hand"; • begin to respond inconsistently to simple questions with "yes" and "no" head nods.
IV: confused, agitated	• be very confused and frightened; • not understand what he feels or what is happening around him; • overreact to what he sees, hears, or feels by hitting, screaming, using abusive language, or thrashing about. This is because of the confusion; • be restrained so he doesn't hurt himself; • be highly focused on his basic needs (i.e., eating, relieving pain, going back to bed, going to the bathroom, or going home); • may not understand that people are trying to help him;

(Continued)

Cognitive Level	The patient will
	• not pay attention or be able to concentrate for a few seconds;
	• have difficulty following directions;
	• recognize family/friends some of the time;
	• with help, be able to do simple routine activities such as feeding himself, dressing, or talking.
V: confused, inappropriate, nonagitated	• be confused and have difficulty making sense of things outside himself;
	• not know the date, where he is, or why he is in the hospital;
	• not be able to start or complete everyday activities, such as brushing his teeth, even when physically able. He may need step-by-step instructions;
	• become overloaded and restless when tired or when there are too many people around; have a very poor memory, he will remember past events from before the accident better than his daily routine or information he has been told since the injury;
	• try to fill in gaps in memory by making things up (confabulation).
VI: confused, appropriate	• be somewhat confused because of memory and thinking problems, he will remember the main points from a conversation but forget and confuse the details. For example, he may remember he had visitors in the morning but forget what they talked about;
	• follow a schedule with some assistance, but become confused by changes in the routine;
	• know the month and year, unless there is a severe memory problem;
	• pay attention for about 30 minutes, but have trouble concentrating when it is noisy or when the activity involves many steps. For example, at an intersection, he may be unable to step off the curb, watch for cars, watch the traffic light, walk, and talk at the same time;
	• brush his teeth, get dressed, feed himself, etc., with help;
	• know when he needs to use the bathroom;
	• do or say things too fast, without thinking first;
	• know that he is hospitalized because of an injury, but will not understand all of the problems he is having;
	• be more aware of physical problems than thinking problems;
	• associate his problems with being in the hospital and believe he will be fine as soon as he goes home.
VII: automatic, appropriate	• follow a set schedule;
	• be able to do routine self-care without help, if physically able. For example, he can dress or feed himself independently; have problems in new situations and may become frustrated or act without thinking first;
	• have problems planning, starting, and following through with activities;
	• have trouble paying attention in distracting or stressful situations. For example, family gatherings, work, school, church, or sports events;
	• not realize how his thinking and memory problems may affect future plans and goals. Therefore, he may expect to return to his previous lifestyle or work;
VIII: purposeful, appropriate	• realize that he has a problem in his thinking and memory;
	• begin to compensate for his problems;
	• be more flexible and less rigid in his thinking. For example, he may be able to come up with several solutions to a problem;
	• be ready for driving or job training evaluation;
	• be able to learn new things at a slower rate;
	• still become overloaded with difficult, stressful, or emergency situations;
	• show poor judgment in new situations and may require assistance;
	• need some guidance to make decisions;
	• have thinking problems that may not be noticeable to people who did not know the person before the injury.

Source: From Rancho Los Amigos National Rehabilitation Center. (n.d.).

the interdisciplinary team but is generally administered by the speech and language pathologist and/or the rehabilitation psychologist. (Case Study 16.1)

CASE STUDY 16.1

R. W. is a 68-year-old man with a history of subarachnoid hemorrhage treated by aneurysm clipping. This is the second aneurysm clipping he has undergone. The first was approximately 1 year ago after the initial hemorrhage and was followed by extended rehabilitation. The second surgery was 1 week prior and was an elective surgery to manage the remaining aneurysm.

The nurse attempts to receive the patient into the rehabilitation unit when he begins to get agitated and tries to get out of the chair. The nurse asks him to sit and he does not respond, except to increase in agitation. He makes guttural noises in response to verbal commands. The nurse attempts to detain him because she has not had the opportunity to assess his mobility status. A nurse aide from the neurosurgery unit has accompanied the patient, and the nurse has a report from the previous nurse. As she detains the patient in his wheelchair, he becomes combative, and after he has been in the wheelchair in his room on the rehabilitation unit for about 5 minutes the nurse becomes frightened and asks for security assistance. Other staff arrive to assist.

The patient is very agitated, sitting with his legs stiff and knees together, and he tries to get out of the chair. A staff member determines that he might need to relieve his bladder due to his body position and offers him the urinal. He pushes the urinal away and tries to get up. A staff member asks the nurse aide from the previous unit if the patient voided recently, and the aide does not know. The next question for the aide is whether the patient can stand and, with an affirmative, brings a nearby commode chair to the patient and assists him to stand. He begins to urinate before he can stand up and exhibits embarrassment and sorrow at this outcome by hanging his head, dropping his shoulders, and groaning.

Questions

1. What is the Rancho Los Amigos level of cognitive functioning of this patient, and how might it apply to the patient's current behavior?
2. Is calling security services the best response to this patient's behavior?
3. Given his severe communicative deficit, what nonverbal cues exist to tell the nurse why the patient might be increasing in agitation?
4. What pieces of information should the rehabilitation nurse obtained from the previous nurse at the time of hand-off to avert this unfortunate outcome?

The **Galveston orientation and amnesia test** is a valid and reliable 10-question test for determination of the extent of posttraumatic amnesia (Levin, O'Donnell, & Grossman, 1979). Each question is assigned an error value given if the patient is unable to accurately answer the question, and the scores are totaled to give a value that is subtracted from 100. The score is reported as "<value> out of 100 points." The test is administered weekly, frequently by the speech and language pathologist. Table 16.4 lists the questions associated with this test.

Other **functional assessment measures** the nurse may see and use include the functional independence measure, functional assessment measure, Craig handicap assessment and reporting technique, community integration questionnaire, and the disability rating scale. All have been tested for validity and reliability with valid results. The functional independence measure (FIM) has excellent reliability and validity, whereas the functional assessment measure attempts to improve cognitive, communicative, and psychosocial assessment. The community integration questionnaire and Craig handicap assessment and reporting technique are reliable and correlate with each

---

TABLE 16.4   Galveston Orientation and Amnesia Test Questions with Error Points

What is your name? (2)

When were you born? (4)

Where do you live? (4)

Where are you now? City? (5) Hospital? (5) (*unnecessary to state name of hospital*)

On what date were you admitted to this hospital? (5)

How did you get here? (5)

What is the first event you can remember *after* the injury? (5)

Can you describe in detail (e.g., date, time, companions) the first event you can recall *after* the injury? (5)

Can you describe the last event you recall *before* the accident? (5)

Can you describe in detail (e.g., date, time, companions) the first event you can recall *before* the injury? (5)

What time is it now? (*1 for each half hour removed from correct time, to maximum of 5*)

What day of the week is it? (*1 for each day removed from correct one*)

What day of the month is it? (*1 for each day removed from correct date, to maximum of 5*)

What is the month? (*5 for each month removed from correct one, to a maximum of 15*)

What is the year? (*10 for each year removed from correct one, to maximum of 30*)

Source: From Levin, O'Donnell, and Grossman (1979).

other. The disability rating scale is simple, brief (takes < 5 minutes to administer), and useful from coma to community reintegration. Box 16.2 provides resources for more information about these functional assessment tools.

BOX 16.2	Resources

The Center for Outcome Measurement in Brain Injury (COMBI) http://www.tbims.org/combi/index.html

FAM Center for Outcome Measurement in Brain Injury (COMBI) http://tbims.org/combi/FAM/index.html

DRS Center for Outcome Measurement in Brain Injury (COMBI) http://tbims.org/combi/drs/index.html

National Institute of Neurological Disorders and Stroke http://www.ninds.nih.gov

Brain Injury Association of America http://www.biausa.org

CDC National Center for Injury Prevention and Control (NCIPC) http://www.cdc.gov/TraumaticBrainInjury/index.html

http://www.cdc.gov/traumaticbraininjury/tbi_ed.html

http://www.braininjury.com/injured.html

FIM® Uniform Data Set (UDS) website http://www.udsmr.org

Craig Handicap Assessment and Reporting Technique http://www.craighospital.org/Research/CHART.asp

Nursing assessments include elements of the physical and functional assessments, such as evaluation of the neurological, pulmonary, cardiovascular, and musculoskeletal systems to monitor for changes in mental status, cognition, respiration, and circulation that can indicate systemic complications of the TBI. In addition, the nurse monitors nutrition, elimination, and safety of the patient and intervenes as indicated. Part II of this text offers more detailed information on these topics.

MEDICAL INTERVENTIONS

Medical interventions include managing the systemic complications and sequelae of the brain injury. In addition, medications are used judiciously to assist the brain to function while the healing process goes on. Antiepileptics may be necessary in the setting of seizures. In addition, some psychopharmacological agents assist in the management of aggression, anxiety, confusion, depression disinhibition, motor restlessness, low attention, and arousal. These include lorazepam, trazodone, propranolol, carbamazepine, buspirone, fluoxetine, amitriptyline, bromocriptine, methyphenidate, and D-amphetamine. Management of these TBI symptoms is not the primary use of many of these drugs; they have gained favor in the practice of rehabilitation. The doses are carefully monitored to minimize sedating side effects and are tapered or titrated after the desired effect is obtained to assess the behaviors. In some circumstances, even in the absence of seizures, anticonvulsants may be necessary to calm brain activity during the most agitated periods. Some commonly used medications such as anticonvulsants, some antihypertensives, antispasmodics, psychoactive agents, and such gastrointestinal medications as cimetidine and metoclopramide are contraindicated or must be used with caution because of the central nervous system effects (sedation, decreased cognition, and memory impairment).

NURSING STRATEGIES

Rehabilitative care of the patient with a TBI includes providing a safe environment and managing the patient with cognitive deficits. Management of the physical needs of the TBI patient is unique. Table 16.5 lists the potential

TABLE 16.5	Nursing Care Strategies
System	**Assessment and Nursing Strategies**
Neurological	Assess cognitive, motor, and sensory status including reflexes and cranial nerves.
	Monitor anticonvulsant drug levels, medication effects, and side effects such as somnolence and dizziness.
	Collaborate with interdisciplinary team to provide cognitive therapies such as use of a memory book to encourage memory and thinking strategies.
Respiratory	Assess airway patency via lung sounds, oxygen saturation, production and character of secretions, and potential for aspiration.
	Provide airway protection and prevent aspiration by positioning with head of bed up to 30 degrees as necessary, administer supplemental oxygen as required, and follow feeding guidelines for consistency of food and oral fluids as appropriate.
	Monitor for respiratory distress, especially in the presence of blood clotting disorder such as deep vein thrombosis.

(Continued)

TABLE 16.5	**Nursing Care Strategies** *(Continued)*
System	**Assessment and Nursing Strategies**
Cardiovascular	Assess blood pressure, heart rate and rhythm at appropriate intervals, and for deep vein thrombosis (swelling warmth and pain in extremities).
	Monitor medication levels and cardiac effects of beta-blockers used to decrease restlessness and agitation in the TBI patient.
	Administer deep vein thrombosis prophylaxis (low-dose heparin or enoxaparin and/or sequential compression devices) as appropriate.
Nutrition	Assess hydration status and dietary intake each day, and monitor weight weekly.
	Provide feedings as appropriate, oral or enteral as needed, and provide hydration as appropriate. Patients may not be able to interpret hunger and thirst signals accurately due to brain injury.
Elimination	Assess preinjury bowel and bladder habits if possible, and compare with current bowel and bladder patterns. Assess continence and effectiveness of elimination interventions.
	Use an active approach to elimination, remembering that the brain-injured patient may not be able to correctly interpret body signals of need to urinate or defecate. Keep in mind that the patient may become constipated due to difficulty expressing the need to use the toilet.
Musculoskeletal	Assess for pain and range of motion deficits (heterotopic ossification), preinjury conditions, fractures, contractures, spasticity, and tone.
	Monitor gait and mobility if appropriate, providing mobility in collaboration with interdisciplinary team, using adaptive equipment as needed.
Communicative Cognitive Behavior	Assess for aphasias, dysarthria, behavioral excess (agitation, disinhibition, impulsivity, restlessness, perseveration, emotional lability, restlessness) and/or deficits (apathy, poor or absent initiation).
	Collaborate with multidisciplinary team to provide cognitive strategies and interventions as appropriate:
	Reorient the individual as appropriate.
	Monitor and adjust stimuli in the environment as appropriate.
	Provide cues and memory strategies as appropriate.
	Keep in mind that the brain is not providing or interpreting input in the usual way. The patient may be frustrated, fearful, and anxious, making the individual difficult to handle.
Safety	Assess for risk for falls (balance disturbance, sensory deficit, polypharmacy, elimination urgency), wandering, impulsivity, and judgment disturbance.
	Provide fall precautions as needed.
	Assess need for restraint and provide least restrictive form of restraint.
	Consider 1:1 supervision.
Psychosocial	Assess family support and coping mechanisms.
	Provide education and support to family in collaboration with interdisciplinary team.
Sexual	Assess level of function related to physical and behavioral deficits.
	Collaborate with the interdisciplinary team to provide education and support in the area of intimacy and sexuality.
Vocational	Assess the individual's potential for returning to work or school and reintegration to the community.
	Provide strategies such as neuropsychological testing and interventions to assist the individual and family with planning.

Sources: Dufour, Williams, and Coleman (2001) and Hoeman (2002).

care needs of the patient with TBI and associated nursing interventions. Use of a standard language for describing our work in nursing has been widely encouraged (Ozbolt, 2000). Box 16.3 lists primary areas of intervention and common nursing diagnoses.

BOX 16.3   Nursing Diagnoses and Core Interventions

Selected NANDA Nursing Diagnosis

- Impaired verbal communication
- Acute confusion
- Chronic confusion
- Risk for injury
- Disturbed thought process

Selected Core Interventions for Rehabilitation Nursing

- Behavior management
- Communication management: speech deficit
- Emotional support
- Environmental management: home preparation
- Environmental management: safety
- Family support
- Health education
- Memory training
- Socialization enhancement
- Swallowing therapy
- Unilateral neglect management

Strategies for working with patients at the various Ranchos Los Amigos cognitive levels work well during the time the brain is healing. (Case Study 16.2) These are discussed further here.

CASE STUDY 16.2

R. S. is a 54-year-old man who was the victim of an assault and has suffered severe brain injury. He is at Rancho level 4 most of the time and has been for some time. His speech is barely intelligible at times, and his eyesight is impaired, but the degree is unknown because he is not cooperative with testing. He recognizes his sister at times, but then often believes staff members are his mother or others. He occasionally has flashbacks to his assault but does not always recognize that he was assaulted. He occasionally tries to get out of bed and leave the room but does not react well to restraints. He has a one-on-one sitter present at the bedside most of the time and occasionally yells at them. He is more cooperative during the day when he can get up and about and more agitated at night when staff want him to stay in bed. He has been getting lorazepam PRN, usually one or two doses a night, and frequently is placed in locked limb restraints during the night.

At approximately 0430 hours staff hear glass breaking and furniture crashing. The sitter calls for help. On arrival the staff find that the patient lunged out of bed toward the door, pushed the overbed table out of his way, causing it to knock a glass item off the windowsill. The sitter is frightened. Staff become frightened as Mr. S. again lunges toward the door and peers menacingly at staff. His nurse reports that she had given lorazepam at 0130 hours and he had been sleeping soundly since.

Security is summoned, and Mr. S. is forced into bed and held as locked limb holders are applied. He agrees to have an injection to make him feel better, but he is fighting against the restraints. He begins to cry. About 10 minutes after the medication, he settles down but does not go to sleep, and he begins to converse with staff. Later in the day physicians titrate up his antiepileptic drug and add a beta-blocker.

Questions

1. What could staff do to mitigate the problems they experience with R. S.'s behavior at night?
2. How does it make you feel when you read that he begins to cry?
3. Was restraint necessary in this case? When should restraint be removed in this case?
4. Why is he on an antiepileptic and a beta-blocker?

Levels I, II, and III

- Explain to the individual what you are about to do. For example, "I'm going to move your leg."
- Speak in a normal tone of voice.
- Keep comments and questions short and simple, using plain language. For example, instead of "Can you turn your head toward me?" say, "Look at me." Instead of "Do you need the urinal?" say "It is time to go to the bathroom."
- Reorient the individual to time, place, person, and situation.
- Limit the number of visitors to two to three people at a time.
- Keep the room calm and quiet.
- Allow the person extra time to respond.
- Give the individual rest periods.

Level IV

- Reorient the individual to time, place, person, and situation and reassure her that she is safe.
- Take extra precautions for patient safety, because this is often a period of greater agitation.
- Increase activity as appropriate for safety.
- Allow family to take the individual for rides in a wheelchair as appropriate.
- Experiment to find familiar activities that are calming to her, such as listening to music, eating, and so on.

- Do not force her to do things.
- Because she often becomes distracted, restless, or agitated, give the individual rest periods and change activities frequently.
- Keep the room quiet and calm. For example, turn off the television and radio, don't talk too much, and use a calm voice.
- Limit the number of visitors to two to three people at a time.

Level V

- Repeat things as needed. Don't assume the individual will remember what you tell him.
- Reorient the individual to time, place, person, and situation often.
- Keep comments and questions short and simple.
- Help him organize and get started on an activity.
- Allow/encourage family to bring in pictures and personal items from home.
- Limit the number of visitors to two to three at a time.
- Give the individual rest periods when he has problems paying attention.

Level VI

- Use a memory book to assist with recall of the day's events.
- Assist the individual to initiate and continuing activities.
- Encourage the individual to participate in all therapies even though she provides logical and convincing arguments that she is not impaired.

Levels VII and VIII

- At this point the patient is getting ready for discharge from the acute rehabilitation setting.
- Provide guidance and assistance in decision making.
- Talk with the individual using adult language.
- Use caution when joking or using slang because the individual may misunderstand the meaning.
- During familiar activities help the individual to recognize the problems he has in thinking, problem solving, and memory.
- Encourage the individual to continue to participate in all therapies.
- Encourage the individual to continue to use memory aids he has learned.

For all the preceding interventions/strategies, be sure to communicate with the interdisciplinary team (Table 16.6) and set reasonable goals in the team conference.

TABLE 16.6   Traumatic Brain Injury Rehabilitation Team

Patient
Family
Physician
Nurse
Dietitian
Occupational therapist
Physical therapist
Recreational therapist
Rehabilitation psychologist/neuropsychologist
Rehabilitation engineer
Social worker
Speech-language pathologist
Vocational rehabilitation counselor

Involve family members as much as possible, and provide education to them about what to expect in the recovery/rehabilitation phase.

PATIENT AND FAMILY EDUCATION

The diagnosis of TBI and the cognitive features that are displayed by the patient can be devastating to the patient and the family. Care does not end at discharge from the rehabilitation facility to the next level of care. Patients and families need support and education to succeed in the next setting. Nurses should educate the patient/family on the persistent nature of the deficits and the slow and steady nature of recovery. They should be reassured that the recovery will wax and wane, and reversions can be expected as the recovery continues.

In the area of safety, encourage families to adhere to safety recommendations from the interdisciplinary team. Often, as patients recover they are perceived by those close to them as "normal." This is a common feature at higher Rancho cognitive levels and can put the individual at risk of harm if it is not recognized. Encourage family members to continue strategies used by the nurse to assist the patient to recognize his or her deficits.

SUMMARY

Traumatic brain injury can be present in various levels of severity. Several tools and scales were discussed in this chapter that can assist rehabilitation nurses in assessment and management of persons with brain injury. Educating clients and family members is essential to positive outcomes for those with brain injury, and nurses should be aware of resources in their communities that can assist those requiring long-term interventions.

CRITICAL THINKING EXERCISES

1. Have you ever cared for a person with a brain injury? If so, what level of severity did the patient have? What difficulties did you encounter in providing care? How was the family educated to help the person with recovery and rehabilitation? Were the outcomes positive?
2. Explore the resources in your own community for persons with brain injury. What types of support is available to patients and families after return home? What is the closest outpatient day treatment center near your home? What would patients and families do if there was a lack of help within the community to care for a person with moderate to severe TBI?

PERSONAL REFLECTION

- Do you understand the need for quiet and controlled stimulation in the environment of the brain-injured patient? How would you handle the situation in which the significant other of a brain-injured patient at Rancho level IV with emerging level V behaviors arrives with three of his or her friends to cheer the individual? How would you respond if they wanted to turn on the television set or the CD player?
- Have you ever taken care of a patient who has had a stroke or a brain hemorrhage who has exhibited anger and frustration, trying to push you away and do something for himself? How does that make you feel as a healthcare provider trying to care for the patient?

REFERENCES

Becker, D. P., & Povlishock, J. R. (Eds.). (1988). *Central nervous system trauma status report, 1985* (pp. 271–280). Washington, DC: U.S. Government Printing Office.

Centers for Disease Control and Prevention (NCIPC) Office of Noncommunicable Diseases. (n.d.). Glasgow coma scale. Retrieved May 16, 2010, from http://www.bt.cdc.gov/mass-casualties/gscale.asp

Chestnut, R. M., Marshall, L. F., Klauber, M. R., Blunt, B. A., Baldwin, N., Eisenberg, H. M., Jan, J. A . . . Foulkes, M. A. (1993). The role of secondary brain injury in determining outcomes from severe head injury. *Journal of Trauma, 34*(2), 216–222.

Corrigan, J. D., Selassie, A. W., & Orman, J. A. (2010). The epidemiology of traumatic brain injury. *Journal of Head Trauma Rehabilitation, 25*(2), 72–80.

Dowling, G. A. (1985). Levels of cognitive functioning: Evaluation of interrater reliability. *Journal of Neurosurgical Nursing, 17*(2), 129–134.

Dufour, L., Williams, J., & Coleman, K. (2001). Traumatic injuries: TBI and SCI. In P. A. Edwards (Ed.), *The specialty practice of rehabilitation nursing: A core curriculum* (4th ed., pp. 189–210). Glenview, IL: Association of Rehabilitation Nurses.

Ferullo, S. M., & Green, A. (2010). Update on concussion: Here's what the experts say. *Journal of Family Practice, 59*(8), 428–433.

Greer, D. M. (2006). Mechanisms of injury in hypoxic-ischemic encephalopathy: Implications to therapy. *Seminars in Neurology, 26*(4), 373–379.

Hagen, C., Malkmus, D., & Durham, P. (1979). *Levels of cognitive functioning. Rehabilitation of the head injured adult. Comprehensive physical management.* Downey, CA: Professional Staff Association of Rancho Los Amigos National Rehabilitation Center.

Hall, K. M., & Johnston, M. V. (1994). Outcomes evaluation in TBI rehabilitation, Part II: Measurement tools for a nationwide data system. *Archives of Physical Medicine and Rehabilitation, 75*, SC10–SC18.

Hoeman, S. P. (Ed.). (2002). *Rehabilitation nursing: Process, application and outcomes* (3rd ed.). St. Louis, MO: Mosby.

Katayama, Y., Kawamata, T., & Tsubokawa, T. (1995). Rise of excitatory amino acid-mediated ionic fluxes in traumatic brain injury. *Brain Pathology, 5*(4), 427–435.

Langlois, J. A., Kegler, S. R., Butler, J. A., Gotsch, K. E., Johnson, R. L., Reichard, A. L., & Thurman, D. J. (2003) Traumatic brain injury-related hospital discharges: Results from a 14-state surveillance system, 1997. *MMWR Surveillance Summaries, 52*(SS04), 1–18. Retrieved May 16, 2010, from http://www.cdc.gov/mmwr/preview/mmwrhtml/ss5204a1.htm

Levin, H. S., O'Donnell, V. M., & Grossman, R. G. (1979). The Galveston orientation and amnesia test: A practical scale to assess cognition after head injury. *Journal of Nervous and Mental Diseases, 167*(11), 675–684.

Lovasik, D., Kerr, M. E., & Alexander, S. (2001). Traumatic brain injury research: A review of clinical studies. *Critical Care Nursing Quarterly, 23*(4), 24–41.

Ozbolt, J. (2000). White paper: Terminology standards for nursing: Collaboration at the summit. *Journal of the American Informatics Medical Association, 7*(6), 517–522.

Rancho Los Amigos National Rehabilitation Center. (n.d.). Family guide to the Rancho levels of cognitive functioning. Retrieved May 16, 2010, from http://www.rancho.org/research_home.htm

Reinert, M., Khaldi, A, Zauner, A., Doppenberg, E., Choi, S., & Bullock, R. (2000). High extracellular potassium and its correlates after severe head injury: Relationship to high intracranial pressure. *Neurosurgical Focus, 8*(1), 1–8.

Rowley, G., & Fielding, K. (1991). Reliability and accuracy of the Glasgow coma scale with experienced and inexperienced users. *Lancet, 337*, 535–538.

Teasdale, G., & Jennett, B. (1974). Assessment of coma and impaired consciousness. *Lancet, 304*(7872), 81–84.

CHAPTER 17

Spinal Cord Injury

Marsha Branche-Spelich
Ivy Ann Reyes
David Miller

LEARNING OBJECTIVES

At the end of this chapter, the reader will be able to

- State general anatomy and physiology of the spinal cord and common causes of spinal cord injuries.
- Recognize common presentations and complications of spinal cord injuries and identify appropriate nursing interventions.
- Identify functional outcomes and goals for a patient with spinal cord injury.
- List common risk factors by body system impacted for a patient with a spinal cord injury.
- Discuss the signs and symptoms of autonomic dysreflexia and appropriate treatment.

KEY CONCEPTS AND TERMS

Activity-based restorative therapies	Cauda equina	Poikilothermic
Allodynia	Central cord syndrome	Pressure relief
Anterior cord syndrome	Conus medullaris	Psychogenic erection
ASIA Impairment Scale	Heterotopic ossification	Reflexogenic erection
Autonomic dysreflexia	Lower motor neuron (LMN)	Spinal shock
Bladder tapping	Muscle spasms	Tetraplegia
Brown-Sequard syndrome	Paraplegia	Upper motor neuron (UMN)
	PLISSIT	

Spinal cord injury (SCI) is a disability commonly treated in the rehabilitation environment. SCI may seem to be simple—damage to the spinal cord causes paralysis. However, SCI is actually very complex. In this chapter authors will identify the body systems impacted by SCI, present complications, describe various presentations of SCI, and highlight appropriate nursing care and interventions in the rehabilitation environment.

BACKGROUND

There are an estimated 250,000 or more spinal cord–injured individuals living in the United States, with approximately 12,000 new cases of SCI occurring each year (National Spinal Cord Injury Statistical Center [NSCISC], 2009a). The most common cause of SCI is motor vehicle accidents, followed by falls and violence (NSCISC, 2009) (Figure 17.1).

In the 1970s the average age at the time of injury was 28.7 years, whereas in 2005 the average age at time of injury was 40.2 years (NSCISC, 2009b). It is important to note that the median age of the U.S. population increased by 8 years during this time frame as well. More than 75% of SCIs occur among males (NSCISC, 2009b). Since the

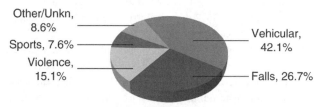

FIGURE 17.1 Causes of SCI since 2005.

1970s the ethnic distribution pattern of SCI has changed, decreasing among Whites and increasing among African Americans and Hispanics. Most persons with SCI are single (NSCISC, 2009b).

The incidence of **paraplegia** (involvement of two limbs) and **tetraplegia** (involvement of four limbs) is evenly split. (Quadriplegia is now referred to as tetraplegia, according to the Paralyzed Veterans Association.) Less than 1% of SCI individuals regain full neurological recovery by the time of hospital discharge (NSCISC, 2009a). Mortality rates are highest among individuals with SCI in the first year after injury (NSCISC, 2009a). Overall, life expectancy has improved for persons with SCI, but it is still less than that of persons without SCI. Two major factors that impact life expectancy after SCI are severity of injury and age at time of injury. Pneumonia, pulmonary embolism, and septicemia are leading causes of death after SCI (NSCISC, 2009a).

ANATOMY AND PHYSIOLOGY OF SCI

The spinal cord is a fibrous bundle of nerves, housed within the vertebral column and extending from the skull to the pelvic girdle. It is the communication highway from the brain to organs and muscles. The vertebral column is grouped into five regions: 7 cervical vertebrae, 12 thoracic vertebrae, 5 lumbar vertebrae, 5 bones fused together to form the sacrum, and 3 to 5 bones fused together to form the coccyx. The spinal cord is identified according to its location within the vertebral column; however, it ends below L1–2, where it becomes a loose collection of nerves that resembles a horse's tail; thus, the term "**cauda equina**" is used to describe this section of the spinal cord.

SCI occurs when the axons of the spinal cord are damaged. Traumatic injury can be caused by displaced bone fragments, disc material, or ligaments that cause pressure, bruises, or tear into the spinal cord tissue. This is often the result of a sudden blow or force, which causes vertebral fracture, compression, or dislocation. Nontraumatic causes of SCI include spinal tumors, degenerative changes, infections, embolic events, or congenital abnormalities.

ACUTE PHASE OF SCI

The acute treatment phase for SCI focuses on stabilization of respiratory, cardiac, and musculoskeletal systems. Often, corticosteroids are given during this acute phase, preferably within 4 to 8 hours of injury. The goal in stabilizing the fracture is to decompress the spinal cord and realign the vertebrae. This may require orthopedic surgery with pins, rods, or screws to stabilize the vertebral body. Odontoid cervical fractures may be stabilized with a halo brace. Other fractures may be treated with a variety of braces, such as a hard cervical collar or a thoracic-lumbar-sacral orthosis.

Spinal shock is observed in the initial phases of SCI. It is defined as the absence of spinal reflex activity below the level of the injury. Spinal shock can result in disruption of the autonomic system and can lead to hypotension and bradycardia. Spinal shock can last 8 to 12 weeks after injury. Return of reflexes below the level of injury signals the resolution of spinal shock.

Systems and function impacted by SCI include the bowel and bladder, the respiratory system, sensation, muscle tone, circulation, and sexuality and fertility. Secondary complications of SCI include urinary tract infections, pressure ulcers, pain, depression, spasticity, pneumonia, autonomic dysreflexia, heterotopic bone ossification, and renal damage.

EVALUATION AND ASSESSMENT

The American Spinal Cord Injury Association (ASIA) developed a classification system for the evaluation and assessment of SCI (available at http://www.asia-spinalinjury.org/publications/2006_Classif_worksheet.pdf). The **ASIA Impairment Scale** defines the function of motor and sensation below the level of injury. ASIA A indicates a "complete" injury—no motor or sensory function below the level of injury. ASIA B through D indicates levels of "incomplete" injury. Thus, an SCI will have a two-part label, for example, "C-4, ASIA A." The first part indicates a level, "C-4" (for damage at the fourth cervical vertebral level), and the ASIA rating, "ASIA A," in this case indicating a complete injury.

LEVEL OF INJURY

SCI presents as either an **upper motor neuron (UMN)** injury or **lower motor neuron (LMN)** injury. The clinical pictures between UMN and LMN injuries are markedly different.

UMN injuries represent damage to the motor pathways between the cerebral cortex and the conus medullaris, which is the distal end of the spinal cord. UMN injuries typically demonstrate a reflexic (spastic) motor pattern. Injuries sustained at T-11 to L-1 and above (cervical and thoracic injuries) are considered to be UMN injuries.

LMN injuries represent damage to the motor neurons connecting the spinal cord to muscle fibers. LMN injuries typically demonstrate an areflexic (flaccid) motor pattern. Injuries at L-1 and below (lumbar and sacral injuries) are considered to be LMN injuries.

Paraplegia is the impairment or loss of motor and/or sensory function in the trunk, legs, and pelvic organs. It occurs in injuries at or below T-2. Tetraplegia is the impairment or loss of motor and/or sensory function in trunk, legs, pelvic organs, and arms. It occurs in injuries at or above T-1.

LEVEL OF INJURY AND FUNCTIONAL OUTCOMES

The degree of return of function after an SCI depends on many factors, including the extent of direct destruction and secondary damage (hemorrhage and edema). Resolution of edema may produce an improvement of one to two levels. It is important to note that spasticity does not signify a return of function. Other factors that can influence functional outcome include level of injury, degree of completeness of the injury, personal motivation, preexisting conditions, level of fitness at time of injury, and anthropometric characteristics. Extrinsic factors that may influence functional outcomes include funding and the care setting—both during the acute and rehabilitative phases. There are no hard and fast rules for expected functional outcomes after SCI. However, presented below are some very general guidelines for potential movement, patterns of weakness, and impact on the level of independence according to the level of injury (Paralyzed Veterans of America, 1999).

An injury at level C1–3 is considered a UMN injury. Potential movement after this level of injury includes the preservation of neck flexion, extension, and rotation. Patterns of weakness with a C1–3 injury include total paralysis of trunk and upper and lower extremities. A person with a C1–3 injury typically presents as ventilator dependent due to the extent of respiratory involvement (the diaphragm may be paralyzed) and inability to clear secretions. Generally, total assistance is needed in all realms of daily care; however, the person with a C1–3 level SCI may be able to operate a power/tilt wheelchair with a "sip 'n puff" assistive device. Sip 'n puff technology allows the user to control devises such as a wheelchair by inhaling or exhaling through a straw. Global goals of rehabilitation include bladder care, bowel regulation,

pulmonary care, increasing sitting tolerance, determining and providing appropriate equipment and technology, and educating the patient to direct care needed. Twenty-four-hour care is typically needed.

A C-4 injury is also considered a UMN injury. Possible movements remaining after a C-4 injury include neck flexion, extension and rotation, and scapular movement. Patterns of weakness with a C-4 injury include trunk, upper and lower extremity weakness, inability to cough, and the respiratory reserve may be diminished secondary to paralysis of the intercostal muscles. Total assistance is needed in all realms of daily care; however, the person with a C-4 injury may be able to breathe without a ventilator. The person with a C-4 injury may also be able to operate a power/tilt wheelchair. Global goals of rehabilitation for this level of injury include bladder care, bowel regulation, pulmonary care (including cough assist), increasing sitting tolerance, determining and providing appropriate equipment and technology, and educating the patient to direct care needed. Twenty-four-hour care is typically needed.

After a C-5 injury possible movements remaining at this level include shoulder and elbow movements. Patterns of weakness for the person with a C-5 injury include the absence of elbow extension/supination and all wrist/hand movements as well as total paralysis of the trunk and lower extremities. The person with a C-5 injury may be able to perform self-feeding with equipment and set-up as well as some grooming tasks, turning pages, writing, and pressing buttons with adaptive equipment. Respiratory endurance and vital capacity are diminished, and the person with a C-5 injury may require assistance to clear secretions. They will remain dependent with bowel and bladder care. Global goals of rehabilitation include bladder care, bowel regulation, pulmonary care (including cough assist), increasing sitting tolerance, determining and providing appropriate equipment to allow performance of activities of daily living (ADLs) as able, and technology and educating patient to direct care needed. Personal and home care are required.

Possible movement remaining after a C-6 (UMN) injury includes C-5 movements plus wrist extension and forearm supination. Patterns of weakness include absence of wrist flexion, elbow extension, and hand movement. There is total paralysis of trunk and lower extremities. The person with a C-6 injury may be able to empty a leg bag, assist with level transfers, feed self with minimal assistance, bath and dress upper body, and drive a car from wheelchair level. They should be able to propel a wheelchair manually on indoor surfaces. Respiratory endurance and vital capacity remains diminished, and they may continue to require assistance to clear secretions. Global goals of rehabilitation include bladder care, bowel regulation, pulmonary care (including cough assist), increasing sitting tolerance, determining and providing appropriate equipment to allow performance of ADLs as able, and prescribing technology and educating patient to direct care needed. Some personal and home care are needed.

A C7–8 injury is still considered to be a UMN injury. Possible movements remaining after a C7–8 injury include C-6 movements plus elbow/wrist extension and finger and thumb movements. Patterns of weakness include limited hand dexterity and paralysis of trunk and lower extremities. The person with a C7–8 injury may require some assistance with bladder, bed mobility, and lower extremity dressing activities but can use the triceps arm muscles and thus perform manual pressure relief independently. The person will be independent with eating, grooming, level transfers, and upper extremity dressing and may be able to drive a car from a modified captain's chair. The patient will also be able to propel a manual wheelchair on even outdoor terrain. Respiratory endurance and vital capacity remain low, and the person with a C7–8 SCI may continue to require assistance to clear secretions. Global goals of rehabilitation include modification of the environment to allow maximal independence, bladder care (may be able to self-catheterize), bowel regulation (may be able to assist), pulmonary care (including cough assist), increasing sitting tolerance, building endurance, determining and providing appropriate equipment to allow performance of ADLs as able, and technology and education to direct care as appropriate.

A T1–9 level SCI is considered to be an LMN injury. Possible movement remaining after a T1–9 injury includes fully intact upper extremities with limited upper trunk stability. Patterns of weakness include lower trunk and lower extremity paralysis. The person with a T1–9 injury is expected to be independent in most realms of self-care, in car with hand controls, with light housekeeping, and with management of wheelchair. Vital capacity and endurance remain compromised, and the person with a T1–9 injury remains wheelchair dependent. Global goals of rehabilitation include instruction for independence in bladder and bowel care, wheelchair and transfer management on both even and uneven surfaces (including shower chair), increasing sitting tolerance, independence with manual pressure relief, building endurance, determining and providing appropriate equipment to allow perfor-

mance of ADLs as able, and technology and educating patient to direct care needed. Minimal home-making assistance is required.

A T10–L1 SCI is considered to be an LMN injury. Possible movement remaining after a T10–L1 injury includes good trunk stability and upper extremity movement. Patterns of weakness include paralysis of lower extremities. Expected functional outcomes are as above for T1–9 but also includes intact respiratory function.

An L2–S5 SCI is considered to be an LMN injury. Possible movements include partial to full control of lower extremities. Patterns of weakness may include partial paralysis of lower extremities. Expected functional outcomes include bathing with a tub bench, standing and heavy housekeeping, and functional ambulation with appropriate orthotics or assistive device. The person with an L2–S1 injury may still require hand controls for driving.

INCOMPLETE SCI SYNDROMES

SCIs can be classified as complete or incomplete. Complete injuries indicate total damage to the spinal cord nerve pathways. Incomplete injuries can present with varying degrees of sensory, motor, and autonomic function and varying degrees of recovery from partial to complete.

Central cord syndrome usually involves a hyperextension injury to the cervical region in older adults. Motor deficits with central cord syndrome are greater in the upper extremities than in the lower. Therefore, an individual with central cord syndrome presents with a gait that is less affected but with difficulty in feeding self, performing hygiene needs, and dressing. The degree of bowel and bladder dysfunction is variable. The functional goal of walking is usually achieved in these individuals.

Approximately 2% to 4% of SCIs result in **Brown-Sequard syndrome** (Vandenakker-Albanese & Zhao, 2008). Brown-Sequard syndrome is usually due to a penetrating injury or tumor. It occurs when there is damage to one side of the spinal cord. On the damaged side there is loss of motor function, proprioception, and vibratory sense below the level of the injury. On the opposite side there is loss of pain and temperature sensation. A patient with this type of syndrome can only feel pain on one side of body. In general, patients with this syndrome (Coggrave & Wilson-Barnett, 2008) may experience more return of function than most with SCI (Vandenakker-Albanese & Zhao, 2008).

Anterior cord syndrome is rare. Anterior cord syndrome occurs when there is damage to the anterior spinal artery. Typical causes are from bone fragments or a herniated disc. This results in paralysis and loss of pain, temperature, and touch sensation. However, position sense is preserved. Ten percent to 20% of patients affected by anterior cord syndrome experience return of motor function.

The **conus medullaris** is the distal end of the spinal cord. Most common causes of this SCI syndrome are due to lumbar stenosis, disc herniation, trauma, tumors, and spina bifida (Dawodu & Lorenzo, 2009). Conus medullaris syndrome may present with both UMN and LMN symptoms. Onset is usually sudden and presents bilaterally. Damage to this area (usually around L-1) may cause distal leg paresis, saddle anesthesia, erectile dysfunction, urinary retention, and fecal incontinence. Hypertonicity is typically present with UMN involvement. Recovery is variable and correlates to the ASIA impairment scale grading.

The cauda equina contains nerve roots from L1–5 to S1–5 and is housed in the subarachnoid space distal to the conus medullaris. Causes of cauda equina syndrome include trauma, disc herniation, tumors, and spinal stenosis (Eck, Hodges, & Humphreys, 2009). Cauda equina symptoms typically present gradually and unilaterally (Dawodu & Lorenzo, 2009). An injury to this area can result in loss of bowel, bladder, and sexual functions. Cauda equina injury presents with severe radicular (nerve root) pain with asymmetrical areflexic paraplegia, unilateral or asymmetrical paresthesia, and impotence. In many cases recovery depends on effectiveness of surgical decompression to relieve pressure on the nerves (Eck et al., 2009).

SYSTEM FUNCTIONS

Bowel

Neurogenic bowel is a common consequence of SCI and occurs when there is damage to the nerves that control bowel function. This condition presents both medical implications and quality of life issues. Bowel dysfunction has a significantly greater impact than other aspects of SCI (Coggrave & Wilson-Barnett, 2008). Bowel accidents (incontinence) are major contributor to psychological distress and represent a limitation factor in independence and resumption of normal activities, including sex. An evaluation of bowel function should be performed at the onset of SCI and then annually. Gastrointestinal symptoms tend to increase over time after SCI (Paralyzed Veterans of America, 1998b).

Assessment of bowel function after SCI should begin with a bowel history to assess for preexisting conditions that may affect bowel function and consequently bowel regulation. A physical examination is required and should include

- Abdominal assessment
- Rectal examination
- Assessment of anal sphincter tone
- Elicitation of the bulbocavernous and anocutaneous reflexes to determine UMN/LMN bowel pattern

In designing a bowel management program, the following factors should be considered:

- Assessment of function
  - Ability to learn and direct others
  - Sitting balance and tolerance
  - Upper extremity strength and function
  - Transfer skills
  - Anthropometric characteristics
- Equipment needs
- Home accessibility and environment
- Presence of attendant care
- Personal goals and lifestyle of the individual

Bowel management programs are usually a lifelong consequence of SCI. In managing neurogenic bowel, the development of a safe, effective, realistic bowel program is essential. The goals of a bowel program are to do away with unplanned elimination and to prevent long-term complications. A successful bowel program should produce predictable results on a regular schedule within 60 minutes of initiation of program. A successful bowel program should be scheduled at the same time every day, within 30 minutes of ingestion of food or warm liquids (to stimulate gastrocolic reflex). Once regulated, the bowel program can be scheduled every other day, as long as regulation is maintained and no other complications occur. The elements of a bowel program should begin with the least noxious stimulant(s) that creates effectiveness.

Neurogenic bowel in SCI typically presents either as a reflexic (UMN) or areflexic (LMN) bowel pattern. Reflexic and areflexic bowel programs are distinctly different and should be based on the type of neurogenic bowel pattern present. See Chapter 9 for more information on neurogenic bowel and bladder function.

A reflexic bowel program usually consists of the following:

- Putting patient in side-lying position.
- A rectal check and manual removal if needed to remove any stool in the rectum.
- Insertion of a chemical stimulant, such as a suppository.
- Digital stimulation (may cause **autonomic dysreflexia**).
- Assuming an upright position, if possible for evacuation.
- Rectal check postevacuation.
- Repeat of program if no results or if stool present postevacuation.

Stool consistency goal for reflexic bowel programs should be soft formed.

An areflexic bowel program usually consists of the following:

- Putting the patient in upright position, if possible, and side-lying position if not.
- If possible, encourage patient to perform Valsalva maneuver or lean forward while bearing down (bladder should be empty before performing this maneuver) to encourage evacuation.
- If evacuation does not occur, perform manual removal.
- Digital stimulation may or may not be effective.
- Repeat manual removal until rectum is cleared.

Stool consistency goal for areflexic bowel programs should be firm but not hard stool.

Adjunctive medications may be used in either type of program. Suppositories may be glycerin or contain medications such as bisacodyl. Oral medications such as stool softeners, laxatives, and fiber may also be used to obtain the desired stool consistency and improve effectiveness of program.

Adaptive equipment, based on the individual's functional capability, may be used. General mobility/transfer equipment such as rolling shower chairs/commode chairs and transfer boards are typically used. In addition, digital stimulators, suppository inserters, and adaptive equipment for clothes management may be used.

Monitoring the effectiveness of the bowel program is essential. A daily log that includes unplanned evacuation events as well as total time required for bowel program is helpful in determining success of the current regimen. If revision of the bowel program is required, only one element at a time should be changed. At least three to five cycles of the bowel program should take place

before another revision is made (Paralyzed Veterans of America, 1998b).

When revising a bowel program, consider the following components:

- Diet (foods that caused gastric distress before injury, such as beans or greasy foods, may cause bowel accidents after injury)
- Fluids
- Schedule of bowel program (consider frequency as well as time of day)
- Positioning
- Type of rectal stimulant
- Addition of digital stimulation
- Oral medications

A major role the nurse in the initial phases of rehabilitation it to educate the patient. Many times bowel accidents are misinterpreted as return of function. Additionally, the nurse must perform a detailed, comprehensive assessment and partner with the patient to develop a bowel program that promotes optimal results, is safe, and is easily replicated in the community (Box 17.1).

BOX 17.1   Web Exploration

An evidence-based clinical practice guideline for neurogenic bowel management in adults with SCI can be found at http://guideline.gov/content.aspx?id=850

Bladder

The overwhelming majority of patients with SCI experience voiding dysfunction. Bladder management differs between genders. After SCI 16% of males and 20% of females experience normal micturition at time of discharge (NSCISC, 2009a). The most common bladder management program for females at time of discharge is indwelling urinary catheter (NSCISC, 2009a). The most common bladder management program for males at time of discharge is an intermittent catheterization program (NSCISC, 2009a).

For normal micturition to occur, the detrusor muscle which surrounds the walls of the bladder contract and the sphincter relaxes. The sacral micturition center is located at S2–4; therefore, most SCIs result in some type of bladder/voiding involvement. The primary function of this reflex center is to cause the bladder to contract. The pontine micturition center is primarily responsible for relaxation of the urinary sphincter when the bladder contracts.

SCI above the level of the sacrum results in uninhibited bladder contractions. These individuals may also experience detrusor-external sphincter dyssynergia. In this case the bladder muscle, which contracts to force urine out, and the sphincter, which is supposed to relax to let the urine out, do not work in a coordinated fashion. This can result in high voiding pressures which can lead to hydronephrosis and renal deterioration (Paralyzed Veterans of America, 2006). This is also known as a reflexic bladder.

SCI at or below the level of the sacral cord results in an areflexic bladder pattern. The detrusor muscle is affected to a greater degree than the sphincter. This creates a flaccid bladder with a relatively intact sphincter, which leaders to bladder over-distention.

Intermittent catheterization programs are appropriate for those who have sufficient hand movement to allow self-catheterization or have a caregiver willing to perform the catheterization. The goal is to create a program that results in catheterization volumes consistently less than 500 mL. This usually requires the individual to wake at night to perform catheterization. Monitoring of fluid intake is an element of success for this program. Males are generally more successful with this type of program than females. For those without a strong pinch grasp, there are adaptive equipment devices to assist with this type of program. Complications with this type of program may be noncompliance with catheterization times, recurrent urinary tract infections, urethral irritation, and development of a false urethral passage (Box 17.2).

BOX 17.2   Web Exploration

Evidence-based clinical practice guideline for bladder management in adults with SCI can be found at http://www.pva.org/site/DocServer/Bladder.WEB.pdf?docID=1101

Browse these guidelines and compare them with the guideline from The Consortium for Spinal Cord Medicine found at http://www.ncbi.nlm.nih.gov/pmc/articles/PMC1949036

Indwelling urethral catheterization programs are appropriate for those with little or no hand movement, high fluid intake, high detrusor muscle pressures, or limited caregiver assistance. Individuals with long-term use of indwelling catheters may opt for the insertion of a suprapubic catheter, especially if a urethral fistula or recurrent urethral catheter obstructions have occurred. Complications with this type of program are clogged catheters, urethral erosions, recurrent urinary tract in-

fections, and epididymitis. Additionally, recurrent bladder infections and bladder stones are risk factors for bladder cancer. Individuals using this type of program should have frequent cystoscopic evaluations because these complications are also associated with indwelling catheters (Paralyzed Veterans of America, 2006). Reflex voiding can occur in those with an intact sacral micturition reflex. In this case involuntary bladder contractions occur, but the sphincter relaxes intermittently (detrusor muscle dyssynergia)—not in a coordinated fashion. This can result in involuntary voiding, with little to no warning. Those individuals may require a collecting device, such as an external catheter, to stay dry. Interventions to overcome detrusor sphincter dyssynergia such as **bladder tapping**, sphincterotomy, or urethral stents may be effective. Complications with external catheter programs are penile skin breakdown, failure of device, and poor compliance with fluid restrictions.

A sphincterotomy may be an option to reduce the voiding pressures associated with detrusor sphincter dyssynergia. This goal of this procedure is to improve bladder emptying. It results in permanent incontinence and 30% to 60% may have to have the procedure repeated (Paralyzed Veterans of America, 2006).

Skin

Maintaining intact and healthy skin is extremely important to a person with SCI, more so than for almost any other population when considering all the additional risk factors present. Depending on the level of the injury sensation is affected, and mobility, nutrition, and circulation may also be affected (Mauk, 2007).

The primary reason SCI patients are more at risk is their forced immobility due to the restrictions of their level of injury. Sensation is altered, and the most problematic for skin is decreased sensation because the person cannot respond to the normal sign of tissue damage, which is pain. Patients are comfortable staying in one position for an extended period of time but must be educated in the importance of **pressure relief**. Turning while lying in bed is the most common form of pressure relief. It is important to make sure the weight of the person's body is now on a completely different location to give the area that was just receiving pressure a chance to recover.

The way in which movement of the patient is accomplished is also important. Friction and shearing of the skin can occur when a patient is moved across a surface. To prevent this, two people should assist in moving the patient so they may lift the patient instead of dragging him or her. Raising the knee portion of the bed when raising the head of the bed also reduces shearing. Use of a lift sheet or mechanical lifts are also helpful to prevent injury. Despite these preventive measures, a wound may develop to such a size that it will not heal in a reasonable amount of time. In these cases skin flap surgery can be done. During this surgery the skin is pulled over the open wound area and then surgically closed. Skin grafts may also be involved. Chapter 8 provides more detailed information about skin and wound care.

Respiratory System

Four major muscles help an individual breathe: the intercostal muscles, neck muscles, diaphragm, and abdominal muscles (Figure 17.2). After SCI a patient's breathing and lungs are not normally affected; however, the muscles mentioned above might be. The patient's ability to effectively breathe in and out will depend on the level of injury and extent of muscle weakness. Injuries above T-12 maintain the function of the four respiratory muscle groups. The higher the injury, the greater the loss to respiratory muscle controls.

> *Respiratory complications after SCI remain the number one cause for morbidity and mortality in acute and chronic SCI.*

Respiratory complications after SCI remain the number one cause for morbidity and mortality in acute and chronic SCI. It is very important to lessen the complication associated with this problem. No matter what level of

SCI a person has, it is still important to treat respiratory infections aggressively. Serious respiratory complications include pneumonia, atelectasis, and even death (Zimmer, Gosgarian, & Kwaku, 2007). Although more problems are seen in patients with high level injuries compared with the low level injuries, the primary cause of death after SCI, regardless of level of injury, is respiratory insufficiency and complications associated with impaired respiratory function.

Spasms and Spasticity

Muscle spasms generally begin to occur after spinal shock and are an exaggeration of normal reflexes. They are triggered primarily by range of motion and stretching. Increased muscle spasms have also been associated with urinary tract infections, bowel fullness, or other medical complications. Because of this muscle spasms can be used as an early warning sign before regular signs and symptoms occur. Spasms are not necessarily something that needs to be completely rectified; many patients find a way to use their spasms once they figure out there is a predictable trigger and response. For instance, it may assist them with eating, transferring, or walking. Spasticity should not be confused with the return of function or seizures. Though involuntary, due to their intensity muscle spasms take a lot of the body's energy and can leave a person who has frequent spasms tired.

Baclofen is a common medication used to decrease muscle spasms, and its main side effect is drowsiness. Muscle spasms can be extremely painful, even though

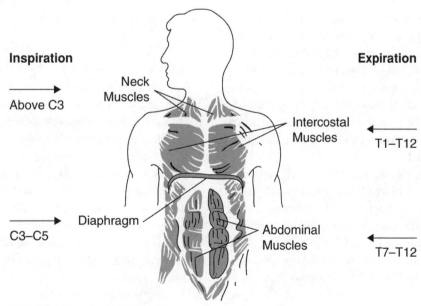

FIGURE 17.2   Muscles and spinal levels involved with breathing.

the patient may not have sensation below their level of injury. This can also make baclofen an effective pain reliever. However, using too high a dose of muscle relaxant can leave the person unable to participate in therapy due to the loss of what tone they did have. There is often a therapeutic balance that must be found between pain, usefulness, and the side effects of medications used to decrease spasms (Nesathurai, 2000).

Heterotopic Ossification

Heterotopic ossification, the development of bone outside the skeleton, tends to occur in 10% to 20% of SCI patients, most commonly in the first 2 months after the injury. It becomes rarer past 6 months. Heterotopic ossification generally occurs in the joints below the level of injury, most commonly the hips and knees. Manifestations may include decreased range of movement, pain, swelling, and erythema (Nesathurai, 2000).

Treatment for heterotopic ossification must take into consideration the effect it has on the patient's functional ability. If there is no negative impact on the patient, then no treatment may be necessary. If the patient's ability to function is impaired, then most cases can be managed with physical therapy or anti-inflammatory medications. If range of motion cannot be improved or maintained, then surgery may be needed to remove the ossification. Removal of the affected area can only occur after the mass has stopped growing. If it is removed before the termination of growth, it will continue to grow again after the surgery.

Autonomic System

Autonomic dysreflexia is unique to the SCI population and is a medical emergency. If left untreated it can cause seizures, brain hemorrhage, and death. Autonomic dysreflexia occurs in up to 90% of those with SCIs at or above T-6. It is also more common in males than in females. Autonomic dysreflexia is caused by anything the body interprets as a noxious stimulus below the level of injury (Paralyzed Veterans of America/Consortium for Spinal Cord Medicine, 2001).

Autonomic dysreflexia is most commonly caused by a distended bladder or bowel. Other triggers include ingrown toenails, tight clothing, wounds, infection, sexual activity, pregnancy, fractures, and deep vein thrombosis. The primary symptom of dysreflexia is a rise in blood pressure of 20 to 40 mm Hg above the patient's baseline and an accompanying headache. Other symptoms of autonomic dysreflexia include bradycardia, flushing, goose bumps, nasal congestion, flushing, and sweating above the level of injury. Every patient manifests autonomic dysreflexia differently, so it is important to note each patient's symptoms to help make identification of future episodes easier (Paralyzed Veterans of America/Consortium for Spinal Cord Medicine, 2001).

Treatment for autonomic dysreflexia is finding and removing the irritating stimulus. The first step is to check the patient's blood pressure. If autonomic dysreflexia is confirmed, the patient's head should be raised and their legs lowered to decrease the blood pressure. The next step is to remove any tight or constricting clothing. These actions help to lower the blood pressure further and may be the cause. The third step is to find the cause. Empty the bladder and bowel and also look for any other cause. If the cause cannot be found quickly, then medical treatment may be necessary to keep the blood pressure under control. Nitro-paste or nitro-pills are often used to bring the blood pressure down rapidly while the cause is found. Surgery may also be needed if the cause is internal, such as kidney stones. Prevention is the key and can most easily be accomplished with excellent bladder, bowel, and skin care.

After the initial blood pressure confirms an episode of autonomic dysreflexia, the nurse should notify the physician and continue to monitor the blood pressure every 5 minutes. In the meantime the nurse should be looking for the cause and administering any medication ordered by the medical doctor to keep the blood pressure close to the patient's normal levels. The family or caregivers can assist the patient to get undressed as needed and to reduce external stimuli. Turning lights off, turning of the television, and remaining calm all contribute to keeping the patient's blood pressure down.

Orthostasis

An additional result of SCI at the T-6 level that is a result of autonomic system dysfunction is orthostatic hypotension. The patient is not able to adapt to changes in position as readily as a person without SCI. Orthostatic hypotension is a result of the interruption in the control of vasopressor reflexes below the level of injury that controls the narrowing of the blood vessels. There is also a lack of muscle contraction in the extremities and abdomen that accounts for the slow and insufficient blood flow to the heart. The result is decreased cardiac output, low blood pressure, venous pooling, and decreased blood flow to the brain. These symptoms manifest as lightheadedness, blurred vision, faintness, weakness, and dizziness. If symptoms do occur, the head of the bed is lowered or the wheelchair is reclined and the legs elevated (Love, 2001).

In most cases the patient may be able to retrain the body and strengthen its response to positional changes. To aid the body, compression stockings should be applied to the lower extremities and an abdominal binder can be used to help increase venous return. Other preventive measures include drinking adequate amounts of water, slowly changing position, and doing ankle pumps depending on the patient's level of injury. ProAmatine is a common medication used to help maintain blood pressure. Adequate fluid intake and a balanced diet also help to maintain proper blood pressure. It is important, however, to remember that blood is diverted to the process of digestion after a large meal, and extra time may be needed for a patient safely attempt movement after eating.

One type of therapy aimed directly at increasing the body's tolerance of orthostasis is using a tilt table. After a person with SCI is able to tolerate sitting up in bed and then sitting up in a chair, the tilt table may be applicable. It is used to simulate a standing position by securing the patient to the table when it is flat and then increasing the incline as tolerated. Tolerance is measured by the person's self-report of symptoms of hypotension and by measuring the blood pressure with each increase in angle. The blood pressure reading is compared with the person's baseline. The eventual goal is to have the patient reach the vertical position while being asymptomatic of hypotension.

Thermoregulation

Thermal regulation is the body's ability to maintain temperature within normal limits of 97.0 to 100.0°F. In the SCI patient the autonomic system may be impaired in such a way that it interrupts the normal regulatory functions of the body. Functions like vasoconstriction, vasodilatation, shivering, and sweating may not occur appropriately. The person with an SCI then becomes "**poikilothermic**," meaning they have a body temperature that varies with the temperature of their environment. The most common way to lower the environmental temperature of a person is by the use of a fan or application of ice packs if not contraindicated through decreased sensation. Because of this body temperatures above 100°F can occur in the summer heat or in an overly heated room. Elevated temperatures due to environment can be managed by removing blankets or heavy clothing, spritzing the body with cool water, staying in the shade, or drinking cool liquids. Body temperatures below 97°F that occur in cooler environments—air-conditioned rooms or winter cold—can be managed by adding coverings or covering the head and changing the environmental temperature by adjusting the ambient temperature, but hot and cold liquids should be used with caution because of the risk of burns. Do not place hot packs or cold packs directly on the skin of the person with an SCI. This is important for people without SCI but especially for SCI patients because of their altered sensation (Love, 2001).

> *Persons with an SCI may have difficulty with body temperature regulation, resulting in becoming "poikilothermic," in which the body temperature varies with the temperature of their environment.*

It is always important to rule out other causes of a high or low temperature reading of an SCI patient before assuming the current body temperature is due to the environment. It is also important that people with SCI dress appropriately for the environment.

Pain

Pain ranks among the most difficult problem after SCI, together with other problems that may or may not exist depending on the level of injury, such as spasticity, altered bowel and bladder functions, and sexual dysfunctions.

After SCI, patients often experience different kinds of pain, including neuropathic and musculoskeletal pain. The chronic pain that SCI patients experience is from the abnormal communication and processing between the brain and the rest of the body. Musculoskeletal pain results from overuse of tissues in the body such as bones, joints, and muscle. This type of pain is usually relieved with narcotics and nonsteroidal anti-inflammatory drugs. Neuropathic pain is unrelated to movement and often worsens with infections. This pain is often described as "pins and needles." Neuropathic pain is associated with **allodynia** (pain from something that is not usually painful) and hyperalgesia (extreme pain caused by something that normally causes a little pain) and does not usually respond to opioids; however, certain anticonvulsants or antidepressants may help to manage it.

It is important for the rehabilitation nurse to be proactive with pain management for the person with SCI. Timely pain management interventions enable the patient to attend and progress in therapies.

Conventional and alternative complementary treatments are commonly used in treatment of pain for the person with SCI. Medications used in the treatment of pain after SCI include nonsteroidal anti-inflammatory medications such as Motrin or Advil, antiseizure medications like Lyrica and Neurontin, narcotics such as codeine and morphine, muscle relaxants and antispasticity medications such as baclofen and tizanidine (Zanaflex), and topical local analgesics like the Lidoderm patch for allodynia (Paralyzed Veterans of America, 2010). Alternative treatments include Transcutaneous Electical Nerve Stimulation (TENS), acupuncture, massage, and relaxation techniques. Depression and other psychosocial problems such as anxiety and stress are often seen in persons with SCI who have had chronic pain.

Sex and Reproduction

Sexuality is consistently identified as one of the most important topics for individuals after SCI (Widerstrom-Noga, Felipe Cuervo, Broton, Duncan, & Yezierski, 1999). SCI affects individuals and their relationships in multiple domains. As medical science has advanced, researchers have made great strides in understanding and restoring an individual's ability to function after a devastating trauma such as SCI It is adamantly held that intimacy, irrespective of level of injury, can be maintained (Paralyzed Veterans of America, 2010).

New nurses often feel uncomfortable when patients ask questions regarding sex and sexual function. The role of the healthcare provider is to ensure that people with SCI have access to the information they need regarding these topics.

One of the tools that can help in providing education regarding sexuality is the **PLISSIT** model. The PLISSIT model stands for **P**ermission, **L**imited **I**nformation, **S**pecific **S**uggestions, and **I**ntensive **T**herapy (McBride & Rines, 2000; Annon, 1976). Because many sexual problems are caused by anxiety, guilt feelings, or inhibitions, in addition to the physiological reasons like SCI and stroke, the nurse therapist can use her or his professional authority to simply "give permission" to do what the patient is already doing, alleviating unnecessary suffering. The intervention of limited information is to simply give patients correct anatomical and physiological information to restore their sexual functioning. It is not at all uncommon that patients have erroneous notions about the functioning of their own body after SCI and thus fall victim to unrealistic expectations. In such cases a little more factual information and education is necessary. The intervention of specific suggestions requires practical hints or exercises tailored to the individual case. Only the last intervention, intensive therapy, requires a long-term plan to address complex underlying causes such as SCI. This type of therapy is often done by an expert therapist who specializes in addressing sexual function in this population. Thus, the whole PLISSIT model represents a graduated system of therapeutic sieves in which the easy cases are caught and eliminated first, and the more difficult cases sink to the bottom in steadily diminishing numbers.

Annon's (1976) pragmatic and practical model is a useful reminder for all therapists and their clients that not every sexual problem requires the whole therapeutic arsenal. When planning for education and intervention on this topic it is important to determine the patient's readiness to learn about sexual function and expression after his or her SCI and that the utmost privacy and respect is afforded to the patients.

It is important to maintain an open discussion about sexuality and to provide access to education about sex in both formal and informal settings throughout the patient's stay. Team members can take an active role in providing assurance to the individual that basic information about sexuality will be provided and that more extensive information will be available throughout care. The topic of sexuality should be introduced in a straightforward and nonjudgmental manner. Open-ended questions that encourage an ongoing dialogue should be used. Providing opportunities for patients to include their partners in discussions regarding intimacy, sexuality, and fertility is helpful (Annon, 1976). If underlying problems regarding sexuality, intimacy, and fertility are not addressed, the patient and his or her significant other will experience some degree of difficulty when the patient goes back to the community. A male with SCI may or may not be able to achieve erection. The level, severity, time elapsed, and type of the injury may determine this (NSCISC, 2009a):

- *Level:* Generally, a complete lower level injury precludes the ability to have erections. However, persons with an upper level injury usually can have erections. In general, the higher the injury, the more chance of achieving and maintaining a complete erection.
- *Severity:* If the injury is incomplete, there is a better chance for a complete erection.
- *Time elapsed since injury:* Men who are unable to have an erection shortly after the injury may regain the capability during the first year.
- *Type:* Spastic paraplegics, for example, have a much greater chance of achieving an erection than individuals with flaccid paraplegia.

Male SCI patients experience changes in their sexual function and ability to biologically father children. In addition to these changes, most men also experience emotional issues that often affect their overall sexuality.

Two types of erections are discussed below. The brain is the source of psychogenic erections. The process begins with sexual stimulation or arousing. Signals from the brain are then sent through the nerves of the spinal cord down to the T10–L2 levels. The signals are then relayed to the penis and trigger an erection. A reflexogenic erection occurs with direct physical contact to the penis, is involuntary, and can occur without sexually stimulating thoughts. The nerves that control a man's ability to have a reflex erection are located at S2–4 of the spinal cord. Men with complete injuries are less likely to experience psychogenic erections. However, most men with SCI are able to have a reflexogenic erection with physical stimulation regardless of the extent of the injury if the S2–4 nerve pathways are not damaged.

- **Psychogenic erections** result when messages are passed down the spinal cord from the brain to the sacral area. Depending on the level and completeness of the injury to the spinal cord, men with SCI may or may not experience psychogenic erections (Spinal Cord Injury Information Network, n.d.). In men with lower level injuries, researchers report that up to 83% with *incomplete* lower level injuries had psychogenic erections and up to 26% of men with complete lesions have psychogenic erections. In men with incomplete upper level injuries, up to 25% can achieve psychogenic erections.
- **Reflexogenic erections** result from direct stimulation of the genital area. They are called reflexogenic because they are controlled by a reflex arc between the genital area and the spinal cord. In men with upper level injuries, researchers report that up to 98% of men with *incomplete* upper level injuries have reflexogenic erections and up to 93% of men with *complete* upper level injuries have reflexogenic erections; 7% do not have erections.

Females with SCI will discover that sexuality is still an important part of their lives. It may take some time for a newly injured woman to become comfortable with her body and resume natural feelings of sexuality. Healthy adjustment begins with knowing the facts about the impact of SCI on sexual issues.

In actuality, few physiological changes after injury prevent women from engaging in sexual activity. Some women have decreased vaginal lubrication. This problem is likely the result of the interruption in normal nerve signals from the brain to the genital area. Although most women with SCI maintain some degree of lubrication, a water-based lubricant (never use oil lubricants), such as K-Y jelly, can facilitate sexual activity. Another change that women with SCI may notice is that it takes longer for an orgasm to occur. A vibrator may help women with injury below the T-6 level. It may also helpful to speak to the physician to see if medications could be adjusted to minimize impact on sexual responses.

It is normal for most women to experience a brief pause in their menstrual cycle after SCI. This pause may last as long as 6 months after injury. However, the ability of women to have children is not usually affected once their period resumes (PVA, 1999).

Areas of concern regarding sexual activity usually center around

- Urinary accidents
- Bowel accidents
- Not satisfying a partner

Psychological

It is not uncommon for an SCI patient to feel depressed and to be in denial after being diagnosed with SCI. SCI is a life-changing event. One can be walking one day and the next minute is paralyzed due to an accident. The impact is sudden, and patients and their families are often not ready to face the circumstances surrounding it. Therefore, it is a must for the interdisciplinary team to be sensitive to the needs not only of the patient but to the whole family as well. Chronic pain sufferers often experience depression; because of this it is important to alleviate pain to help with a patient's psychological well-being (Paralyzed Veterans of America, 1998a).

ROLES OF THE CAREGIVER

Caregivers are important in the rehabilitation of the person with SCI. The caregiver may be a family member, a close friend, or a hired assistant. The role of the caregiver is to provide assistance to the person with SCI but not to impede his or her progress toward independence. Ideally, the patient will be able to teach any given caregiver the proper way to care for him or her, making the caregiver an extension of the patient's independence (Burdsall, 1999).

Hiring a Caregiver

Many times a caregiver is needed after a patient with an SCI leaves the acute care setting. If more skilled services are needed, such as with a higher level SCI, then the caregiver may have to be specially trained before the patient leaves the rehabilitation setting. The amount of time required for this process varies with who is being taught. Teaching family members with no medical background or experience working with people who require intensive care will take longer to train. Many professional caregivers are also not familiar with the unique needs of a person with an SCI (Case Study 17.1).

CASE STUDY 17.1

Jacob is a 19-year-old man who is on the acute rehabilitation unit after a motorcycle accident in which he sustained a complete SCI at T-6. Jacob was previously active in motocross racing and was an exceptional athlete with a full scholarship to Navy for football. He is experiencing depression and has many questions about his condition.

Questions

1. What are the most important issues to address with Jacob?
2. How can the rehab nurse help Jacob adjust to his physical limitations?
3. What education needs to be done with Jacob's family and significant others?
4. In terms of realistic expectations, what do you say to Jacob when he says he expects that his life will go on just as it was going to as soon as he recovers?
5. What team members should be consulted regarding his depression?

A caregiver's skills and resources they can offer must be compatible with the patient's needs. Interviews and background checks are suggested; however, these require time and money. The patient, family, hospital, care manager, or employer may search for and hire the caregiver. A caregiver may not always be available, so it is important to have at least one backup helper. Abuse is another risk. A person with an SCI is vulnerable and can be subject to various forms of abuse similar to that of an elderly person because of their dependence on others for care (Burdsall, 1999). With this in mind it is always important to stress to patients while in the inpatient unit that abuse or any abusive behavior should not be tolerated by them, especially when it happens in the confines of their home after their discharge from the unit. Patients should be given resources and tools they can use to report any abuse accurately and in a timely fashion.

AGING WITH AN SCI

As the life span of persons with SCI increases, there is a growing focus on successful aging. There are two pictures of aging with SCI: the person who acquires an SCI

at a young age and the person who acquires an SCI at an advanced age. The two pictures are different, yet both are important. Consider the following.

John was injured at age 38 during a football game. A C-6 tetraplegic, before the injury he was the perfect picture of health. All body systems—renal, cardiac, pulmonary, musculoskeletal—were in perfect condition. His cholesterol, blood pressure, and blood sugar were all normal. John worked a physically demanding job and was also very athletic, playing competitive sports in his community. He belonged to a gym and had the much dreamed of "six-pack" abdominal muscles. John took no medications, no illicit drugs, and drank only moderate alcohol during social occasions.

Gary was injured at age 7, when his brother pushed him down the stairs. Now 38, Gary has been a complete C-6 tetraplegic since that time. Sedentary for the past 31 years, he just feels old. His cholesterol is elevated, and he takes statins for this problem. His weight has been creeping up, and he has a chronic sacral pressure ulcer. Gary has repeated urinary tract infections from his catheterization program and has had a colostomy for the past 5 years for bowel management. The doctors are watching Gary's lab work related to his kidneys, suspecting that chronic use of multiple medications has affected his renal function. Gary's shoulders have started to hurt when he propels the wheelchair, and he can no longer assist with transfers due to shoulder pain. He is concerned that his wrists will soon show signs of overuse as well.

Although these men are the same age, it is clear that the effect of SCI over time can affect the overall health. Now consider how each of their health pictures might look at age 55, 65, and 75.

Normal signs of aging are superimposed upon SCI and complicate the picture. These include aging changes in the cardiac, pulmonary, renal, musculoskeletal, and integumentary systems.

CURRENT RESEARCH AND EMERGING TRENDS

The concept of an irreparable central nervous system is slowly being challenged with interventions and modalities designed to promote repair and regeneration. Repair of the spinal cord and recovery of neurological function are fairly new concepts in spinal cord medicine, which has traditionally been focused on maximizing function through therapies and adaptive equipment. For instance, the use of stem cell therapy is a new and controversial intervention for SCI repair. Stem cell therapy represents the potential to limit damage or repair the spinal cord. **Activity-based restorative therapies** are evidence-based tools used for neurological recovery, thought to promote recovery through regeneration of nerve cells. Diaphragm muscle pacing, phrenic nerve pacing, and combined intercostals and unilateral diaphragm pacing techniques are currently being used to wean patients from ventilators and reduce the incidence of respiratory complications.

Another area of development and intense research is in the use of robotics either in the treatment/rehabilitative phase or to provide function in lieu of voluntary movement. Functional electrical stimulation has been used to stimulate grasp in tetraplegia, and new research has focused on integrating robotic orthosis to accomplish functional lower extremity movement.

Implantable devices to stimulate function have been another emerging trend. The sacral anterior root stimulator has been available for use with neurogenic bladders (Anthem, n.d.). Recent research has suggested it may be useful for neurogenic bowel as well. Independence from ventilators is now possible through use of an implantable device: Electrodes are surgically implanted onto the diaphragm and then a small electric current stimulates contraction of the diaphragm, which initiates inspiration (Rehabilitation Institute of Chicago, 2009). This procedure is replacing the phrenic nerve stimulator.

SUMMARY

The major focus for nursing is to provide support and education to the patient and family. Because of the sudden impact of SCI the patient and family need thorough guidance and education from the nursing staff. Most patients come to the rehabilitation unit with many questions they might have not asked while they were in the acute setting or were afraid to ask at all because of uncertainty. Family members are also the same; they are afraid and bewildered at times because of the suddenness of the situation. It is not uncommon for patients to have never set foot in a hospital before this event. Then, suddenly, loss of function occurs in a matter of minutes. The suddenness and scope of change is overwhelming to the patient and family.

The nurse must carefully assess readiness for learning and then involve the patient and family in all aspects of care, providing opportunities for learning and practicing needed skills. At times one of the challenges the nurse may face is denial by the patient and family and subsequent refusal to be taught: "I won't need to learn how to do _____, because I won't need that by the time I go home." Developing a therapeutic relationship with the patient and family and partnering as a team are critical to creating a successful and safe discharge.

CRITICAL THINKING

1. Consider the ASIA impairment scale. What is the difference between the various levels of injury?
2. Using the PLISSIT model, what level of involvement in sexuality education are you comfortable with at this point in your career? If you continue to work as a rehabilitation nurse, what level of education in this model do you believe you should aspire to?
3. What types of teaching are needed for a 29-year-old woman who is paraplegic but whose partner is pressuring her to have children before she is ready?

PERSONAL REFLECTION

- Imagine that you are enjoying a good time at the community swimming pool, playing with your friends. You dive in the deep end and hit your head on the bottom of the pool unexpectedly. Suddenly, you cannot move on your own. What would be going through your mind? Let's say that the lifeguard at the pool pulled you out of the water, but you still cannot feel anything below your neck. How would your life change in that instant? What changes would occur if you have a complete cervical SCI?
- Have you ever cared for a person who had an SCI? What challenges did he or she face? How was life different for him or her than for you?

REFERENCES

Annon, J. (1976). The PLISSIT model: a proposed conceptual scheme for the behavioural treatment of sexual problems. *Journal of Sex Education Therapy 2*, 1–15.

Anthem. (n.d.). Sacral nerve stimulation as a treatment of neurogenic bladder secondary to spinal cord injury. Retrieved September 1, 2010, from http://www.anthem.com

Burdsall, D. (1999). Hiring and management of personal care assistants for individuals with spinal cord injury. Santa Clara Valley, California: Spinal Cord Injury Project. Retrieved September 1, 2010, from www.tbi-sci.org/pdf/pas.pdf

Coggrave, M., & Wilson-Barnett, J. (2008). Management of neurogenic bowel dysfunction in the community after spinal cord injury: A postal survey in the United Kingdom. *Spinal Cord*, 323–330. Retrieved April 1, 2010, from http://pubget.com/search?q=doi:10.1038%2Fsc.2008.137

Dawodu, S. T., & Lorenzo, N. (2009). Cauda equina and conus medullaris syndromes. Retrieved December 1, 2010, from http://emedicine.medscape.com

Eck, J., Hodges, S., & Humphreys, C. (2009). Cauda equina syndrome. Retrieved December 1, 2010, from http://emedicine.medscape.com

Love, L. (2001). Cardiovascular and thermoregulatory control. In *Nursing practice related to spinal cord impairment: A core curriculum* (pp. 145–158).

Mauk, K. (2007). *The specialty practice of rehabilitation nursing. A core curriculum* (5th ed.). Glenview, IL: Association of Rehabilitation Nurses.

McBride, K. E. & Rines, B. (2000). Sexuality and spinal cord injury: A roadmap for nurses. *SCI Nursing, 17*(1), 8–13.

National Spinal Cord Injury Statistical Center (NSCISC). (2009a). NSCISC 2009 annual statistical report. Retrieved December 1, 2010, from http://www.nscisc.uab.edu

National Spinal Cord Injury Statistical Center (NSCISC). (2009b). Facts and figures at a glance. Retrieved September 1, 2010, from https://www.nscisc.uab.edu

Nesathurai, S. (2000). *The rehabilitation of people with spinal cord injury* (2nd ed.). Boston, MA: Blackwell.

Paralyzed Veterans of America. (1998a). *Depression following spinal cord injury: A clinical practice guidelines for primary care physicians.* Washington, DC: Author.

Paralyzed Veterans of America. (1998b). *Neurogenic bowel management in adults with spinal cord injury.* Washington, DC: Author.

Paralyzed Veterans of America. (1999). *Outcomes following traumatic spinal cord injury: A clinical practice guideline for health care professionals.* Washington, DC: Author.

Paralyzed Veterans of America/Consortium for Spinal Cord Medicine. (2001). *Acute management of autonomic dysreflexia: individuals with spinal cord injury presenting to health-care facilities.* Washington, DC: Author.

Paralyzed Veterans of America. (2006). *Bladder management for adults with spinal cord injury: A clinical practice guideline for health-care providers.* Washington, DC: Author.

Paralyzed Veterans of America. (2010). *Pain management after SCI: Consumer guide.* Washington, DC: Author.

Rehabilitation Institute of Chicago. (2009). RIC offers diaphragm pacing system to help patient with spinal cord injury regain independence, thrive in life. Retrieved December 1, 2010, from http://www.ric.org

Spinal Cord Injury Information Network. (n.d.). Sexual function for men with spinal cord injury. Retrieved August 15, 2010, from http://www.spinalcord.uab.edu/show.asp?durki=22405

Vandenakker-Albanese, C., & Zhao, H. (2008). Brown-Sequard syndrome. Retrieved August 15, 2010, from http://emedicine.medscape.com

Widerstrom-Noga, E. G., Felipe Cuervo, E., Broton, J. G., Duncan, R. C., & Yezierski, R. P. (1999). Perceived difficulty in dealing with consequences of SCI. *Archives of Physical Medicine Rehabilitation, 80*(5), 580–6.

Zimmer, M., Gosgarian, & Kwaku, N. (2007). Effect of spinal cord injury on the respiratory system. *Basic Research and Current Clinical Treatment Option, 30*(4), 319–330.

CHAPTER 18

Total Joint Replacement

Laura Horman
Ethan Roberts

LEARNING OBJECTIVES

At the end of this chapter, the reader will be able to

- Recognize the implications for total joint replacement.
- Identify major potential complications after total joint replacement.
- Discuss care-planning needs after total joint replacement.
- Describe aspects of rehabilitation care after total joint replacement.

KEY CONCEPTS AND TERMS

Active assistive range of motion	Extracellular matrix (ECM)	Shoulder arthroplasty
Active range of motion	Hip arthroplasty	Synovial joint
Articular cartilage	Hip precautions	Synovial membrane
Avascular necrosis	Knee arthroplasty	Total joint replacement
Chondrocytes	Passive range of motion	Weight bearing as tolerated (WBAT)
	Rheumatoid arthritis	

The goal of **total joint replacement** is to decrease pain and to increase or restore function. Conservative treatments of joint pain and decreased function are attempted first, but when they fail surgical intervention is considered. The surgeon considers level of pain, functional limitations, and risk versus benefit (Brander & Stulberg, 2006). With the advancements in surgical techniques, longevity of implants, and surgeon experience, these procedures are being performed on patients who may not have been candidates years ago (Brander & Stulberg, 2006). Total hip, knee, and shoulder replacements are being performed on persons of all ages with multiple medical issues and disabilities in an attempt to improve quality of life.

Attempts to treat painful hips surgically date back to at least 1826, where soft tissue, wood, and gold foil were used (Zimmerman, 1998). The first attempt at replacing a hip joint was performed by Wiles in 1938 (Zimmerman, 1998). According to the American Academy of Orthopedic Surgeons (2009a), the first successful hip replacement was performed in 1960, and today there are 193,000 performed in the United States annually.

The first attempt at replacing a knee joint was in the 1950s with a hinged design by Wallidus (Zimmerman, 1998). According to the American Academy of Orthopedic Surgeons (2009b), the first successful knee replacement was performed in 1968, and today there are 581,000 performed in the United States annually. Knee replacements are expected to increase to more than 3.4 million by 2030 (Topp, Swank, Quesada, Nyland, & Malkani, 2009).

The first attempt at replacing a shoulder joint was performed by Pean in 1893 (Wilcox, Arslanian, & Millett, 2005). In the 1990s approximately 5,000 shoulder replacements were performed annually (Wilcox et al., 2005). The American Academy of Orthopedic Surgeons (2009a) cites 27,000 shoulder replacements are performed in the United States annually.

PATHOPHYSIOLOGY REVIEW

Synovial Joint

A **synovial joint** is a joint that allows for movement. Most joints in the human body are synovial joints. A typical synovial joint is composed of two moving bony surfaces, synovial membrane and synovial fluid within a joint space, joint capsule with ligamentous and/or muscular attachments, and sometimes other intra-articular structures (Gould & Hettings, 1985).

Although the synovial joint is designed for movement, it must have an underlying amount of stability. Some joints are inherently unstable to allow for function. A comparison of the shoulder and hip joints illustrates this. Although similar in structure (both a "ball and socket" type), the shoulder allows significantly more movement than the hip. Stability in a joint is provided by the bony configuration of the joint, joint capsule, ligamentous, and muscular structures. Optimal movement at a synovial joint could be described as controlled mobility, or mobility within stability.

A thin layer of articular cartilage covers the bony surfaces of a synovial joint. This articular cartilage is connected to the bone by a subchondral plate. The articular cartilage is essentially avascular. The combination of normal healthy articular cartilage in concert with synovial fluid within the joint space allows movement with minimal frictional resistance. The articular cartilage also helps with load disbursement to the underlying bone and acts as a shock absorber (Merck & Company, 2001)

Synovial Membrane

The **synovial membrane** is located on the inner surface of the joint capsule, which encloses the synovial capsule. It covers any ligaments or tendons that may pass through the joint. It does not cover the articular surfaces of the joint. The synovial membrane has essentially two layers: the intima, or synovial lining, and the subsynovial tissue. The intima is a thin layer of tissue approximately one to three cells in depth. Its major functions include the synthesis of hyaluronic acid that helps provide the joint lubrication properties of synovial fluid as well as assisting in nutritional and waste exchange with other structures of the joint (Gould & Hettings, 1985). The subsynovial tissue is a layer of fibrous connective tissue that is highly vascularized. This also facilitates the exchange of waste and nutrients.

Articular Cartilage

The primary components of **articular cartilage** are the **extracellular matrix (ECM)** and **chondrocytes**. The ECM consists of water, collagen, and aggrecan. The chondrocytes are the main cells within the articular cartilage. They are responsible for the synthesis and breakdown of the ECM, which is a continuous process in normal joint function. Because the articular cartilage is avascular, the chondrocytes rely on diffusion to receive nutrients and eliminate waste. This is achieved via synovial fluid, as well as through blood vessels in the synovial membrane and subchondral bone. Joint movement encourages diffusion, so some degree of movement is vital to overall joint health.

Articular cartilage gains its strength and mobility by way of its components and their arrangement. Although the ECM is primarily water, aggrecan in combination with collagen fibrils provide tensile strength yet allow for force disbursement and deformation. Aggrecan is a macromolecule consisting of small highly charged glycosaminoglycan chains that are interwoven with the collagen. The natural electrostatic repulsion of the aggrecan gives cartilage compressive stiffness (Felson, 2004). In early osteoarthritis, degradation of the ECM exceeds synthesis, which in turn leads to increased water uptake and cartilaginous swelling (Felson, 2004).

As mentioned previously, healthy articular cartilage is constantly remodeled. This process is facilitated by the chondrocytes. The chondrocytes are stimulated by and secrete enzymes that facilitate both synthesis and breakdown of the ECM. These abilities are limited in comparison with other connective tissues throughout the body (Merck & Company, 2001).

IMPLICATIONS FOR TOTAL JOINT REPLACEMENT

Osteoarthritis

Osteoarthritis is the most common form of arthritis. It is present in 13.9% of adults aged 25 and older and 33.6% of adults aged 65 and older (Centers for Disease Control and Prevention [CDC], 2009a). Typical symptoms include joint edema, pain, and stiffness. Rest usually relieves symptoms. X-rays find joint space narrowing, osteophytes, and bony sclerosis.

In the initial phases of osteoarthritis, chondrocytes become more metabolically active. Exactly why this occurs is unknown. Certain physical stresses may act in conjunction with genetic and other factors to initiate this process. This eventually leads to collagen breakdown and subsequent alteration of the ECM. This in turn leads to deterioration of cartilage strength and elasticity. The cartilage surface loses its smooth, slick surface as roughened areas and cracks may appear. Eventually, erosions in the cartilage extend to the level of subchondral bone. In the subchondral bone increasing quantities of bone grow, producing denser bone. There may be some evidence that this leads to decreased force attenuation and accelerates cartilage loss (Radin, 1986). In addition, chondral structures begin to form at the joint space in response to increased stress and tension. These are known as osteophytes and lead to further irregularities in the joint surface, although it is thought they may contribute to joint stability (Felson, 2004).

Synovial hypertrophy and fibrosis occur in most joints affected by osteoarthritis. This process may lead to further degradation of the articular cartilage by encouraging development of cytokines which in turn inhibit chondrocytes-mediated ECM synthesis, being a site for nocioceptive fibers, and by secreting excess synovial fluid, which may increase joint instability (Felson, 2004).

Multifactorial Aspects of Osteoarthritis

Exactly how and why osteoarthritis begins is unknown. There appears to be a complex interaction between many factors. Age, genetics, gender, previous injury, joint laxity, muscle weakness, obesity, and activity are major contributory factors that play a part in the susceptibility of developing osteoarthritis. Genetics plays a greater role in the development of hand and hip arthritis compared with that of the knee joint (Spector, Cicuttini, Baker, Loughlin, & Hart, 1996). Previous injury of a joint may damage structures within the joint and lead to secondary or traumatic arthritis. There appears to be evidence that age at the time of injury may play a part in the development of arthritis. Major injury to the knee after age 30 produces osteoarthritis more readily than in younger subjects (Roos, Adalberth, Dahlberg, & Lohmander, 1995). Normal movement is beneficial for joint health because it facilitates movement of synovial fluid through the joint and promotes nutrient and waste exchange throughout the avascular articular cartilage. However, it has been shown that certain occupations with repetitive movement have higher incidences of osteoarthritis development. Repetitive heavy lifting or squatting may predispose individuals to the development of osteoarthritis, especially in the knees. Obesity increases the amount of mechanical load across a joint.

Rheumatoid Arthritis

Rheumatoid arthritis is a systemic autoimmune disease that affects the synovial joints. In 2005, according to the CDC (2009b), 1.293 million adults, or 0.6% of the population, was suffering from rheumatoid arthritis in the United States. It typically affects women more than men in a ratio of approximately 2 to 3 to 1 (CDC, 2009b). It is typically diagnosed by a combination of physical evaluation of symptoms, laboratory tests, and radiographic results (CDC, 2009b).

Disease Process

T cells appear to initiate the disease, the reason for which is not completely understood. In a normal inflammatory response, the human body responds by increasing the production of blood vessels, lymphocytes, and macrophages to provide additional nutrition and production of new cellular material as well as the removal and digestion of dead and or foreign matter. Believing the body has been injured and healing needs to take place, an inflammatory process begins that includes the breakdown of supposed "foreign" matter. Unfortunately for the rheumatoid arthritis patient, this "foreign" matter is in actuality healthy joint tissue. The inflammatory response results in development of a thickened synovial lining as well as subintimal layer. These areas become infiltrated with inflammatory cells such as T and B lymphocytes, macrophages, and mast cells and the development of new blood vessel growth (Bathon, n.d.). The hypertrophied synovium, known as a pannus, covers the articular surfaces of the joint. The pannus spreads to cover the articular surfaces and propagates joint destruction through release of enzymes and the facilitation of the above listed cells in "attacking" and degrading the previously healthy articular surface.

Avascular Necrosis

According the American Academy of Orthopedic Surgeons (2009c), 10,000 to 20,000 people develop **avascular necrosis** per year. Diagnosis is typically made through a physical examination and use of diagnostic testing such as x-ray, magnetic resonance imaging, bone scan, and computed tomography (National Institute of Arthritis and Musculoskeletal and Skin Disease, 2009).

Avascular necrosis is the death of bone tissue due to ischemia or loss of blood supply. It may occur due to major trauma, such as hip fracture or dislocation or proximal humorous and/or glenoid fracture, or through other means including intraluminal obliteration, increased marrow pressure, or cytotoxicity (Lafforgue, 2006). Risk factors for the development of this disease include glucocorticoid (steroid) therapy, endogenous hypercorticism, organ transplant, systemic lupus erythematosus, alcohol abuse, pregnancy, dyslipidemia, Caisson disease, sickle cell disease, Gaucher disease, HIV, and idiopathic reasons. In addition to the above, other risk factors specific to the hip include femoral neck fractures, septic hip, decompression sickness, slipped capital femoral epiphysis, and Legg-Calvé-Perthes disease (Dudkiewicz et al., 2004). Typically, necrosis develops first in the area of yellow marrow. Due to alteration in blood flow as listed above and/or cytotoxic reasons, blood flow to bone tissue is interrupted, leading to cell death. Healing response through granulation tissue occurs, as this is laid down at the sight of injury. However, this response is inadequate in healing the initial destruction. The necrotic area becomes further weakened, resulting in eventual small compression fractures and, if unchecked, bone collapse (Lafforgue, 2006).

BRIEF REVIEW OF SURGICAL APPROACHES: EXPOSURE TO THE JOINT

The goal of joint replacement surgery is to provide function of the joint and to relieve pain. Several approaches are possible depending on the joint undergoing surgery.

Hip Arthroplasty

There are two primary approaches used for modern **hip arthroplasty**: anterior lateral and posterior lateral. Recently, a "mini-anterior" approach has also been popularized but has not yet been widely accepted. In the posterior-lateral approach the patient in positioned in a lateral decubitus position with the involved hip facing up. The leg is prepped and draped free to allow for full mobility. The skin incision centers over the greater trochanter extending laterally down the shaft of the femur and posterior over the gluteal muscles. The size of the incision usually depends on the size of the patient. The key component of any incision is to provide adequate exposure of the relevant anatomy. The fascia lata on the lateral aspect of the femur is then divided and the gluteus maximus is then split in the line of its fibers by blunt dissection. This then exposes the short external rotators of the hip. The tendon attachments of these muscles can then be tagged with a stay suture divided at the attachment and retracted posterior to protect the sciatic nerve. The sciatic nerve runs longitudinally emerging from the pelvis to innervate the leg. Once the short external rotators are divided the capsule can be divided, exposing the joint. The leg is the flexed, adducted, and internally rotated to dislocate the hip. A resurfacing arthroplasty of the hip can then begin at this point. If a total hip arthroplasty is to be performed, the femoral head is the removed, the leg is brought down to the table, and the acetabulum is exposed by placing retractors to hold the femur anteriorly.

The anterior-lateral approach to the hip is begun with the patient supine on the operating table. The leg is prepped and draped free and then flexed and brought across midline. A straight longitudinal incision is made laterally. Like the posterior-lateral approach the fascia is then divided, but in this approach it curves anteriorly in the interval between the gluteus medius and tensor fascia lata. A small portion of the gluteus medius tendon is released and the gluteus minimus is incised to expose the joint capsule. The capsule is then divided, and the hip is externally rotated to dislocate the hip and expose the femoral head. A resurfacing hip arthroplasty can then be performed or the head can be resected to expose the acetabulum for total hip arthroplasty.

Knee Arthroplasty

Total **knee arthroplasty** surgery begins with a midline anterior incision. The patient is positioned supine on the operating table. Once the skin incision is made the patella, patellar tendon, and quadriceps muscle can be seen. Approach to the joint can be made via a standard, subvastus, or midvastus incision in the quadriceps muscle–tendon unit. The standard approach follows the medial border of the patellar tendon and patella and divides the quadriceps tendon longitudinally in its medial one-third for a distance of a few centimeters. Retractors are then placed exposing the distal femur and the proximal tibia. As the name implies, the subvastus approach starts off like the standard approach, but instead of dividing the quadriceps tendon it runs beneath the vastus medialis tendon obliquely. Similarly, the midvastus approach divides through the body of the vastus medialis muscle instead of dividing the quadriceps tendon. Proponents of the subvastus and midvastus approach believe it hastens rehabilitation by not dividing the quadriceps tendon, whereas proponents of the standard approach stress the wide surgical exposure as a benefit.

Shoulder Arthroplasty

In **shoulder arthroplasty** a partial replacement such as a humeral head arthroplasty or a total shoulder replacement is performed through an anterior approach to the shoulder. This approach allows for full visualization of the bony anatomy of the humeral head and glenoid fossa of the scapula. This approach is also useful in other open procedures of the shoulder such as fixation of shoulder fractures.

The patient is positioned on the operating table in a "beach chair" position with the head of the table elevated about 30 degrees. The clavicle and humeral head can easily be palpated. The incision is made in the deltopectoral groove, the area where the deltoid muscle, which covers the top of the shoulder, blends with the pectoral muscle, which originates from the chest to attach to the proximal portion of the humerus. In this groove runs the cephalic vein, which is protected by retracting it either medially or laterally. Once the interval is opened and the fascia divided, the coracoid process of the scapula is seen with the biceps and coracobrachialis tendons running longitudinally from the top of the shoulder to the elbow. Lateral to these tendons is the subscapularis tendon, which lies directly across the shoulder joint. A stay suture (a suture used to identify, retract, or retrieve a structure) is placed and the subscapularis tendon and underlying joint capsule is divided longitudinally to expose the joint. Extending the capsular incision inferiorly, with care to avoid injury to axillary vessels and nerves, and externally rotating the arm provides full exposure to the humeral head. For total shoulder arthroplasty, once the humeral head has been resected, retractors are placed to expose the glenoid fossa.*

PROSTHETICS

The surgeon determines the type and size of a prosthetic needed during arthroplasty. The surgeon has several options: metal, ceramic, porous coated, and cemented versus noncemented. Prosthetics can be affixed in several ways. Zimmerman (1998) describes several fixatives and devices. Polymethylmethacrylate bone cement is a putty-like substance that is packed into the bone that hardens to hold the prosthetic in place. A porous coated prosthesis can be used in the hopes a healing response will occur, to allow the body to develop its own bone and adhering the prosthetic into place. Hydroxyapatite coating is a bioactive ceramic substance that allows the body to generate new bone growth to hold the prosthetic into place. In press-fit stabilization, the prosthesis is the same size or smaller than the surface being replaced. The surgeon hammers the components into place, allowing the prosthesis to stay in place.

Knowing and understanding the types of prosthesis and fixative is important for rehabilitation care. It allows the healthcare professional to determine and estimate precautions related to the healing and efficacy of the materials used. An example is the use of a cemented or noncemented prosthetic, because this could potentially influence weight-bearing status (Brander & Stulberg, 2006).

---

* A special thanks to Dr. Ralph T. Salvagno, M.D., orthopedic surgeon, for helping to write this section.

MAJOR POSTOPERATIVE COMPLICATIONS

It is important to understand potential postoperative complications with joint replacements. Several complications need to be monitored, not only immediately postoperatively but also for weeks and months after surgery.

Loosening and Dislocation of Prosthesis

The most common cause of painful or increased dysfunction of a joint is due to loosening of the prosthetic. Aseptic loosening is the most common cause of failed joint replacement; it may appear years after the initial surgery by wear and tear on the prosthetic devices (Brander & Stulberg, 2006).

Hip dislocation is the number one reason for reoperation. The rate of dislocation is as high as 10% (Brander & Stulberg, 2006). Posterior hip dislocations are the most common and happen from flexion, adduction, and internal rotation of the hip joint (Brander & Stulberg, 2006). Anterior hip dislocations are not as common but happen from extension and external rotation (Brander & Stulberg, 2006). Dislocation can happen within the early postoperative period, but more than half occur within the first 4 to 6 weeks (Brander & Stulberg, 2006). During rehabilitation, the rate of hip dislocation was found to be 2.1% (Brander & Stulberg, 2006). Patients and families need to be taught about the risk, proper positioning techniques, and use of adaptive equipment. Patients often complain of immediate pain and describe hearing a "pop." Confirmation of a dislocation is often visualized on x-ray.

Aseptic loosening of the shoulder prosthesis is estimated to be at 2% and accounts of one-third of all complications (Canniggia, Fornara, Franci, Maniscalco, & Picinotti, 1999). Dislocation of a shoulder is usually related to the stability of the prosthetic device. Instability can be classified as anterior instability, posterior instability, superior instability, and inferior instability (Canniggia et al., 1999). Instability is usually related to the humeral component.

Infection

According to the American Association of Orthopedic Surgeons (2009b), infections happen in less than 2% of total joint replacements. Several factors have been attributed to joint infections, including the presence of certain diseases (such as diabetes and alcoholism), use of immunosuppressant drugs, obesity, the presence of infections such as skin or in the urinary tract, and non-healing ulcers (Brander & Stulberg, 2006). Infection of the joint capsule is usually confirmed by a needle aspiration. The microorganisms responsible for infection are usually gram-positive bacilli (Canniggia et al., 1999). The ultimate outcome is preserving the joint prosthetics. In the event of infection that cannot be treated, removal of hardware, prolonged antibiotic treatment, and a repeat joint replacement may occur. To prevent infection, the surgeon may recommend prophylactic antibiotics before dental procedures and other invasive treatments.

Blood Clots

A major concern and potentially life-threatening complication is that of deep vein thrombosis and pulmonary emboli. Virchow's triad is a physiological bodily response; when all are met, a blood clot can occur. Patients who have had a joint replacement may meet all the triad criteria: local vessel wall damage, hypercoagulability, and venous stasis exist after surgery. Surgeons usually order some form of anticoagulant such as Coumadin, low-molecular-weight heparin, or unfractionated heparin postoperatively. It is common to administer anticoagulants immediately postoperatively and up to 14 days after surgery (Eikelboom, Quinlan, & Douketis, 2001).

MUSCULOSKELETAL ASSESSMENT

Comprehensive nursing assessment of the patient having joint replacement considers both preoperative and postoperative factors. Preoperative assessment focuses on obtaining a thorough history and physical. Postoperative assessment considers surgical wound healing, prevention of infection, pain management, and rehabilitation to regain mobility.

Preoperatively-Focused Assessment

Interdisciplinary team members all contribute to a comprehensive assessment. Nurses should particularly note the following:

- *Past medical history:* general health, pervious surgeries, hospitalizations, illnesses, immunizations, medications, allergies, history of blood transfusions, functional status and ability to complete activities of daily living (ADLs), transfers, and ambulation
- *Personal history:* cultural and religious background, economic issues, home environment, occupation, tobacco, alcohol, and illicit drug use, diet, exercise regimen
- *Pain:* chronic versus acute, location, intensity, exacerbation, medications, and home treatments

- *Musculoskeletal:* inspection and palpation of surgical extremity, posture, alignment, symmetry, muscle tone, and range of motion
- *Vital signs:* blood pressure, temperature, pulse, respiratory rate, and pulse oximetry

Postoperatively-Focused Assessment

Assessment after joint replacement surgery should address the following areas:

- *Musculoskeletal:* frequent visualization of surgical area; monitor incision line for intactness, redness, warmth, amount of drainage, amount of edema, sensation, pulses
- *Pain:* frequent assessment of pain intensity, location, radiation, and evaluation of previous interventions to treat pain
- *Vital signs:* frequent vital signs until stable
- *Function:* assess amount of help needed for bed mobility, transfers, ambulation, and ADLs.

REHABILITATION: THERAPEUTIC MODALITIES

Many programs include a multidisciplinary team of professionals including nursing, physical therapy, occupational therapy, social work, and physician. Exercise for a total joint replacement often begins in a preoperative setting. Instruction is given to patients depending on their level of need. Several team members may offer therapeutic modalities at various stages during the rehabilitation phase.

Total Joint Replacements: Hip and Knees

Preoperative

Nursing staff may complete a comprehensive review of the medical management of a total joint replacement. This could include a complete patient medical history, coordinating necessary preoperative testing, a tour of the medical facility, instruction in proper dressing changes, signs and symptoms of infection, and review of the surgical procedure itself. Programs such as these have been shown to decrease patient anxiety about their upcoming procedure (Brander & Stulberg, 2006). Physical therapy intervention at this stage may include a musculoskeletal evaluation of the patient and instruction in the completion of a preoperative home exercise program; proper transfers in and out of bed, chairs, and vehicles; instruction in use of assistive devices such as canes and walkers; and information regarding postoperative rehabilitation. There is some evidence that "prehabilitation exercise" may have long-term benefits for the patient (Topp et al., 2009). Occupational therapists may provide evaluation and instruction in the use of assistive devices to improve completion of ADLs. For example, proper use of a long-handled sponge or sock donner can allow a patient to safely complete necessary activities without risk of injury. Social workers can help coordinate the program by facilitating evaluation of home needs and initiating discharge planning.

Postoperative

Coordinated rehabilitation during recovery after joint replacement is essential to successful recovery. Therapeutic exercise begins shortly after surgery and continues until the patient has reached his or her maximal functional recovery.

Inpatient Rehabilitation.

The primary focus of initial postoperative rehabilitation is safe mobility. At most facilities most patients are transferred out of bed and stand on day 1 after surgery. Early movement in combination with other prophylactic measures is essential in diminishing the risk of postoperative deep vein thrombosis. Rehabilitation and nursing personnel may both play an active part in this process via safe transfers Proper transfer techniques can reduce the risk of aggravation of symptoms and injury for the patient and professional.

Depending on the type of procedure and surgical technique, certain precautions and/or weight-bearing restrictions may need to be followed. Choice of prosthetic components may affect weight-bearing status. For example, some surgeons may restrict weight bearing of patients with noncemented THA components. Cemented components generally allow immediate full weight bearing or what is often referred to as **weight bearing as tolerated (WBAT)**. Other surgical complications or processes may limit weight bearing. Bone grafting or inadvertent fracture during surgery may also call for limitations on weight bearing. Communication between all health professionals—physician, nursing, and rehab staff—is essential to ensure safe, effective treatment.

During the inpatient stay, physical therapy consists primarily of general range of motion (ROM) and strengthening exercise, transfer, and gait training. Patients must demonstrate a certain level of independence before they can be safely discharged home. Instruction in use of an appropriate assistive device, usually a walker or crutches, with proper gait pattern helps ensure patients are safe to be discharged. This includes walking on level surfaces as well as stairs and ramps. Patients also need to be able to safely transfer from sit to stand, in and out bed, and in and out vehicles if indicated. Depending on surgeon and/or facility preference, a continuous passive motion (CPM) machine may be used by patients with total knee replacements while in bed in an effort to improve range of motion. There is some controversy as to how effective these devices are. For hip replacement patients, this can be more challenging because **hip precautions** must be maintained at all times. For example, hip precautions for a posterolateral THA may include no hip flexion beyond 90 degrees, no crossing of midline with the operated leg, and no rotation (Figure 18.1). Despite the difficulties, this is usually completed rather rapidly. Inpatient stays of 2 to 3 days (e.g., surgery Monday and discharge Thursday) for patients with uncomplicated stays have become the norm. This is significantly different from 15 years ago, when patients routinely stayed 2 weeks. Appendix 18.1 provides examples of exercises for patients after total hip and total knee replacement.

Posthospital Rehabilitation.

Rehabilitation continues upon discharge from the hospital. A patient may be discharged home or, if medical or other care needs dictate, to a nursing home or subacute rehab facility. Therapy continues to focus on addressing functional deficits the patient may have. For example, a patient with total knee replacement will typically exhibit lower extremity edema, muscle weakness, especially in the quadriceps, range of motion limitations in the operated knee, and gait deficits requiring the use of an assistive device. Treatment will focus on addressing these deficits. Gait training, progressive resistive exercise, balance training, patellar mobilization, soft tissue (nonjoint) mobilization, electrical stimulation for quadriceps strengthening and edema control, and range of motion and stretching exercises are all typical interventions for this patient. Modalities, including ice and later moist heat, are commonly used to minimize edema and pain and to facilitate stretching and exercise. Instruction in an appropriate comprehensive home exercise program is also essential for optimal patient outcome.

Similar deficits may be found in a total hip replacement patient. However, rather than the significant quadriceps weakness found with knee replacement, a hip replacement patient often has significant weakness in the hip abductor musculature. This is especially evident in anterolateral and direct-lateral surgical approaches. The posterolateral approach has less direct effect on the abductor musculature but may be associated with a higher

Total hip replacement precautions

1. Do not bend operated hip greater than 90 degrees

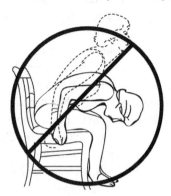 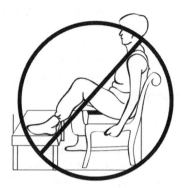

2. Do not cross legs or bring operated leg past the midline of the body

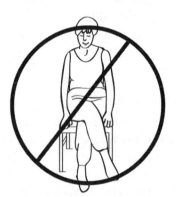 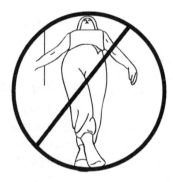 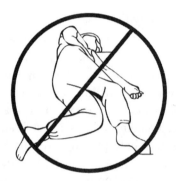

3. Do not turn or twist operated leg inward

FIGURE 18.1   Example of a teaching sheet for patients about total hip replacement.

Source: Used with permission of Total Rehab Care of Washington County Hospital, Hagerstown, Maryland.

dislocation rate (Brander & Stulberg, 2006). Weakness in the hip abductor musculature leads to significant gait deviation, known as a Trendelenburg gait pattern. A patient with this deficit will laterally deviate his or her trunk to the weakened side in an effort to decrease pelvic drop due to the hip weakness. Patients should be encouraged to use appropriate assistive devices to avoid this deviation. As with the total knee replacement patient, range of motion exercises, progressive resistive exercises, soft tissue (nonjoint) mobilization, and balance and gait training are standard interventions. Again, a comprehensive home exercise program is essential.

Total Shoulder Replacement

As with lower extremity joint replacements, which are far more common, shoulder replacement requires a good deal of rehabilitation to regain function. Total shoulder replacements are less frequently seen. Surgery may be a total shoulder replacement, meaning involvement

of both the humeral head and the glenoid fossa of the scapula, or a hemiarthroplasty, meaning replacement of one of the two. Indications for this procedure include osteoarthritis, rheumatoid arthritis, rotator cuff tear arthropathy, osteonecrosis, and humeral head fracture (Roos et al., 1995).

Inpatient Rehabilitation

Patients are typically in a sling for approximately 1 month or more after total shoulder replacements. Exercise begins day one with **passive range of motion**, eventually progressing to **active assistive range of motion**, **active range of motion**, and strength training. Active range of motion and strength training typically begin 4 or more weeks after surgery. Inpatient rehabilitation typically focuses on initiating the passive range of motion process and ensuring safe transfers and completion of ADLs without injury. Passive range of motion into external rotation is typically limited to avoid excessive stress on the anterior capsule and or subscapularis, the latter of which is often reflected by the surgeon to allow access to the joint for the procedure. Average length of stay for a total shoulder replacement is 2 days.

Outpatient Rehabilitation

Rehabilitation expectations differ with respect to indication for surgery. For example, a patient with osteoarthritis and an intact rotator cuff may expect a significantly different outcome than one with advanced rheumatoid arthritis, poor bone quality, and a deficient rotator cuff. It is beneficial for all healthcare professionals to communicate reasonable expectations for patients to help them plan for life after surgery and subsequent rehabilitation. Exercise is progressed to active range of motion and strength training as noted above. Electrical stimulation may be used for facilitation of muscle strengthening, and ice and heat are commonly used as well. As with other joint replacements, an appropriate and comprehensive home exercise program is essential for achieving optimal functional outcome.

EVALUATION OF OUTCOMES

For any type of joint replacement surgery, expected outcomes depend on a variety of factors, as previously discussed (see Case Study 18.1). However, general outcomes for patients include the following:

- Pain management, with pain under control
- Adequate range of motion
- Return of functional mobility
- Increased quality of life

CASE STUDY 18.1

Mr. Eberle is a 47-year-old man in generally good health, status post left total knee arthroplasty from 3 days ago after a 20-year course of worsening osteoarthritis precipitated by a fall at the age of 27. He had been working full time on his farm before surgery and has maintained an overall active lifestyle. He has been progressing without incident, completing exercises and ambulating with axillary crutches, weight bearing as tolerated. As he is being prepared for discharge, you notice he seems to be breathing harder then he normally would. He reports that "it is no big deal," attributing it to many years of smoking in combination with the demands of recovering after surgery. He denies any chest pain, just the feeling of being "unable to catch my breath." He denies any excessive erythema or pain in the left lower extremity or calf, no report of fever or malaise. More than anything, he is eager

to get home where he states he can "finally get some rest." You do a quick physical examination of the left knee, and the lower extremity does not reveal any significant findings; lungs clear, no oxygen, pulse ox. is 95% on room air. Vital signs are as follows: pulse rate is 105 beats per minute at rest, respiratory rate of 20 per minute, blood pressure 135/95.

Questions
1. What do you suspect is happening with this patient? Should you be concerned?
2. What course of action would you recommend? Should you let this patient go home, or ask him to wait until you speak to the doctor?
3. What other tests would be helpful to definitively determine the proper course of treatment for this patient?

In addition, program outcomes provide an indication of the success and quality of rehabilitative care services. Desired program outcomes are as follows:

- Successful patient outcomes
- Low complication rates, such as low rates of infections, low rates of blood clots, and low rates of dislocations
- Successful patient flow through care-map and program
- Low rate of revisions (surgery again to fix a problem)

Rehabilitation nurses can play an important role in the successful recovery of persons after joint replacement surgery. By applying the information in this chapter and engaging in meaningful teaching using evidence-based practice tools (Boxes 18.1 and 18.2), nurses can facilitate continuity of care after discharge.

BOX 18.1   Evidence-Based Practice Teaching Resources

Review the resources available at www.orthonurse.org. These publications can be printed and distributed as needed to patients undergoing total joint replacement. They may be copied and reproduced without permission.

BOX 18.2   Client–Family Teaching

The National Association of Orthopedic Nurses (NAON) Patient Education Series (2009), "Total Hip Replacement & Total Knee Replacement," is an excellent resource for patient and family teaching. It is designed as a workbook for all aspects of care preoperatively and postoperatively. Teaching includes general information and introduction to total joint replacement, before surgery education and checklists, day of surgery and hospital care, caring for yourself at home, exercises and self-care guidelines, and a section for additional information of your healthcare team.

SUMMARY

The content in this chapter provided an overview of joint replacement surgery, post-operative interventions, and desired rehabilitation outcomes. Joint replacement of the hip and knee are more common than those of the upper extremities. For all persons with joint replacement, successful outcomes are measured in terms of return to maximum mobility and range of motion, with a low incidence of complications. Rehabilitation nurses can facilitate these positive outcomes by actively preventing common complications and reinforcing what patients are taught in physical therapy. Educating patients and families about the healing process after joint replacement is a key nursing intervention to promote recovery.

CRITICAL THINKING

As a group, consider these situations and discuss ethical implications for total joint surgery.

1. An 85-year-old man lives in a nursing home. He has been bed-bound for 6 to 7 months due to pain and decreased mobility. This man is not oriented to place and time but knows his name and can interact minimally with his family. His family has searched out an orthopedic surgeon to consider doing a total hip replacement to help with pain management and with transfers to get from a bed to a wheelchair. What are the ethical considerations for this case? What is the risk-to-benefit of total joint surgery for this man?

2. As a nurse you have encountered a patient who has gone through a total hip replacement, has cerebral palsy, and is unable to follow directions or follow the tenants of a joint replacement program. You must consider the safety implications a patient must follow after this type of surgery. Are there any ethical considerations for this patient? If so, what are they and why?

PERSONAL REFLECTION

- Have you ever cared for a patient with a joint replacement? If so, what type of joint replacement was it? Think about the major nursing issues you addressed with this patient? How was his or her pain managed? What was the level of activity? What was the person's discharge status? Were there any areas that might have been improved with more of a focus on rehabilitation?

- Using the nursing diagnoses listed in Table 18.1, which do you believe would take priority in caring for each of the following patients:
  - A 92-year-old woman with a complicated total hip arthroplasty (THA) after a fall

TABLE 18.1	Nursing Diagnoses and Care Planning	
Nursing Diagnoses	**Outcomes**	**Interventions**
Pain, acute	Alleviation of pain or a reduction to a level that is acceptable to the patient	• Proper positioning, ice to extremity, guided imagery, music therapy, distraction • Use of IV and PO medications, patient-controlled analgesia as prescribed by physician, administer before any activity
Infection, potential for	No infection at surgical site	• Hand washing • Universal precautions • Appropriate wound care techniques • Assessment of wound: color, temperature, drainage • Appropriate antibiotic use, as prescribed by physician • Teaching patient/family of proper techniques of wound care and dressing changes
Mobility, physical, impaired	Increase mobility and advancement to independence with or without a device	• Use of adaptive equipment as necessary • Active, active-assisted, and passive range of motion exercises • Mobilize as soon as possible • Teaching patient/family of proper mobilization techniques

(Continued)

TABLE 18.1   Nursing Diagnoses and Care Planning *(Continued)*

Nursing Diagnoses	Outcomes	Interventions
Tissue perfusion, potential for ineffective	Maintain adequate tissue perfusion to extremities; be free of thrombosis	• Encourage range of motion exercises • Teach ankle pumps, circular motion of feet • Use TED hose as appropriate • Use sequential devices as appropriate • Frequent assessment of extremities for pulses, color, temperature, and sensation • Administer anticoagulants as ordered by physician • Monitor lab values as ordered by physician
Constipation	Maintenance of regular bowel pattern as per patient	• Encourage activity as soon as possible • Encourage fluid intake • Encourage proper diet • Assess bowel sounds, monitor nausea and vomiting • Administer laxatives, stool softeners as ordered by physician
Breathing pattern, ineffective	Maintain proper ventilation	• Oxygen support as needed • Teach coughing and deep breathing exercises • Teach use of incentive spirometry • Teach proper positioning for effective breathing, sitting position, slightly forward, and shoulders relaxed • Assess lung sounds and pulse oximetry

Sources: Dochterman & Bulecheck (2004), Johnson et al. (2006), and McCourt, Mumma, & Tracey (1995).

- A 32-year-old male baseball player requiring a total shoulder replacement
- A 66-year-old woman with a history of severe rheumatoid arthritis who needs multiple joint replacements to regain functional movement

REFERENCES

American Academy of Orthopedic Surgeons. (2009a). Total hip replacement. Retrieved January 15, 2009 from http://ortho-info.aaos.org/topic.cfm?topic=A00377&return_link=0

American Academy of Orthopedic Surgeons. (2009b). Total knee replacement. Retrieved December 1, 2010, from http://ortho-info.aaos.org/topic.cfm?topic=A00389

American Academy of Orthopedic Surgeons. (2009c). Osteone-crosis of the hip. Retrieved September 15, 2010, from http://orthoinfo.aaos.org/topic.cfm?topic=A00216

Bathon, J. (n.d.). Rheumatoid arthritis pathophysiology. Retrieved April 1, 2010, from http://hopkins-arthritis.org/arthritis-info/rheumatoid-arthritis/rheum_clin_path.html

Brander, V., & Stulberg, S. (2006). Rehabilitation after hip and knee joint replacement: An experience and evidence-based approach to care. *American Journal of Physical Medicine and Rehabilitation, 85*(Supplement), S98–S118.

Canniggia, M., Fornara, P., Franci, P., Maniscalco, P., & Picinotti, A. (1999). Shoulder arthroplasty: Indications, contraindications, and complications. *Paanminerva MED, 41,* 341–349.

Centers for Disease Control and Prevention (CDC). (2009a). Osteoarthritis. Retrieved December 1, 2010, from http://www.cdc.gov/arthritis/basics/osteoarthritis.htm

Centers for Disease Control and Prevention (CDC). (2009b). Rheumatoid arthritis. Retrieved September 1, 2010, from http://www.cdc.gov/arthritis/basics/rheumatoid.htm

Dochterman, J. M., & Bulecheck, G. M. (Eds.). (2004). *Nursing Interventions Classifications* (4th ed.). St. Louis, MO: Mosby.

Dudkiewicz, I., Covo, A., Salai, M., Israeli, A., Amit, Y., & Chechik, A. (2004). Total hip arthroplasty after avascular necrosis of the femoral head: Does etiology affect the result? *Archives of Orthopedic and Trauma Surgery, 124,* 82–85.

Eikelboom, J. W., Quinlan, D. J., & Douketis, J. D. (2001). Extended-duration prophylaxis against venous thromboembolism after total hip or knee replacement: A meta-analysis of the randomised trials. *Lancet, 358* (9275), 9–15.

Felson, D. (2004). An update on the pathogenesis and epidemiology of osteoarthritis. *Radiologic Clinics of North America, 42*(1), 1–9.

Gould, J., & Hettings, D. (1985.). Inflammatory response of synovial joint structures. In J. Gould and G. Davies (Eds) *Orthopedic and Sports Physical Therapy* (2nd ed., pp. 87–117). Philadelphia, PA: Mosby.

Johnson, M., Bulechek, G., Butcher, H., Dochterman, J. M., Maas, M., Moorehead, S., & Swanson, E. (Eds.). (2006). *NANDA, NOC, and NIC Linkages* (2nd ed.). St. Louis, MO: Mosby.

Lafforgue, P. (2006). Pathophysiology and natural history of avascular necrosis of bone. *Joint Bone Spine, 73*, 500–507.

McCourt, A., Mumma, C., & Tracey, C. (Eds.). (1995). *21 Rehabilitation nursing diagnosis*. Glenview, IL: Rehabilitation Nursing Foundation.

Merck & Company (2001). Pathophysiology: Function and structure of normal articular cartilage. Retrieved April 1, 2010, from http://merckmedicus.com/pp/us/hcp/diseasemodules/osteoarthritis/pathophysiology

National Institute of Arthritis and Musculoskeletal and Skin Disease. (2009). Osteonecrosis. Retrieved September 1, 2010, from http://www.niams.nih,gov/Health_Info/Osteonecrosis/default.asp

Radin, E. (1986). Role of subchondral bone in the initiation and progression of cartilage damage. *Clinical Orthopedics, 213*, 34–40.

Roos, H., Adalberth, T., Dahlberg, L., & Lohmander, L. (1995). Osteoarthritis of the knee after injury to the anterior cruciate ligament or meniscus: the influence of time and age. *Osteoarthritis Cartilage, 3*, 261–267.

Spector, T., Cicuttini, F., Baker, J., Loughlin, J., & Hart, D. (1996). Genetic influences on osteoarthritis in women: A twin study. *British Medical Journal, 312*, 940–944.

Topp, R., Swank, A., Quesada, P., Nyland, J., & Malkani, A. (2009). The effect of prehabilitation exercise on strength and functioning after total knee arthroplasty. *American Academy of Physical Medicine and Rehabilitation, 1*, 729–735.

Wilcox, R., Arslanian, L., & Millett, P. (2005). Rehabilitation following total shoulder arthroplasty. *Journal of Orthopedic & Sports Physical Therapy, 35*(12), 821–836.

Zimmerman, J. (1998). Rehabilitation of total hip and total knee replacements. In J. Delisa & B. Gans (Eds.), *Rehabilitation medicine: Principles and practice* (3rd ed., pp. 1677–1693). Philadelphia: Lippincott-Raven.

APPENDIX 18   EXERCISES FOR PATIENTS AFTER HIP OR KNEE SURGERY

Ankle Pumps: Bend ankles to move feet up and down, alternating feet. Repeat this exercise several times throughout the day.

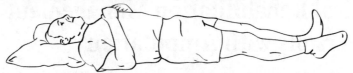

Quad Sets: Slowly tighten muscles on thigh of straight leg while counting to 5; repeat with the other leg.

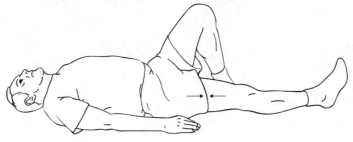

Short Arc Quad: Place large can or rolled towel under leg. Straighten knee and leg. Hold for 5 seconds; repeat with other leg.

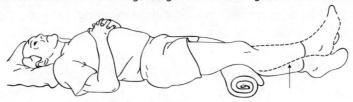

Straight Let Raise: Bend uninvolved leg. Keep other leg as straight as possible and tighten muscles on top of thigh. Slowly lift straight leg 6–8 inches from bed and hold for 5 seconds; lower. Relax.

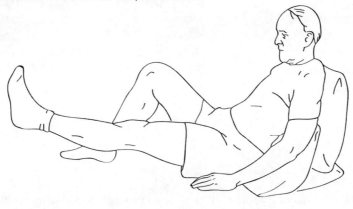

Heel Slides: Bend knee and pull heels toward buttocks. Hold for 5 seconds, return to starting point. Repeat with other knee.

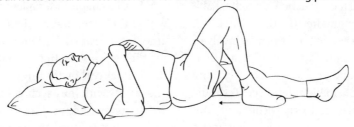

Source: Washington County Hospital Association, Total Joint Replacement Program, Hagerstown, Maryland.

CHAPTER 19

Clinical Rehabilitation Management for Persons with Amputation

Elizabeth Yetzer
Edward Hansen
Yolanda Haskell
Sharleen Koenig
Judy Kapton
Edmond Ayyappa

LEARNING OBJECTIVES

At the end of this chapter, the reader will be able to

- Discuss three client/family education topics related to limb amputation.
- Identify the signs and symptoms of depression in the client with a limb amputation.
- Recognize comorbidities that can affect the client's candidacy for prosthetic use and gait training.
- Describe major components of an artificial limb and describe its function.

KEY CONCEPTS AND TERMS

Ace wrapping	Grieving	Residual limb
Alteration in comfort	Impaired physical mobility	Rigid dressing
Ambulatory aids	Knee immobilizer	Self-care deficit
Amputation	Knowledge deficit	Shrinker
Assistive devices	Liner	Suction socket
Body image disturbance	Peer visitor	Transfemoral
Contracture	Phantom limb pain	Transhumeral
Dynamic alignment	Prehension	Transradial
Dysvascular	Proning	Transtibial
Edema	Proprioception	
Gait	Prosthesis	

Amputation is defined as the partial or complete surgical removal of a limb as the result of an injury, intolerable pain, gangrene, vascular obstruction, uncontrollable infection, or congenital anomalies (birth defects). It is without doubt a devastating event for the person involved. The rehabilitation team can make a significant difference in the quality of life and preservation of health for those with limb amputation. Rehabilitation goals should include providing the client with the knowledge and skills needed for physical, emotional, and social adjustment. The rehabilitation nurse is a key member of the team and provides specific interventions to assist the client in reaching those goals.

In this chapter we review rehabilitation of the client with a limb amputation, including the major causes of amputation; the educational needs of the client and family; the common feelings about amputation; and factors that influence those feelings. Measures to assist the client and family with the psychological aspects of amputation are discussed. Physical therapy evaluation, positioning, and the **gait** training program for the amputee are also presented, and criteria for identifying candidacy for a

TABLE 19.1	Major Causes of Amputations
Causes	**Examples**
Medical	Diabetes, peripheral vascular disease, cancer, gangrene, and infection
	Usually of lower extremity
	Accounts for 74% of amputations
Trauma	Accidents: crushing injury, burns, frostbite
	Often of upper extremity
	Accounts for 23% of amputations
Congenital anomalies	Can be upper or lower extremities or birth defects
	Accounts for 3% of amputations

prosthetic are outlined. Prosthetic components for both upper and lower limb loss are discussed.

CAUSES OF AMPUTATION

Amputation is the 11th most common procedure performed on the lower extremities. There are nine lower extremity amputees for every one upper extremity amputee in the United States. The National Center for Health Statistics estimates that 1 in 200 people in the United States have a lower extremity amputation (ACA, 2007, 2008a).

There are several major causes for amputations, some of which are summarized in Table 19.1. Seventy-four percent of amputations are due to medical causes. Medical causes of amputation include diabetes, vascular obstruction, cancer, gangrene, and uncontrollable infections. These amputations are usually of the lower extremity (ACA, 2006, 2007; Johannesson et al., 2009).

Accidental or traumatic amputations account for 23% of amputations. Most of these amputations are of the upper extremities. The causes of these amputations include occupational injuries, motor vehicular accidents, farm machinery, and armed conflicts.

Congenital anomalies, or birth defects, account for 3% of amputations and can be of the upper or the lower extremities. In 2007 the number of amputations in the United States was estimated at 1.7 million: 102,000 upper extremity and 256,000 lower extremity amputations (ACA, 2007, 2008a).

INCIDENCE AND STATISTICS RELATED TO AMPUTATION

Ziegler-Graham, Mackenzie, Ephraim, Travison, and Brookmeyer (2008) estimated that 1.6 million persons

were living with loss of a limb in the United States in 2005; 1 in 190 persons is currently living with the loss of a limb. The number of people with loss of a limb is expected to more than double by the year 2050 to 3.6 million. The increase in the number of people living with amputation is thought to be related to the aging population and the increase in **dysvascular** conditions such as diabetes.

Thirty-eight percent of amputations in diabetics are due to dysvascular disease (compromised circulation). and 64% of amputations due to dysvascular disease occur in persons over the age of 65. African Americans with diabetes have 1.5:1 to 3.5:1 and Hispanic Americans 3.6:1 amputation rates compared with Whites with diabetes (ACA, 2007, 2008b; Johannesson et al., 2009;). See Box 19.1.

BOX 19.1	Research Update Related to Amputation

Although there has been a great deal of research concerning amputation, much remains to be done. For example, there are still gaps in knowledge about phantom limb pain and its causes, prevention, and treatment. Outcome studies compare inpatient rehabilitation, home care, and outpatient rehabilitation as to which facilitates the client to become more functional faster. Inexpensive prosthetic components such as the Jaipur Foot and the Jaipur Knee need to be developed for use for amputees in developing countries.

Traumatic amputations, according to Ziegler-Graham et al. (2008), account for 45% of cases of limb loss. Two-thirds of these amputations occur among adolescents and adults younger than age 45 years (ACA, 2007).

The surgeon determines the level of amputation depending on the reason for the amputation (e.g., gangrene, cancer, infection). Circulation in the limb is evaluated for ample blood flow to support wound/incision healing. As much of the length of the limb as possible is saved to increase the client's ability to use the prosthesis. It is easier for clients to use a prosthesis if they have their own knee joint (a transtibial amputation versus a transfemoral amputation).

RISK FACTORS

Obesity often results in diabetes and contributes to dysvascular disease. Because of changes in circulation and sensation related to diabetes, a minor injury to the lower extremities of the diabetic can result in infection and amputation. With the increase in the incidence of diabetes, estimated to be 7.8% of the population (National Diabetes Fact Sheet, 2007), an increase in the number of amputations is anticipated. In 1999 the American Diabetes Association estimated that 15% of diabetics would develop a foot ulcer during the course of their disease and about 14% to 24% would require a lower extremity amputation (Markowitz, Gutterman, Magee, & Margolis, 2006).

PREVENTION

Amputation prevention for the diabetic focuses on control of diabetes, proper foot care, and foot screening. Nurses in a variety of settings can offer effective interventions such as education for diabetes self-management, foot care education, and foot screening programs to reduce the risk of foot ulcers and amputation (Ziegler-Graham et al., 2008). Proper foot care begins with daily foot inspection for discoloration and open areas of the skin. Foot screening by a healthcare provider at least every 6 months includes the use of a monofilament to detect changes in sensation of the feet. Semmes-Weinstein 5.07 (10-g) monofilament is applied to several locations on the bottom of the foot with enough pressure to bend the filament. With eyes closed, the client is asked to indicate if they can feel the monofilament. Lack of feeling indicates lack of sensation and possible diabetic neuropathy. Other circulation studies include foot and ankle systolic blood pressure, vibration perception threshold, and thermal sense testing (Boughton, 2003). A decrease in circulation may also result in subsequent or sequential amputations involving the same limb.

If lack of circulation in a limb is a major problem, a vascular surgery procedure such as a bypass may be done to improve blood flow. It is important to note that clients with poor circulation are at risk for amputation of the remaining leg within 3 to 5 years of the first leg (Izumi, Lee, Satterfield, & Harkless, 2006).

SPECIAL CONSIDERATIONS

Additional factors can affect the risk of amputation and influence the recovery potential. These include advanced age, young age, and polytrauma.

Geriatric Considerations

For an amputee older than 65 years of age, the effects of aging will impact their rehabilitation. The following are common effects of aging that could affect success with rehabilitation of the older adult with an amputation:

- Changes in cardiopulmonary capacity
- Reduced neuromuscular coordination
- Visual and hearing impairments
- Weakened musculature
- Limited range of motion
- Changes in memory, learning, executive function, and behavior

Other considerations for the older adult include multiple comorbidities, such as heart failure and pulmonary disease, which decrease available energy that may affect rehabilitation outcomes. These clients may also have dual diagnoses, such as amputation and blindness, or one-sided weakness due to stroke or traumatic brain injury. Often, these problems are a factor in determining if the client will be a prosthetic candidate or not. Because of these clients are at increased risk for amputation of the remaining leg. A geriatric client with bilateral amputations may not be a candidate for bilateral prostheses due to the energy required to walk and a higher risk for falls. They may, however, be fitted with a prosthesis to enable transfers. Geriatric clients are at higher risk for complications such as depression, pressure ulcers, falls, and infections (Lehman, 2008).

Pediatric Considerations

Amputations in pediatric clients are usually due to birth defects resulting in either a missing or a nonfunctioning limb. The parents must make the decision about surgical amputation for the child and often go through the stages of grief for the lost limb and the future consequences this will have for their child. The rehabilitation team works with both the parents and the child to help them develop the knowledge and skills needed to use a prosthesis. Depending on the age of the child, training can be incorporated into play therapy. The child will require multiple evaluations and changes in prosthetics as dictated by individual growth and development.

Trauma/Polytrauma Considerations

Polytrauma is defined by the Veterans Administration as two or more injuries to physical regions or organ systems, one of which may be life threatening, resulting in physical, cognitive, psychological, or psychosocial impairments and functional disability (Lehman, 2008). The client with polytrauma may have more than one amputation.

Clients with a traumatic amputation should be evaluated for other injuries that will affect their ability to participate in rehabilitation (see Box 19.2). According to Lehman (2008), the types of injuries sustained by service members in Afghanistan and Iraq include not only amputation but closed head injury, hearing loss, other tissue injury, and posttraumatic stress disorder. The rehabilitation nurse caring for these clients needs to assess for complications such as delayed onset of infection, pain, internal injuries, deficits in hearing and vision, brain injury, and swallowing function. Civilian clients in severe accidents may also have these complications.

> ### BOX 19.2 Ethical Considerations
>
> Ethical issues related to amputations occasionally arise when the client is at risk for loss of life due to septicemia and is refusing the amputation, thus loss of life versus loss of limb. This may require the formation of an ethics panel to make a recommendation for amputation surgery to save the client's life.

PSYCHOLOGICAL ASPECTS OF AMPUTATION

There is a heavy psychological impact related to amputation. Persons with amputation experience many present and future losses. Depression, fear, anxiety, changes in body image, and role alterations are some of the common issues faced by those with new amputation.

Depression

Depression is an illness that involves the mood, body, and thoughts. Depression can affect the way a person eats and sleeps, feels about oneself, and thinks of oneself. Causes of depression after limb loss may be due to poor body image, concerns of being a burden on the family, or feelings of uselessness (Singh et al., 2009).

The client may exhibit signs of depression before or after the amputation. Some signs are more obvious than others. Outward signs include anger, crying, tremors, clenched fists, and pursed lips; less obvious signs include withdrawal, denial and grief, loss of appetite, insomnia, decreased energy, weight gain or loss, headache, chronic pain, and thoughts of suicide. Singh, Hunter, and Philip (2007) reported a reduction in the incidence of psychological symptoms after limb loss while the client was learning new skills to adjust to life after rehabilitation but found the incidence of depression and anxiety sometimes rose again after discharge.

The client is often grieving not only the loss of a body part but also the loss of function and the loss of independence. Clients express fear and go through a grieving process: denial, anger, bargaining, and acceptance. There may be decreased energy, fatigue, weight gain or loss, restlessness, irritability, chronic pain, and fear of intimacy.

Body Image

After surgery the client may be afraid to look at his or her residual limb. A person's self-concept, physical characteristics, and abilities include feelings, attitudes, and self-worth. Body image has a profound effect on self-esteem. After amputation the person must adjust to a new body image. Persons are often reluctant to look at the surgical site after amputation, and some may refuse to participate in their own care. There may be a fear of nonacceptance by their spouse or significant other. The client may not want his or her significant other to view the wound. Nurses should be alert to persons who continue to express nonacceptance of this body image change and consult with the rehabilitation psychologist as needed (Houston, 2005).

Cultural Sensitivity

Persons of many different cultures and ethnic backgrounds may experience amputation. The healthcare provider must always be aware of the potential for cultural differences between the client and the provider. For instance, many cultures are very private and do not want others, except for hospital personnel, to know their medical records. A handshake in one culture may be like a hug or a bow in another culture. In one culture direct eye contact is expected, and in another it may be a sign of disrespect and hostility. Likewise, gender and age equality in one culture may be in contrast to defined roles in another culture.

The nurse should be aware of body language and facial expressions (ACA, 2004). Recognize cultural diversities. Avoid yes or no questions. A yes or a nod may mean "yes, I heard you" rather than "yes, I agree." Take cues from others regarding distance and touch. Be open to including family in most discussions, unless the client does not want the family involved at this time.

The National Multicultural Institute recommends that healthcare professionals maintain their sense of humor and patience, because it is not always easy to communicate effectively across cultures. Try to see things from another person's perspective (ACA, 2004). Ask for clarification. Check frequently for understanding. Recognize your own communication style and acknowledge when it may clash with the new amputee. Be aware of your own biases and stereotypes and work at controlling them.

Family Issues

Families will likely have numerous questions about their loved one's amputation, including details about the doctors, rehabilitation nurses, therapists, social workers, psychologists, and other professionals connected with the client. The client may or may not want their family informed. Healthcare professionals should remember the rules of Health Insurance Portability and Accountability Act, or HIPAA, in maintaining client confidentiality. Some psychological issues of amputation may be the same for the family as they are for the client: signs and symptoms of depression, feelings of sorrow or pity, and symptoms of grief, anger, and sadness. Common questions center around how to care for the loved one and whether the loved one will be able to walk or work again. It is important to know if the family has the willingness, resources, and abilities to help meet the needs of the client.

It is important that the rehabilitation nurse listens to the client and family. Sometimes the client just wants to talk. The nurse may ask the client if he or she would like to see a peer visitor. A **peer visitor** is an amputee who has had training by the ACA in peer support. The ACA maintains a list of peer visitors and tries to match visitors with the same type of amputation and gender as the client, if possible. Other amputee support teams are often available, and the ACA will share that information with the client or social worker (ACA, 2004; Fitzgerald, 2000; Marzen-Groller and Bartman, 2005).

ROLE OF THE REHABILITATION TEAM

The role of the amputation rehabilitation team is to assist the client and family to cope and adapt to the life changes of an amputation and to provide the knowledge and skills necessary for self-care. The rehabilitation team can help the client to maintain relationships by encouraging socialization with friends and family, promoting community reintegration, and attending a local support group (Amputation Rehabilitation Team, 2010).

Members of the rehabilitation team vary depending on the needs of the client. Examples of members of a rehabilitation team and their roles are shown in Table 19.2. (See Chapter 5 for more information on roles and team goal setting.)

Physical Therapy

Physical therapists (PTs) are clinicians with an established theoretical and scientific base (American Physical Therapy Association, 2003). PTs diagnose and manage dysfunctional movement to enhance an individual's physical and functional abilities. Physical function, health, and fitness are optimized to restore and maintain optimal quality of life. Prevention of functional limitations, progression of impairments, and symptoms or onset of disabilities from injuries, disorders, diseases, or conditions are imperative.

TABLE 19.2   Rehabilitation Team Members and Their Roles

- **Client and family or significant other:** Key members of the team whose participation should be encouraged.
- **Rehabilitation Doctor (Physiatrist):** Monitors medical stability of the client, prescribes a therapy program, and assesses if or when client is ready for a prosthesis.
- **Rehabilitation Nurse:** Provides orientation to the rehabilitation program, gives emotional support to client and family, helps client manage pain, participates in pre- and postoperative teaching, and supports the therapy interventions.
- **Therapists: Physical and Occupational:** Educates the client in edema control, skin inspection, donning and doffing prosthesis, gait and transfer training, fall prevention, contracture prevention and energy conservation. Evaluates the need for home equipment.
- **Prosthetist:** Provides information about the prosthesis, designs and aligns the prosthesis to fit the individual client, and educates the client in prosthetic care.
- **Social Worker or Case Manager:** Coordinates discharge planning and posthospital care and secures entitlements and benefits.
- **Psychologist:** Addresses the stress associated with limb loss and its effects and provides the client and family with techniques for stress management and coping.
- **Dietitian:** Instructs client and family in proper diet to meet energy requirements and control weight.

Source: Adapted from Amputation Rehabilitation Team, 2010, Rusk Institute of Rehabilitation Medicine, 2009.

Physical Therapy Evaluation

The physical therapy evaluation of the client, both pre-operative and postoperative amputation, provides the PT with an assessment of the client's functional mobility, muscle strength, range of motion, balance, and skin integrity (i.e., potential pressure areas, areas of abnormal tissue degeneration) (Magee, 2002; Veterans Affairs/Department of Defense [VA/DoD], 2008). Most often, physical therapy evaluations are done postoperatively; however, when given the opportunity it is helpful to assess a client who is scheduled for amputation preoperatively. Client education during the preoperative period may include bed mobility, use of **ambulatory aids** (such as walker, crutches, or wheelchair), and care of the **residual limb** to prevent **contractures** and pressure sores (Magee, 2002).

The physical therapy evaluation begins with a client history, which should include the client's past medical and surgical history as well as his or her prior level of function (for upper and lower limbs and ambulatory level). Information regarding the client's pain, stressors, and psychiatric history is also important to obtain during the assessment (Magee, 2002). The client's social history such as recreational activities, occupation, home environment, and living arrangements (i.e., determining whether the client lives alone or in a home that requires access via stairs, etc.) helps the therapist develop a treatment plan to enable the client to return to his or her prior living arrangement if possible.

Observation and functional assessment of the client is obtained in sitting, standing, and walking (when safe to do so). Assessment of balance in sitting and standing can be obtained as well as the client's current level of mobility. Both the residual limb and the remaining sound limb are also examined for skin condition, temperature, circulation, and sensation. The residual limb examination should include palpation and measurements (limb length and girth). Skin ulcers should also be measured and monitored closely to ensure proper wound healing. If a **prosthesis** is available, the client is observed with and without the prosthesis. Gait deviations should be noted and any prosthetic issues identified should be corrected by either the PT (i.e., adding socks for proper socket fit) or by the prosthetist (i.e., adjusting alignment) (Magee, 2002; VA/DoD, 2008).

The examination includes objective measurements that are obtained as a baseline of the client's status and used to identify any barriers that may interfere with the client's functional outcome. The PT examiner performs a manual muscle test to determine the client's strength in addition to active and passive range of motion measurements of both limbs (Magee, 2002; VA/DoD, 2008). The deficits identified during the examination are useful in developing a therapeutic program that is suitable for the client. Reassessments are performed by PTs, and the client's program is modified as necessary throughout the course of therapy to ensure the client is making progress.

Client and Caregiver Education

Client education is one of the most important aspects of treatment the PT can impart to a client. The client with an amputation must regard what he or she learns and adhere to it for the rest of his or her life.

Functional Mobility

Functional training is one of the key components a client undergoes while participating in physical therapy. Bed mobility is one of the very first things assessed by the PT. To be able to roll and lay prone independently can essentially determine the client's prognosis in terms of other higher level activities, such as walking. Transfers to the bed, toilet, tub, and car are all tasks that need to be practiced by the client to live as independently and safely as possible.

Other Issues for the Interdisciplinary Team

In addition to physical therapy considerations, many team members work together to promote positive patient outcomes in a variety of areas. Adaptation after amputation is truly a task for an interdisciplinary team.

Care of the Residual Limb

Clients are taught skin checks of the residual limb soon after their amputation, especially once they are in the gait training phase while using a prosthesis. This is particularly important for those individuals with diabetes because they may be unable to feel pain and other types of sensation in their limb. All team members should enforce appropriate principles of skin care, although it may be the rehabilitation nurse who primarily does this teaching with the patient and family.

A **knee immobilizer** is often first issued by the surgeon to the **transtibial** (below the knee) amputee to help prevent knee flexure contractures and to protect the limb in case of fall or impact (i.e., knocking against an object or hitting the limb while in their wheelchair). A knee immobilizer is a long, orthopedic brace that prevents both medial/lateral movement and flexion/extension. It is donned by using Velcro straps that run the length of the brace. A **rigid dressing** is a hard plastic device that also serves to protect the freshly sutured limb while maintaining knee extension (DeLuccia, Anderson, & Berlet, 2007; Miklos, 2007).

Managing Edema

One of the challenges facing the treatment team can be edema of the residual limb. **Edema** is present to some extent in all cases, and it makes fitting of the prosthesis challenging. However, certain measures can be taken to reduce edema. If the person with an amputation has a rigid dressing and it has been removed, compression of the limb before a prosthesis is provided prepares the residual limb. The use of elastic soft dressing is often used in lieu of a shrinker sock to manage edema. When using a soft dressing or elastic bandage, care should be taken to reapply at regular intervals, generally about every 4 hours. Shrinker socks generally maintain their position and thus function for a longer period. The residual limb is said to have a "mature" shape when soft tissues have been reduced after prosthetic wear and proper use of a shrinker sock. If the clinic team determines that a prosthesis is safe and appropriate for a given client, they are typically referred to a specialty clinic for amputation treatment.

Ace wrapping is performed once the client is out of the rigid dressing. Rewrapping of the limb should occur every 3 to 4 hours (Pugh, Yetzer, & Naden-Blucher, 2007). Once there is no longer drainage and the incision is healed, **shrinkers** for the residual limb, sometimes termed "stump shrinkers" on some manufacturers' packaging, are ordered for edema control and for reshaping the limb. They are made of elastic and should be washed daily with warm water; therefore, two shrinkers are needed. Shrinkers are worn all day until liners are issued. A **liner** is shaped like the residual limb and is of a thicker material; it is donned with the prosthesis. Once the client begins to use a liner and starts gait training using a prosthesis, he or she is instructed to wear the liner during the day and the shrinker at night. Clients are encouraged to buy a handheld mirror so they can continually monitor their limb for any redness or abrasions.

PT and nurses are also trained in wound care as part of their educational curriculum. Upon initial evaluation the PT assesses the incision, takes longitudinal and circumferential measurements of the residual limb, checks the patient's sensation, and palpates for pain and bony prominences. Incision dressing changes and assessments may also be performed throughout the course of therapy and by the rehabilitation nurse during nursing care. If a client develops a wound on the residual limb for whatever reason, they are not to wear their prosthesis. This will only delay, or make worse, the condition of their existing wound.

Exercise Program

Physical therapy is initiated when the client is medically stable. Generally, lower extremity exercises are given to both the sound side and the amputated side. Strengthening exercises primarily focus on the extensors of the hip and knee and the hip abductors, which act to stabilize the pelvis during gait (O'Sullivan, 2007). Examples of initial exercises include, but are not limited to, quad sets, bridges (using a bolster to support the limbs), supine hip abduction, adductor pillow squeezes, single knee-to-chest stretch, and supine hip internal rotation.

Positioning

Positioning refers to the positions of the body that both should be avoided and should be emphasized. Imagine sitting at a 90-degree angle in a wheelchair for hours on end, day after day, or laying in bed with the head of the bed elevated and the foot of the bed also slightly elevated for comfort. You are too weak to stand into full trunk extension, at least not yet. What happens? Contractures of the hip and knee develop.

Positions to avoid for the client with a transtibial (below the knee) amputation include prolonged flexion and external rotation at the hip and knee flexion and for a transfemoral (above the knee) amputation are flexion, abduction, and external rotation of the hip (O'Sullivan, 2007). **Proning** is essential to prevent hip flexure contractures. Clients are urged to lie prone (lie on their stomach), beginning for 5 minutes at a time. A pillow under the hips may be added for greater comfort to the low back. Clients are to progress proning as tolerated, up to 20 minutes three or four times a day (Pugh et al., 2007). Laying supine, and especially sleeping, with their affected leg on a pillow should be avoided. For a person with a transtibial amputation, this only encourages knee flexure contractures. For a person with a **transfemoral** (above the knee) amputation, hip flexure contractures will develop. The client with a hip or knee flexion contracture may not be able to use a prosthesis. A hip or knee flexion contracture of less than 15 degrees is not usually a problem (O'Sullivan & Schmitz, 2001). Even so, contractures are to be prevented, because it is very difficult to reduce moderate to severe contractures through manual stretching, especially in the hip (O'Sullivan & Schmitz, 2001).

DETERMINING IF CLIENT IS A CANDIDATE FOR PROSTHETIC USE

Simply because a person receives an amputation does not mean a prosthesis will automatically be fabricated for them. Decisions about the appropriateness of a prosthesis are based on the following questions (Table 19.3): What was the client's prior level of function? Do they have

hip and/or knee flexure contractures severe enough to interfere with gait? Do they have good enough cognition to understand how to care for their limb and prosthesis? What other comorbidities do they have that will prevent them from walking? Are they motivated to learn the skills necessary and will they follow the therapist's instructions?

Just because a person is not a candidate for gait training with a prosthesis does not mean he or she will not receive any physical therapy. PTs can work with clients to help increase their functional independence as much as possible. Prostheses can even be fabricated for cosmetic purposes and/or transfers-only. A trial period with use of temporary prosthesis can be used to assess for candidacy (Tables 19.4 and 19.5), especially in the elderly (O'Sullivan, 2007).

PAIN MANAGEMENT

Phantom limb pain (the feeling of pain in a limb, or portion of a limb, that is no longer there) has been reported to have a 50% to 76.9% prevalence rate in clients with amputation (Richardson, Glenn, Nurmikko, & Horgan, 2006).

TABLE 19.3 Criteria for Evaluation of Prosthetic Use

Client is motivated to learn and has the skills necessary for self-care.

Client and/or family are able to learn and have the skills for self-care.

There is an absence of hip or knee contractures.

Other medical problems, such as respiratory, cardiac, stroke, or visual problems, will not interfere with use of prosthetic limb.

TABLE 19.4 Example of a Good Candidate for a Prosthetic

Prior Level of Function	Contractures	Motivation/ Cooperation	Cognition	Any Comorbidities that May Interfere with Progress	Other Barriers
Previous community ambulator, ran for exercise	None	Goal is to be able to run again; very motivated to return to his prior level of function; attentive to the therapist	Intact, alert, and oriented ×3; no psych history, memory loss, etc.	None	None

TABLE 19.5 Example of a Poor Candidate for Prosthetic Use

Previous Level of Function	Contractures	Motivation/ Cooperation	Cognition	Any Comorbidities that May Interfere with Progress	Other Barriers
Has not walked in 4 years, independent with ADLs at a wheelchair level	15-degree hip and knee flexion contracture	Depressed and does not appear motivated to perform exercises; does not comply with wearing knee immobilizer, proning, etc.	History of mild dementia	PMH of diabetes, CAD, CHF; is obese	Alcohol abuse; peripheral nerve damage to right axillary nerve

ADLs, activities of daily living; CAD, coronary artery disease; CHF, congestive heart failure; PMH, past medical history.

Methods to help reduce phantom pain include massage, gentle stroking of the limb, tapping the residual limb, and ice. Clients are referred to their doctor for medication to reduce phantom pain. According to Bhuvaneswar, Epstein, and Stern (2007), classifications of medications that could be used for phantom pain relief include opioid analgesics, antidepressants, anticonvulsants, and benzodiazepines, along with such alternative modalities as biofeedback, transcutaneous electrical nerve stimulation, hypnosis, and acupuncture.

There may also be residual limb pain, especially to palpation. Other bodily pains can also affect a person's gait and functional ability.

COMPLICATIONS OF LIMB HEALING

Cardiac disease, diabetes, renal disease, smoking, and other physiological problems can influence wound healing (O'Sullivan & Schmitz, 2001). Ischemia or infection may result in residual limb skin breakdown. Dependant positioning of the limb can decrease circulation to the area and cause edema (Yetzer, 1998). Uncontrolled diabetes is also a contributor toward poor wound healing (Yetzer, 1996). Poorly healing and necrotic wounds can lead to higher amputations if surgical debridement is not a viable option. Any delay in wound healing delays using a prosthesis.

COMORBIDITIES

Cardiopulmonary deconditioning may result from bed rest even before any amputation surgery. Deconditioning refers to a decline in ability to perform functional daily activities due to a prolonged period of inactivity. Past medical histories of any cardiac or pulmonary disease can affect outcomes after amputation, and a diagnosis of peripheral vascular disease will affect the level of amputation required. This is significant because studies have shown that the age of the patient and the level of amputation are the two most significant predictors of functional outcomes (Kelly & Dowling, 2008).

PREVENTING SECONDARY COMPLICATIONS

Secondary complications are not uncommon after amputation. These may include falls, skin breakdown, and additional complications related to prosthetic use (Pauley, Devlin, & Heslin, 2006).

Fall Prevention

One in five clients with lower extremity amputations will experience at least one fall during inpatient rehabilitation, with 18% sustaining injury (Pauley et al., 2006). Balance training and fall recovery is therefore incorporated into physical therapy. It is vital to the client that he or she does not sustain a fall; if the client does fall, it is important for him or her to know how get up as independently as possible. A fall early in the recovery process can lead to the opening of the sutures and the need for a revision by the surgeon. Other injuries may also be sustained in a fall, such as a factures and concussion. Protecting the residual limb is of utmost importance. Thus, clients are given a rigid protector to protect the limb when they are out of bed.

Skin Inspection

Skin inspection is important for the client with amputation. Redness (purplish in those with higher melanin content), rashes, and skin lesions must be treated seriously. Clients are taught to inspect their skin before and after donning/doffing the prosthesis. It should be noted if their skin integrity is compromised, especially along bony prominences and weight-bearing areas. The prosthesis can be modified by the prosthetist to accommodate any changes in socket fit.

REASSESSING THE CLIENT

The client is constantly being reassessed for progress throughout the course of physical therapy. The client usually is first gait trained in the parallel bars and then advanced to a front-wheeled walker. Sometimes, that is all a client will be able to use. If the client ambulates well, he or she may progress to bilateral axillary crutches, a single crutch, a single point cane, and finally to no **assistive devices**.

Because rehabilitating the amputee is a long process, outpatient care is commonly used. This might mean that a person goes home at a wheelchair level and comes back to therapy for prosthetic training to achieve a normalized gait. Some clients may want to be able to perform higher level activities, such being able to dance and play golf again. Task-specific training is then incorporated by the PT to accommodate the client's goals, so the client can live the best quality of life as possible.

PROSTHETICS

Though most amputees are candidates for a prosthesis, many are not. The amputee must have adequate strength, range of motion, and control of the proximal joints of both limbs. Balance, fear, pain, attitude, and **proprioception** (knowledge of the position of limb and joint in space) each play a role in determining the appropriateness of a prosthesis. Other key factors in the decision to use a prosthesis include the level of amputation, the condition of the residual limb, and overall health and fitness. The individual goals of the person with an amputation must also be considered. In general, it can be said that if a person with an amputation is able to ambulate on crutches or walker before the amputation, he or she will be able to function with a prosthesis. Moderate flexion contractures may present complications in ambulation but can be overcome (Lusardi & Nielsen, 2007; Smith, Michael, & Bowker, 2004).

Preparatory Prosthesis

A preparatory prosthesis is the initial prosthesis provided. Fitting a prosthesis soon after the suture line has healed helps to combat edema, reduces the possibility of contracture, generally improves overall physical condition, and improves psychological well-being. The temporary limb is frequently used for several weeks or even months until the residual limb volume has stabilized before the definitive prosthesis is provided. Figure 19.1 provides a picture of an above-the knee prosthesis and Figure 19.2 shows a below-the-knee prosthesis.

Prosthetic Interface

The socket of the prosthesis is the part that contacts and contains the residual limb. It provides a means for transferring the weight of the body to the ground through the prosthesis. In some cases a secondary role of the socket is to assist in the suspension of the prosthesis. The shape of the socket is critical to both comfort and function. The socket must not restrict circulation, yet it cannot be loose. Most sockets cover the entire residual limb. This is referred to as a total contact or total surface bearing socket (Fergason, 2005). Several designs are available to take maximum advantage of the muscles in the residual limb for control of the prosthesis and for transferring weight to the floor.

The socket is made specifically to fit the residual limb so that it fits intimately with the anatomy of the residual limb. The prosthetist creates a model of the residual limb

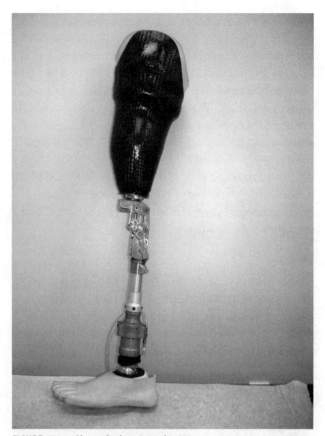

FIGURE 19.1   Above the knee prosthesis.

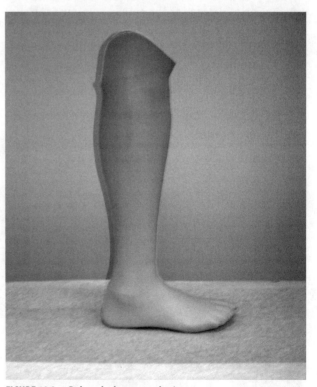

FIGURE 19.2   Below the knee prosthesis.

to fabricate a socket that is intimate enough to be effective. This is typically done with plaster, but in some cases a computer scanner is used. The prosthesis can be held in place by "suction," a vacuum provided by a close fit between the residual limb and socket. This is known as a **suction socket**. Variations of socket design include methods of suspending the limb and of providing cushion and comfort to the limb (Michael, 2005). The physician, prosthetist, and client typically work closely together to determine the most appropriate and comfortable design. A liner made of silicone or other soft material which rolls onto the residual limb is often used. One function of the liner is to provide suspension of the prostheses.

Socks

A prosthetic sock (Figure 19.3) is typically worn between the socket and residual limb to provide for ventilation and general comfort. Most prosthetic socks are woven of virgin lamb's wool, but socks of synthetic yarns are also used. Prosthetic socks are available in varying thickness, most commonly one-, three-, five-, and six-ply. Socks should be laundered daily according to the manufactures' instructions. As the number of ply increases, the sock becomes thicker. Socks can be used to compensate for residual limb shrinkage if the amount of shrinkage is limited. The prosthetist works with the person with an amputation to determine the optimal type and number of socks. When a 10-ply sock fit is reached, typically the socket may need to be replaced and sometimes, depending on wear, the entire prosthetic limb as well.

Prosthetic Knee

A prosthetic knee unit is required for all transfemoral amputations. To provide optimal ambulation and in-

creased safety, the prosthesis may have special design features that increase stability during weight bearing and allow for knee flexion and extension in gait. A prosthetic knee has various design features intended to provide the most efficient and safe walking pattern matched to the person with an amputation (Figure 19.4). In some cases they may incorporate hydraulic, pneumatic, magnetic, or microprocessor functions (Michael, 2005). With advances in technology, sophisticated mechanisms are now available, but there can still be limitations, including increased prosthetic weight and reduced durability.

Pylon

The pylon is the means of attachment of the prosthetic socket to the prosthetic foot. It is a lightweight titanium or carbon tube or strut. Most pylons are designed so that the alignment of the foot with respect to the socket can be changed by the prosthetist as needed to optimize the gait characteristics. The prosthetist adjusts the alignment to make walking as effortless and natural as possible. This process is called **dynamic alignment** (Laferrier, 2010).

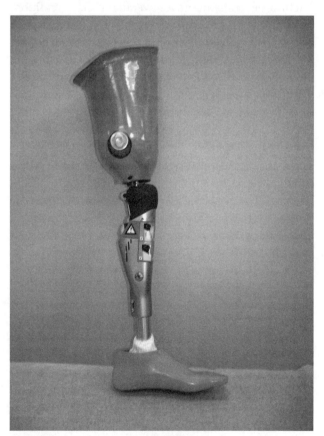

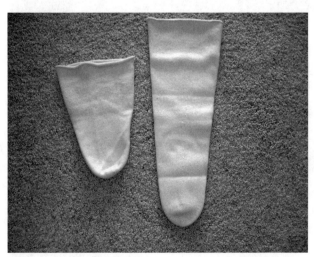

FIGURE 19.3   Prosthetic socks.

FIGURE 19.4   Above the knee prosthetic knee.

Foot

A variety of prosthetic foot designs is available (Figure 19.5), each having its advantages and disadvantages. Prosthetic feet may have an ankle joint with a significant amount of motion or have less motion and provide more forward momentum during weight bearing. Other options are available and are intended to match the activity level or gait velocity potential of the person with an amputation (Sleeth & Ayyappa, 2001).

Shoe

The shoe is an integral part of the prosthesis. Different shoes can be used by an amputee with the prosthetic foot, as long as the heel heights are consistent in all shoes. The prosthetist takes into account the shoe design, including heel height, when preparing the alignment of the prosthetic components. For women who wear different types of shoes with various high heels, an adjustable prosthetic foot or ankle is available. Men who wear boots can also use this feature.

Fitting the Prosthesis

Regardless of the functions provided by the prosthetic design, the most important factors in successful use of a prosthesis are fitting of the socket and achieving proper

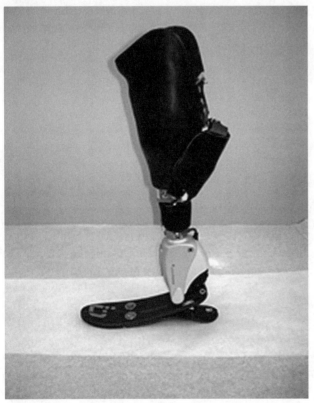

FIGURE 19.5   Foot and ankle for below the knee.

alignment of the various parts with respect to the each other. Fitting and alignment are not simple procedures and require a great deal of skill on the part of the prosthetist. The client also needs to have cooperation, patience, and communication with the prosthetist and clinic team. Fitting a prosthesis may take 2 to 6 weeks with a half dozen or so appointments. During prosthetic fitting and alignment the prosthetist provides initial training in the basic principles of standing and walking. Socket comfort affects alignment, alignment affects socket comfort, and both affect the gait or ability to walk effectively. To achieve an optimal gait and prosthetic function, training in the use of the prosthesis is necessary.

For a new amputee, a PT provides additional training as required. Any new prosthesis should be worn initially for short periods of several hours and wearing time increased as appropriate. When receiving a new prosthesis, the residual limb should be inspected several times a day. A significant problem in obtaining the best possible performance and comfort is excessive weight gain. Small fluctuations in body weight are reflected in the residual limb where changes in volume can result in poor fit, discomfort, and consequently poor performance.

High Activity or Special Use Prostheses

For seasoned individuals with an amputation who have achieved an appropriate level of performance that requires a special prosthetic design, there are many options. Examples include skiing, swimming, climbing, running, and golfing prostheses. Other applications are available for bilateral and multilateral amputees.

Walking with a transtibial prosthesis requires 40% more energy and with a transfemoral prosthesis 60% more energy when compared with a self-propelled wheelchair requiring 12% more energy. Even more dramatic is the increase in oxygen consumption by the dysvascular amputee using the prosthesis. If the client also has chronic obstructive pulmonary disease or other respiratory problems the increase in energy and oxygen needs may preclude the client from being a prosthetics candidate (Walters, 2005).

Cost for a transtibial prosthesis is typically $8,000 to $10,000 and can increase with specialized components, whereas cost for a transfemoral prosthesis start at $15,000 and can go as high as $80,000 depending on the design features selected (A. Ayyappam, personal communication, July 29, 2010).

Upper Limb Prosthetics

Upper limb amputation is relatively rare. According to Marathon Medical Communications Inc. (2009) about

3% of amputees have lost an arm or part of an arm. Twenty-two percent of new military amputees have lost an arm or part of an arm, but the number of military trauma-related amputees (<1,000 over the last decade) is dwarfed by the number of dysvascular lower limb amputees; thus, the overall percentage of upper limb has not appreciably changed. That is because, as noted, most amputations are caused by vascular disease, and upper limb amputation is almost never the result of vascular disease. Further, the rejection rate of a prosthesis for upper limb amputation is much higher than that of lower limb.

Prehension is the ability to use one or more digits or replacement digits against an opposing thumb or replacement thumb. One does not need to have sensation to function well with a lower limb prosthesis, but the lack of sensation in upper limb amputees requires that the individual use direct line of sight for prehension, limiting the function of all prosthetic hands, regardless of the level of technology used.

The primary challenges to be met in upper limb prostheses are providing a comfortable socket design and achieving the appropriate components and alignment for effective placement in space of the hand or hook (Kelly, Pangilinan, Rodriguez, Mipro, & Bodeau, 2009; Smurr, Gluck, Yancosek, & Ganz, 2008) See Figure 19.6.

Amputation Levels and Socket Design

Partial hand amputations are those that involve the distal 10% of the forearm. Socket design is based on the need to achieve a secure suspension framework on which an opposition bar can be fashioned to allow prehension of some digit or hand remnant. The wrist disarticulation has little or no available space to attach the hand or hook in a way

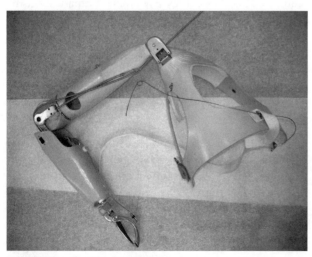

FIGURE 19.6   Shoulder disarticulation.

that is bilaterally symmetrical. Additionally, the boney styloid processes must be precisely relieved of contact within the socket. A goal for all wrist disarticulations is to capture forearm pronation and supination within the socket. Forearm pronation occurs in the proximal and distal articulations of the radioulnar joints. Distorting the socket in a "screwdriver fit" to lock onto the forearm permits the amputee much increased forearm rotation (Meier & Atkins, 2004).

Below elbow (**transradial**) amputations are classified by length, a condition that influences the type of prosthetic design used. The medium to long transradial amputation, like the wrist disarticulation, requires a "screwdriver fit" to capture all available forearm rotation. Flexible sockets have been increasingly popular for the management of transradial amputations. Many transradial amputees receive a socket that extends up to the cubital fossa anteriority and just proximal to the olecranon process posteriorly.

When less than 10% of the humerus remains, the amputee is often treated as an elbow disarticulation. Here the expansion area around the epicondyles of the humerus is sometimes used for suspension. A flexible socket design may be particularly appropriate, because it is cool and gives way slightly with muscular expansion, increasing comfort. When 50% to 90% of the humerus remains, the amputation is classified as a standard **transhumeral**. A short transhumeral is one in which 30% to 50% of the humerus is remaining. All these levels may be addressed with either a total contact rigid or flexible socket (Kelly et al., 2009; Marathon Medical Communications Inc., 2009; Smurr et al., 2008).

Componentry

Except for bilateral upper limb amputees, children, and high level amputees (i.e., shoulder disarticulation), every terminal device prescription should include both a hook and a hand. Prosthetic hands are often referred to as "functional hands," a deceptive description. Hands provide negligible function. The main problem with all prosthetic hands, whether mechanical or electric, is that the fingers get in the way of the line of vision. The amputee loses proprioception, full visual feedback, and tactile sensation. For these reasons there are significant functional limitations to using a hand with broad fingers compared with a hook with relatively thin fingers. Hands, although more cosmetic (Figures 19.7 and 19.8), are not as efficient as hooks. Most hooks are offset, which permits a better line of vision for small object manipulation. The alternative lyre shape allows a straight ap-

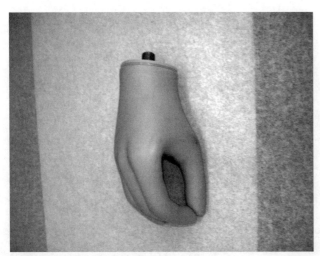

FIGURE 19.7   Hand prosthesis.

proach for improved control of larger round objects. Both hooks and hands are available in large and medium adult sizes and in child sizes. Transradial amputees who are quite active use stainless steel hooks. Any amputation that is more proximal than the transradial uses an aluminum hook to reduce weight (Smurr et al., 2008).

Special hooks with serrated holding surfaces are available for farmers, factory workers, and others involved with significant physical labor. Special devices are also available for improved control of a broom, shovel, or other garden tool. There are also task specific devices for sports, such as baseball, basketball, bowling, archery, hunting, and fishing. Some hooks are lined with neoprene to prevent slippage.

The vast majority of terminal devices are voluntary opening, using the body motion or arm flexion to achieve.

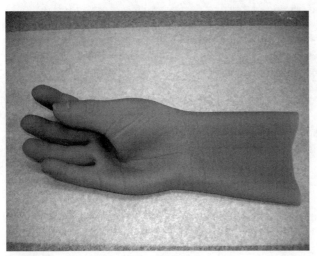

FIGURE 19.8   Cover for hand prosthesis.

Amputees with limited range of arm flexion may not be successful using body-powered limbs and may need external power (myoelectric or electric). Closing action of most hands and hooks is provided by either rubber bands, springs, or, in the case of myoelectric, a small electric motor (Kelly et al., 2009).

Children typically use plastic-coated hooks to avoid injuring their friends in play. The baby mitt is useful as a crawling assist for children up to age 4. Other options for children include a series of hooks, all plastic-coated aluminum, which may be more cosmetic and sometimes "wafered" or flattened to prevent injury to the amputee or his or her playmates.

A Quick Disconnect wrist design is most appropriate for the unilateral transradial amputee who uses both a hand and hook. This enables the client to interchange a hand for social engagements with a hook for increased function. A flexion-friction wrist permits the positioning and locking of the terminal devices in three different attitudes of flexion. Some version of the flexion wrist must always be incorporated in the prescription for the bilateral amputee who must reach the midline of the body for toileting and eating purposes.

The main advantage of electric and myoelectric for the transradial amputee is a reduction and simplification in the suspension mechanism and a faster learning curve in operating the device. The prosthetic hand always remains a singular challenge without sensation. Bilateral upper limb amputees, who must truly depend on the prosthesis for function, typically choose body-powered hooks and, unlike unilateral amputees, rarely reject their prosthesis.

EDUCATIONAL OBJECTIVES FOR THE CLIENT WITH AN AMPUTATION

The client facing an amputation is dealing with the physical, social, and psychological impact of the amputation. They also have a lack of knowledge about how their life will be altered by the amputation. They often lack the skills to deal with these major bio-psycho-social changes. The primary goal of the rehabilitation team is to assist the client and family in learning the knowledge and skills necessary for maxim independence and self care. Tables 19.6 and 19.7 provide goals for teaching clients and family both preoperatively and postoperatively. Table 19.8 gives a summary of rehabilitation goals. Educational topics that should be covered during these teaching times are also provided in these tables.

TABLE 19.6 Preoperative Teaching
Goals are to assist the client to:
• Verbalize feelings about amputation and what the loss means to them.
• Define phantom limb sensation as a normal sensation that the amputated part is still there.
• Describe the dressings used after surgery.
• Describe pain control after surgery.
• Identify the goals for rehabilitation.
• Develop a plan for discharge.
Education should include the following:
• The opportunity and encouragement for the client and family to discuss their feelings and fears.
• Discussion about how the surgical incision will look.
• Description of the soft or rigid dressings that will be used. Assure the client that the staff will be routinely checking the dressings.
• Provide pain management education. The client is evaluated for the need for pain medication in the postoperative period and is encouraged to request medication when needed. The use of the pain scale will be described. Phantom limb sensation should also be discussed.
• Discuss rehabilitation goals. Although rehabilitation should begin before surgery, often the client is too ill to participate. The client will be evaluated for therapy, which includes activities such as transfer training, ambulation using crutches or walker, evaluation for home equipment as shower chair, gait training, and learning to walk with the prosthesis if the client is a prosthetic candidate.
• Have the client and family participate in discharge planning. Often, the client is ready for discharge from the acute ward about a week after surgery. There are several questions to be discussed with the client and family: Does the client live alone, and are they able to care for themselves? If the client is going home, is there wheelchair access into the home and the living areas such as the bathroom? Is there transportation for the client to come to therapy as an outpatient? Is there a need for equipment for the activities of daily living? Should an extended care or rehabilitation facility be considered?

TABLE 19.7 Postoperative Teaching
Goals are that the client will be able to:
• State the purpose of the residual limb dressing.
• Explain the purpose of proper positioning of the residual limb.
• Explain the purpose of and demonstrate the prone position.
• Demonstrate safe transfer techniques.
Education should include the following:
• *Residual limb dressing:* If a soft or rigid dressing is used, it can be changed frequently to inspect the suture line. The purposes of a rigid dressing are to prevent edema, prevent knee flexion contracture, decrease pain, and provide protection (Pugh et al., 2007).
• *Limb positioning:* Proper positioning of the residual limb is important to prevent edema of the limb and contractures of the knee and hip. For the first 24 to 48 hours after surgery the residual limb is elevated on pillows to prevent edema. After 24 hours the lower limb is positioned flat on the bed or supported straight when the client is in the wheelchair to prevent contractures of the hip and knee.
• *Prone positioning:* The client with a lower extremity amputation should lie prone for 15 to 20 minutes twice a day to help prevent hip contractures. If hip or knee flexion contractures develop, they may prevent the client from using the prosthesis
• *Safe transfer techniques:* Although the client receives instructions in proper use of the wheelchair, walker, and crutches, the nursing staff should observe and remind the client of safety instructions to prevent falls.

Educational Objectives for Family Education

The family is also involved in the physical, psychological, and social changes that affect the client. They need to understand what has happened to the family member and how they can assist the person through these changes. The family should be able to verbalize their feelings about the amputation, the client's reaction to the amputation, and the changes in the family structure. They need to

TABLE 19.8   Rehabilitation Teaching

Goals are that the client will be able to:

- Demonstrate residual limb inspection and care.
- State purpose of residual limb wrapping or use of shrinker.
- Demonstrate residual limb wrapping or use of shrinker.
- Demonstrate proper care of prosthesis.
- Describe the purpose of a liner or special socks.
- Demonstrate proper donning and doffing of prosthesis.
- Demonstrate proper foot care.
- Describe signs and symptoms of infections and actions if infection is noted.

Education should include the following:

- The residual limb should be inspected daily for any discolorations, open areas, or skin irritation. A mirror may be needed to view the end or back of the residual limb. The limb should be cleaned with soap and water the dried thoroughly.
- The purpose of residual limb wrapping or use of a shrinker is to reduce edema and shape the limb for the prosthesis. A shrinker is used in place of ace wrapping. Shrinkers must be hand washed and dried thoroughly before use. Wrapping or use of a shrinker will be needed for up to 4 months after surgery to control edema. The client should become independent in wrapping or use of the shrinker.
- Proper care of the prosthesis includes cleaning the socket with a damp cloth when the prosthesis is removed for the day. The prosthesis is inspected daily for any cracks or rough areas inside the socket and unusual noise or movement in the joint or foot.
- A liner or specially shaped socks of different thicknesses are used to maintain proper fit between the residual limb and socket of the prosthesis. The liner and socks should be cleaned according to manufacturer's instructions.
- Donning and doffing of the prosthesis correctly is important to prevent injury to the residual limb. If there is an opening in the skin, the prosthesis should not be worn to prevent possible infection. A new prosthesis should be worn for short periods, removed, and the residual limb inspected for any skin problems. The wearing time and use of the prosthesis should be increased slowly.
- Proper care of the remaining foot consists of daily inspection for open areas, blisters, and discolorations. Skin care includes washing and drying well. Lotion can be used for dry skin, but not between the toes because the moisture may lead to skin breakdown. Wearing shoes that fit properly is important to prevent open areas.

Source: From Carpenito-Moyet (2008), Kelly & Dowling (2008), Lusardi & Nielsen (2007), Pugh et al. (2007), and VA/DoD (2008).

understand the client's feelings, their own feelings, and how to use coping skills (Pugh et al., 2007). In addition, the nurse's teaching should focus on helping family members and significant others to

- Define phantom limb sensation and understand that these feelings are very real to the client.
- Identify the goals of rehabilitation and how they can enable the client to be independent.
- Be involved in the discharge plan for the client.

NURSING DIAGNOSES, OUTCOMES, AND INTERVENTIONS

Several nursing diagnoses related to the client with an amputation are easily identified. These include knowledge deficit, self-care deficit, impaired mobility, body image disturbance, grieving related to loss of body part, and alteration in comfort due to phantom pain or operative stump pain. Other nursing diagnoses may also be identified for use with these clients, such as fall prevention (Carpenito-Moyet, 2008).

Knowledge deficit is the absence of information or skills for disability management usually due to the lack of previous experience with the disability. It could also be related to a lack of knowledge of available community resources. Interventions for the nursing diagnosis of knowledge deficit include the following (Association of Rehabilitation Nurses & Rehabilitation Nursing Foundation, 2006):

- Develop educational objectives and goals with client and family.
- Build information on what client and family already know.

- Provide information and demonstration of skills while providing client care.
- Have the client and family demonstrate skills and verbalize knowledge to evaluate their understanding.
- Document assessments, teaching, and outcomes of education.

The nurse would expect, after providing education in the area of knowledge deficit, that the client and family could demonstrate the skills and knowledge for self-care, such as residual limb care, demonstrating limb wrapping, donning and doffing prosthesis, and demonstrating care of the other foot.

CASE STUDY 19.1

Your client is learning to use the prosthesis. He has developed a small open area on the residual limb. What would you teach him concerning the following?

1. Inspection of the residual limb?
   {Answer: He should daily inspect the residual limb for any discolorations and open areas. He may need to use a mirror to inspect all areas}
2. Wearing the prosthesis?
   {Answer: He should not wear the prosthesis while there is an open area because the area could become infected}

Self-care deficit is the decreased ability to perform activities of daily living. Persons with amputation may experience many changes in the ability to perform activities of daily living and may require instruction in adapting to changes in physical ability (Pugh et al., 2007). The rehabilitation nurse may use some of the following interventions to address self-care deficit:

- Involve client, family, and caregiver in setting goals.
- Reinforce therapist's instructions and activities for adapted activities of daily living.
- Encourage the client's independence and assist family to understand to provide only assistance necessary.

Expected outcomes could include that the client and family are able to demonstrate adapted techniques and equipment to meet self-care needs. If the patient is unable to meet his or her own self-care needs, the client should be able to direct care given by others.

Impaired physical mobility is the impaired physical ability for independent movement within the environment. In the case of amputation, this is related to balance difficulties due to change in body's center of gravity

from loss of lower limb (Carpenito-Moyer, 2008; Pugh et al., 2007).

Nursing interventions are as follows:

- Teach home safety and fall prevention.
- Discuss need to adapt environment for independence.
- Educate regarding the need to pace activities.
- Encourage use of adaptive equipment for safety and energy conservation.

Reasonable outcomes that the nurse would expect to see after patient/family education include the patient's ability to perform activities, as transfers, using safety precautions. The patient should also be able to demonstrate the safe use of adaptive equipment and positions to prevent joint contractures (Carpenito-Moyet, 2008; Pugh et al, 2007; Yetzer, 1998).

Body image disturbance occurs when there is a change in how the client perceives him- or herself. Certainly, this is a major consideration with amputation of any body part. According to Gallagher, Horgan, Franchignoni, Giordano, and MacLachlan (2007) there are several changes in body image for the client with an amputation: the body before amputation, the traumatized body, the healing body, and the extended body, including the prosthesis and assistive devices (Gallagher et al., 2007; Houston, 2005).

Nursing interventions for the client with body image disturbance are as follows:

- Encourage client and family to express feelings about loss and change in body image.
- Provide support by actively listening.
- Assist client and family to explore sources of support as professional and peer support groups.
- Assist client and family to identify and use helpful coping techniques.

Several outcomes are expected when addressing the nursing diagnosis of body image disturbance. The client should be able to express feelings about self-concept and changes in body image. Clients should begin the process of adapting to the changes in body image. They would be expected to participate in social activities without hiding residual limb and resume role-related responsibilities in family and community. Maintaining positive relationships with significant others is also a desired outcome.

In addition to body image changes, **grieving** related to loss of a body part and the resulting changes in body functioning, self-image, and usual lifestyle and roles is also common after amputation (Hanley et al., 2005). To help clients and families with the grieving process, the nurses could use these strategies (Bhuvaneswar et al., 2007):

- Provide support by active listening.
- Encourage client and family to express and share their feelings about the loss.
- Discuss the grief process and that it is an expected response to loss or change.
- Provide information about support groups, peer visitors, and counseling services (see Box 19.3).

- Encourage client and family to discuss their perception of the short- and long-term effects of the disability.

Expected outcomes are the client and family being able to express grief and begin to work through their feelings. They should be able to use available support systems and positive coping mechanisms.

Alteration in comfort is due to phantom pain or postoperative residual limb pain. Residual limb pain can be caused by the surgical incision, can be an expression of grief and altered body image, can result from postop-

---

BOX 19.3   Additional Helpful Resources

Journals

Amputee Coalition of America / National Limb Loss Information Center Fact Sheet. (2008). Financial assistance for prosthetic services, durable medical equipment, and other assistive devices. Retrieved from http://www.amputee-coalition.org/fact_sheets/assist_orgs.html

Hakimi, K. (2009). Pre-operative rehabilitation evaluation of the dysvascular patient prior to amputation. *Physical Medicine and Rehabilitation Clinics of North America, 20*(4), 677–688.

Highsmith, M. J. (2008). Barriers to the provision of prosthetic services in the geriatric populations. *Topics in Geriatric Rehabilitation, 24*(4), 325–331. Retrieved from http://www.amputee-coalition.org/first_step_2005/altered_states.html

Johnson, M., Newton, P., Jiwa, M., & Goyder, E. (2005). Meeting the educational needs of people at risk of diabetes-related amputation: a vignette study with patients and professionals. *Health Expectations, 8*, 324–333.

Kadel, N. J., Campbell, K., Phelps, E., Ehde, D., & Smith, D. G. (2008). Prosthesis use in persons with lower- and upper-limb amputation. *Journal of Rehabilitation Research & Development, 45*(7), 961–972.

MacKenzie, E. J., Snow Jones, A., Bosse, M. J., et al. (2007). Health-care costs associated with amputation or reconstruction of a limb-threatening injury. *Journal of Bone and Joint Surgery, 89*, 1685–1692.

National Amputation Foundation. (n.d). Tips for the new amputee and their families and friends. Retrieved from http://home.comcast.net/-n2fc/natamp/tips.html

Rogers, L. C., Lavery, L. A., & Armstrong, D. G. (2008). The right to bear legs—an amendment to healthcare: How preventing amputations can save billions for the US health-care system. *Journal of American Podiatric Medical Association, 98*(2), 166–168.

Smurr, L. M., Gulick, K., Yancosek, K., & Ganz, O. (2008). Managing the upper extremity amputee: A protocol for success. *Journal of Hand Therapy, 21*(2), 160–176.

Uustal, H. (2009). Prosthetic rehabilitation issues in the diabetic and dysvascular amputee. *Physical Medicine & Rehabilitation Clinics of North America, 20*(4), 689–704.

Books

National Limb Loss Information Center. (2005). *First step: A guide for adapting to limb loss.* Knoxville, TN: Amputation Coalition of America.

Meier, R. H., & Atkins, D.J. (Eds.). (2004). *Functional restoration of adults and children with upper extremity amputation.* New York, NY: Demos Medical Publishers.

Kirkup, J. (2006). *A History of Limb Amputation.* New York, NY: Springer.

Cristian, A. (2005). *Lower limb amputation: A guide to living a quality life.* New York, NY: Demos Publishing.

Muzumdar, A. (2004). *Powered upper limb prosthesis.* Berlin, NY: Springer.

Gallagher, P., Desmond, D., & MacLaachlan, M. (2007). *Psychoprosthetics.* New York, NY: Springer.

National Limb Loss Information Center. (2004). *Senior step: A Guide for adapting to limb loss.* Knoxville, TN: Amputation Coalition of America.

erative complications, or can be caused by phantom limb pain. Surgical incision pain is usually time limited and controlled by analgesics. Pain due to the expression of grief and alteration of body image may not be changed by analgesics. Severe pain due to complications must be reported to the surgeon for treatment of its cause. Phantom limb pain is usually due to severed nerves that continue to send pain impulses and give the sensation of the limb's presence (Ephraim, Wegener, MacKenzie, Dillingham, & Pezzin, 2005; Hanley et al., 2005; Richardson et al., 2006).

The nurse can assist the person with pain through these interventions:

- Assist the client to identify the nature of the discomfort and assess the need for pain medication or other measures to decrease discomfort.
- Administer appropriate pain medications as needed. Assess effectiveness of pain relief measures and document.
- Assist client to find comfortable position and support the limb during movement.
- Instruct client in other pain management techniques, such as tapping, massaging, and contracting and relaxing muscle groups of the residual limb.
- Encourage client to report phantom limb sensation and pain.

The specific outcomes the nurse should look for in relation to pain management include the client experiencing the absence of pain as evidenced by appearing relaxed and by verbalizing comfort. The client should participate in self-care and mobility activities without complaints of pain and be able to demonstrate techniques for management of phantom limb sensation and/or pain. Clients should also be able to explain the differences between phantom limb sensation and phantom limb pain.

SUMMARY

As the general population ages and the many complications of diabetes and vascular disease become more prevalent, the numbers of clients facing amputation will increase. The client with an amputation tends to be older with more concomitant and complicating medical problems. A major function of the rehabilitation team is to assist these clients and their families in dealing with everyday life after an amputation (see Box 19.4). This chapter presented information on the rehabilitation of the client with an amputation. The roles of members of the rehabilitation team, such as the nurse, PT, and

prosthetist, were described. Patience from everyone on the team, especially the client, is key in the rehabilitation of an amputee, because it can be a very long process from the initial amputation surgery to the final fit of a prosthesis.

BOX 19.4   Recommended Readings

Fischman, J. (2010). A better life with bionics. *National Geographic, 217*(1), 34–53.

Fitzgerald, D. (2000). Peer visitation for the preoperative amputee patient. *Journal of Vascular Nursing, 18*(2), 41–46.

Marzen-Groller, K., & Bartman, K. (2005). Successful support group for post-amputation patients. *Journal of Vascular Nursing, 23*(2), 42–45.

Mayo Clinic Staff. Phantom pain. Retrieved from www.mayoclinic.com/health/phantom-pain/DS00444/METHOD=print

---

CRITICAL THINKING

1. How is the level of amputation determined?
   (Answer: Where there is circulation to support healing the amputation)
2. How will a positive psychological outlook influence the functional outcome of the person with an amputation?
   (Answer: A positive psychological outlook will assist the client to participate in therapy and learn the knowledge and skills necessary for self-care.)
3. What factors are evaluated to determine if the client will be a prosthetics candidate?
   (Answer: Motivation and ability to learn the knowledge and skills needed for self-care. The absence of hip or knee contractures of the residual limb. The presence of any comorbidity that interfere with the use of a prosthesis.)
4. What are three comorbidities that can affect the client's candidacy for using a prosthesis?
   (Answer: Changes in memory and learning that affect client's ability to learn skills and knowledge to use prosthesis. Presence of cardiac and/or pulmonary diseases that affect the client's ability to meet energy requirements to use a prosthesis.)
5. Identify the parts of a prosthesis and describe their function.
   (Answer: The socket: contains the residual limb; Pylon: attaches the socket to the knee/foot; Prosthetic knee: for use in trans-femoral amputations to provide optimal ambulation; Prosthetic Foot/ankle joint: to enable walking.)

6. What should the client be taught about care of the remaining foot?
(Answer: Daily inspection for open areas, blisters, and discolorations. Skin care of washing and drying well. Lotion applied on top and bottom of the foot, but not between the toes. Wearing shoes the fit properly.)
7. Which of the following is the proper positioning of the residual limb when the client is in bed?
   a. Limb elevated on pillows
   b. Limb externally rotated
   c. Limb with knee flexed over end of bed
   d. Limb straight and flat on the bed.
(Answer: Limb straight and flat on the bed. This is to avoid contractions and promote full extension.)

PERSONAL REFLECTION

- Have you ever worked with a client with an amputation? How did you feel about the experience? How did the client cope with the changes in body image and the effects of the amputation? How did the family cope with the changes in family dynamics such as the client at this time may not be able to bring in income? What were their coping strategies?
- How do you define depression? What are four signs of depression?
- Imagine that you are in a serious car accident and lose your right arm above the elbow and the left leg below the knee. How would this change your life as you live at this point in time? What modifications would you have to make in your living situation? Housing? Transportation? Education? Vocation or job? How would this affect your body image and self-esteem? How would such losses affect your current relationship with family, significant others, and friends?

REFERENCES

American Physical Therapy Association. (2003). *Guide to physical therapy practice* (2nd ed., p. 13). Alexandria, VA: Author.

Amputee Coalition of America (ACA). (2004). *Peer visitor manual.* Knoxville, TN: National Limb Loss Information Center.

Amputee Coalition of America (ACA). (2006). Fact sheet: Peripheral arterial disease (PAD) and limb loss. Retrieved July 24, 2010, from www.amputeecoalition.org/fact_sheet/dysvascular.html

Amputee Coalition of America (ACA). (2007). Fact sheet: Limb loss in U.S. Retrieved from www.aca.org/fact_stat/limbloss_us.html

Amputee Coalition of America (ACA). (2008a). Fact sheet: Amputation statistics by cause. Retrieved November 1, 2009, from www.amputee-coalition.org/factsheet/amp_stats_cause.html

Amputee Coalition of America (ACA). (2008b). Fact sheet: Minorities, diabetes, and limb loss. Retrieved February 24, 2010, from www.amputee-coalition.org/fact_sheets/multicultural/all_groups.html

Association of Rehabilitation Nurses & Rehabilitation Nursing Foundation. (2006). Evidence-based rehabilitation nursing: Common challenges and intervention. Knowledge deficit, mobility. Glenview, IL: Author.

Bhuvaneswar, C., Epstein, L., & Stern, T. (2007). Reactions to amputation: Recognition and treatment. *Journal of Clinical Psychiatry, 9*(4), 303–308.

Boughton, B. (2003). Practitioners look beyond monofilaments for neuropathy screening. *Biomechanics, 11*(1), 51–57.

Carpenito-Moyet, L. (2008). *Nursing care plans and documentation: Nursing diagnosis and collaborative problems* (5th ed.). Philadelphia: Lippincott Williams & Wilkins.

DeLuccia, D. M., Anderson, J., & Berlet, G. C. (2007). Postoperative management for the trans-tibial amputee: Part 1. *Techniques in Foot & Ankle Surgery, 6*(3), 162–165.

Ephraim, P. L., Wegener, S. T., MacKenzie, E. L., Dillingham, T. R., & Pezzin, L. E. (2005). Phantom pain, residual limb pain, and back pain in amputees: Results of a national survey. *Archive of Physical Medicine and Rehabilitation, 86,* 1919–1919.

Fergason, K. (2005). Transtibial amputation: Prosthetic management. In D. Smith, J. Michael, & J. Howker (Eds.). *Atlas of amputations and limb deficiencies* (pp. 507–508). Rosemont, IL: American Academy of Orthopaedic Surgeons.

Fitzgerald, D. (2000). Peer visitation for the preoperative amputee patient. *Journal of Vascular Nursing, 18*(2), 41–46

Gallagher, P., Horgan, O., Franchignoni, F., Giordano, A., & MacLachlan, M. (2007). Body image in people with lower-limb amputation: A Rasch analysis of the Amputee Body Image Scale. *American Journal of Physical Medicine and Rehabilitation, 86*(3), 205–215.

Hanley, M. A., Jensen, M. P., Ehde, D. M., Hoffman, A. J., Patterson, D. R., & Robinson, L. R. (2005). Psychological predictors of long-term adjustment to lower-limb amputation and phantom limb pain. *Pain Practice, 5*(2), 146–147.

Houston, S. (2005). Altered states: Our body image, relationships and sexuality. First Step, 4. Retrieved August 29, 2009, from www.amputee-coalition.org/first_step/altered_states.html

Izumi, Y., Lee, S., Satterfield, K., & Harkless, L. B. (2006). Risk of reamputation in diabetic patients stratified by limb and level of amputation. *Diabetes Care, 29*(3), 566–570.

Johannesson, A., Turkiewicz, A., Larsson, G., Wirehn, A., Ramstrand, N., & Atroshi, I. (2009). Incidence of lower-level amputation in the diabetic and nondiabetic general population. *Diabetic Care, 32*(2), 275–280.

Kelly, B., Pangilian, P., Rodriguez, G., Mipro, R., & Bodeau, V. (2009). Upper limb prosthetics. *Physical Medicine and Rehabilitation.* Retrieved February 2, 2010, from emedicine. medscape.com/article/317234-print.

Kelly, M., & Dowling, M. (2008). Patient rehabilitation following lower limb amputation. *Nursing Standard, 22*(49), 35–40.

Laferrier, J. (2010). Advances in lower-limb prosthetic technology. *Physical Medicine and Rehabilitation Clinics of North America, 21*(1), 87–110.

Lehman, C. (2008). Mechanisms of injury in wartime. *Rehabilitation Nursing, 33*(5), 192–197, 205.

Lusardi, M., & Nielsen, C. (2007). *Orthotics and prosthetics in rehabilitation* (2nd ed.). St. Louis, MO: Saunders/Elsevier.

Magee, D. (2002). Assessment of the amputee. In D. Magee (Ed.), *Orthopedic physical assessment* (4th ed., pp. 905–925). Philadelphia: W.B. Saunders.

Marathon Medical Communications Inc. (2009). Upper limb amputees: The real advance lies in the future. *U.S. Medicine: The Voice of Federal Medicine.* Retrieved August 1, 2010, from www.usmedicine.com.

Marzen-Groller, K., & Bartman, K. (2005). Building a successful support group for post-amputation patients. *Journal of Vascular Nursing, 23*(2), 42–45.

Meier, R., & Atkins, D. (2004). *Functional restoration of adults and children with upper extremity amputation.* New York: Demos Medical Publishing.

Michael, J. (2005). Prosthetic suspensions and components. In D. Smith, J. Michael, & J. Bowker (Eds.), *Atlas of amputations and limb deficiencies* (pp. 409–423). Rosemont, IL: American Academy of Orthopaedic Surgeons.

Miklos, C. (2007). Physical therapy for the transtibial amputee with a removable rigid dressing: A program outline. *Techniques in Foot & Ankle Surgery, 6*(3), 166–169.

National Diabetes Fact Sheet. (2007). Retrieved November 1, 2009, from www.cdc.gov

O'Sullivan, S. (2007). Functional training and orthotic, prosthetic, supportive devices. In S. O'Sullivan (Ed.), *National physical therapy examination and study guide* (10th ed., p. 322). Evanston, IL: International Education Resources.

O'Sullivan, S., & Schmitz, T. (2001). Assessment and treatment of individuals following lower extremity amputation. In M. Schnee (Ed.), *Physical rehabilitation assessment and treatment* (4th ed., pp. 622–633). Philadelphia: F.A. Davis.

Pauley, T., Devlin, M., & Heslin, K. (2006). Falls sustained during inpatient rehabilitation after lower limb amputation: Prevalence and predictors. *American Journal of Physical Medicine and Rehabilitation, 85*, 521–532.

Pugh, S., Yetzer, E., & Naden-Blucher, B. (2007). Musculoskeletal and orthopedic disorders. In K. Mauk (Ed.), *The specialty practice of rehabilitation nursing: A core curriculum* (5th ed., pp. 208). Glenview, IL: Association of Rehabilitation Nurses.

Richardson, C., Glenn, S., Nurmikko, T., & Horgan, M. (2006). Incidence of phantom phenomena including phantom limb pain 6 months after major lower limb amputation in patients with peripheral vascular disease. *Clinical Journal of Pain, 20*(4), 353–358.

Rusk Institute of Rehabilitation Medicine. (2010). Amputation Rehabilitation Team. Retrieved August 1, 2010, from http:// amputee-support.med.nyu.edu/resources/healthcare-team

Singh, R., Hunter, J., & Philip, A. (2007). The rapid resolution of depression and anxiety symptoms after lower limb amputation. *Clinical Rehabilitation, 2*(8), 754–759.

Singh, R., Ripley, D., Pentland, B., Todd, I., Hunter, J., Hutton, L., & Philip. A. (2009). Depression and anxiety symptoms after lower limb amputation: The rise and fall. *Clinical Rehabilitation, 23*, 281–286.

Sleeth, J., & Ayyappa, E. (2001). *Prosthetics reference guide* (pp. 26–29). Long Beach, CA: Prosthetics Services Line, VISN.

Smith, D., Michael, J., & Bowker, J. (2004). *Atlas of amputations and limb deficiencies: Surgical, prosthetic, and rehabilitation principles* (3rd ed.). Rosemont, IL: American Academy of Orthopedic Surgeons.

Smurr, L., Gluck, K., Yancosek, K, & Ganz, O. (2008). Managing the upper extremity amputee: A protocol for success. *Journal of Hand Therapy, 21*(2), 160–176.

Veterans Affairs/Department of Defense (VA/DoD). (2008). Clinical practice guideline for rehabilitation of lower limb amputation. Retrieved September 1, 2010, from www.09P.med. va.gov/cpg.htm

Walters, R. (2005). Energy expenditure of walking in individuals with lower limb amputations. In D. Smith, J. Michael, & J. Bowker (Eds.), *Amputation and limb deficiencies* (pp. 395–407). Rosemont, IL: American Academy of Orthopaedic Surgeons.

Yetzer, E. (1996). Helping the patient through the experience of an amputation. *Orthopaedic Nursing, 15*(16), 45–49.

Yetzer E. (1998). Care of the client with an amputation. In P. Chin, D. Finocchiaro, & A. Rosebrough (Eds.), *Rehabilitation nursing practice* (pp. 375–392). New York; McGraw-Hill.

Ziegler-Graham, K., MacKenzie, E.J., Ephraim, P.L., Travison, T. G., & Bookmeyer, R. (2008). Estimating the prevalence of limb loss in the United States: 2005 to 2050. *Archive of Physical Medicine and Rehabilitation, 89*, 422–428.

CHAPTER 20

Polytrauma

Lucille Raia
Lisa Perla

LEARNING OBJECTIVES

At the end of this chapter, the reader will be able to

- Define polytrauma.
- Discuss the impact of polytrauma on the delivery of nursing care.
- Describe the Veterans Health Administration system of polytrauma care.
- Recognize the unique injuries and symptoms associated with blast injury.
- Understand the nursing challenges in caring for the blast-injured service member.

KEY CONCEPTS AND TERMS

Ambiguous loss
Blast injury
Burns
Compassion fatigue
Conflicts of death
Department of Defense
Improvised explosive devices
 (IEDs)

Operation Enduring Freedom
 (OEF)
Operation Iraqi Freedom (OIF)
Polytrauma
Polytrauma rehabilitation
 center
Polytrauma–TBI system of care
Polytrauma triad

Posttraumatic stress disorder
 (PTSD)
Veterans Health Administration
 (VHA)
Wars of disabilities

The **Operation Enduring Freedom (OEF)** and **Operation Iraqi Freedom (OIF)** conflicts have dramatically changed nursing care in the **Veterans Health Administration (VHA)**. Through a unique alliance between the **Department of Defense** (DOD) and the VHA, active-duty injured soldiers who have sustained catastrophic injuries from blasts are now being transferred from military hospitals to continue care and begin rehabilitation at designated Veterans Administration (VA) hospitals.

The VA healthcare team, especially the rehabilitation nurse, has been confronted with new and unique challenges in caring for patients with **blast injury** and subsequent **polytrauma**. The VHA defines polytrauma as follows (VHA, 2010, p. 3):

Two or more injuries sustained in the same incident that affect multiple body parts or organ systems and result in physical, cognitive, psychological, or psychosocial impairments and functional disabilities. TBI frequently occurs as part of the polytrauma spectrum in combination with other disabling conditions, such as amputations, burns, pain, fractures, auditory and visual impairments, PTSD, and other mental health conditions. When present, injury to the brain is often the impairment that dictates the course of rehabilitation due to the nature of the cognitive, emotional, and behavioral deficits related to TBI.

The challenges presented by greater numbers of service members with polytrauma have necessitated the development of new practice patterns not seen in traditional rehabilitation units, closer relationships within the rehabilitation teams, and stronger partnerships with families, significant others, and advocacy organizations.

POLYTRAUMA AND BLAST INJURY CARE: NEW PRACTICE CHALLENGES FOR NURSES

Historically, mortality rates in past wars were significantly higher than in the OEF and OIF initiatives (U.S. Department of Defense, 2010). The sophisticated resuscitative efforts in the Joint Theater Trauma System have been instrumental in this increase in survival rates. Past wars were mainly **conflicts of death**, whereas OEF and OIF are thought of as **wars of disabilities**. Because of these survival rates, rehabilitation has become as important in the care received as in the initial stabilization phase (Eshel, 2009; Fecura, Martin, Martin, Bolenbaucher, & Cotner-Pouncy, 2008). Blast injuries, mainly from **improvised explosive devices (IEDs)**, are responsible for many of the injuries and the changes seen in patterns of injury.

Scott, Vanderploeg, Belanger, and Scholten (2005) describe the injuries sustained by blast as profound and multifactorial. A blast creates pressure changes within the body (especially in cavities that are air filled), causes items in the environment to become lethal projectiles, propels the body in space, and exposes the body to other toxins, burns, and trauma from falling debris (Defense and Veterans Brain Injury Center, n.d). Because of the complexity and the unpredictable nature of the injuries, practitioners are challenged in diagnosing, treating, and evaluating care. According to Lew et al (2009), the care of blast-injured individuals who subsequently sustain polytrauma injury involves a wide range of medical and psychosocial interventions throughout the continuum of care. Therefore, polytrauma/blast-injured individuals warrant a different care delivery paradigm, both from a medical and a nursing perspective. Rehabilitation care for the polytrauma/blast-injured service member encompasses physical and occupational therapies, medical interventions, cognitive and behavioral approaches, and certainly family and significant other participation on a more extensive scale than previously seen in the VA setting. Moreover, because of the complexity and number of injuries, the vagueness of presentations, and the uncommon manifestations of illness, the nurse's role in the rehabilitation setting becomes critical in identifying the early signs and symptoms of acute illness, psychosocial needs, the trajectory of functional impairments, and interpreting how all these impact the daily lives of their patients and families.

Presentations of illness and disability in the polytrauma patient can be masked by confounding factors, such as an unknown physiological and psychological baseline, or by insignificant manifestations such as gait changes or vague generalized complaints (Almogy et al., 2006). Polytrauma/blast-injured individuals and their families may also experience many changes secondary to perceived and real losses. Behavioral changes may include apathy, depression, anger, and disruptive relationships that may affect the outcome of medical treatment.

POLYTRAUMA SYSTEM OF CARE

"In 2004, Congress passed Public Law 108-422, The Veterans Health Programs Improvement Act of 2004, Section 302, which directed the Department of Veterans Affairs (VA) to designate an appropriate number of cooperative centers for clinical care, consultation, research, and education activities on complex TBI and Polytrauma associated with combat injuries" (VHA Directive 2009-028, 2.d). Further, the Conference Report for Public Law 108-447 (Conference Report on H.R. 4818, Report 108-792) directed the Department of Veterans Affairs to implement a new initiative to ensure that returning war veterans with loss of limb and other severe and lasting injuries have access to the best of both modern medicine and integrative holistic therapies. In 2008, to further meet the needs of service members and veterans in combat operations, Title 38 U.S. Code sections 1710D, and 1710E, addressing rehabilitation of traumatic brain injury, were enacted.

Because polytrauma and TBI can also occur as a result of noncombat events, such as motor vehicle accidents, to ensure that the needs of both combat- and noncombat-injured service members and veterans are met and in response to the above legislation, the VHA developed a **polytrauma–TBI system of care** that provides specialized rehabilitation care for veterans and service members with polytrauma and TBI. This system integrates specialized rehabilitation services at regional centers, veterans integrated service sites, and local VA medical centers. Polytrauma and TBI rehabilitation care is provided at the facility closest to the veteran's home that has the expertise necessary to manage the veteran's or service member's rehabilitation and physical and mental health needs.

The VA polytrauma system is designed to balance the need for highly specialized expertise with the need for accessibility. Persons with severe TBI often have functionally devastating injuries that may cause impairments that require lifelong assistance with activities of daily living. Therefore, early and specialized care can reduce acute and long-term medical and functional impairments.

Implications for Nurses Working in Polytrauma

As previously stated, the role of the rehabilitation nurse has taken on greater importance within new polytrauma treatment systems. More specialized knowledge and skills are required to meet the challenges of caring for persons with polytrauma (MacLennan et al., 2008). In this section of the chapter, general nursing implications are discussed, with more specific strategies for interventions following later in the chapter.

Effects of Blast Injury

Many returning polytrauma/blast-injured individuals from OEF and OIF have been injured by IEDs. Blasts cause displacement of organs, a stress and shear pressure to the body, subsequent injury from flying objects, and propulsion of the body into solid objects (Belanger, Scott, Scholten, Curtis, & Vanderploeg, 2005; Taber, Warden, & Hurley, 2006; Warden, 2006). These forces damage vital internal organs, causing TBI, skull compression, blindness from eye trauma, loss of limbs and multiple fractures, or **burns** (Spotswood, 2006; Taber et al., 2006; Warden, 2006). Table 20.1 provides more information on injuries caused by blasts.

The blast-injured are also at a greater risk for developing infections, not only because of the multiple traumas they have sustained, but also as a result of bacterial exposure in the field (Holcomb, 2005; Schecter & Fry, 2005). Many times these organisms are indigenous to the country at war and may pose a challenge for infectious disease management in our country. For individuals injured by blast, stabilization at the battlefront is the first level of treatment.

Stabilization

Medical care at the battlefront has evolved from single-response medical personnel to comprehensive hi-tech surgical theatres. Polytrauma/blast-injured individuals who sustain extensive injuries can now be stabilized and surgically treated at the battlefront before being triaged to overseas military installations. At the military sites these individuals undergo further stabilization and acute management before they are finally transferred to military hospitals in the United States. After this course, many of those requiring rehabilitation or further management are transferred to a VA Medical Center Level I acute rehabilitation facility.

Rehabilitation

Nursing care of the blast-injured individual poses many challenges. The concept of rehabilitation usually indicates that an individual at the end of a hospital course is medically stable and is nearly ready for discharge to his or her home (Delisa, Currie, & Martin, 1998). Web explorations 20.1, 20.2, and 20.3 provide some excellent websites and resources for healthcare professionals that could be used to educate patients and family members.

Polytrauma/blast-injured individuals who have multiple injuries, particularly TBI, differ from the usual rehabilitation patient. Notably, the injuries of polytrauma/

TABLE 20.1 Blast-Related Injuries	
System	**Injury or Condition**
Auditory	Tympanic membrane rupture, ossicular disruption, cochlear damage, foreign body. If tympanic membrane rupture, consider at risk for pulmonary viscous injury.
Eye, orbit, face	Perforated globe, foreign body, air embolism, fractures. Up to 10% of all blast survivors have significant eye injuries.
Respiratory	Blast lung, hemothorax, pneumothorax, pulmonary contusion, and hemorrhage.
Digestive	Bowel perforation, hemorrhage, ruptured liver or spleen.
Circulatory	Cardiac contusion, myocardial infarction from air embolism, shock, vasovagal hypotension, peripheral vascular injury, and air embolism–induced injury.
Central nervous system	Concussion, closed and open brain injury, stroke, spinal cord injury, and air embolism–induced injury.
Renal	Renal contusion, laceration, and acute renal failure.
Extremity	Traumatic amputation, fractures, crush injuries, compartment syndrome, burns, cuts, lacerations, acute arterial occlusion, and air embolism–induced injury.

Source: From Centers for Disease Control and Prevention (2008).

blast-injured individuals are multiple and severe, and the acute signs of illness can be masked. Moreover, rehabilitation teams may be unfamiliar with the expected course of recovery of the polytrauma/blast-injured individual. Compounding the challenges in the rehabilitation phase is the brief time period between injury and rehabilitation, which can be just a few short weeks. Given the devastating and systemic injuries, the cognitive and behavioral changes, the social and political implications, and a changing reality of rehabilitation, a new framework of care is needed that is patient and family centered and underscores the diversity of cultures and philosophical beliefs, with a fluidity of roles among all stakeholders in an environment of learning and with a new script for nurses.

The first area to address within a new framework of care is the need for specialized education for the rehabilitation team member. A comprehensive educational program has been developed by the VA polytrauma system in which the manifestations of acute illness, concepts of rehabilitation, and psychosocial approaches are reviewed. For example, a polytrauma/blast-injured individual's only complaint could be a change in gait, when in fact a diagnosis of a more serious condition like meningitis may be the etiology. It is well known that in the elderly population, infection many times manifests in a fall (Gosney, 2007; Lopez et al, 2002; Tinetti, 2003) or cardiac ischemia manifests in shortness of breath or may present as a gastrointestinal upset (Gallo, Fulmer, Paveza, & Reichel, 2000). Similarly, polytrauma/blast-injured individuals may exhibit understated presentations when in fact the underlying pathology is more serious.

Psychosocial Nursing Issues

The results of injury can be devastating to both polytrauma/blast-injured individuals and their families. Because nurses are at the forefront of the service member's hospital care, nurses may personally feel the impact of such devastating injuries through interactions with families, friends, and visitors. Because of the intense family and visitor presence, it may appear that the nursing care of the polytrauma/blast-injured serviceperson is being scrutinized by "outsiders." For instance, a military liaison who is a representative of the Department of Defense is assigned to the **polytrauma rehabilitation center** (PRC) and oversees the care of the serviceperson. Additionally, many family members are frequently at the serviceperson's bedside throughout the day, sometimes spending up to 24 hours each day with their loved ones Therefore, nurses face the challenge of caring for service members with medical and surgical presentations that are unfamiliar, dynamic, and evolving within an environment of family and military presence and oversight.

Nursing practice for polytrauma/blast injury has been evolving since the establishment of the VA polytrauma centers. Historically, it has been the nurse who offers emotional support. Service members and families continue to expect the nurse to understand both their physical and emotional losses. Moreover, it is nurses at the bedside that the serviceperson and the family expect to understand their feelings of anger and powerlessness. Therefore, nurses need to be skilled in managing difficult situations when the dynamics are not ideal. Additionally, nurses need be aware of their own feelings and how their feelings may have an impact on their own well-being.

Emotional Support

Emotional support and empathy for loss underscore the nurses' role in the delivery of holistic care. It is what caregivers offer even when there is nothing else available. Empathy is a basic nursing tool that may become less sharp when the nurse is under stress, has increased scrutiny, or is in an extremely challenging situation. Emotional support involves developing rapport, listening with an empathetic ear, appreciating the serviceperson's and the family's values, and assessing and responding to their daily needs. Bond, Draeger, Mandleco, and Donnelly (2003), in a qualitative study of family members of servicepersons with TBI in an intensive care unit (ICU), reported the needs of families with TBI differ significantly from the needs of families of servicepersons who did not have such injuries. The authors identified a need to know and a need for consistent information and involvement in care for the families to make sense of the situation that may deal with the probability of death. These needs carry over to the rehabilitation setting. The nurse can help empower the family through education and support. The

time to begin the process of offering emotional support is at the onset of an admission. Emotional support can be as simple as listening with a projection of concern. Offering emotional support can revolve around the everyday task of performing the nursing assessment.

Moreover, according to Boss (1996) a newly emerging concept of **ambiguous loss** occurs. Ambiguous loss consists of feelings of not being certain of a person's absence or presence. Boss (1996, 2006) contends that as humans, we seek certainty and accept death more easily than continuing with doubt: doubt if a loved one is dead or alive, dying, or recovering. Boss (1996, 2006) reports that similar feelings of ambiguous loss were seen post-9/11 whereby significant others reported their loved ones who had survived this terrible nightmare were not the same people they knew before. Or conversely, ambiguous loss might exist for families with loved ones whose bodies were never recovered from the destruction and still remain missing. Parallel to this experience, spouses of individuals with dementia report feelings of ambiguous loss as they care for a loved one who no longer resembles the person they knew, who is now perceived as absent, but is physically present. Ambiguous loss, if not diagnosed early, can lead to symptoms similar to posttraumatic stress disorder (PTSD), which compounds the stress for polytrauma families.

To complicate the situation, there may also be the loss of a family's primary financial source, established careers or career goals, dreams, aspirations, place in the family, and possessions. Situational losses are not always obvious to others, yet they can affect the rehabilitation process, recovery trajectory, and family health. Families may struggle with these losses and the accompanying feelings of anger, guilt, helplessness, confusion, and depression. The anger is often displaced and frequently masks their feelings of helplessness and confusion and uncertainty about the future. Family and patient education is paramount in addressing these issues.

Compassion Fatigue

Nurses who care for servicepersons with traumatic injuries may be further challenged by the phenomenon of **compassion fatigue**. Compassion fatigue is the emotional residue from caring for those who have suffered from traumatic events. According to Collins and Long (2003) compassion fatigue is sudden and acute. In the instance of caring for servicepersons with traumatic injuries, the nurse is also working with family members who have sustained a devastating emotional experience. Compassion fatigue is sometimes thought of as "secondary posttraumatic stress" (Sabo, 2006). The nurse may experience low morale, anxiety, anger, blaming, complaining, and an overall decline in job performance. If unchecked, compassion fatigue can lead to a decline in general health. In an effort to combat compassion fatigue the nurse needs to remember to avoid over-identification with the serviceperson and/or his or her family members, work closely with the interdisciplinary team to manage difficult situations, recharge batteries every day, take breaks off the unit, and keep the caring process within boundaries of care.

Confronting Psychosocial Nursing Needs

In summary, care of polytrauma/blast-injured servicepersons warranted a paradigm shift in the VA system of care. Moreover, the partnerships that evolved created a challenging departure from the traditional family involvement.

Nurses caring for this dynamic population have been confronted with the need to learn new practice parameters and to develop expertise in assessing subtle nuances of critical illness in a rehabilitation setting. The psychological needs necessitated a new model of care underscored by caring for self. This approach created opportunities for staff to grow and heal each other as they provided support to patients and families.

A host of physical, psychological, social, and emotional factors characterized by blast injury are manifested throughout the continuum of care. Providers at all levels have been called on to develop evidence-based practice, conduct research, create opportunities for independence, and thread the goals of the team, injured person, and family in a integrated horizontal pattern to support wellness and function in any setting.

COMMON INJURIES SEEN IN POLYTRAUMA

The following overview of polytrauma sequelae is an attempt to illustrate the number and severity of the injuries. Understanding these and appreciating the differences that may exist between those who were injured from a blast to other injuries sustained by nonblast causes may pose a challenge to nurses when assessing, identifying nursing diagnoses, determining goals, and correlating the appropriate interventions and evaluations. After this overview a list of general nursing implications is included as well as some that are imbedded into the subject matter when appropriate. These implications aim to provide general considerations that are salient to all, specifics that

are applicable to some, and with caveats that imply the vagaries of the complexity of each presentation.

Traumatic Brain Injury

TBI is defined as traumatically induced structural injury or physiological disruption of brain function as a result of an external force. Injuries can be penetrating or closed and can be classified as mild, moderate, or severe. Severity level of the TBI is determined by using the following measurements at the time of the injury: Glasgow coma scale (GCS) score, length of loss of consciousness (LOC), and length of posttraumatic amnesia (PTA).

The spectrum of TBI injuries is highly variable (see Chapter 16 for a more thorough discussion about brain injury). Most TBIs due to blast or other mechanisms are mild, and most patients recover within days or weeks. When rapidly and appropriately managed, mild TBI, often called concussion, tends to resolve with no or only minimal functional sequelae. A small percentage of persons with mild TBI have symptoms that require specialized rehabilitation services to manage acute problems and to prevent long-term sequelae. These ongoing symptoms might include headache, dizziness, visual changes, difficulty with maintaining balance, and changes in behavior.

On the other hand, persons with moderate to severe TBI generally require intensive inpatient rehabilitation. Many of these individuals may have some permanent functional sequelae that can be significantly reduced with timely and appropriate services.

> *When present, injury to the brain is often the impairment that dictates the course of rehabilitation due to the nature of the cognitive, emotional, and behavioral deficits related to TBI.*

Military and Civilian Statistics

Among civilians, TBI is the leading cause of death and disability among children and young adults. Approximately 1.4 million TBIs occur in the United States in the civilian sector (Centers for Disease Control and Prevention [CDC], 2006). Additionally, annually more than 80,000 individuals are left with lifelong disabilities from TBI. Currently, approximately 5.3 million people are living with a brain injury in the United States. The leading causes of TBI are falls (28%), motor vehicle accidents (20%), struck by/against events (19%), and assaults (11%). Males are 1.5 times as likely as females to sustain a TBI (CDC, 2006). There is a bimodal age distribution for increased risk of TBI between the ages of 0 to 4 and 15 to 19 years of age (CDC, 2006). Direct medical costs and indirect costs such as lost productivity after TBI are estimated at $60 billion per year. Additionally, the costs associated with lifetime treatment for TBI are estimated to be between $600,000 and $1.8 million (Brain Injury Association of America, 2007; www.va.gov, 2004; Zaloshnja, Miller, Langlois, & Selassie, 2008).

For military personnel, the Department of Defense's Report to Congress in Accordance with Section1634(b) of the National Defense Authorization Act for Fiscal Year 2008, the Military Health U.S. Military Casualty Statistics Congressional Research Service System (MHS) has recorded 43,779 patients who have been diagnosed with a TBI in calendar years 2003 through 2007. The MHS has spent an estimated $100 million on direct and purchased care for TBI patients and $10.1 million on prescription costs for those with the diagnosis of TBI (Defense and Veterans Brain Injury Center, n.d.).

TBI Level of Severity

Mild TBI or concussion is the most prevalent type of TBI, accounting for about 75% of TBIs that occur each year. A mild TBI is a result of the forceful motion of the head or impact causing a brief change in mental status (confusion, disorientation, or loss of memory) or loss of consciousness for less than 30 minutes. Often missed at time of initial injury, 15% of people with mild TBI have symptoms that last 1 year or more. Postinjury symptoms are often referred to as postconcussive syndrome. Recognizing the implications of these shear numbers and the nuances with which individuals present, the nurse's role becomes paramount in identifying cognitive and behavioral changes that may indicate a TBI was indeed sustained. Table 20.2 provides a summary of grading the severity of brain injuries. Nursing implications for care of the person with TBI appear in Chapter 16.

Burns

Challenges associated with TBI and polytrauma in the rehabilitation of patients with burns are, by definition, not confined to just skin care. There are several types or degrees of burns. A first-degree burn is superficial and causes local inflammation of the skin. Sunburns often are categorized as first-degree burns. The inflammation is characterized by pain, redness, and mild swelling. The skin may be tender to touch. Second-degree burns are deeper, and in addition to the pain, redness, and inflammation there may be blistering of the skin. Third-degree burns are deeper still and involve all layers of the skin and cause damage to the nerves and blood vessels. The skin appears white and leathery and tends to be relatively painless. Burns are not static and can continue to evolve and mature.

Incidence

Burns are a significant problem in the ongoing conflicts in Iraq and Afghanistan. Five percent to 10% of combat casualties result in thermal injuries. Inhalation injury is also relatively common with blast, affecting 18% of individuals who are near to or in a confined space (CDC, 2008).

> Patient quote: "The tightness of my skin made it feel like I was being squeezed by a boa constrictor. It was suffocating."

Typical Treatments and Interventions for Burns

Medical, nursing, and rehabilitative care for persons with burns may be complex and ongoing and may include the following:

- Timely wound closure and staged grafting
- Escharotomies/fasciotomies
- Dressings for protection from infections

TABLE 20.2 Classifying Severity of Brain Injury		
Grade 1 (Mild)	**Grade 2 (Moderate)**	**Grades 3 and 4 (Severe)**
Altered or LOC < 30 min with normal CT +/– MRI	LOC < 6 hr with abnormal CT +/– MRI	LOC > 6 hr with abnormal CT +/– MRI
GCS 13–15	GCS 9–12	GCS < 9
PTA < 24 hr	PTA < 7 days	PTA > 7 days

CT, computed tomography; GCS, Glasgow coma scale; LOC, loss of consciousness; MRI, magnetic resonance imaging; PTA, posttraumatic amnesia.

Source: Department of Veterans Affairs. (2004). Traumatic brain injury independent study course. Veterans Health Initiative. Retrieved from www.va.gov

- Collection of drainage to aid in proper extremity and digit position to reduce water loss and to protect injured areas sensitive to air currents
- Coordination of medications with dressing changes and therapy times
- Topical antibiotics, moisturizing agents
- Splinting and alignment
- Elevating injured limbs or digits
- Stretching exercises
- Pressure garments
- Skin grafts

Patient/Family Education

The increased presence of family members during the recovery process presents an ideal opportunity for rehabilitation nurses to act in the role of teacher. Key components for patient and family education are

- Need for use of extremities
- Limiting the use of adaptive equipment
- Stretching exercises
- Good skin care and protection
- Observing skin changes that may indicate infections
- Making life changes to sustain and improve function and independence

Nurses also need to understand the dynamics of the family in promoting the individual's self-care and enhancing their abilities versus having the family intervene without giving the loved one opportunity to achieve the skills and abilities for independence (Hall, 2005).

Psychosocial Considerations

The psychological and neuropsychological impact of burn injuries includes anxiety, mood disturbance, increased suicidal ideations, PTSD, anger, fear, body image/social stigma, adjustment, and coping issues. Table 20.3 provides a complete list of potential psychological and psychosocial symptoms commonly seen after burn injury.

Orthopedic Injuries and Fractures

Blast injuries may result in traumatic-limb, dissolving, or partial-limb amputation; soft tissue and crush injuries; and fractures. Traumatic or dissolving amputations are often caused by the primary effects of the pressure waves from the blast on the shaft of the bone as compared with other types of orthopedic injuries, which are commonly

TABLE 20.3   Emotional and Psychological Symptoms for Victims Coping with Burn Injuries

- Apathy
- Preoccupation with trauma
- Perfectionism
- Anxiety
- Depression
- Fatigue
- Sleep disturbances
- Guilt
- Numbness
- Misplaced anger
- Emotional exhaustion
- Being accident prone
- Anger with god (loss of faith)
- Lack of purpose
- Negativity
- Impatience
- Nightmares
- Substance overuse/abuse

caused by penetrating or impact trauma. The latter are usually a result of the tertiary and quaternary effects of the blast (CDC, 2008). Because of the advances in medicine and the protective armor worn in battle, survival is enhanced with many returning service members presenting with lifelong functional disabilities from loss of limb.

Heterotopic ossification is an abnormal growth of bone in soft tissue such as muscle. Heterotopic ossification often appears after traumatic injury, but the causes are not known. Heterotopic ossification can restrict range of motion, cause pain, and impact basic activities of daily living. For patients who may also have a TBI, the functional impairments that heterotopic ossification and other orthopedic injuries produce can be as life-threatening as the injury itself.

Patient/Family Education

Patient and family education is critical after any injury. The rehabilitation process and discharge plans are interwoven, carefully evaluated, and can be dynamic. A change or loss of function alters the plans for the discharge setting; therefore, teaching the patient and family about what complaints warrant immediate action versus those that may just require a watch and wait strategy is important.

Wounds

The care of wounds related to polytrauma is also a unique challenge for the rehabilitation nurse. The types of wounds might range from simple abrasions to burns, skin ulcers, staphylococcal infections, and gaping wounds with attached closure devices. Therefore, the care of wounds is prioritized according to the individual's needs. The priority for the rehabilitation nurse is to recognize and minimize the occurrence of infection, help eliminate existing infections, and promote expedited healing through diligent wound care. The assignment of private rooms, bathrooms, and showers should be used when necessary to avoid cross-contamination (Hall, 2005). It is well known that mortality rates reach 75% among those individuals who have subsequent bacteremia (Spanholtz, Theodorou, Amini, & Spilker, 2009). These rates necessitate the careful attention and monitoring of wound healing. The use of a specially trained wound care nurse can be a great asset for the patient with the challenging wounds often seen with polytrauma. The relief of pain associated with wounds and traumatic injury is imperative during the healing process and can be an important factor in the patient's recovery and overall sense of well being. Chapter 8 provides additional information about skin and wound care.

Patient/Family Education

Patient and family education surrounding wound healing includes dietary factors they can implement, especially surrounding protein stores, vitamins necessary for wound healing, and, when appropriate, frequent shifting of body positions and aligning extremities. Families can be the eyes of the patient when observing potential sites for breakdown and work in collaboration with the therapy team to ensure optimal wound healing (Hall, 2005; Long, 2007)

Posttraumatic Stress Disorder

PTSD is a severe anxiety disorder that can develop after exposure to any event that results in psychological trauma, such as those events involved in war. The event may involve the threat of death to oneself or to someone else and may overwhelm the individual's ability to cope. Diagnostic symptoms for PTSD include reexperiencing the original trauma(s) through flashbacks or nightmares, avoidance of stimuli associated with the trauma, and increased arousal, such as difficulty falling or staying asleep, anger, and hypervigilance. Nurses should minimize high-pressure situations for patients with the diagnosis of PTSD. Patience, tolerance, and acceptance are also important communication styles when assisting patients with PTSD.

Patient/Family Education

PTSD is not only an individual burden but also a family, community, and system one. As with nursing interventions, families can seek to minimize situations that are laden with emotionally charged issues, take serious threats of harm to self or others, and use open and continuous communication with members of the rehabilitation team (Lew et al., 2009b).

Sensory, Vision, and Hearing Impairments

As a result of IEDs and stateside injuries, both ocular and auditory trauma rates have increased for patients with and without a TBI. According to the National Alliance for Eye and Vision Research (2009), approximately 16% of war-related injuries affect the eyes. More specifically, optic nerve trauma is the most severe. Furthermore, of those servicepersons who have sustained a TBI in Iraq secondary to blast, 85% have visual symptoms.

According to Lew and colleagues (2009a), frequencies and effects of recovery of auditory and vision impairment in individuals with blast-related injury are not well documented. In a preliminary study of 175 patients admitted to a polytrauma rehabilitation center, hearing and visual examinations were obtained at admission and discharge for 62 patients with blast-related TBI. This study revealed a diagnoses of hearing impairment only, vision impairment only, and dual sensory impairment in 19%, 34%, and 32% of patients, respectively. Understanding the long-term consequences of sensory impairments and the functional recovery of patients with blast-related TBI is ongoing.

Patient/Family Education

Individuals who have deficits in either vision or hearing may at first rely on family members to act as their eyes and ears. Moving the individual from dependence to independence necessitates that families are ready to allow this transition, much like parents do for smaller children when they first learn to walk. Strong family support systems need to be in place and the rehabilitation team needs to be cohesive and supportive as they recognize the struggle families may have in letting go and in trusting the team and the individual to take risks and take charge of his or her future.

Pain and Polytrauma

With the extreme forces found in combat and civilian trauma the resultant physical injuries and pain from trauma or injury can be a significant problem. Lew et al. (2009b) reported on the prevalence of a triad of symptoms, chronic pain, PTSD, and postconcussive syndrome, also known as the **polytrauma triad**. According to Clark, Bair, Buckenmaier, Gironda, and Walker, (2007), comprehensive assessment and reassessment of pain is the cornerstone of optimal pain management for all pain conditions. Tengvall, Wickman, and Wengstrom (2010) found in their study that memories of pain after burn injury were clearly remembered, as were their experiences surrounding pain management along the trajectory of their care. They further contend that patients carry these memories and that these memories could worsen or contribute to depression or to PTSD. Thus, the rehabilitation team, but especially nursing, needs to be aware of the lingering effects of the pain experiences from acute through the rehabilitation phase of care. Managing pain requires nursing diligence to ensure adequate pain medications are offered and that the use of diversionary management has been encouraged. The nurse should also offer thorough education regarding pain management to the patient as well as their family and/or significant others. Psychosocial support should also be offered in the form of mental health providers and/or a pain care team whenever possible. (Case Study 20.1)

CASE STUDY 20.1

A 19-year-old male, active-duty service member transferred to Bethesda Naval Medical Center (NNMC) after sustaining a blast injury from an IED in Iraq (OIF). His injuries and medical/surgical history are as follows:

- Coma times 6 days, with initial Glasgow coma scale score of 9 (moderate TBI)
- Posterior fossa fracture
- Left frontoparietal subdural hematoma
- Diffuse axonal injury
- Splenic laceration, s/p splenectomy
- Pancreatic laceration with history of a pancreatic fistula
- Fractures of the left tibia, fibula, and femur, s/p ORIF of tib/fib and IM rod to the femur
- Third-degree burns to the left leg and buttocks, s/p debridement and grafting

Sixty-four days after injury the patient was transferred from NNMC to a polytrauma rehabilitation center. On the third day of admission a low grade fever was noted with elevated white blood counts and abdominal pain. Abdominal x-rays revealed free fluid adjacent to the liver. Also noted was a left iliac thrombus which was treated with anticoagulation therapy.

The mother has been at the patient's side for several months. Now that the patient is at the polytrauma rehabilitation center the mother arrives on the unit at 7 a.m. before the breakfast trays are served. She keeps constant vigil and seldom leaves the room, even for meals.

Physical Exam

VS: T, 99.5; P, 102; RR, 22; BP, 162/95; pain, 2 (on 0–10 scale)
GEN: alert and oriented to name and place but not date
HEENT: no lymphadenopathy
CV: tachycardic with no murmurs, rubs, gallops
Lungs: clear to auscultation bilaterally
Abdomen: bowel sounds present, abd firm, nontender, non-distended
MS: decreased strength in LLE
Ext: no RE edema

Laboratory Values

WBC	18.7 H
HGB	12.9 L
HCT	38.1 L
PLT	255.0 H
K	3.1 L
NA	126 L
CL	89 L
CO2	24

Nurse's Notes

S: Mother at bedside. They note increased confusion since the weekend & an episode of urinary incontinence.
Patient complaining & moaning. Also C/O "ringing in ears, weakness, & back pain."
O: Skin: pale, warm, dry. Stage 1 pressure ulcer on L heel
CV: BP @ 160/84, HR @ 128
Resp: RR 28, Color pale
GI: Vomited x 1 after eating 25% of his dinner. Diarrhea x 3.
GU: Voided x 1 this shift-180cc
Pain: Unable to get comfortable or lay still in bed.
Musculoskeletal: LLE remains immobilized and elevated when in wheelchair
Mobility: Wheelchair—most of day
Psych: Appears to be anxious, received Xanax x 2 for restlessness. During this tour unable to sleep.
A: s/p TBI, change in mental status and low grade fever
P: Consult & collaborate with MD regarding change in mental status and new incontinence (x 1 episode)
Administer PRN analgesic

Results

The MD assessed the patient and offered the following orders, results, and interventions:

- Obtain blood, urine, and wound cultures
  - Findings *Acinetobacter* of blood, all other cultures were negative
  - Intravenous antibiotics were started
- Computed tomography of the abdomen
  - Findings significant for hepatic pseudocyst
  - Percutaneous drain placed

Patient/Family Education

Chronic pain can be a disabling issue for patients and families. Families may question the therapy, the management of pain, as well as the individual's perception. Furthermore, pain may mask acute illness, and families need to be astute in distinguishing changes from a baseline or an ongoing chronicity of symptoms.

Nursing Implications

The nursing implications needed to care for polytrauma are considerable and are emerging as we move from unknowns to identifying patterns of care. Individuals who have sustained burns, grafting, and donor site harvesting may complain of tightness, joint stiffness, contractures, scarring, and pain from compression neuropathies that may present after the acute phase of injury (Ferguson, Franco, Pollack, Rumbolo, & Smock, 2010; Spanholtz, Theodorou, Amini, & Spilker, 2009). Some of the other common issues associated with burns that dictate the need for specialized nursing care and staff training are as follows:

- Importance of protecting the individual from extremes in temperature and damage from exposure to the sun and other environmental effects.
- Management of acute pain that may still be present from the ongoing cleansing, dressing changes, the donor and graft site, and general skin care. Many times the pain is accompanied by inflammation with or without itching.
- Nutritional deficits related to increased metabolic needs, especially during the initial phase of burn treatment.
- Necessity of recurrent reconstructive surgeries.
- Immobilization resulting in deconditioning, muscle atrophy, stiffness, and contractures.
- Disfiguring scars and heterotopic ossification.
- Infection of donor and graft sites and open wounds.
- Temperature regulation (depends on thickness and loss of sweat glands).
- Peripheral neuropathy.
- Pulmonary scarring and inhalation injuries.
- Self-concept and body image.

The nursing indications surrounding care for the unusual and devastating orthopedic injuries sustained from a blast include the practice standards of assessing limbs for circulation, sensation, and motion deficits. Because of the destructive nature of blast, bone injury and traumatic amputations are common and many times are compounded by infection. The organisms that have been discharged into these open wounds and bone shafts are indigenous to the area or foreign country from where they were sustained. Therefore, careful observation for signs of infection and/or changes in a limb status, gait change, or other nuances from the individual's baseline need to be carefully worked up and followed through to all settings.

General skin and wound care also includes ongoing consultation with a skin care specialist or at the very least referring to evidence-based practices that have been well established in treating a variety of patients and conditions. Paramount is the thorough, ongoing, and complete assessment of the skin. Many times, the open wounds from the trauma may overshadow pressure ulcer formation or other preventable conditions. If this occurs, patients have poorer outcomes and added comorbidities (Harrow, Rashka, Fitzgerald, & Nelson, 2008).

Nursing implications for other more common presentations like PTSD and pain warrant vigilance, especially because the incidence of suicide is higher among veterans than the general population and among individuals with chronic pain (Kaplan, McFarland, & Huguet, 2009; McDonald, 2010). For pain management the nurse's role becomes vital, especially when the types of pain differ widely because of the complexity of injuries. The four major pain categories are somatic, visceral, neuropathic, and nociceptive. Some examples include phantom pain, musculoskeletal, joint, neuralgias, psychogenic, and complex regional pain syndrome (Bruckenthal, Reid, & Reisner, 2009; Pain Management Guide, 2010).

The nurse working in polytrauma learns to observe and interpret the dynamics of the patient–family relationship, the patient's response pattern, and the full range of abilities within contextual situations. This observation and interpretation assists the entire team in understanding the whole person and the patient–family system. These insights not only optimize therapies from all providers but provide a more proactive approach to treatment.

Polytrauma Multi-/Interdisciplinary Team

Because of the complexity and number of injuries involved in polytrauma and TBI and the sometimes vague presentation associated with complications and comorbid illness, the nurse's role in the rehabilitation setting becomes critical in identifying the early signs and symptoms of acute illness, supporting and exploring the psychosocial needs, and understanding the trajectory of functional impairments and how all these impact the daily lives of their patients and families. This also requires the skill set and knowledge base of a comprehensive interdisciplinary team of consultants, including physical and occupational therapists, speech-language pathologists, recreational and vocational therapy specialists, psychologists, neuropsychologists, psychiatrists, infectious disease specialists, orthopedic surgeons, neurologists, neurosurgeons, dieticians, rehabilitation specialists for the blind and vision impaired, audiologists, and, most importantly, the patient and family. This team depends on nurses to be their eyes and ears, respond to the patient's and family's immediate needs, identify gaps in plans of care, and facilitate the overall progression toward optimal function and independence.

Chapter 5 discussed the roles of the interdisciplinary rehabilitation team. Box 20.3 provides suggested references for rehabilitation nurses and other team members. Two professionals on the polytrauma team who are newer additions to this arena bear additional discussion here: rehabilitation psychologist and the family therapist. Historically, the VA healthcare system recognized veterans as their primary patients, thus the rules and regulations that emerged prohibited treatment, except in humanitarian conditions, to any others. Since OEF/OIF engagements it became blatantly clear that families were also their primary patients. As well, it became evident that a new kind of rehabilitation system was needed that addressed the psychology of rehabilitation. Rehabilitation was no longer providing training to patients with orthopedic replace-

ments to function but now was so laced with multifaceted labyrinthine of injuries, vagueness, and unknowns that the traditional approaches and providers needed to address them were insufficient. With this discovery, the polytrauma system of care made great strides in introducing these new roles to the rehabilitation setting.

Rehabilitation Psychologist

The polytrauma team includes the rehabilitation psychologist who is a licensed mental health provider trained and experienced in understanding the behavioral, medical, and emotional components of rehabilitation. Common concerns that the rehabilitation psychologist can address are as follows:

- Understanding the physical and emotional changes that occur after an injury
- Coping with adjustment to disability
- Getting motivated for rehabilitation therapies
- Understanding medical jargon
- Working with the rehabilitation team

The rehabilitation psychologist is available to help with any of these concerns and serves as an adjunct to nursing.

Many times the nurse is privy to the fears of both the individual and the family early in the process. The rehabilitation psychologist and the nurse can identify strategies to move the person and family to a functional, accepting, and open phase. The nurse needs to be aware of nonverbal communication as well as any expressions of anger, doubt, and myths surrounding injuries. Nursing plays a supportive role with the family rehabilitation therapist by following the plan of care, helping the family and the patient review goals, and offering a positive encouraging milieu for families to express anger in a constructive way, recognizing the dichotomy of feelings from anger to love and by helping them gain a sense of control over the course of treatment.

Family Therapist

The family therapist is a licensed mental health provider who is trained and experienced in understanding the issues that families face in the treatment and recovery of their loved one with brain injury. The family therapist can address the following common concerns:

- Improving family communication
- Developing healthy lifestyle habits
- Stress management
- Parenting issues

BOX 20.3   Suggested Readings and Resources

Mansfield, S. (2005). *Faith of the American soldier.* New York: Tarcher/Penguin.

Swanson, K. L. (1999). *I'll carry the fork!* Scotts Valley, CA: Rising Star Press.

Osborn, C. L. (2000). *Over my head: A doctor's own story of head injury from the "inside looking out."* Kansas City, MO: Andrews McMeel.

Lloyd, D. J., & Kehoe, S. L. (2001). *Smile and jump high!* Monroe, GA: Starlight Press.

Karp, G. (2008). *Disability and the art of kissing.* Sebastopol, CA: Life on Wheels Press.

Crimmins, C. (2000). *Where is the mango princess?* New York: Alfred A. Knopf.

Bryant, B. (2001). *In search of wings: A journey back from traumatic brain injury.* South Paris, ME: Wings.

- Marital problems
- Family support groups
- Family planning

Nursing plays a supportive role with the family rehabilitation therapist by following the plan of care, helping the family and the patient review goals, and offering a positive encouraging milieu for families to express anger in a constructive way, to recognize the dichotomy of feelings from anger to love, and to help them gain a sense of control over the course of treatment.

NEW MILITARY EFFORTS AT MEETING POPULATION NEEDS

In 2007 the Army created warrior transition units to provide ongoing support for wounded soldiers. The U.S. Army Wounded Warrior Program (AW2) is a program developed and implemented by the U.S. Army Warrior Transition Command that assists severely wounded soldiers and their families throughout recovery. The U.S. Army created the AW2 program in response to the needs of the most severely wounded, injured, or ill soldiers from the Global War on Terrorism. This initiative was a response to the growing number of soldiers wounded in operations in the Iraq and Afghanistan wars. AW2 is a key component of the Army's commitment to wounded warriors and their families. All wounded, ill, and injured soldiers who are expected to require 6 months of rehabilitative care and the need for complex medical management are assigned to a warrior transition unit to focus on healing before returning to active duty or transitioning to veteran status.

SUMMARY

The U.S. government and the VA have made great strides in the provision of rehabilitation services to the polytrauma/blast-injured service member. Changes in philosophy as well as care settings have meant changes for the nurses who care for the wounded warriors. VA polytrauma nurses are working with very complicated, younger veterans and servicepersons with injuries never before seen in the VA system. Overall, they have coped well with the changes and in many cases initiated new practice patterns, added to the evidence-based literature, and improved team functioning. However, they realize that more research, innovation, and sharing needs to be done as the healthcare system learns more about the

nature and treatment of polytraumatic injuries (MacLennan et al., 2008).

CRITICAL THINKING

1. Of the various effects of polytrauma mentioned in this chapter, what are the topics with which you are least familiar?
2. Review Web Exploration 20.3 and evaluate the forms/sheets for the following components: a) reading level for patients and families, b) clarity of information, c) reliability of information, and d) visual appeal. How could the rehabilitation nurse use these tools in clinical practice?
3. Visit the Bob Woodruff Foundation and explore the site at http://remind.org/about_us. Consider how one man's journey has made an impact on the lives and recovery of soldiers.

PERSONAL REFLECTION

- Do you know anyone who has acquired a service-related disability? If so, would that persons' injury be classified as polytrauma? Why or why not?
- Consider the various components of polytrauma. Which do you believe would be the most difficult? And why?
- If you had a loved one who experienced polytrauma injuries due to an IED in a foreign war, how would you feel? What do you believe would be your most significant struggles physically, emotionally, and spiritually?

REFERENCES

Almogy, G., Mintz, Y., & Zamir, G. (2006). Suicide bombing attacks: Can external signs predict internal injuries? *Annals of Surgery, 243*(4), 541–546.

Belanger, H., Scott, S., Scholten, J., Curtis, G., & Vanderploeg, R. (2005). Utility of mechanism of injury based assessment and treatment: Blast injury program case illustration. *Journal of Rehabilitation Research & Development, 42*(4), 403–412.

Bond, A., Draeger, C., Mandleco, B., & Donnelly, M. (2003) Needs of family members of patients with severe traumatic brain injury: Implication for evidenced based practice. *Critical Care Nurse, 23*(4), 63–72.

Boss, P. (1996). *Ambiguous loss: Learning to live with unresolved grief.* Cambridge, MA: Harvard Press.

Boss, P. (2006). *Loss, trauma, and resilience: Therapeutic work with ambiguous loss* (1st ed.). New York: Norton.

Brain Injury Association of America. (2007). *The essential brain injury guide.* Washington, DC: Author.

Bruckenthal, P., Reid, M., & Reisner, L. (2009). Special issues in the management of chronic pain in older adults. *Pain Medicine, 10*(supplement 2), 67–78.

Centers for Disease Control and Prevention (CDC). (2006). Injury prevention and control: Traumatic brain injury. Retrieved December 1, 2010, from http://www.cdc.gov/traumaticbrain-injury/tbi_ed.html

Centers for Disease Control and Prevention (CDC). (2008). Statistics on blast injury. Retrieved September 1, 2010, from www.cdc.gov/masstrauma/preparedness/primer.pdf

Clark, M., Bair, M., Buckenmaier, C., Gironda, R., & Walker, R. (2007). Pain and combat injuries in soldiers returning from Operations Enduring Freedom and Iraqi Freedom: Implications for research and practice. *Journal of Rehabilitation Research and Development, 44*(2), 179–194.

Collins, S., & Long, A. (2003). Too tired to care? The psychological effects of working with trauma. *Journal of Psychiatric and Mental Health Nursing, 10*(1), 17–27.

Defense and Veterans Brain Injury Center. (n.d.). Military blast injuries. Retrieved September 1, 2010, from www.dvbic.org/TBI---The-Military/Blast-Injuries.aspx

Delisa, J. A., Currie, D. M., & Martin, M. (1998). Rehabilitation medicine: Past, present, and future. In J. A. Delisa & B. M. Gans (Eds.), *Rehabilitation medicine: Principles and practice* (pp. 3–22). Philadelphia: Lippincott-Raven.

Eshel, D. (2009). IED blast related brain injuries: The silent killer. Retrieved December 1, 2010, from htpp://www.defense-up-date.com/analysis

Fecura, S. E., Martin, C. M., Martin, K. D., Bolenbaucher, R. M., & Cotner-Pouncy, T. (2008). Nurses' role in the Joint Theater Trauma System. *Journal of Trauma Nursing, 15*, 170–173.

Ferguson, J., Franco, J., Pollack, J., Rumbolo, P., & Smock, M. (2010). Compression neuropathy: A late finding in the post-burn population. A four-year institutional review. *Journal of Burn Care & Research, 31*, 458–461.

Gallo, J. J., Fulmer, T., Paveza, G. J., & Reichel, W. (2000). *Handbook of geriatric assessment.* Gaithersburg, Maryland: Aspen.

Gosney, M. (2007). Diagnosis of UTI amongst elderly patients in hospital. *Age and Ageing, 36*(3), 353.

Hall, B. (2005). Wound care for burn patients in acute rehabilitation settings. *Rehabilitation Nursing, 30*(3) 114–117.

Harrow, J., Rashka, L., Fitzgerald, S., & Nelson, A. (2008). Pressure ulcers and occipital alopecia and Operation Iraqi Freedom, polytrauma casualties. *Military Medicine, 173*(11), 1068–1072.

Holcomb, J. (2005). The 2004 Fitts lecture: Current perspective on combat casualty care. *Journal of Trauma: Injury, Infection, and Critical Care, 59*, 990–1002.

Kaplan, M., McFarland, B., & Huguet, N. (2009). Firearm suicide among veterans in the general population: Findings from the national violent death reporting system. *Journal of Trauma, 67*, 503–507.

Lew, H. L., Garvert, D. W., & Pogoda, T. K. (2009a). Auditory and visual impairments in patients with blast-related traumatic brain injury: Effect of dual sensory impairment on Functional Independence Measure. *Journal of Rehabilitation Research and Development, 46*(4), 819–826.

Lew, H., Otis, J., Tun, C., Kerns, R., Clark, M., & Cifu, D. (2009b). Prevalence of chronic pain, posttraumatic stress disorder, and persistent postconcussive symptoms in OIF/OEF veterans: Polytrauma clinical triad. *Journal of Rehabilitation, Research, & Development, 46*(6), 697–702.

Long, MA. (2007). Clinical consultations; Deep tissue injury. *Rehabilitation Nursing, 32*(4), 135–136.

Lopez, M., Delmore, B., & Ake, J. (2002). Implementing a geriatric resource nurse model. *Journal of Nursing Administration, 32*(11), 577–585.

MacLennan, D., Clausen, S., Pagel, N., Avery, J., Sigford, B., MacLennan, D., & Mahowald, R. (2008). Developing a polytrauma rehabilitation center: A pioneer experience in building staffing, and training. *Rehabilitation Nursing, 33*(5), 198–205.

McDonald, P. (2010). Caring for the older person. *Practice Nurse, 3*(39), 14–16.

National Alliance for Eye and Vision Research. (2009). FY2009 increase of at least $230 million in NIH and Defense vision funding emphasizes research quality, public health need, and impact of NAEVR advocacy. Retrieved April 2, 2010, from http://www.eyeresarch.org

Pain Management Guide. (2010). Retrieved July 12, 2010, from http://www.webmd.com/pain

Sabo, B. (2006) Compassion fatigue and nursing work: can we accurately capture the consequences of caring work? *International Journal of Nursing Practice, 12*(3), 136–142.

Schecter, W. P., & Fry, D. E. (2005). The governor's committee on blood borne infection and environmental risk of the American College of Surgeons. The surgeon and acts of civilian terrorism: chemical agents. *Journal of the American College of Surgeons, 200*, 128–135.

Scott, S. G., Vanderploeg, R. D., Belanger, H. G., & Scholten, J. D. (2005). Blast injuries: Evaluating and treating the postacute sequelae. *Federal Practitioner, 22*(1), 66–75.

Spanholz, T., Theodorou, P., Amini, P., & Spilker, G., (2009). Severe burn injuries: Acute and long term treatment. *Deutsches Arzteblatt International, 106*(38), 607–613.

Spotswood, S. (2006). Military surgeons study prevalent blast injuries. *U.S. Medicine, 42*(12), 1–31.

Taber, K. H., Warden, D., & Hurley, R. (2006). Blast-related traumatic injury: What is known? *Journal of Neuropsychiatry Clinical Neuroscience, 18*(2), 141–145.

Tengvall. O., Wickman, M., & Wengstrom, Y. (2010). Memories of pain after burn injury-the patient's experience. *Journal of Burn Care & Research, 31*(2), 319–327.

Tinetti, M. E. (2003). Preventing falls in the elderly people. *New England Journal of Medicine, 348*(1), 42–49.

U.S. Department of Defense. (2010). Blast injury. Retrieved December 1, 2010, from http://www.dod.gov

Veterans Health Administration Directive. (2009). Retrieved December 1, 2010, from www1.va.gov/vhapublications/ViewPublications.asp?pub_ID=2032

Veterans Health Administration (VHA). (2010). *VHA Handbook 1172.1.* Washington, DC: Department of Veteran Affairs.

Warden, D. (2006). Military TBI during the Iraq and Afghanistan wars. *Journal of Head Trauma Rehabilitation, 21*(5), 389–402.

Zaloshnja, E., Miller, T., Langlois, J., & Selassie, A. (2008). Prevalence of long-term disability from traumatic brain injury in the civilian population of the United States, 2005. *Journal of Head Trauma Rehabilitation, 23*(6), 394–400.

CHAPTER 21

Cardiac and Pulmonary Disease

Catherine Biviano

LEARNING OBJECTIVES

At the end of this chapter, the reader will be able to

- List the risk factors for cardiac disease.
- Describe the signs and symptoms of coronary heart disease and heart failure.
- Identify diagnoses appropriate for cardiac rehabilitation.
- Delineate the phases of cardiac rehabilitation.
- Recognize risk factors for pulmonary disease.
- Discuss the goals of pulmonary rehabilitation.
- Describe the components of a pulmonary rehabilitation program.

KEY CONCEPTS AND TERMS

Angina pectoris	Coronary artery bypass graft surgery	Functional capacity
Asthma		Heart failure (HF)
Chronic bronchitis	Coronary artery disease (CAD)	Lung cancer
Chronic obstructive pulmonary disease (COPD)	Coronary heart disease	Myocardial infarction (MI)
Coronary angioplasty	Cystic fibrosis (CF)	
	Emphysema	

Cardiovascular diseases are conditions that involve the heart or blood vessels. These conditions include **coronary artery disease (CAD)**, **heart failure (HF)**, cardiomyopathy, and congenital cardiac conditions. More than one in three Americans has some sort of cardiac disease. The American Heart Association (AHA, 2010a) provides the following estimates:

- 74,500,000 Americans have hypertension.
- 17,600,000 Americans have coronary heart disease.
- 5,800,000 Americans have HF.
- Between 650,000 and 1,300,000 Americans have a congenital heart condition.

Cardiovascular diseases are more prevalent in older adults and in certain races or ethnic groups. For example, African Americans have higher rates of hypertension (31.8%), more Whites, American Indians, and Alaska Natives have heart disease (12.1%), and Asians have the lowest rates of coronary heart disease (2.9%). Box 21.1 provides a web link to more statistics on heart disease.

> **BOX 21.1   Web Exploration**
>
> Go to http://americanheart.org/downloadable/heart/1265665152970DS-3241%20HeartStrokeUpdate_2010.pdf for more statistics on heart disease.

Rehabilitation can assist persons with cardiovascular disease to improve their health condition. In particular, cardiac rehabilitation can (1) prevent progression of disease/disability, (2) improve physical functioning, and (3) improve quality of life. In this chapter, cardiac and pulmonary rehabilitation are discussed.

CORONARY ARTERY DISEASE

CAD, also called **coronary heart disease**, is caused by atherosclerosis, with narrowing of the coronary arteries due to the build up of plaque (Crowley, 2004). CAD is the single leading cause of death in the United States. **Angina pectoris** or **myocardial infarction (MI)** may be the result of CAD. Angina pectoris is chest pain or discomfort due to a temporary interruption of blood to the heart muscle. MI, also known as a heart attack, is the interruption of blood supply to part of the heart, causing heart cells to die. In 2010, the AHA reported an estimated 1.26 million Americans will have a new or recurrent cardiac event. In fact, it is estimated that in 2010 alone 785,000 Americans will have a new heart attack and about 470,000 will have a recurrent attack. It is also estimated that an additional 195,000 silent heart attacks occur each year (AHA, 2010a).

> CAD is the single leading cause of death in the United States (AHA, 2010a).

The coronary arteries supply blood to the heart and, when functioning normally, ensure adequate oxygenation of the myocardium at all levels of cardiac activity. CAD causes changes in both structure and function of the blood vessels. Atherosclerotic processes cause an abnormal deposition of lipids in the vessel wall, leukocyte infiltration and vascular inflammation, plaque formation, and thickening of the vessel wall. These changes lead to a narrowing of the lumen, which restricts blood flow (Figure 21.1). There are also subtle yet functionally important changes that can occur before overt changes in structure are observed.

When CAD restricts blood flow to the myocardium there is an imbalance between oxygen supply and demand. When oxygen supply is insufficient to meet the oxygen demand, the myocardium becomes hypoxic. This is often associated with angina or chest pain and other clinical symptoms (Figure 21.2). Severe ischemia can lead to infarction, or death, of the tissue.

HEART FAILURE

HF is the inability of the heart to supply the blood and oxygen needed to the body; it may be left or right sided. Left-sided HF results in increased fluid building up in the pulmonary vessels. Right-sided HF leads to fluid buildup in the abdomen and extremities. Both types of HF have systemic implications.

In HF the heart becomes increasingly unable to fill with or eject blood due to structural or functional cardiac conditions. There is a change in heart muscle structure that impairs the heart's ability to pump efficiently. This can be due to long-standing hypertension, CAD, poor blood supply to the heart muscle, valvular disease, or cardiomyopathy. Some causes of HF include CAD,

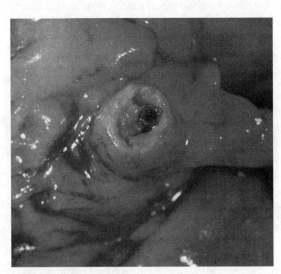

FIGURE 21.1   Severely sclerotic coronary artery in cross section. Note that the lumen is almost completely blocked.

Source: Photo courtesy of Leonard V. Crowley.

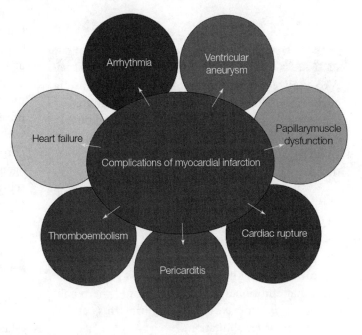

FIGURE 21.2   Possible complications of myocardial infarction.

Source: Crowley, Introduction to Human Disease, (2004)

hypertension, diabetes, arrhythmia, congenital heart disease, valvular heart disease, and medications.

HF is the fastest-growing clinical cardiac disease entity in the United States. "According to the American Heart Association, heart failure is a condition that affects nearly 5.7 million Americans of all ages and is responsible for more hospitalizations than all forms of cancer combined. It is the number one cause for hospitalization among Medicare patients. With improvement in survival of acute myocardial infarctions and a population that continues to age, heart failure will continue to increase in prominence as a major health problem in the United States" (Dumitru & Maker, 2010, para. 1).

OTHER CARDIAC DISEASES

Cardiomyopathy is a disease that weakens and enlarges the heart muscle. Restrictive cardiomyopathy can be caused by infections, medications, radiation therapy, chemotherapy, sarcoidosis, or genetic factors. Dilated cardiomyopathy, on the other hand, can be caused by CAD, diabetes, obesity, thyroid disease, cocaine, pregnancy, viral infection, and alcohol use. Hypertrophic cardiomyopathy is usually inherited.

There are also congenital cardiac disorders. But no matter the cause of the cardiovascular disease, all can result in symptoms and complications that reduce activity, decrease oxygenation, and cause a decline in the quality of life of the individual affected (Case Study 21.1).

CASE STUDY 21.1

A 65-year-old obese male smoker with hypertension complains of chest pain and calls 911. He is admitted to the hospital and taken for a cardiac catheterization. It reveals arthrosclerosis, and angioplasty is performed. Upon discharge the nurse reviews instructions with the patient.

Questions

1. What lifestyle modifications would be included in the discharge instructions?
2. Is this patient a good candidate for outpatient cardiac rehabilitation?
3. What additional information would the rehab nurse wish to have before admitting this patient to cardiac rehabilitation?

TREATMENT

Cornary Artery Disease

The goal in treating CAD is to restore normal coronary perfusion or, if that is not possible, to reduce the oxygen demand by the heart (i.e., normalize the oxygen supply-to-demand ratio) to minimize myocardial hypoxia. In severe CAD, in which one or more coronary arteries is very stenotic, some patients will have a stent implanted within the coronary artery to open up the lumen and restore blood flow. Other patients may undergo **coronary artery bypass graft surgery** in which the diseased segment is bypassed using an artery or vein harvested from elsewhere in their body. If the coronary artery is occluded by a blood clot, a thrombolytic drug may be administered to dissolve the clot. **Coronary angioplasty** is a percutaneous coronary intervention in which a balloon is inflated within the coronary artery to crush the plaque into the walls of the artery.

The vast majority of CAD patients, however, are treated with medications that reduce the myocardial oxygen demand by decreasing heart rate, contractility, afterload, or preload. Table 21.1 summarizes commonly used cardiac medications.

Heart Failure

Symptoms associated with HF include varying degrees of dyspnea, acute pulmonary edema, chest pain, peripheral edema, palpitations, fatigue, nocturia, and mental status changes. Dyspnea is less prominent in right-sided failure, but right-sided failure can lead to hepatic congestion, ascites, anasarca, and abdominal pain. Treatment is aimed at stopping progression of the disease, treating acute symptoms, maximizing medication and diet management, patient education, and developing a heart-healthy lifestyle. Medical treatment includes fluid management with diuretics, management of hypertension and other chronic diseases, management of arrhythmias, pain management, ensuring adequate oxygenation, and diet counseling. Box 21.2 provides a web link to clinical guidelines from the AHA for management of HF.

BOX 21.2   Web Exploration

The American Heart Association has published clinical practice guidelines for medical management of HF, available at http://www.americanheart.org/presenter.jhtml?identifier=3004550

TABLE 21.1   Common Categories of Cardiac Medications

Beta-Blockers

Examples: Atenolol (Tenormin), metoprolol (Lopressor), propanolol (Inderal)

Action: Block the effects of catecholamines epinephrine and norepinephrine

Indications*: Cardiac arrhythmias, angina, hypertension

Calcium Channel Blockers

Examples: Amlodipine (Norvasc), nifedipine (Procardia)

Action: Work by blocking calcium channels in cardiac muscle and blood vessels

Indications: Hypertension, control heart rate, reduce angina

Angiotensin-Converting Enzyme Inhibitors

Example: Enalapril (Vasotec)

Action: Prevent the formation of angiotensin II rather than by blocking the binding of angiotensin II to muscles on blood vessels

Indications: Hypertension, heart failure

Angiotensin II Receptor Blockers

Example: Losartan (Cozaar)

Action: Block the action of angiotensin II by preventing angiotensin II from binding to angiotensin II receptors on blood vessels

Indications: Hypertension, heart failure

Nitrates

Example: Nitroglycerin

Action: Aid in the dilation of arteries

Indications: Angina, heart failure

Anticoagulants

Example: Enoxaparin (Lovenox), warfarin (Coumadin), heparin

Action: Decrease the clotting ability of the blood

Indications: Prevention of blood clots

Antiplatelet

Example: Ticlopidine, aspirin

Action: Prevents blood clots from forming

Indications: unstable angina, strokes, transient ischemic attacks

Diuretics

Example: Furosemide (Lasix), bumetanide (Bumex)

Action: Relieve heart work load by removing excess fluid

Indications: Hypertension, edema

*Beta-blockers may also be indicated in a variety of other noncardiac diagnoses.

RISK FACTORS AND WARNING SIGNS

Modifiable risk factors are responsible for about 80% of cardiac disease and cerebrovascular disease (stroke). The most common causes of cardiac disease are unhealthy diet, physical inactivity, and tobacco use. The effects of unhealthy diet and physical inactivity may present in individuals as elevated blood pressure, elevated blood glucose, hypercholesterolemia, and obesity. Also, a number of underlying determinants of chronic diseases are a reflection of the major forces driving social, economic, and cultural change, such as globalization, urbanization, and population aging. Table 21.2 lists the risk factors for cardiovascular disease.

PREVENTION

Many modifiable risk factors can be eliminated for prevention of cardiac disease. Following a diet low in saturated fats with moderate exercise is a good way to prevent cardiac disease. It is also important to keep alcohol consumption to a minimum, and smoking should be avoided.

The AHA recommends a minimum of 30 minutes of exercise daily 5 days a week. Running, biking, and all types of aerobic activity have both cardiovascular and psychological benefits for wellness. A well-balanced diet of fruits and vegetables helps to maintain a healthy weight, resulting in a normal blood pressure and cholesterol level. Older adults can accumulate the effects of exercise so that even daily activities that provide continuous movement (such as cleaning house, gardening,

TABLE 21.2   Risk Factors for Cardiovascular Disease

- Heredity
- Race
- Gender
- Age
- Smoking
- Hypertension
- Cholesterol
- Diabetes
- Sedentary lifestyle
- Stress
- Birth control pills
- Alcohol
- Obesity

walking, and shopping) may count as exercise (Mauk & Hanson, 2010).

EFFECTS OF CARDIAC DISEASE

Cardiac disease can result in many symptoms. Dysrhythmias are not unusual and can be fatal. Ischemia leading to angina and/or MI is very concerning. Poor tissue perfusion can lead to vascular changes in the extremities, renal failure, and cognitive changes. Exercise intolerance and deconditioning are a result of poor cardiac response and resultant poor oxygenation. Pain from angina, dyspnea, and edema from HF are common symptoms. Malnutrition evolves over time. Rehabilitation can help address many of these symptoms.

CARDIAC REHABILITATION

Rehabilitation in the cardiac patient population is an important step to help decrease the risks associated with the cardiac disease process. Cardiac rehabilitation aims to reverse the limitations experienced by patients who have suffered the adverse physiological and psychological consequences of cardiac events. Cardiac rehabilitation can benefit any patient with heart problems, including heart attack, angina, HF, angioplasty, or coronary artery bypass surgery. About 400,000 patients who undergo coronary angioplasty each year make up a subgroup that could benefit from cardiac rehabilitation. Approximately 4.7 million patients with HF are also eligible for a slightly modified program of rehabilitation, as are the ever-increasing number of patients who have undergone heart transplantation (AHA, 2010b).

Cardiac rehabilitation is a medically supervised program to help heart patients recover quickly and improve their overall physical, mental, and social functioning. The goal is to stabilize, slow, or even reverse the progression of cardiovascular disease, thereby reducing the risk of heart disease, another cardiac event, or death (AHA, 2010b).

Cardiac rehabilitation includes education about how to be more active and make lifestyle changes. These changes may include smoking cessation and weight loss through diet modification and exercise. The following are some of the components of a cardiac rehabilitation program:

- Medical evaluation
- Prescribed exercise
- Education on nutrition
- Counseling of patients with cardiac disease
- Emotional support

Cardiac rehabilitation programs have been consistently shown to improve exercise tolerance and psychosocial well-being without increasing significant complications.

Cardiac rehabilitation has changed a great deal over the years. In the past, fewer patients were considered appropriate candidates for therapy. Today, with the advancements in the management of CAD, more patients qualify and are being sent by their physicians. Participation in a cardiac rehabilitation program may act as a catalyst for behavior modification that can lower their risk factors. Combining all aspects of cardiac rehabilitation in appropriate patients improves functional capacity and quality of life, reduces risk factors, and may create a sense of well-being and optimism about the future.

Functional capacity is an important factor in deciding who is appropriate for cardiac rehabilitation. Some of the factors that influence functional capacity are

- Age
- Precardiac event physical capacity
- Treatments and bed rest during the event
- Fluid volume
- Left ventricular dysfunction
- Residual myocardial ischemia
- Skeletal muscle performance
- Autonomic function
- Peripheral vascular status
- Pulmonary status
- Other systemic illnesses, such as orthopedic conditions that limit mobility

Box 21.3 describes the types of patients who may benefit from cardiac rehabilitation.

Although many patients may benefit, cardiac rehabilitation services are contraindicated in patients with the following conditions:

- Severe residual angina
- Uncompensated HF
- Uncontrolled arrhythmias
- Severe ischemia, left ventricular dysfunction, or arrhythmia during exercise testing
- Poorly controlled hypertension
- Hypertensive or any hypotensive systolic blood pressure response to exercise
- Unstable concomitant medical problems (e.g., poorly controlled or "brittle" diabetes, diabetes prone to hypoglycemia, ongoing febrile illness, active transplant rejection)

BOX 21.3   Persons Who May Benefit From Cardiac Rehabilitation

Patients eligible for a cardiac rehabilitation program fall into the following categories:

- Lower risk patients after an acute cardiac event
- Patients who have undergone coronary bypass surgery
- Patients with chronic, stable angina
- Patients who have undergone heart transplant
- Patients who have had percutaneous coronary angioplasty
- Patients who have not had a cardiac event but are at risk because of an unfavorable risk factor
- Patients with stable HFe
- Patients with previous stable heart disease who have become seriously deconditioned by an illness

Patients with these conditions may also benefit from cardiac rehabilitation:

- Arrhythmia
- Heart valve surgery
- Hypertension
- Hyperlipidemia
- MI
- Obesity
- Stroke

CARDIAC REHABILITATION PROGRAM

A cardiac rehabilitation program has several phases. These are summarized in Box 21.4 and discussed in this section.

Phase 1

This phase begins while patients are still in the hospital. Phase 1 includes a visit by a member of the cardiac rehabilitation team, education regarding the disease and the recovery process, personal encouragement, and inclusion of family members in classroom group meetings (Singh, Schocken, & Williams, 2008).

Phase 1.5

This phase begins after the patient returns home from the hospital. Team members work with patients and family members. Emphasis is placed on how to keep the heart healthy and strong. Team members check the patient's medical status and continuing recovery and offer reassurance as the patient regains health and strength. This phase of recovery includes low-level exercise and physical activity as well as instruction regarding changes for the resumption of an active and satisfying lifestyle (Singh et al., 2008).

Phase 2

Phase 2 of a cardiac rehabilitation program is initiated based on the results of exercise testing, and the exercise prescription is individualized. There are three main components of an exercise training program:

- Frequency: The minimum frequency for exercising to improve cardiovascular fitness is three times weekly.
- Time: Patients usually need to allow 30 to 60 minutes for each session, which includes a warm-up of at least 10 minutes.
- Intensity: The intensity prescribed is in relation to the patient's target heart rate. Aerobic conditioning is emphasized in the first few weeks of exercise. Strength training is introduced later. The Borg scale of rate of perceived exertion is used as a measure to gauge the intensity of treatment. Patients usually should exercise at a rate of perceived exertion of 13 to 15.

Phase 2 includes supervised exercise. Patients who have completed hospitalization and 2 to 6 weeks of recovery at home can begin phase 2 of their cardiac rehabilitation program. The physician and cardiac rehabilitation staff members formulate the level of exercise necessary to meet an individual patient's needs. Exercise treatments usually are scheduled three times a week at the rehabilitation facility. Constant medical supervision is provided; this includes supervision by a nurse and an exercise specialist as well as the use of exercise electrocardiograms. Phase 2 includes education on stress management, smoking cessation, nutrition, and weight loss and may last 3 to 6 months (Singh et al., 2008).

Phase 3

Phase 3 of cardiac rehabilitation is development of a maintenance program designed to continue for the patient's

BOX 21.4   Phases of Cardiac Rehabilitation

- Phase 1: Initiated while the patient is still in the hospital.
- Phase 2: A supervised ambulatory outpatient program spanning 3–6 months.
- Phase 3: A lifetime maintenance phase in which physical fitness and additional risk-factor reduction are emphasized.

lifetime. The exercise sessions usually are scheduled three times a week. Activities consist of the type of exercises the patient enjoys, such as walking, bicycling, or jogging. A registered nurse supervises these classes. Electrocardiographic monitoring usually is not necessary (Singh et al., 2008).

Goal Setting

Cardiac rehabilitation encompasses short- and long-term goals that are to be achieved through exercise, education, and counseling. The interdisciplinary team of cardiac rehabilitation professionals works with each patient to help attain mutually established goals. Short-term goals include the following (Singh et al., 2008):

- Reconditioning enough to allow the patient to resume customary activities
- Limiting the physiological and psychological effects of heart disease
- Decreasing the risk of sudden cardiac arrest or reinfarction
- Controlling the symptoms of cardiac disease

Long-term goals are as follows (Singh et al., 2008):

- Identification and treatment of risk factors
- Stabilizing or reversing the atherosclerotic process
- Enhancing the psychological status of the patients
- Relieving cardiac symptoms

CARDIAC DISEASE SUMMARY

The National Institutes of Health website at www.nih.gov reports evidence that suggests a survival benefit for patients who participate in cardiac rehabilitation. The lifestyle modification learned through education in cardiac rehabilitation is a contributing factor. Patient compliance is the most important factor in the long-term success of any cardiac rehabilitation program.

Cardiac rehabilitation nurses work with adults with cardiovascular disease or those who are at risk. Nurses in this specialty promote cardiac wellness by helping patients alter their lifestyles (such as decreasing stress; eating low-fat, low-cholesterol meals; exercising; smoking cessation) to lessen the risk of cardiovascular disease and its complications and to minimize the lasting effects of past cardiac incidents. Some cardiac rehabilitation settings must require electrocardiogram proficiency for telemetry monitoring of patients.

There is no longer an American Nurses Credentialing Center (ANCC) certification for this specialty.

This exam has been retired, but certifications can be renewed if professional development and practice hour requirements have been met. Testing is not an option for this certification renewal. For information about other nursing certifications, visit the ANCC website at www.nursecredentialing.org/certification.aspx.

PULMONARY DISEASE

Pulmonary diseases affect a significant number of Americans. These diseases include asthma, chronic obstructive pulmonary disease (COPD), cystic fibrosis, pulmonary fibrosis, lung cancer, asbestosis, and sarcoidosis, among others. According to the American Lung Association (2008), 400,000 Americans die each year from lung disease. Lung disease is the number 3 killer in the United States, and lung disease death rates are increasing. More than 35,000,000 Americans have a chronic lung disease.

Pulmonary diseases cause many symptoms, including dyspnea, cough, sputum production, and weight loss. The ability to participate in society decreases, as does the overall quality of life. Table 21.3 delineates the symptoms of the most common pulmonary diseases.

Risk Factors for Lung Disease

Risk factors for lung disease include age (very young or very old), genetics, exposure to air and environmental pollution, smoking, and a history of childhood respiratory infections. Radiation and chemotherapy can contribute to lung disease. Living in low socioeconomic conditions also seems to be a contributing factor. Allergens contribute to diseases such as asthma.

Consequences of Lung Disease

Lung disease can have both local and systemic consequences. For instance, there can be both peripheral muscle dysfunction and respiratory muscle dysfunction. Nutritional abnormalities can develop. Lung disease can also cause cardiac impairment, skeletal disease, sensory deficits, and psychosocial dysfunction. The effects of lung disease stem from a variety of sources, both acute and chronic (Sharma & Arneja, 2010):

- Deconditioning
- Malnutrition
- Chronic effects of hypoxemia
- Steroid myopathy or intensive care unit neuropathy
- Hyperinflation
- Diaphragmatic fatigue

TABLE 21.3	Symptoms of Pulmonary Diseases
Disease	**Symptoms and Complications**
COPD	• Complications
	• Pulmonary hypertension
	• Cor pulmonale
	• Chronic respiratory failure
	• Symptoms
	• Dyspnea
	• Cough
	• Sputum
	• Weight loss (COPD)
	• Obesity (chronic bronchitis)
Asthma	• Wheezing
	• Bronchitis
	• Coughing
	• Chest tightness
	• Respiratory failure
	• Dyspnea
	• Sleep disturbances
	• Pneumonia
	• Respiratory infections
Cystic fibrosis	• Reproductive sterility
	• Pancreatic duct obstruction
	• Bile duct obstruction
	• Blocked sweat glands
	• Bronchial obstruction
	• Intestinal obstruction
	• Malabsorption
	• Esophageal varices
	• Pulmonary hypertension
	• Cor pulmonale
	• Lung abscess
	• Pulmonary insufficiency
	• Atelectasis
	• Pneumonia
Lung cancer	• Cough
	• Hemoptysis
	• Wheezing
	• Pain
	• Hoarseness
	• Weight loss
	• Fever of unknown origin
	• Dyspnea
	• Infections
	• Effects of radiation and chemotherapy

- Frequent hospitalizations
- Effects of various medications
- Psychosocial dysfunction resulting from anxiety, depression, guilt, dependency, and sleep disturbance

Disability that results from pulmonary disease also stems from a variety of sources, such as muscle dysfunction, primary skeletal or cardiopulmonary pathology, poor endurance, inadequate finances, inadequate family support or education, and public policies.

Rehabilitation and Lung Disease

A structured rehabilitation program can benefit the individual with pulmonary disease in a number of ways. Both peripheral and respiratory muscles can be strengthened, helping with both mobility and breathing. Medications can be adjusted, resulting in better breathing, which also helps to decrease anxiety and depression. Nutrition can be addressed to help with weight gain and intake of proper nutrients. Goals of pulmonary rehabilitation include improvements in overall and exertional dyspnea, improvements in health-related quality of life, and significant increases in maximal exercise capacity, as measured during exercise testing (Ferreira, Feuerman, & Spiegler, 2006).

Indications for Pulmonary Rehabilitation

Pulmonary rehabilitation is indicated for people with chronic lung disease who have received optimal medical management but are still symptomatic, with dyspnea, poor exercise tolerance, or restricted activities. Admission to a pulmonary rehabilitation program is not based on the severity of lung impairment but rather the persistence of symptoms, disability, and handicap. Pulmonary rehabilitation can take place in the inpatient, outpatient, or home setting (Sharma & Arneja, 2010).

Pulmonary Rehabilitation Program

A cornerstone of a pulmonary rehabilitation program is smoking cessation. Interventions include counseling, support, and medications where indicated. Medications used for smoking cessation are nicotine replacement therapy, bupropion, or Chantix. Another important aspect of rehabilitation is maximizing medication therapy for the lung disease. This might include inhaled steroids, bronchodilators, beta-2 agonists, long-acting bronchodilators, and anticholinergics, as well as steroids, antibiotics, and mucolytics, depending on the disease. Oxygen is considered to be a medication, and its use is included in the program. Other routine medications include flu vaccine and Pneumovax (Sharma & Arneja, 2010).

Exercise training is a core intervention, targeted at increasing endurance. This consists of both walking exercises and arm exercises. Nutritional assessment and related counseling are also included. Patient education centers on medications, recognizing and treating symptoms and exacerbations, and energy conservation. Psychosocial support addresses coping, anxiety management, and depression. Respiratory techniques are taught, such as chest physiotherapy (CPT) for bronchiectasis, purse-lipped breathing for COPD, and postural drainage for cystic fibrosis (Sharma & Arneja, 2010).

Pulmonary rehabilitation therapy can last for more than 12 weeks. Outcome assessments for a pulmonary rehabilitation program include dyspnea ratings, exercise tolerance, health status, and activity levels.

CHRONIC OBSTRUCTIVE PULMONARY DISEASE

COPD is a term that is used for two closely related diseases of the respiratory system: chronic bronchitis and emphysema. In many cases these diseases occur together, although there may be more symptoms of one than the other. COPD gets gradually worse over time. At first, there may be only a mild shortness of breath and occasional coughing. Then, a chronic cough develops with clear, colorless sputum. As the disease progresses, the cough becomes more frequent, and more effort is needed to get air into and out of the lungs. In later stages of the disease the heart may be affected. Eventually, death occurs when the function of the lungs and heart is no longer adequate to deliver oxygen to the body's organs and tissues. COPD often develops in people at the height of their productive years, disabling them with constant shortness of breath. It destroys their ability to earn a living, causes frequent use of the healthcare system, and disrupts the lives of the victims' family members for as long as 20 years before death occurs. The American Lung Association reports that COPD is the fourth leading cause of death in the United States.

Chronic bronchitis, one of the two major diseases of the lung grouped under COPD, is diagnosed when a patient has excessive airway mucous secretion leading to a persistent, productive cough. An individual is considered to have chronic bronchitis if cough and sputum are present on most days for a minimum of 3 months for at least 2 successive years or for 6 months during 1 year. In chronic bronchitis there may also be narrowing of the large and small airways, making it more difficult to move air into and out of the lungs.

In **emphysema**, there is a permanent destruction of the alveoli, the tiny elastic air sacs of the lung, because of irreversible destruction of a protein in the lung called elastin, which is important for maintaining the strength of the alveolar walls. The loss of elastin also causes collapse or narrowing of the smallest air passages, called bronchioles, which in turn limits airflow out of the lung. COPD is the fifth leading cause of death in the United States.

Risk Factors

Most patients with COPD have a history of heavy cigarette smoking. Cigarette smoking is the most important risk factor for COPD, both for disease development and for disease exacerbation.

Other risk factors for COPD include age, heredity, exposure to air pollution at work and in the environment, and a history of childhood respiratory infections. Living in low socioeconomic conditions also seems to be a contributing factor.

Prevention

COPD can be prevented through smoking cessation, avoiding exposure to secondary cigarette smoke, avoiding exposure to chemical fumes and dust, avoiding air pollution, and avoiding exposure to coal dust, silica, and asbestos.

Assessment

In people with COPD, a mild cough that produces clear sputum develops by around age 45. The cough usually occurs when the person first gets out of bed in the morning. Cough and sputum production persist. Shortness of breath may occur with exertion. Sometimes, shortness of breath first occurs only with a lung infection, during which time the person coughs more and has an increased amount of sputum. The color of the sputum changes from clear or white to yellow or green.

By the time people with COPD reach their middle to late 60s, especially if they continue smoking, shortness of breath with exertion becomes more troublesome. Pneumonia and other lung infections occur more often. They may result in severe shortness of breath even when the person is at rest and may require hospitalization. Shortness of breath during activities of daily living, such as toileting, washing, dressing, and sexual activity, may persist after the person has recovered from the lung infection.

About one-third of people with severe COPD experience severe weight loss, in part because shortness of breath makes eating difficult and in part because of increased levels in the blood of a substance called tumor necrosis factor. People with COPD may intermittently cough up blood, which is usually due to inflammation of the bronchi but which always raises the concern of lung cancer. Morning headaches may occur because breathing decreases during sleep, which causes increased retention of carbon dioxide.

Goals for rehabilitation for the patient with COPD include slowing the progression of disease, reducing the amount of secretions, preventing complications like infection, maximizing oxygenation, reducing factors that precipitate exacerbations, and smoking cessation.

ASTHMA

Asthma is a chronic respiratory disease characterized by recurring attacks of labored breathing, chest constriction, and coughing. Associated with allergies in many cases, nearly 23,000,000 Americans have been diagnosed with this illness. Asthma is categorized as a reversible obstructive lung disease and is a frequent cost of lost days at school and work due to exacerbations.

Asthma causes many symptoms. Wheezing is most recognizable. Also associated are coughing, chest tightness, bronchitis, and sleep disturbances. Persons with asthma are more likely to get pneumonia and other infections and are at risk for respiratory failure. Goals for treatment include identifying and controlling triggers, maximizing medications, and teaching stepped interventions. Asthma camps for children have been formed, such as Camp RAD in Galveston, Texas, which teaches the principles of asthma management to children during a week long camp.

Rehabilitation for asthmatics focuses on self-care and self-disease management. You can learn more about developing an action program for management of asthma symptoms at http://www.nhlbi.nih.gov/health/public/lung/asthma/asthma_actplan.pdf

CYSTIC FIBROSIS

Cystic fibrosis (CF) is an inherited disease that causes thick, sticky mucus to be formed, affecting the lungs, pancreas, and other organs. People with CF have a shortened life span. CF is the second most inherited disease in the United States. Approximately 30,000 people in the United States have CF, and there are about 1,000 new cases every year (American Lung Association, 2010a).

Symptoms of CF are related to the thick sticky mucus that block airways and makes breathing difficult. Mucus also clogs the pancreas, interfering with digestive processes and contributing to malnutrition. People with CF are at higher risk for infection, as mucus is an ideal medium in which to grow bacteria. Symptoms include salty-tasting skin, persistent wheezing, coughing or shortness of breath, foul, greasy stools, and good appetite with poor weight gain (American Lung Association, 2010a).

Treatment for CF is focused on preventing infection, promoting drainage of mucus, maximizing medications, and promoting activity and community integration. Parents of children with CF must be taught about postural drainage techniques, medications and nebulizers, symptoms management, and promoting growth and development (American Lung Association, 2010a).

Aging with CF is a new field of knowledge. Almost 45% of the population with CF is 18 or older. Diseases associated with CF and aging are CF-associated diabetes, osteoporosis, and male infertility (American Lung Association, 2010a).

LUNG CANCER

Lung cancer is the second most commonly diagnosed cancer in males and females. It is the most common cause of cancer death, and about 162,000 people die from it annually (American Lung Association, 2010b). In some European countries where the legal age for tobacco use is younger than that in the United States, lung cancer is even more prevalent. Although not often thought of as a condition that requires rehabilitation, pulmonary rehabilitation has much to offer persons with lung cancer.

Symptoms that accompany lung cancer can include pain, coughing, hemoptysis, wheezing, hoarseness, weight loss, dyspnea, fever, infections, and the effects of radiation and chemotherapy treatments. Rehabilitation goals such as these can benefit the patient with lung cancer:

- Maximizing breathing
- Maintaining/improving functional status
- Enhancing coping
- Maintaining/improving nutrition
- Educating about disease

Strengthening muscles to assist in mobility and self-care can be of benefit, as can nutritional management, training about energy conservation, and prevention of infection.

NURSING INTERVENTIONS FOR PULMONARY DISEASE

- Assess the patient for signs and symptoms of respiratory distress.
- Administer and educate about medications.
- Promote adequate rest.
- Provide psychosocial support for patient and family (social work, physical therapy, occupational therapy).
- Patient teaching including lifestyle modification and smoking cessation.

CLIENT–FAMILY TEACHING

Patient teaching for patients with lung disease includes acute care activities such as reporting chest pain or dyspnea and wellness teaching such as smoking cessation, stress reduction, weight reduction, heart-healthy diet, drug regimen, and relaxation (Case Study 21.2). Other patient teaching activities include teaching the patient home blood pressure, pulse, and weight monitoring.

EVALUATION OF OUTCOMES

Patients with cardiac and pulmonary diseases should be evaluated on a routine basis to determine whether the plan of care should be changed. During outpatient visits to rehabilitation programs, there is an ongoing assessment of the patient's progress that should be communicated to their primary doctor. Patients receiving rehabilitation for other problems but who also have cardiac and/or pulmonary diseases will likely have modified outcomes based on their maximal potential in light of existing co-morbidities.

ETHICAL CONSIDERATIONS

Some of the ethical considerations associated with cardiac and pulmonary disease include the patient population at the highest risk for CAD and COPD. Economic status plays an important role in healthcare education and lifestyle choices. Eating a well-balanced diet and having the opportunity to engage in exercise are often not a priority for the economically challenged. Many community programs have been established in lower economic status areas and in the public school system to increase healthcare literacy throughout the United States. The goal of these programs is to reduce the modifiable risk factors for cardiac and pulmonary disease.

NURSING COMPETENCIES

Nurses working in cardiac and pulmonary rehabilitation focus on patient education and improving or maintaining their activity level. Reducing modifiable risk factors associated with cardiac and pulmonary disease have a direct impact on the patient outcome. Nurses working with this patient population should be clinically competent and highly motivated to guide the patient toward life change. Working in a cardiac or pulmonary rehabilitation setting can be a rewarding experience, knowing there is a great benefit to patients' lives.

SUMMARY

Rehabilitation patients often have comorbidities related to cardiac and pulmonary function. As the population ages, the number of persons seen in rehabilitation who also have cardiopulmonary limitations may also increase. Patients with disorders such as HF, CAD, or COPD may find physical rehabilitation after any other problem more difficult. Cardiac rehabilitation has been shown to be beneficial to persons after MI. In addition, pulmonary rehabilitation programs may be useful for persons with lung cancer or for those attempting smoking cessation after a long period of tobacco use. Rehabilitation nurses should be aware of available resources related to these services in their own communities.

CASE STUDY 21.2

A 70-year-old woman with a history of smoking one pack of cigarettes a day for the past 20 years is diagnosed with emphysema. She wears oxygen at home and tolerates activity, including going for short walks and going to the bingo.

Questions

1. Is this patient a good candidate for a pulmonary rehabilitation program? Why or why not?
2. What additional information should the nurse ask about to best assist this patient?
3. What would a typical respiratory program look like for this patient if she was admitted to a pulmonary rehabilitation program?

CRITICAL THINKING

1. Go to the AHA website www.americanheart.org. Check the guidelines listed for healthy eating and exercise. Poll friends and family and see how many are aware of these guidelines and currently follow them. How many do you follow?
2. Go to the American Association of Cardiovascular and Pulmonary Rehabilitation website at www.aacvpr. Locate a cardiac or pulmonary rehabilitation program in your area. Ask them about short- and long-term goals for their patients. What kind of education is provided to these patients?
3. Think about the people in your life who are at a high risk for cardiac or pulmonary disease. What can you do to help them reduce these risk factors? What resources are available for them?

PERSONAL REFLECTION

- Do you or someone you know have risk factors for cardiac or pulmonary disease? What risk factors are the most serious?
- What are some changes you can make right now to ensure keeping your risk factors for cardiac and pulmonary disease low?
- Look at Figure 21.2. Which of the possible complications of MI have you seen most frequently in your rehabilitation patients?
- If you had a loved one with coronary heart disease, what steps would you take to help them gain knowledge about associated morbidities and mortality?

WEBSITE RESOURCES

American Association of Cardiovascular and
Pulmonary Rehabilitation
http://www.aacvpr.org

American Lung Association
http://www.lungusa.org

American Heart Association
http://www.americanheart.org/ or
http://www.eart.org

REFERENCES

American Heart Association (AHA). (2010a). Heart disease and stroke statistics: 2010 Update at-a-glance. Retrieved July 15, 2010, from http://americanheart.org/downloadable/heart/1265665152970DS-3241%20HeartStrokeUpdate_2010.pdf

American Heart Association (AHA). (2010b). Cardiac rehabilitation. Retrieved June 1, 2010, from http://www.americanheart.org/presenter.jhtml?identifier=4490

American Lung Association. (2008). Lung disease data, 2008. Retrieved December 10, 2010, from http://www.lungusa.org/assets/documents/publications/lung-disease-data/LDD_2008.pdf

American Lung Association. (2010a). Cystic fibrosis. Retrieved June 1, 2010, from http://www.lungusa.org/lung-disease/cystic-fibrosis

American Lung Association. (2010b). Lung cancer. Retrieved August 15, 2010, from http://www.lungusa.org/lung-disease/lung-cancer

Crowley, L. (2004). *An introduction to human disease: Pathology and pathophysiology correlations*. Sudbury, MA: Jones and Bartlett.

Dumitru, I., & Maker, M. (2010). Heart failure. Retrieved December 1, 2010, from http://emedicine.medscape.com/article/163062-overview

Ferreira, G., Feuerman, M., & Spiegler, P. (2006). Results of an 8-week, outpatient pulmonary rehabilitation program on patients with and without chronic obstructive pulmonary disease. *Journal of Cardiopulmonary Rehabilitation, 26*(1), 54–60.

Mauk, K. L., & Hanson, P. (2010). Management of common illnesses, diseases, and health conditions. In K. L. Mauk (Ed.), *Gerontological nursing: Competencies for care* (pp. 382–453). Sudbury, MA: Jones and Bartlett.

Sharma, S., & Arneja, A. (2010). Pulmonary rehabilitation. Retrieved December 1, 2010, from http://emedicine.medscape.com/article/319885-overview

Singh, V.N., Schocken, D.D., & Williams, K. (2008). Cardiac rehabilitation. Retrieved August 15, 2010, from http://emedicine.medscape.com/article/319683-overview

CHAPTER 22

Neurological Disorders

Matthew R. Sorenson

LEARNING OBJECTIVES

At the end of this chapter, the reader will be able to

- Identify the major physiological concepts underlying the most common neurological diseases seen in rehabilitation.
- Describe the risk factors associated with neurological disease.
- Name the main medical and nursing treatment options for patients with neurological disease in the rehabilitation setting.
- Discuss the major health issues faced by patients with various neurological diseases.
- Explain the potential impact of neurological disease for the patient and family.

KEY CONCEPTS AND TERMS

Afferent	Eaton-Lambert syndrome	Multiple sclerosis (MS)
Autoimmune disorders	Efferent	Parkinson's disease
Charcot-Marie-Tooth (CMT) disease	Guillian-Barré syndrome (GBS)	Post-polio syndrome (PPS)
	Immune mediated	Ptosis
Clasp knife phenomenon	Innervation	Receptor
Degenerative disorders	Lewy body	Scotomas
Demyelination	Lower motor neuron	Spasticity
Diplopia	Motor neurons	Tremor
Dysphonia	Myasthenia gravis	Upper motor neuron

Neurological diseases comprise a significant proportion of the conditions encountered in rehabilitation settings. These diseases have a chronic and often degenerative nature that can result in significant care burden. The uncertain or progressively degenerative course of these diseases can generate a state of stress for both patient and family members. As the diseases progress, there are resultant functional limitations and the risk of complications from immobility. Quality of life is adversely affected, and there is a high rate of depression associated with neurological disorders (Rickards, 2006). Associated costs of neurological diseases include rehabilitative therapies, pharmacological agents, and psychological burden.

The intent of this chapter is to provide an overview of select neurological disorders from the perspective of the rehabilitation nurse. Disorders were selected based on their incidence and the likelihood of the rehabilitation nurse encountering patients with these conditions. This chapter divides neurological disorders into two pathogenic categories: **autoimmune disorders** and **degenerative disorders**. Autoimmune-mediated neurological disorders are those in which autoimmune antibodies destroy receptors or peripheral myelin and include myasthenia gravis, Easton-Lambert syndrome, and Guillain-Barré syndrome (GBS). The immune system is also implicated in the course of **multiple sclerosis (MS)** through a process of **immune-mediated** central **demyelination**. Degenerative neurological disorders include **Parkinson's disease**, amyotrophic lateral sclerosis (ALS), Huntington's disease, post-polio syndrome (PPS), and Charcot-Marie-Tooth (CMT) disease.

INCIDENCE AND PREVALENCE

Of the neurological disorders discussed in this chapter, the most common are Parkinson's disease and MS. About 1.5 million people in the United States are believed to have Parkinson's disease (American ParkinsonDisease Association, 2010), with increasing incidence over age 65 (Alves, Forsaa, Pedersen, Dreetz Gjerstad, & Larsen, 2008). The estimates for MS range from 300,000 to 500,000 people in the United States, with an earlier age at onset between 20 and 40 years. Available data on the other disease states are quite variable, depending on geographical location, gender, and racial background.

Prevalence and incidence numbers do not reflect those at risk for disease. As an example, approximately 150,000 individuals in the United States are believed to have a 50% probability of developing Huntington's disease, whereas around 15,000 individuals actually have the disease. Additionally, there are approximately 400,000 polio survivors living in the United States, and as many as 60% of these people are at risk for the development of PPS. It is thus important to consider not only the actual prevalence of a disease but the potential incidence. For a sense of scope regarding the epidemiology of these diseases, see Table 22.1.

PATHOPHYSIOLOGY REVIEW

A few select physiological mechanisms underlie the development of the neurological diseases covered in this chapter. One is the degeneration or loss of **motor neurons**, leaving muscles without the necessary **innervation**. The other primary mechanism is an inappropriate activation of the immune system with or without the production of autoimmune antibodies.

Autoimmunity, Immune Activation, and Neurological Diseases

The immune system surveys cells through a variety of mechanisms and clears cells that are damaged from the body. Through a process of self-tolerance, the immune system recognizes cellular markers and **receptors** present on healthy cells. In autoimmune disease self-tolerance is lost and the immune system begins to produce antibodies against cellular components, basically attacking the body. Autoimmune antibodies can seek out and destroy receptors (myasthenia gravis) or synaptic channels (**Eaton-Lambert syndrome**) and even contribute to the destruction of peripheral myelin (GBS). Separate from this process, inappropriate activation of the immune system can lead to destruction of central myelin (MS). These immunological-mediated neurological disorders are generally characterized by patterns of remission and exacerbation.

Eaton-Lambert Syndrome

Neurotransmitters provide the means for the conduction of an impulse across the neuromuscular junction. This requires the release of neurotransmitter from presynaptic storage vesicles and the presence of an adequate number of receptors on the receiving muscle cell. In Eaton-Lambert syndrome, autoimmune antibodies destroy presynaptic calcium channels. This leads to a loss of functional channels and a decrease in the release of acetylcholine. Acetylcholine is the main neurotransmitter associated with muscle contraction. The loss of acetylcholine is then

TABLE 22.1 Incidence and Prevalence of Neurological Disorders in the United States			
Disorder	Age Most At Risk	Incidence	Prevalence
Parkinson's disease	Over 60	19:100,000	1.5 million
Multiple sclerosis	20–40	10:100,000	400,000
Post-polio syndrome	20–40 years after polio exposure	5–60:100,000	200,000
Charcot-Marie-Tooth	15–30	10–30:100,000	125,000
Myasthenia gravis	30–70	20:100,000	60,000
Huntington's disease	30–50	7: 100,000	15,000
Amyotrophic lateral sclerosis	40–60	2:100,000	5,000
Gullain-Barré syndrome	15–35	1:100,000	2,700
	50–75		
Eaton Lambert syndrome	40–60	1:100,000	1,500

associated with muscle weakness and decreased deep tendon reflexes. Because the presence of acetylcholine within presynaptic vesicles is not affected, it is possible to elicit its release through movement.

> A common complaint among those with neurological disease is the presence of a crushing level of fatigue in the afternoon that significantly reduces activities of daily living.

A significant finding in Eaton-Lambert syndrome is the loss or significant diminishment of deep tendon reflexes after a period of muscle contraction, due to consumption of available acetylcholine within the synapse. The symptoms of Eaton-Lambert syndrome can be improved with exercise or stimulation of the muscles, a finding that does not occur in other neurological disorders. Clinical presentation in this disease involves upper extremity weakness. The ocular and bulbar muscles are not affected, and those with Eaton-Lambert syndrome do not display the respiratory and swallowing complications seen with myasthenia gravis. There is a strong relationship between Eaton-Lambert syndrome and the development of carcinoma (Wirtz, Smallegange, Wintzen, & Verschuuren, 2002).

Myasthenia Gravis

Myasthenia gravis is a condition in which antibodies destroy postsynaptic acetylcholine receptors, leading to a slow decrease in the number of receptors and eventually reaching the point at which acetylcholine can no longer bind effectively. Without effective receptor binding, acetylcholine can no longer elicit muscular contraction. Initial symptoms of myasthenia gravis involve the ocular muscles, manifesting as **diplopia** (double vision) and **ptosis** (drooping eyelids) (Figure 22.1). This is followed by weakness of facial muscles, swallowing and voice impairment (**dysphonia**), fatigue, and generalized weakness (Howard, 2008).

Guillain-Barré Syndrome

Exposure to infectious agents or vaccinations triggers development of antibodies. Certain infectious agents display an affinity for antigens that appear similarly to receptors present on neurons. In those with **GBS**, there seems to be a process of molecular mimicry in which the body begins to produce antibodies that attack peptides contained within peripheral myelin. The rapid accumulation of autoimmune antibodies results in an acute attack on peripheral nerve myelin. This process of rapid demyelination may also produce respiratory failure and

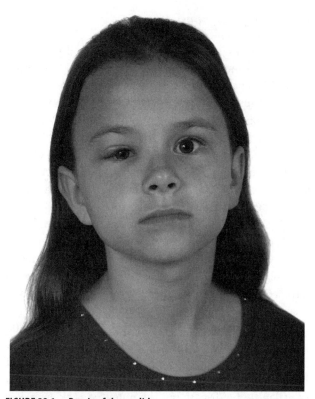

FIGURE 22.1   Ptosis of the eyelids.
Source: © Stacy Barnett/Dreamstime.com

autonomic nervous system dysfunction along with a classic pattern of ascending weakness. Manifestations are variable and include ascending weakness, paralysis, pain, diminished or absent reflexes starting with the lower extremities and progressing upward, bulbar weakness, cranial nerve symptoms, tachycardia, bradycardia, hypertension, or hypotension. In certain variants of GBS, a pattern of descending weakness may be seen (Snyder, Rismondo, & Miller, 2009; Vucic, Kiernan, & Cornblath, 2009).

Multiple Sclerosis

MS is a disorder that evolves from an immune-mediated inflammatory demyelinating process that leads to progressive and degenerative changes in neurological function. The process of demyelination in MS is accompanied by an inflammatory infiltrate composed primarily of activated T cells and macrophages that have crossed the blood–brain barrier. These cells are associated with production of inflammatory mediators (cytokines and chemokines) that contribute to the death of oligodendrocytes and the loss of myelin. The pharmacological agents used in the treatment of MS attempt to mediate this process of inflammation. Active inflammatory infiltrate can be detected in the brain and spinal cord through the use of gadolinium-enhanced magnetic resonance images for a period of approximately 3 months. Areas of prior damage can be detected using other planes and magnetic resonance imaging (MRI) techniques, to the point that MRI evidence can satisfy diagnostic criteria. Figure 22.2 provides an image of a brain with multiple MS plaques.

Although controversial, the cause of MS is believed to be related to the combination of a genetic susceptibility and precipitating environmental factors such as infection, physical injury, pregnancy, or emotional stress. Symptom presentation varies but generally includes fatigue, **tremor**, visual disturbances, and ataxia along with bladder or bowel dysfunction (Polman, Thompson, Murray, Bowling, & Noseworthy, 2006).

The course of MS has a degree of unpredictability. Individuals with MS are diagnosed with a particular "form" or subtype based on the observed disease course. There are five common types or patterns of disease progression (Polman et al., 2006):

1. In the benign form the individual commonly displays little disability.
2. With the relapsing-remitting form the individual displays a circular pattern of disease exacerbation generally followed by a distinct period of remission. This is the most common form of MS. In these first two forms of MS, there is little continual progression of disease.
3. With progressive-relapsing MS, the individual experiences continued progression of the disease, intermixed with periods of relapse.
4. In secondary-progressive MS the individual initially displays a pattern of remission and relapse but then eventually experiences continued progression of disease with little remission.
5. With the primary-progressive form of MS, the individual may have a slower period of symptom onset, yet the disease gradually progresses with little remission.

Figure 22.3 provides a graphic representation of the most common clinical patterns of MS. Case study 22.1 may assist the reader to apply practical information to a patient scenario.

Degenerative Neurological Disease

Degenerative neurological diseases are generally associated with the impairment or loss of motor neurons. Unlike autoimmune-mediated conditions that exhibit

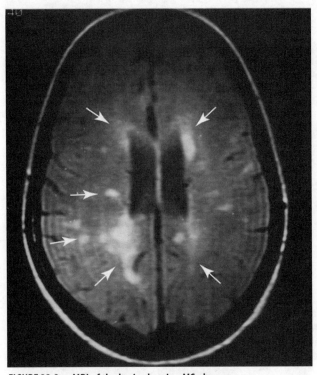

FIGURE 22.2   MRI of the brain showing MS plaques.

Source: Photo courtesy of Leonard V. Crowley.

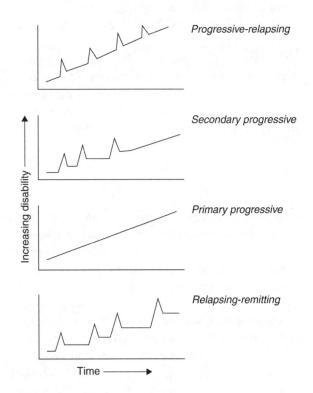

FIGURE 22.3   Clinical patterns of MS.

CASE STUDY 22.1

A 29-year-old woman, J.D., initially presented 2 years ago with tingling in her right fingers and toes along with occasional shooting pain in the right hip with gait ataxia lasting for a period of 2 to 3 weeks. She was diagnosed with MS based on MRI and treated with a disease-modifying therapy.

History of Present Illness

Two weeks ago J.D. awoke with numbness on the right side of her face. She also could not feel the right side of her face with her fingers. Over a period of 3 days the numbness extended to her right hand and foot and she experienced intermittent double vision lasting several minutes. She was admitted for 10 days to an acute care setting with significant lower extremity weakness (1/5), peripheral neuropathy, and double vision. Treatment included intravenous Solu-Medrol and interferon-beta injections. She was referred to acute rehabilitation for strengthening.

Physical Examination

At present, J.D.'s extraocular movements are full with no nystagmus, and speech, language, and mentation are normal. She is unable to stand without assistance and reports feelings of restlessness and anxiety. She is experiencing urinary urgency with fine kinetic tremor.

Discussion

A patient with MS can display a variety of symptoms. Visual disturbances, bowel/bladder dysfunction, neuropathies, and gait disturbance are common. However, the presence of symptoms compatible with MS is not sufficient for diagnosis. A number of other conditions may evoke similar symptomatology and require careful evaluation. The most current diagnostic guidelines are based on the use of MRI. To evaluate for the presence of demyelination, an MRI study of the brain and spinal cord with and without gadolinium enhancement needs to be ordered and preferably compared with previous images. The presence of lesions that take up gadolinium is considered a primary hallmark of MS-associated lesions.

The presentation of MS varies across patients, with the most common complaints being fatigue and visual disturbances along with gait imbalance. These symptoms can vary across the course of disease in the patient with MS, demonstrating the need for close follow-up and monitoring. Here J.D. initially presented with gait disturbance and then with neuropathy. That presentation was followed by visual disturbances and ultimately again neuropathy. The issue of patient compliance with injectable medication is also of import. The experience of adverse side effects often leads to cessation of therapy or inconsistent administration.

Questions

- What might be some teaching needs in this case?
- Is there enough information to determine the possible clinical pattern or type of MS?
- Can you identify some ways of reducing the incidence of medication-related side effects?
- What options are available for this patient is she lacks the fine motor skills necessary to administer the prescribed injections?

patterns of remission and exacerbation, degenerative conditions worsen over time without a return to baseline symptomatology. Two classes of motor neurons are affected by this pathogenic process: upper and lower motor neurons. These neurons differ in terms of function and location.

Upper motor neurons are confined to the central nervous system. These neurons carry impulses within the brain or convey impulses from the brain down the spinal cord in a variety of tracts such as the pyramidal. These nerves, however, do not leave the central nervous system and do not directly innervate muscle. Instead, **upper motor neurons** influence the muscle through connections with lower motor neurons (McCance & Huether, 2002). Upper motor neuron disease is associated with muscle weakness and spastic paralysis. Clinically, those with upper motor neuron disease can exhibit hyperactive deep tendon reflexes with clonus in the face of decreased superficial reflexes (abdominal and cremasteric), in conjunction with a positive Babinski reflex. **Clasp knife phenomenon** is a finding observed in those with upper motor neuron disease and is characterized by rigidity on contraction of a muscle. A positive result is demonstrated by finding increased tone on rapid passive flexion or extension of an extremity (Sheean, 2008). In other words, if the extremity is quickly moved passively, the nurse might encounter a significant degree of rigidity. If the rigidity suddenly abates and the extremity moves out easily, a positive finding for clasp knife phenomenon exists.

Lower motor neurons have cell bodies within the brain or brainstem and enervate muscle. This group of neurons includes the cranial nerves, which have both **efferent** and **afferent** properties. Lower motor neuron disease is associated with the development of fasciculation and muscle weakness that often progresses to flaccid paralysis. The lack of muscle tone manifests as decreased deep tendon and superficial reflexes and muscle atrophy (McCance & Huether, 2002).

Amyotrophic Lateral Sclerosis

ALS, also known as Lou Gehrig's disease, is a degenerative disorder of both the upper and lower motor neurons that occurs without inflammation. Neurons are lost throughout the spinal cord, brainstem and cerebral cortex, with sparing of select cranial nerves (III, IV, and VI). As the nerves degenerate, the innervated muscles begin to atrophy. For a diagnosis of ALS, patterns of upper and lower motor dysfunction need to observed (Chio et al., 2009). The pathogenic process appears to be associated with mechanisms of oxidative stress, although this is not definitive (Barber & Shaw, 2010).

Clinical manifestations include weakness that generally starts in one extremity and may be accompanied by fasciculation. As the disease progresses and more motor neurons are lost, atrophy results and is often accompanied by difficulty in chewing and swallowing. Ultimately, respiratory musculature control is lost, resulting in the patient being placed on a ventilator.

Huntington's Disease

The *huntingtin* gene encodes a protein (huntingtin) that appears to be involved in the development of neuronal structures and signaling transcription. Through a chromosomal defect, a mutant version of the gene can have a repeat polyglutamine section, and it is this mutated gene that is associated with the development of Huntington's disease. Although the precise role of the *huntingtin* gene is unclear, the mutated protein appears to interact with other proteins in a manner that contributes to the death of both neurons and gray matter in the brain. In Huntington's disease there is an accumulation of protein fragments within the cell nucleus. This concentration of proteins then contributes to cell death. It is also speculated that huntingtin protein elicits the release of brain-derived neurotropic factor, a protein necessary for the maintenance of the central nervous system. The mutated protein does not have this role, leading to a reduction in the amount of this factor (Walker, 2007).

In Huntington's disease there is significant atrophy of the caudate nucleus and putamen concomitant with neuronal loss and an increase in the number of astrocytes within affected areas of the brain. The caudate nucleus and putamen comprise the dorsal striatum, a white matter tract located in the forebrain. Much of the neuronal loss associated with Huntington's disease occurs in this striatum and involves neurons that project in the substantia nigra. The neuronal loss seen in Huntington's disease is often diffuse, involving several layers of the cerebral cortex. Neuronal loss also occurs within the frontal and temporal lobes of the brain, areas associated with cognition, movement, and memory. Huntington's disease can be graded from zero to four based on the degree of tissue loss and striatal pathology (Walker, 2007).

The clinical manifestations of Huntington's disease are characterized by involuntary movements known as chorea. These movements are uncontrolled and hyperkinetic and are often accompanied by rigidity and abnormal postures. As the disease progresses, memory and cognitive deficits may occur.

Parkinson's Disease

Coordination of movement relies on an intricate reciprocal balance between two neurotransmitters, one inhibitory (dopamine) and one excitatory (acetylcholine). Dopamine is produced in the substantia nigra, which delivers it to the basal ganglia, a section of the brain that coordinates movement. Degeneration of the substantia nigra then leads to a decrease in levels of dopamine. In the absence of dopamine, acetylcholine is not inhibited, resulting in muscle rigidity and tremor. The pathogenic process behind Parkinson's disease is not well understood but is characterized by the accumulation of abnormal proteins known as **Lewy bodies** within neurons. Parkinson's disease can also occur as a result of medication exposure or repetitive blows to the head (Alves et al., 2008).

Clinical manifestations of Parkinson's disease include tremor, bradykinesia, and rigidity. Postural rigidity results in a characteristic gait pattern. A mask-like facial expression is also associated with the muscular rigidity resulting from excessive levels of acetylcholine.

This rigidity also results in difficulty with chewing and swallowing.

Post-Polio Syndrome

Poliovirus is the causative agent behind poliomyelitis, a disease often simply referred to as polio. After the acute illness has passed, a significant number of individuals develop new symptoms such as fatigue, weakness, pain, and atrophy. **PPS** is the term used to describe this process.

During the acute phase of polio the virus invades motor neurons. This invasion can lead to injury or death of the neuron over time, leading to a lack of muscle innervation that manifests as muscle weakness. After the acute phase of illness axonal sprouting can occur, which leads to reinnervation of muscle. The process of reinnervation is often not as complete or as reliable as the original connections and can decay over time, manifesting as new-onset weakness. As well, the growth process leads to an enlargement of the motor neuron, which may result in fatigue. This places the muscle and motor neuron under metabolic stress, which over time can lead to the death of new innervations and perhaps even the corresponding neuron. This loss of innervation manifests as muscle weakness and paralysis.

Clinical manifestations of PPS include fatigue that is often worsened by physical activity. Decreased concentration may occur with a prolonged need for sleep. There may be new-onset weakness in extremities not previously affected. The triad of fatigue, pain, and new weakness serves as diagnostic criteria for PPS (Lin & Lim, 2005).

Inherited Neurological Disease

Genetic factors are associated with the development of many of the neurological diseases discussed in this chapter. Of these conditions, **Charcot-Marie-Tooth (CMT) disease** is the most common inherited neuromuscular disorder (Pareyson & Marchesi, 2009). There are several forms of CMT disease that share the same pathophysiological pathway. CMT disease results from mutations in genes that either code for proteins that comprise peripheral myelin or in proteins that aid in maintaining axonal health.

As a demyelinating disease, CMT is characterized by peripheral neuropathy, which results in ataxia, foot drop, and lower extremity atrophy. Over time, atrophy of the upper extremities may develop with a loss of fine motor skills. Pain is a common symptom with CMT, affecting both motor and sensory neurons (Banchs et al., 2009).

RISK FACTORS AND WARNING SIGNS

Unfortunately, for many neurological diseases little is known regarding controllable risk factors. For several diseases, such as Parkinson's, little information exists even regarding the pathogenic process, making risk identification difficult. There are, however, some general considerations that the rehabilitation nurse needs to keep in mind.

Autoimmune Neurological Disorders

One consideration is that the presence of one autoimmune disease is strongly associated with the development of another autoimmune disease (Dietert, Dietert, & Gavalchin, 2010). In other words, people who have rheumatoid arthritis, autoimmune thyroiditis, or systemic lupus erythematosus are at increased risk for the development of an autoimmune-related neurological disease. For certain diseases there are clear geographical trends and patterns. As an example, with MS there is a clear pattern of geographical distribution. Those living in northern climates have a significantly increased incidence of disease than do those in southern climates.

More significantly, the complications of immobility and disease place the patient at increased risk for the development of disease exacerbation. Infection, immunization, and emotional stress are associated with the exacerbation of myasthenia gravis and Eaton-Lambert syndrome and are implicated in the pathogenic process of MS. Complications of hospitalization for other conditions (such as age-related knee replacement) may then place the patient with a neurological disease at increased risk for disease exacerbation, requiring additional monitoring.

Infection and Immunization

An infectious process or vaccination is clearly a risk associated with GBS due to increased production of antibodies by the immune system. The presence of a degree of physical stress (such as a surgical procedure) or infection can lead to a myasthenia crisis. It is then critical to monitor those patients with skin breakdown or invasive access for the development of infection. Infection can also precipitate a myasthenic crisis as can stress or emotional crisis (Howard, 2008). As well, a history of viral exposure may be associated with the development of MS (Lauer, 2010) and GBS.

Emotional States and Stress

The perception of stressful events leads to activation of a variety of neuroendocrine mechanisms that culminate in the secretion of numerous stress hormones and neuropeptides, many of which have immunomodulatory effects. Because immune cells possess receptors for a multitude of neuroendocrine mediators, the immunological response to a stressful event in vivo is very likely the result of the net sum of effect(s) of a variety of neuroendocrine mediators, including neuropeptides and neurotransmitters. In other words, stress elicits a hormonal cascade that can place the patient with myasthenia gravis into a crisis state or perhaps even contribute to the development of MS. As well, the presence of negative emotionality can have effects on the performance of activities of daily living and on the ability to adhere to treatment prescriptions and recommendations.

Degenerative Neurological Disorders

Aging itself is associated with the development of degenerative neurological diseases such as Parkinson's disease. Some authors have speculated this is due to the cumulative effects of oxidative stress or other inflammatory mediators. The nature of experienced life events may also influence the level of risk; for example, participants in contact sports that may result in repetitive head injuries have an increased risk for the development of Parkinson's disease (Tanner, 2010). In terms of life events, for the development of PPS the patient needs to have first been diagnosed with poliomyelitis. With a pattern of onset 20 to 40 years after disease, those entering the elder years are those most at risk for PPS.

Warning Signs and Symptom Presentation

The warning signs for most neurological diseases are the appearance of initial symptoms. For example, any change in vision or the appearance of unilateral neuropathy may serve as a warning sign for MS. The presence of such symptoms alone is referred to as clinical isolated syndrome and is considered a precursor of MS. Ptosis (lagging eyelids) are one of the initial signs of myasthenia gravis. Generally, initial signs of visual deficits or disturbances are more likely to be associated with immunologically mediated diseases rather than degenerative disorders. Unfortunately, the early identification of symptoms does not prevent disease but rather provides the opportunity for early intervention and treatment. It is hoped that there can then be some mitigation of disease progression.

PREVENTION

Prevention of neurological disorders is a difficult task. Although select risk factors increase the probability of an individual developing certain disorders, as previously mentioned they are generally uncontrollable factors such as gender and familial history. There does appear to be a strong link between genetic variables and the development of neurological disorders.

Role of Genetics

Genetic defects are associated with the loss of peripheral myelin due to issues with the transcription of necessary proteins as with CMT disease or with the degeneration of the central nervous system as in Huntington's disease. Unfortunately, for many neurological disorders although a genetic link has been demonstrated, the precise role of genetic variables in the pathogenic process is not well understood. For example, some individuals have a clearly inheritable risk, as with CMT disease (Banchs et al., 2009), whereas in other cases inherited forms account for a small percentage of known cases, as with Parkinson's disease (Xiromerisiou et al., 2010). For other diseases, such as ALS, genetic predisposing factors are found in approximately 20% of all cases, with the remaining 80% considered idiopathic (Kuzma-Kozakiewicz & Kwiecinski, 2009).

For other disease states genetic variables are strongly suspected, but the precise nature of the genes involved is as yet not fully understood (Giraud, Vandiedonck, & Garchon, 2008). Genetic deficits on certain cell types may interact with infections or vaccinations and result in GBS (Geleijns et al., 2007). The interaction between a gene and a viral etiology could be referred to as epigenetic. Epigenetic modifications include viruses, medications, and other components that can modify genetic expression or regulation. These variables are most likely associated with the development of neurological diseases.

Genetic testing is available to aid in the diagnosis of Huntington's and CMT diseases. It is possible that in the future genetic variables can be used to predict or identify those at risk for neurological disorders. As the number of genes known to be associated with certain conditions increases, the ability to screen for disease improves. As an example, there are several diseases with clinical features that appear identical to Huntington's disease but are associated with different genetic predispositions (Schneider, Walker, & Bhatia, 2007). As genetic testing procedures evolve, it is hoped that all potential variants of a disease could be included within one testing panel.

ASSESSMENT OF NEUROLOGICAL DISORDERS IN THE REHABILITATION SETTING

Neurological diseases are characterized mainly by a course of weakness, often in conjunction with tremor, ataxia, and difficulties with swallowing or breathing. The clinical presentation of each neurological disorder can be distinct. It is thus imperative to be aware of the previous symptom presentation of the patient.

Clinical History

Increasing weakness may be confused with age-associated weakness rather than disease progression. Determining the clinical history can be helpful in distinguishing age-associated change with disease pathology. The main clinical presentation of PPS is slow progression of weakness over a period of years rather than sudden onset of a loss of strength. A pattern of slowly progressing weakness over time is far more characteristic of the degenerative neurological disorders. Changes in limb size related to atrophy may also occur and be noted more by family members or infrequent visitors. Fluctuating patterns of weakness may be noted with MS or myasthenia gravis.

The location and initial presentation of weakness also provides valuable information. Facial weakness is more likely to be associated with myasthenia gravis, whereas ALS generally begins with generalized weakness in one extremity. Lower motor neuron disease is associated with the development of muscle weakness that often progresses to flaccid paralysis. The lack of muscle tone manifests as decreased deep tendon and superficial reflexes.

Vision

Visual difficulties are also helpful to note. Although peripheral field confrontation is not precise, it may help reveal deficits. **Scotomas** (blind spots in the visual field) are common in those with MS and may also be apparent in patients with cardiovascular disease.

Tremor

Tremor is generally intention (kinetic) or resting (postural) in those with neurological disorders. Kinetic tremor is more common in those with MS and can be noted when the patient attempts movement. If a target is provided to the patient (such as touching the nurse's finger) and the target is significantly missed, then a degree of dysmetria is evident. The presence of dysmetria could indicate problems with fine motor control. Many

medications given for the treatment of fatigue can worsen tremor, as can the use of alcohol. Resting tremor is commonplace in those with Parkinson's disease and often is accompanied by cogwheel rigidity. When tremor occurs should be noted, and also if there are any characteristics that worsen as the patient moves an extremity in a purposeful manner. Providing the patient a piece of paper and asking the patient to draw some common figures may also sharpen a low frequency tremor and make it more evident (Smaga, 2003).

Muscle Tone

Neurological disorders are characterized by a lack of tone (flaccidity), increased tone, or decreased muscle tone. **Spasticity** is a common finding in those with upper motor neuron injury, including MS. Increased tone is indicative of Parkinson's disease, whereas a lack of tone is consistent with progressing ALS and GBS. The nature of the neurological disorder then allows the nurse to predict certain findings in terms of muscle control.

Upper motor neuron disease is associated with muscle weakness and spastic paralysis. Those with upper motor neuron disease can exhibit hyperactive deep tendon reflexes with clonus in the face of decreased superficial reflexes (abdominal and cremasteric), in conjunction with a positive Babinski reflex. Clasp knife phenomenon is characterized by rigidity on contraction of a muscle. This finding is observed in those with upper motor neuron disease, and a positive finding is demonstrated by finding increased tone on rapid passive flexion or extension of an extremity (Sheean, 2008).

Fatigue

The development of fatigue is common across the neurological disorders. In those with MS and PPS, energy levels may be high in morning with rapid depletion as the day wears on. A common complaint is the presence of a crushing level of fatigue in the afternoon that significantly reduces activities of daily living. In additional, many of the immunomodulatory medications given in treatment of immune-mediated neurological disease can also induce fatigue as a side effect. Fatigue may also result from the presence of physical activities that may tire weakened skeletal muscles. As part of the history it is thus important to determine the relationship between fatigue and exercise. The presence of alleviating factors can provide significant information as can the relationship of fatigue or weakness to medications. In those with myasthenia for example, fatigue and weakness can be associated with crisis states.

INTERVENTIONS AND MANAGEMENT

Medical Care in the Rehabilitation Setting

During the acute phase of illness, importance is placed on maintaining a patent airway and controlling the process of immune activation. In terms of pharmacological therapies for autoimmune neurological disease, corticosteroids may be used to suppress the production of antibodies or suppress immune-mediated inflammation. Other immunomodulatory medications may be used in an attempt to modify the disease process. For example, in those with GBS, immunoglobulin may used in an attempt to interfere with the disease process by enhancing the clearance of autoimmune antibodies. Immunomodulatory medications are also used primarily as maintenance therapy to prevent disease exacerbation in the case of MS, with steroidal therapies and other immunosuppressant medications used in the treatment of acute exacerbation. For degenerative neurological disorders, the focus is on correcting deficient neurotransmitter balance (Parkinson's disease) or delaying the process of degeneration (ALS). In the rehabilitation setting these therapies may well continue, but the rehabilitation nurse is also faced with managing other disease complications that in the acute care setting may not viewed as significant. Tremor, spasticity, and fatigue all have significant effects on qual-ity of life and the performance of activities of daily living. In the acute care setting the focus is generally on stabilization of the medical condition, and these disease complications are not as high on the priority list.

Tremor

The manifestation of tremor is generally related to the pathogenic process of the particular disease. Therefore, an intention tremor is seen in those with MS, whereas a resting tremor is found in those with Parkinson's disease. In terms of pharmacological therapies, few have been proven effective in the symptomatic management of tremor. The effective therapies target the disease process, as with the administration of anticholinergics or specific anti-Parkinson medications that increase levels of dopamine. The tremor and rigidity present in those with Parkinson's disease is due to stimulation from acetylcholine and increasing the levels of dopamine reduces these effects.

Spasticity

Spasticity is a common occurrence in those with upper motor neuron disease and spinal cord injury. Pharmacology, specifically muscle relaxants, is typically used to control spasticity. Side effects of these therapies include sedation, confusion, and muscle weakness. Alternative options include nerve blocks or transaction and intrathecal therapies such as baclofen pumps. Adjunctive treatments, such as botulism toxin, which are often used in those with traumatic brain injury and spinal cord injury,

TABLE 22.2   Pharmacological Treatment for Spasticity

Generic Name	Trade Name	Action	Dosing
Muscle relaxants			
Baclofen	Lioresal	Gamma-aminobutyric acid analog	5–80 mg
Tizanidine	Zanaflex	Alpha-adrenergic receptor antagonist	2–36 mg
Dantrolene sodium	Dantrium	Interferes with calcium release in skeletal muscle	25–100 mg
Benzodiazepines			
Diazepam	Valium	Facilitates the action of gamma-aminobutyric acid	5–7.5 mg
Anticonvulsants			
Gabapentin	Neurontin	Shares structural similarity with gamma-aminobutyric acid	300–3600 mg
Levetiracetam	Keppra	Possibly binds to unique site on neurons. Appears to halt negative mediation of gamma-aminobutyric acid	500–1500 mg
Pregabalin	Lyrica	Shares structural similarity with gamma-aminobutyric acid	50–100 mg

have a lower frequency of use with other neurological disorders. In those with spasticity the presence of infections may serve to increase the intensity and frequency of spasm, indicating an increased need for infection monitoring in those with spasticity (Table 22.2).

Fatigue

Managing fatigue involves monitoring for the presence of other medical conditions that may contribute to fatigue, such as hypothyroidism. The sleep pattern of the patient should also be evaluated, and keeping a sleep–wake cycle log may be helpful. Pharmacological agents have been shown to be effective in the management of disease-associated fatigue. Yet, several of the pharmacological agents used in the management of fatigue can result in insomnia and restlessness as a side effect, so timing of administration is an important consideration (Table 22.3). Hospitalization also disrupts the normal routine, and aiding the patient in maintaining appropriate sleep hygiene and habits is significant in managing muscular fatigue.

Complications

In the rehabilitation setting nurses should monitor aggressively for the consequences of immobility. Eventually, most of the neurological disorders lead to decreased mobility in conjunction with generalized weakness. This places the patient at an increased risk for immobility, and in conjunction with swallowing disorders, the patient is then at increased risk for the development of infections and pressure ulcers.

In terms of planning nursing care for those with neurological disease, there are several diagnostic considerations to keep in mind. For the patient with any chronic illness, issues of anxiety, coping, and health management are significant considerations. For the patient with MS,

select nursing diagnoses are provided in Table 22.4. In consideration of Parkinson's disease as an exemplar of degenerative neurological disorders, select nursing diagnoses are provided in Table 22.5.

TEACHING AND EDUCATION OF THE CLIENT AND FAMILY

Adherence to treatment recommendations is an issue with all chronic disease conditions. Management of long-term disease states can require complex medication regimens with multiple administration times. Promoting adherence requires anticipating the needs of the patient and family, along with understanding the physical limitations that can influence participation. The presence of cognitive deficits along with comorbid depression can affect patient readiness to participate in therapy and the likelihood of ongoing adherence.

Educational materials and programs should target not only the patient but also the family member or caregiver. In an individual who may be physically weak with difficulty swallowing, family members or other caretakers need to be aware of how to provide medications, nutrition, and other therapies in the home setting. This education is given in the rehabilitation setting.

For those with a degenerative neurological disease, the potential for genetic susceptibility and the relevance of that susceptibility should be discussed with children and spouses as appropriate. The progressive nature of these disease states may lead to higher levels of physical impairment and possible cognitive deficits. Patients and family members need information on disease progression to help plan for future care needs. Those with MS need to be educated on the administration of injectable therapies in the home and information regarding the prevention of

TABLE 22.3 Pharmacological Interventions for Fatigue			
Generic	**Trade**	**Action**	**Dosage**
Antiviral			
Amantadine	Symmetrel	Direct and indirect effects on dopaminergic neurons	100–200 mg
Central nervous system stimulants			
Methylphenidate	Ritalin	Central nervous system stimulant	5–60 mg
Modafinil	Provigil	Binds to several neurotransmitter sites	100–400 mg
Pemoline	Cylert	Central nervous system stimulant	37.5–11.5 mg

TABLE 22.4   Select Nursing Diagnoses Appropriate for the Care of the Patient with MS

Medical Issue	Nursing Diagnosis	Nursing Actions
Fatigue	Fatigue	• Utilize a standard measure for rating of fatigue. • Evaluate sleep pattern and use of naps during the day. • Encourage pacing of daily activities and schedule tasks during times when patient has most energy. • If patient is on pharmacological agents for treatment of fatigue, evaluate effectiveness and effect on sleep pattern. • Be alert to the effect of heat on fatigue level. Consider scheduling outdoor activities in cooler parts of the day.
Ataxia and other gait disturbance	Impaired physical mobility Impaired transfer mobility Iᵃmpaired walking	• Evaluate gait pattern and activity tolerance. • Encourage participation in strength and balance training activities. • Instruct in performance of active and passive range of motion activities as appropriate. • Assess need for assistive devices and provide referral as appropriate.
Tremor	Impaired physical mobility related to lack of muscle control	• Determine effect of tremor on activities of daily living. • Encourage participation in activities of daily living. • Evaluate need for the use of adaptive devices. • If on pharmacological agents, determine effectiveness.

Visual disturbance
  Blurred vision
  Double vision
	Disturbed sensory perception	• Ensure environmental safety.
		• Interact often with patient and explain all activities.
		• Maintain adequate levels of lighting and ensure call devices are within reach.

Bowel/bladder disturbance
  Retention
  Urgency
	Impaired urinary elimination
	Bowel incontinence
	Bowel constipation
		• Evaluate frequency of bowel and bladder movements.
		• Assess potential for retention and ability to use assistive devices.
		• Monitor intake and output.
		• Encourage appropriate levels of fluid intake.

Neuropathy	Acute/chronic pain Impaired comfort	• Evaluate pain level frequently and determine effects on daily activities. • Provide PRN pain medication before daily therapies or activities. • Assist with determining appropriateness of alternative and nonpharmacological pain relief methods.
Cognitive deficits	Confusion Impaired memory	• Provide calm environment that minimizes environmental stimuli. • Employ orientation and reality-based centering as appropriate. • Encourage use of memory tools and aids.

side effects. This informᵃ(ation is often agent-specific. The course of MS is often uncertain, and the patient should be provided information regarding disease course and strategies for coping with cognitive and physical deficits. For those with Parkinson's disease, education needs to be provided regarding the importance of medication adherence and disease prognosis. With any neurological disease, the patient should have the necessary information regarding potential disease progression, providing the opportunity for patient and family planning.

The following recommendations can promote adherence to prescribed treatments for any chronic disease state, not just neurological disorders. It is best to incorporate a variety of strategies and techniques in managing medication and other therapies. Most neurological disorders have online journals that are available to those with select conditions that contain tips for activities of daily living and managing the disease condition. The web links provided in Box 22.1 can provide an avenue to more patient and professional educational materi-

TABLE 22.5	Select Nursing Diagnoses Appropriate for the Care of the Patient with Parkinson's Disease	
Medical Issue	**Nursing Diagnosis**	**Nursing Actions**
Dysphonia	Impaired verbal communication	• Assist patient with identifying alternative communication techniques. • Encourage avoidance of caffeine and smoking. • Discuss need to rest voice and identify peak times in which communication is most likely to occur successfully.
Gait disturbance Rigidity Postural tremor Bradykinesia	Impaired physical mobility Impaired transfer mobility Impaired walking	• Plan for activities during times of peak medication effectiveness. • Encourage participation in activities of daily living. • Utilize passive and active range of motion activities to avoid development of flexion contracture.
Tremor	Impaired physical mobility related to lack of muscle control	• Determine effect of tremor on activities of daily living. • Encourage participation in activities of daily living. • Evaluate need for the use of adaptive devices. • If on pharmacological agents, determine effectiveness.
Dysphagia	Adult failure to thrive Alteration in nutrition: less than bodily requirements Impaired swallowing	• Monitor intake and output. • Provide soft foods and frequent feedings as appropriate. • Ensure appropriate position during feeding. • Ascertain need for referral to speech therapist and instruction in swallowing techniques.
Cognitive deficits	Altered thought process Confusion Impaired memory	• Provide calm environment that minimizes environmental stimuli. • Employ orientation and reality-based centering as appropriate. • Avoid confronting fixed beliefs, instead focusing on activities that allow for reminiscing and provide the opportunity for interaction on the part of the patient.

als that can help enhance quality of life and promote adherence.

The recommendations are as follows:

- Provide pill boxes to allow the patient or caregiver to set up medications ahead of time.
- Medical calendars or diaries with color coding may be of benefit in helping patients keeping track of medications.
- Alarm clocks that allow for multiple time settings can be used to cue patients to take medication.
- Placing reminder notes in highly visible locations may also help cue the patient.
- For injectable agents, the use of self-injecting devices may be helpful, particularly for patients with a loss of fine motor control.
- Ensuring that medications are in a crushable format for those with swallowing disorders is an important consideration.
- It may be beneficial to discuss differing therapies, such as a weekly intramuscular injection instead of a daily subcutaneous injection for those with MS.

- Referring the patient to inperson or online support groups may be of significant benefit.
- Caregivers and family members should also be provided with resources regarding respite care and support groups.

ETHICAL CONCERNS

For most neurological disorders discussed in this chapter, there are no curative treatments. Existing therapies attempt to delay disease progression or reduce the incidence of disease exacerbation. In the face of the significant disease burden associated with these disease states, the patient may be willing to try unproven therapies or feel compelled to participate in clinical trials. In is important to ensure that all participation is informed with the free will of the participant.

This also provides another avenue for patient education. With the availability of material on the Internet, it can be difficult for patients to judge the quality of the material and potential feasibility of use. Nursing can help initiate a discussion regarding ways of judging the qual-

Each condition discussed in this chapter has a national organization that can provide additional information for both patient and family, with the exception of Eaton-Lambert syndrome. The majority of these organizations also have information targeting the needs of healthcare providers.

The National Institute of Neurological Disorders and Stroke provides health information pages for each of the disorders discussed in this chapter at http://www.ninds.nih.gov

The National Multiple Sclerosis Society at http://www.nationalmssociety.org

Specific information on rehabilitation and MS can be found at the Multiple Sclerosis Rehabilitation and Training Center at http://msrrtc.washington.edu

The Veterans Administration has a Center of Excellence dedicated to the care and rehabilitation of those with MS. The website for the center of excellence provides information for patients and healthcare providers. The information for the latter includes several sets of criteria and guidelines: http://www4.va.gov/ms

Myasthenia Gravis Foundation of America: http://www.myasthenia.org

Eaton-Lambert syndrome: Information can be obtained from the Muscular Dystrophy Association at http://www.mda.org/disease/lems.html

The Guillain-Barré Syndrome and Chronic Inflammatory Demyelinating Polyneuropathy Foundation International: http://www.gbs-cidp.org

The Parkinson Alliance: http://www.parkinsonalliance.org

Huntington's Disease Society of America: http://www.hdsa.org

Post-Polio Health International: http://www.post-polio.org

Charcot-Marie-Tooth Association: http://www.charcot-marie-tooth.org/index.php

ity of available material. This also holds true for family members and other care providers.

As well, with several of these diseases cerebral atrophy and dementia can occur, leading to a situation in which a patient may not possess full cognitive capacity. In these cases, encouraging a discussion between patient and family regarding desired care and possible end-of-life

decisions is important before the onset of cognitive deficits. Chapter 25 presents further information on ethical and legal issues.

CRITICAL THINKING

1. Consider the difference in the pathogenic process between degenerative and immune-mediated neurological disorders. Could the difference in time at onset or pathogenic process influence levels of stress or the adaptation process?
2. Pulling from other chapters of this text, enumerate the complications that can be experienced by any patient with a neurological disorder in areas of
   - Immobility
   - Skin integrity
   - Bowel and bladder function
   - Nutrition and swallowing
   - Cognition and behavior
   - Sexuality and disability
   - Psychosocial and spiritual issues

PERSONAL REFLECTION

- If you or a family member underwent a genetic test to determine susceptibility to Huntington's disease, would you want to know the result? Can you give reasons for wanting to be aware of the finding and reasons for not wanting to know? Should genetic counseling be mandatory for families with genetically inherited diseases such as Huntington's disease?
- Have you ever cared for a patient with GBS? ALS? What were the greatest challenges for nursing care? What were the greatest challenges for patients and families?
- In a gathering of older adults, such as at church or a senior center, observe how many appear to have some type of neurological disorder. Were your observations surprising or expected?

REFERENCES

Alves, G., Forsaa, E. B., Pedersen, K. F., Dreetz Gjerstad, M., & Larsen, J. P. (2008). Epidemiology of Parkinson's disease. *Journal of Neurology, 255*(Suppl 5), 18–32.

American Parkinson Disease Association Inc. (2010). Basic information about Parkinson's Disease. Retrieved September 1, 2010, from http://www.apdaparkinson.org/userND/AboutParkinson.asp

Banchs, I., Casasnovas, C., Alberti, A., De Jorge, L., Povedano, M., Montero, J., Martinez-Matos, J. A., & Volpini, V. (2009). Diagnosis of Charcot-Marie-Tooth disease. *Journal of Biomedicine & Biotechnology, 9*(8), 5415.

Barber, S. C., & Shaw, P. J. (2010). Oxidative stress in ALS: Key role in motor neuron injury and therapeutic target. *Free Radical Biology & Medicine, 48*, 629–641.

Chio, A., Logroscino, G., Hardiman, O., Swingler, R., Mitchell, D., Beghi, E., & Traynor, B. G. (2009). Prognostic factors in ALS: A critical review. *Amyotrophic Lateral Sclerosis, 10*(5–6), 310–323.

Dietert, R. R., Dietert, J. M., & Gavalchin, J. (2010). Risk of autoimmune disease: Challenges for immunotoxicity testing. *Methods in Molecular Biology, 598*, 39–51.

Geleijns, K., Emonts, M., Laman, J. D., van Rijs, W., van Doorn, P. A., Hermans, P. W., & Jacobs, B. C. (2007). Genetic polymorphisms of macrophage-mediators in Guillain-Barré syndrome. *Journal of Neuroimmunology, 190*(1–2), 127–130.

Giraud, M., Vandiedonck, C., & Garchon, H. J. (2008). Genetic factors in autoimmune myasthenia gravis. *Annals of the New York Academy of Sciences, 1132*, 180–192.

Howard, J. F. J. (Ed.). (2008). *Myasthenia gravis: An annual for the health care provider.* St. Paul, MN: Myathenia Gravis Foundation of America.

Kuzma-Kozakiewicz, M., & Kwiecinski, H. (2009). The genetics of amyotrophic lateral sclerosis. *Neurologia i Neurochirurgia polska, 43*(6), 538–549.

Lauer, K. (2010). Environmental risk factors in multiple sclerosis. *Expert Review of Neurotherapeutics, 10*(3), 421–440.

Lin, K. H., & Lim, Y. W. (2005). Post-poliomyelitis syndrome: Case report and review of the literature. *Annals of the Academy of Medicine, Singapore, 34*, 447–449.

McCance, K. L., & Huether, S. E. (2002). *Pathophysiology: The biologic basis for disease in adults & children* (4th ed.). St. Louis: Mosby.

Pareyson, D., & Marchesi, C. (2009). Diagnosis, natural history, and management of Charcot-Marie-Tooth disease. *Lancet Neurology, 8*(7), 654–667.

Polman, C. H., Thompson, A. J., Murray, T. J., Bowling, A. C., & Noseworthy, J. H. (2006). *Multiple sclerosis: The guide to treatmnt and management* (6th ed.). New York: Demos Medical.

Rickards, H. (2006). Depression in neurological disorders: an update. *Current Opinion in Psychiatry, 19*(3), 294–298.

Schneider, S. A., Walker, R. H., & Bhatia, K. P. (2007). The Huntington's disease-like syndromes: What to consider in patients with a negative Huntington's disease gene test. *Nature Clinical Practice Neurology, 3*(9), 517–525.

Sheean, G. (2008). Neurophysiology of spasticity. In M. P. Barnes & G. R. Johnson (Eds.), *Upper motor neuron syndrome and spasticity* (pp. 9–63). Cambridge, England: Cambridge University Press.

Smaga, S. (2003). Tremor. *American Family Physician, 68*(8), 1545–1552.

Snyder, L. A., Rismondo, V., & Miller, N. R. (2009). The Fisher variant of Guillain-Barré syndrome (Fisher syndrome). *Journal of Neuroophthalmology, 29*(4), 312–324.

Tanner, C. M. (2010). Advances in environmental epidemiology. *Movement Disorders, 25*(Suppl 1), S58–S62.

Vucic, S., Kiernan, M. C., & Cornblath, D. R. (2009). Guillain-Barré syndrome: An update. *Journal of Clinical Neurosciences, 16*(6), 733–741.

Walker, F. O. (2007). Huntington's disease. *Seminars in Neurology, 27*(2), 143–150.

Wirtz, P. W., Smallegange, T. M., Wintzen, A. R., & Verschuuren, J. J. (2002). Differences in clinical features between the Lambert-Eaton myasthenic syndrome with and without cancer: An analysis of 227 published cases. *Clinical Neurology and Neurosurgery, 104*(4), 359–363.

Xiromerisiou, G., Dardiotis, E., Tsimourtou, V., Kountra, P. M., Paterakis, K. N., Kapsalaki, E. Z., Fountas, K. N., & Hadjigeorgiou, G. Ml. (2010). Genetic basis of Parkinson disease. *Neurosurgical Focus, 28*(1), E7.

CHAPTER 23

Other Chronic Illnesses

Ann Bonner

LEARNING OBJECTIVES

At the end of this chapter, the reader will be able to

- Discuss the stages associated with chronic kidney disease.
- Describe kidney replacement therapy.
- Analyze rehabilitation nursing interventions for clients with chronic kidney disease.
- Recognize the effects of cancer on the body.
- Understand the importance of rehabilitation for the client with cancer.
- State pathophysiological changes occurring during terminal illness.
- Use rehabilitation nursing interventions required for the client in the terminal stages of illness.

KEY CONCEPTS AND TERMS

Anorexia	Continuous ambulatory peritoneal	Kidney transplantation
Automated peritoneal dialysis	dialysis	Palliative care
Cachexia	End-stage renal disease (ESRD)	Peritoneal dialysis
Cancer	Hemodialysis	Predialysis
Chronic kidney disease (CKD)	Kidney replacement therapy (KRT)	Terminally ill

Chronic kidney disease (CKD) is one of the largest growth areas in chronic health globally. The reasons for this growth include the aging population, an increase in chronic disease burden, increasing life expectancies, and increased access to **kidney replacement therapy (KRT)**. Clients with cancer experience longer survival rates than ever before and have a fluctuating clinical course. People with CKD or cancer experience many varied and complex alterations in their health status. As a consequence, rehabilitation is an important aspect of their care. Terminal illness can occur in clients who have cancer or end-stage organ failure. The typical rehabilitation client does not usually have cancer or a terminal illness, but these clients benefit most from rehabilitation that focuses on optimizing the performance of activities of daily living and minimizes the impact of fatigue; both of these alleviate a client's fear of being a burden on others and ensure their quality of life. This chapter describes the different stages of CKD and the rehabilitation nursing interventions required for clients with CKD. The chapter then discusses cancer and reha-bilitation and the importance of rehabilitation for clients who are terminally ill.

RENAL DISEASE

Background, Statistics, and Significance of Problem

CKD is a serious health problem and, in its later stages, requires people to invest considerable time to manage their health, including modifying their diet, managing numerous medications, undergoing KRT (if required), and attending medical and hospital appointments. CKD is classified into five stages, with those in stage 5 classified as end-stage renal disease (ESRD). CKD, its treatment, and concomitant complications have a significant impact on a person's lifestyle, family responsibilities, ability to work, and financial status. The incidence of CKD is rising across the world, and it is estimated that one in three people are at risk of developing CKD. In the United States 26 million people currently have CKD, and there are over 360,000 people receiving dialysis treatment (National

Kidney Foundation, 2009). There is also high prevalence of CKD in Canada, Europe, Australia, and Asia. In 2010 the direct cost of KRT in the United States is expected to be 28 billion dollars. A large investment is therefore required to promote effective long-term health care for people with CKD.

Pathophysiology Review

CKD is due to a progressive and irreversible destruction of renal function that occurs over varying periods of time ranging from a few months to decades. There are five stages of CKD, but the prognosis and course of CKD are highly variable, depending on the etiology and client's condition, age, and adequacy of medical follow-up. CKD results from a number of conditions that cause permanent loss of nephron function and a decrease in glomerular filtration rate (GFR). Based on GFR a five-stage classification system to describe the severity of CKD and to guide clinical actions has been developed. The entire clinical guideline may be accessed at http://www.kidney.org/professionals/kdoqi/pdf/ckd_evaluation_classification_stratification.pdf.

The kidneys have remarkable functional reserve. Up to 80% of the GFR may be lost with few obvious changes in the functioning of the body. In most cases the individual passes through the early stages of CKD without recognizing the disease state because the remaining nephrons hypertrophy to compensate.

CKD is defined as either kidney damage or a GFR $\leq$ 60 mL/min/1.73 m^2 for more than 3 months. Kidney damage is defined as pathological abnormalities or markers of damage, including abnormalities in blood or urine tests or imaging studies (Vassalotti, Stevens, & Levey, 2007). The vast majority of individuals with CKD stages 2 to 3 live normal, active lives, whereas others may rapidly progress to stage 5 (end-stage kidney disease). The major causes of CKD are diabetes mellitus, glomerulonephritis, and hypertension.

> *The major causes of CKD are diabetes mellitus, glomerulo-nephritis, and hypertension.*

Diabetes mellitus may affect the kidneys by causing microangiopathic changes of the glomerulus (glomerulosclerosis), involving thickening of the glomerular basement membrane. Diabetic nephropathy can develop from both type 1 and type 2 diabetes, and it is estimated that 20% to 40% of diabetics will develop CKD within 10 to 25 years after the onset of diabetes (Grover, Gadpayle,

& Sabharwal, 2010; William, Hogan, & Battle, 2005). However, type 2 diabetes causes the majority of those to develop CKD (Mobley, 2009; William et al., 2005). Often, CKD is asymptomatic in the early stages.

In the early stages of CKD, polyuria results from the decreased ability of the kidneys to concentrate urine. This is most noticeable at night, and the client must arise several times to urinate (nocturia). During stage 3, when about 50% of nephron function has been destroyed, hypertension, elevated urea and creatinine levels, and anemia develop (Kilstoff & Bonner, 2006). As CKD progresses the complications of CKD manifest, usually around late stage 3 and stage 4. These complications are as a result of anemia and abnormal bone and mineral metabolism. Management involves medications (iron supplements and erythropoietin-stimulating agents for anemia, calcitriol and phosphate binders for bone and mineral metabolism). Some clients will need sodium bicarbonate to correct acidosis or sodium polystyrene sulfonate (Kayexalate) for hyperkalemia. In stage 5 CKD edema, electrolyte imbalances, metabolic acidosis, and multisystem effects of uremia develop (Case Study 23.1).

For over 15 years the National Institutes of Health has recommended that people with CKD stage 4 be referred to an interdisciplinary **predialysis** team to minimize morbidity and ease the transition to renal replacement therapy (National Institutes of Health, 1994). The benefits of early referral are improved (1) client involvement and compliance, (2) client education, (3) time for dialysis vascular access maturation, (4) ability to delay progression to stage 5 CKD, (5) quality of life, and (6) mortality rates (Brick & Ellis, 2009; Klang, Bjorvell, & Clyne, 1999). Stage 5 CKD is also termed **end-stage renal disease (ESRD)** in which KRT is required to prevent death. In this stage clients may choose not to commence KRT and opt for **palliative care**.

KRT may be provided by hemodialysis, peritoneal dialysis, or a kidney transplant. Briefly, **hemodialysis** involves access to the vascular system (usually an arteriovenous fistula is formed and cannulated), an extracorporeal circuit, dialyzer, and technological equipment. Typically, a client will receive a minimum of 4 hours of treatment on three occasions each week either in a hospital, satellite/free-standing dialysis center, or at home. Nocturnal home hemodialysis is increasing in acceptance: Clients do their hemodialysis overnight—sometimes six nights per week.

Peritoneal dialysis is performed by introducing 2 to 3 liters of a sterile dextrose-containing solution (dialysate)

CASE STUDY 23.1

Arthur Johnson is a 54-year-old African American man diagnosed with type 2 diabetes 3 years ago. His diabetes follow-up health care since then had been erratic because of problems with accessing doctors, paying his medical bills, and his perception that there wasn't much wrong with him. He recently returned to his physician because he was feeling tired, was short of breath, had swollen ankles, and has several "black toes on my left foot." The physician determines that Arthur has renal failure (stage 5 CKD) because his estimated GFR is < 10 mL/min. Arthur is immediately referred to nephrologists and a vascular surgeon and admitted to hospital. Over the next few days Arthur undergoes a left leg below knee amputation, formation of an arteriovenous fistula, and insertion of a temporary vascular catheter (vas-cath). He also commences hemodialysis three times per week in the dialysis unit.

Questions

1. When should Arthur be referred to the rehabilitation unit?
2. What collaborative strategies should the dialysis and the rehabilitation units put in place for Arthur?
3. What rehabilitation nursing interventions are required for Arthur?

into the peritoneal cavity. Although there are several different techniques for peritoneal dialysis, the most common are **continuous ambulatory peritoneal dialysis** and **automated peritoneal dialysis**. Continuous ambulatory peritoneal dialysis requires the individual to manually change the dialysate in the peritoneal cavity four or five times each day, every day of the year. Automated peritoneal dialysis is typically undertaken overnight in which a small machine performs the dialysis exchanges while the person sleeps.

The last type of KRT is **kidney transplantation** and is an option for most clients with ESRD, either before or after the initiation of dialysis. The donor kidney is placed in the iliac fossa and native kidneys are not normally removed (Bonner & Douglas, 2008). Immunosuppression (e.g., prednisone, mycophenolate, and cyclosporin) is required to prevent rejection.

Risk Factors and Warning Signs

Individuals at risk of CKD must be identified. These include people with a history (or a family history) of renal disease, hypertension, diabetes mellitus, and repeated urinary tract infection. Over 90% of ESRD clients have type 2 diabetes (Williams, 2010). There is a very high risk for CKD among African American, Hispanics, Native Americans, and other aboriginal, first nation, or native populations around the world. Other risk factors are obesity, smoking, and physical inactivity.

Prevention

In the United States the National Kidney Foundation has been active in preventing and managing CKD at all stages, and similar activities are occurring in other countries. These activities primarily involve measuring urine albumin levels because albuminuria is associated with early stages of CKD. The Foundation's Kidney Disease Outcomes Quality Initiative has as its goal the development of clinical practice guidelines to manage clients with CKD; one guideline specifically identifies strategies for managing early stages of kidney disease by slowing disease progression, detecting/treating complications, and managing cardiovascular risk factors (Levey et al., 2007). Clients with CKD are far more likely to die from cardiovascular disease than to develop ESRD (Levey et al., 2007).

Interventions to delay progression of CKD are primarily achieving good blood pressure and glycemic control. Although medication may be introduced early, therapeutic lifestyle changes are also an important element of delaying progression and preventing complications (Williams, 2010). Lifestyle changes include cessation of smoking, increased exercise, weight loss, and reduced dietary sodium intake. Clients with CKD and albuminuria should be prescribed an angiotensin-converting enzyme inhibitor or an angiotensin receptor blocker even if their blood pressure is normal. These classes of drugs have been shown to protect the kidneys by reducing albumin loss as well as lowering blood pressure.

Assessment and Use of Screening Tools

An annual kidney health check is recommended for those at risk of CKD. In its simplest form a kidney health check has three components:

1. A urine test for albumin
2. Serum creatinine measurement, leading to an estimated GFR
3. A blood pressure measurement

Further screening is required if the client also has diabetes (or is suspected to have diabetes). The standard multiple urinalysis dipstick is not specific for albumin and only shows positive protein when there is a large amount of albuminuria. In people with diabetes a test for microalbuminuria should always be performed if the urine dipstick for protein is negative.

In CKD stages 4 and 5 often quality of life assessment tools are used in clinical practice to assess functional activity. These tools are the Medical Outcomes Survey Short Form, Kidney Disease Quality of Life, and Choices Health Experience Questionnaire (Unruh, Weisbord, & Kimmel, 2005). However, these tools are not sensitive enough to assess for clients who have a disability, require the use of a wheelchair, or who live in nursing homes where they are not required to perform activities associated with household chores (e.g., shopping, cooking, or cleaning). Rehabilitation-specific assessment and screening tools using the International Classification of Functioning, Disability and Health are not commonly used for clients with CKD and warrant further research to examine their relevance and accuracy for this particular client population.

Nursing Diagnoses

Rehabilitation in nephrology nursing is about assisting the client to achieve an optimal lifestyle so that CKD and KRT do not assume the sole focus of their lives or create an unmanageable burden for clients and their families. A common expression used by nephrology nurses that reflects rehabilitation thinking is "Don't let the dialysis rule your life, incorporate it into your life." Rehabilitative interventions used by nephrology nurses include teaching, coaching, and providing supporting strategies to assist people in increasing their movement along a continuum toward self-management (Pryor, Stewart, & Bonner, 2005). Given the repeated and frequent contact nephrology nurses have with clients with CKD over long periods of time (e.g., years), they are in an ideal position to provide both nephrology and rehabilitation nursing care. Nephrology nurses also need to work collaboratively with specialist rehabilitation nurses.

> A common quote among dialysis nurses is "Don't let the dialysis rule your life, incorporate it into your life."

Interventions

People with CKD live longer and experience functional (Painter, Carlson, Carey, Paul, & Myll, 2000) and psychosocial limitations that ultimately lead to disability (Tawney, Tawney, & Kovach, 2003). Rehabilitation by definition is about the return of lost function, and it seems logical to expect rehabilitation to be an aspect of the services provided to people with CKD. If the aim of dialysis is to correct the physiological imbalance, rehabilitation would focus on ameliorating the consequences of CKD on the person's ability to function normally. The five core principles of rehabilitation therapy for dialysis clients are encouragement, education, exercise, employment, and evaluation. However, people with CKD experience barriers to accessing rehabilitation services (Kutner, 2010), such as lack of recognition that people with CKD become deconditioned, time away from the rehabilitation unit to receive dialysis, being too fatigued after dialysis to benefit from rehabilitation, and not being referred for rehabilitation, particularly cardiac rehabilitation after coronary artery bypass grafting.

As renal function declines, many people experience a wide range of symptoms that cause people either distress and/or disruption to normal daily living (Thomas-Hawkins, 2000). Approximately 90% of clients with CKD experience fatigue, lack of energy, or tiredness. Fatigue is due to a number of factors including physiological alterations, particularly abnormal urea and hemoglobin levels; psychological factors such as depression and sleep dysfunction; and nutritional deficiencies (Jhamb, Weisbord, Steel, & Unruh, 2008). Although it is well known that fatigue is common for hemodialysis clients (Lee, Lin, Chaboyer, Chiang, & Hung, 2007), Bonner, Wellard, and Caltabiano (2008) found that peritoneal dialysis and predialysis (i.e., stage 4 CKD) clients are more fatigued than hemodialysis clients.

Clients with CKD have a reduced capacity to undertake regular daily activities (Periman et al., 2005) and experience poor balance and functional limitations in performing basic mobility tasks (Tawney et al., 2003). There is also a correlation between increasing severity of physical symptoms with a decline in quality of life of people with CKD, especially after the commencement of KRT (Salzberg, 2009). Clients with stage 4 or 5 CKD are less active than the general population and engage in less personal/household work activities, entertainment/social activities, and independent exercise activities (Bonner, Wellard, & Caltabiano, 2009). Nevertheless, exercise programs during hemodialysis have been found to improve functional capacity (strength, balance, and mobility), lower the risk for falls, reduce the incidence of depression, and increase the well-being and overall quality of life (Bennett, Agius, Simpson-Gore, & Barnard, 2007; Ouzouni, Kouidi, Sioulis, Grekas, & Deligiannis, 2009); however, more support from a rehabilitation perspective for specific strategies that can be incorporated into routine care is warranted.

Client–Family Teaching

The rehabilitative continuum typically begins with teaching people about CKD and its management. From the diagnosis of CKD to dialysis and transplantation clients have much to learn in relation to their disease and how to manage it (Bonner & Douglas, 2008). One goal of CKD client teaching is to establish the foundations of positive self-care attitudes and practices that will make the transition to dialysis and transplantation (if required) easier. Client teaching often involves learning how to adhere to dietary and fluid restrictions and administer medications. In some situations teaching involves instructing people about performing their own dialysis at home. Not everyone can self-manage effectively. For clients who are unable or unwilling to engage in self-management, the healthcare team must develop strategies to provide the best possible outcome for the individual. A collaborative interdisciplinary team approach can improve the identification of problems, setting priorities, establishing goals, and creating an individualized treatment plan.

Evaluation of Outcomes

Evaluation of outcomes for clients with CKD involves the client participating in decision-making regarding his or her condition and its treatment as well as demonstrating compliance with the therapeutic regimen. Clients also report developing strategies to regain control of their life and sufficient energy to engage in activities of daily living.

Ethical Considerations

Rehabilitation ethical considerations for clients with CKD are associated with the principle of justice. There are inequalities in renal clients' access to and receipt of rehabilitation services due to socioeconomic status, race, gender, and age (Kutner, 2010). There is also a lack of recognition by both the renal healthcare team and the rehabilitation team that clients with CKD require specialized rehabilitation services.

CANCER

Background, Statistics, and Significance of Problem

Cancer is a chronic and complex set of diseases that affects every age group but more commonly affects people older than 65 years. More than 1.4 million Americans are diagnosed with cancer each year, and it is second only to cardiovascular disease as a leading cause of death in the United States. In order of frequency, the leading causes of cancer deaths in the United States are lung, prostate, and colorectal cancer in men and lung, breast, and colorectal cancer in women (American Cancer Society, 2009). Similar statistics are seen in other developed countries.

Worldwide the population of long-term cancer survivors continues to grow due to improvements in early detection and treatment of cancer. However, cancer and its treatment, including the effects of surgery, chemotherapy, and radiation, have long been recognized to have disabling complications (Franklin, 2007; Vargo & Gerber, 2005), particularly for older clients who often experience lower functional status than younger clients. Cancer can cause significant short- and long-term physiological and psychological complications, including pain, fatigue, difficulties with mobility and self-care, reduced quality of life, and reduced cardiorespiratory capacity. Interventions to manage these complications have the potential to improve both physical and psychological health in the short and long term (Schwartz, 2008). Even today the goals of cancer rehabilitation described by Cromes in 1978 remain relevant. However, the important role of rehabilitation for cancer clients is only beginning to emerge (Guo & Shin, 2005).

> *"Cancer rehabilitation aims to allow the patient to achieve optimal physical, social, physiological and vocational functioning within the limits imposed by the disease and its treatment." (Cromes, 1978, p. 230).*

Pathophysiology Review

Cancer can arise from any cell in the body that is capable of evading normal regulatory processes. It is a complex disease, and knowledge about cancer has become more detailed due to discoveries in molecular biology and genetics. This has in turn suggested new treatments (Corner & Bailey, 2009). Unexpected changes (mutations) in the cellular deoxyribonucleic acid (DNA) are believed to be due to carcinogens. These carcinogens can be internal factors (hormones, immune conditions, and inherited genetic mutations), external factors (chemicals, viruses, radiation), or a combination of these. It is these carcinogens that trigger the development of cancer.

Malignant neoplasms are aggressive growths that do not respond to the body's homeostatic controls. These growths invade surrounding tissues; cause bleeding, inflammation, and necrosis; and travel through the blood or lymphatic system to invade other tissues and organs of the body (American Cancer Society, 2009). This spread of malignant cells is termed "metastasis," and the most common sites of metastasis are the lymph nodes, liver, lungs, bones, and brain.

The pathophysiological effects of cancer vary with the type and location of the cancer. Several effects are typically seen in clients:

- *Disruption of function:* A neoplasm can disrupt normal function by obstructing or causing an increase in pressure in a tissue. For example, a large growth in the bowel can result in a bowel obstruction.
- *Hematological alterations:* Cancer can impair the normal function of blood cells. For example, leukemia compromises the function of the bone marrow.
- *Infection:* A tumor could destroy surrounding viable tissue, resulting in necrosis and infection.
- *Hemorrhage:* Tumors can erode through blood vessels and cause extensive bleeding.
- *Cachexia:* In many clients unexplained weight loss is the first symptom of a cancer. Weight loss can also be due to pain, infection, side effects of cancer treatment, as well as the effect of the cancer on normal body metabolism
- *Pain:* Direct tumor involvement is the primary cause of pain experienced by people with cancer. Pain can be due to metastatic bone disease, nerve compression, and involvement of visceral organs.
- *Psychological stress:* The diagnosis of cancer can affect a wide range of psychological and emotional responses in people such as grief, guilt, anger, powerlessness, fear, concerns about body image, sexual dysfunction, and death.

Regardless of the type of cancer, a range of functional impairments can occur, and these impairments may be due to the cancer itself, to treatment effects, or to other comorbidities. Common issues across many types of cancer include pain, fatigue, and deconditioning (Smith & Vargo, 2007). Other problems requiring rehabilitation services include neurological deficits (peripheral neuropathies, nerve root, spinal cord or brain involvement); musculoskeletal (amputation, deformities, and contractures), communication, and swallowing problems; cognitive deficits; and limb edema.

Risk Factors and Warning Signs

Several risk factors are strongly linked to cancer. Cancer is a disease associated with aging. Over 75% of cancer diagnoses occur after the age of 55. As a person gets older there is the increased likelihood of genetic mutations, long-term exposure to substances that cause cancer, and immune system alteration with aging (American Cancer Society, 2009). Other risk factors for cancer are inherited genes, gender, stress, diet, tobacco use, alcohol use, obesity, sun exposure, and occupation. The poor are also at a higher risk for cancer due to inadequate access to health care, particularly preventative screening and counseling.

Prevention

The World Health Organization (2007a) claims that we now have sufficient knowledge to prevent approximately 40% of all cancers. This is due to the effectiveness of interventions to modify behavioral risk factors such as tobacco control, diet, physical inactivity, overweight and obesity, reduction in alcohol consumption, and environmental substances.

Assessment and Use of Screening Tools

For most cancers screening programs and early detection improve client outcomes. Population screening programs such as cervical cancer screening, mammography, and fecal occult blood testing as well as opportunistic and diagnostic screening can be used to detect for cancer.

After diagnosis and treatment of cancer, performance rating scales are used in oncology clinical practice. The Karnofsky Performance Status scale, developed in 1948, is still routinely used in the assessment of functional outcome specifically for cancer clients and can be used to compare effectiveness of different therapies and to assess the prognosis in individual clients (Karnofsky & Burchenal, 1949; Zimmermann et. al., 2010). The lower the Karnofsky score, the worse the survival for most serious illnesses (Table 23.1). Typically, cancer clients who require rehabilitation services have Karnofsky scores between 30 and 70 (Smith & Vargo, 2007). Common functional limitations such as generalized deconditioning, exertional intolerance, motor deficits, and inability to independently perform activities of daily living can be determined.

The Eastern Cooperative Oncology Group Performance Status Scale (Table 23.2) is also used to assess how a client's disease is progressing, assess how the disease affects the daily living abilities of the client, and determine appropriate treatment and prognosis (Oken et al., 1982). Often, both the Karnofsky and the Eastern Cooperative Oncology Group performance status scales

TABLE 23.2   Eastern Cooperative Oncology Group (ECOG) Performance Status Scale

Grade	ECOG Score
0	Fully active, able to carry on all predisease performance without restriction.
1	Restricted in physically strenuous activity but ambulatory and able to carry out work of a light or sedentary nature, e.g., light housework, office work.
2	Ambulatory and capable of all self-care but unable to carry out any work activities. Up and about more than 50% of waking hours.
3	Capable of only limited self-care; confined to bed or chair more than 50% of waking hours.
4	Completely disabled. Cannot carry on any self-care. Totally confined to bed or chair.
5	Dead.

Source: From Oken et al. (1982).

TABLE 23.1   Karnofsky Performance Status Scale

Category	Score	Ability
Able to carry on normal activity and to work; no special care needed	100	Normal, no complaints; no evidence of disease
	90	Able to carry on normal activity; minor signs or symptoms of disease
	80	Normal activity with effort; some signs or symptoms of disease
Unable to work; able to live at home and care for most personal needs; varying amount of assistance needed	70	Cares for self; unable to carry on normal activity or to do active work
	60	Requires occasional assistance, but is able to care for most personal needs
	50	Requires considerable assistance and frequent medical care
Unable to care for self; requires equivalent of institutional or hospital care; disease may be progressing rapidly	40	Disabled; requires special care and assistance
	30	Severely disabled; hospital admission is indicated although death not imminent
	20	Very sick; hospital admission necessary; active supportive treatment necessary
	10	Moribund; fatal processes progressing rapidly
	0	Dead

Source: From Karnofsky and Burchenal (1949).

are used together to assess the functional status of clients with cancer (Zimmermann et al., 2010).

Nursing Diagnoses

The rehabilitation team should be introduced to clients early in the decision-making processes and treatment of cancer as part of the interdisciplinary team (Mikkelsen, Sondergaard, Jensen, & Olesen, 2008; Vargo & Gerber, 2005). The expectation that optimal function is possible and that cancer rehabilitation is an important part of holistic treatment ought to be communicated to clients (Cheville, 2005). Slowing functional decline and preserving a client's self-care capability with routine activities of daily living have been shown to preserve quality of life in clients with cancer (Axelsson & Sjoden, 1998; Korstjens, Mesters, & Gijsen, 2007).

The rehabilitation nurse provides a number of important roles for clients with cancer. Planning, exploring, coaching, and supporting clients are useful rehabilitation nursing strategies in assisting clients with cancer (Eades, Chasen, & Bhargava, 2009). The role also includes providing ongoing information, evaluating functional needs, brokering the complex interdisciplinary plan of care, and providing supportive care to clients in acute inpatient setting, outpatient care, long-term facilities, nursing homes, palliative care units, hospices, and in the home. Table 23.3 provides rehabilitation nursing diagnoses for clients with cancer.

TABLE 23.3   Rehabilitation Nursing Diagnoses for Clients with Cancer

- Anxiety related to uncertainty about outcomes, feelings of helplessness and hopelessness, and insufficient knowledge about cancer and treatment
- Acute/chronic pain related to direct tumor involvement and/or cancer therapy
- Powerlessness related to feeling of loss of control and life style restrictions
- Activity intolerance related to fatigue

Interventions

Rehabilitation from cancer involves regaining strength, recovering from surgery or chemotherapy, learning to live with an altered body image, and recovering from psychological and emotional turmoil. Guo and Shin (2005) identify common problems experienced by cancer clients that could be managed by the rehabilitation team (Table 23.4). Rehabilitation interventions should focus on pain relief, preservation or restoration of function, optimizing performance of activities of daily living, education about planning and prioritizing life activities to assist with quality of life, and psychosocial support (Mikkelsen et al., 2008; Vargo & Gerber, 2005).

Cancer rehabilitation goals are challenging to set and should be determined by effectively assessing the client's age, type and stage of cancer, comorbid medical conditions, and baseline functional status. Dietz (1969)

TABLE 23.4   Common Problems Associated with Cancer

- Generalized weakness
- Psychological/psychiatric impairments
- Lymphedema management
- Musculoskeletal impairments
- Neurological impairments
- Swallowing dysfunction
- Impaired communication
- Impairments in activities of daily living
- Impaired gait/ambulation
- Impaired nutrition
- Pain
- Skin management
- Disposition/housing issues
- Vocational assessment

Source: From Guo and Shin (2005, p. 84).

first introduced these goals as restorative, supportive, preventative, and palliative; each of these goals can be applied to each stage of cancer treatment, from physical rehabilitation in the acute stage, to physical and psychosocial rehabilitation in the terminal stage. Cheville (2005) more recently describes each of these goals as follows:

1. Restorative rehabilitation refers to the effort to return clients to their predisease functional status when little or no long-term impairment is anticipated.
2. Supportive rehabilitation attempts to maximize function after permanent impairments caused by cancer and/or its treatment.
3. Preventative rehabilitation attempts to preclude or mitigate functional morbidity caused by cancer or its treatment.
4. Palliative rehabilitation applies to clients with advanced cancer.

Given the dynamic nature of cancer, it is important to regularly review goals with clients.

It is estimated that 70% of clients with cancer have cancer-related pain and that approximately 90% of clients with advanced disease will have pain (Vargo & Gerber, 2005). Evaluation of the location, severity, and quality of pain requires careful assessment. Treatment of pain may include pharmacological and nonpharmacological agents, radiation, or surgery (Franklin, 2007). In acute pain, nonopioid analgesia is the first line of treatment. These agents include aspirin, acetaminophen, and nonsteroidal anti-inflammatory drugs. If these agents fail to control acute pain, then opioids (codeine, oxycodone, morphine, fentanyl, etc.) are used. Routes of administration include oral, rectal, parenteral, transdermal, and intrathecal (Franklin, 2007). Adjuvant agents (antidepressants, psychostimulants, corticosteroids, etc.) may be added for better control. Nonpharmacological interventions such as heat, cold, ultrasound, and nontraditional therapies (relaxation, massage, acupuncture, aromatherapy, etc.) have also been shown to be useful in relieving acute pain. Chronic pain is also common and requires regular and systematic assessment. Similar agents are also used to control chronic pain, although alternative methods of delivery are often needed such as longer-acting preparations, nerve blocks, and other neurosurgical procedures.

Fatigue is the most common and significant side effect for clients receiving cancer treatment; it is a symptom that persists long after treatment ends (Braun, Greenberg, & Pirl, 2007). Contributor factors for fatigue include anemia, cachexia, chronic pain, infection, psychological stress, and side effects of cancer treatment (Vargo & Gerber, 2005). Nursing interventions and client education about maximizing energy conservation, minimizing deconditioning, and exercise are important strategies to deal with cancer-related fatigue (Saarik & Hartley, 2010).

Maintaining some exercise during and after cancer treatment has been shown to benefit functional capacity, decrease fatigue, prevent muscle wasting, and improve quality of life (Spence, Heesch, & Brown, 2010). Although there are no established exercise guidelines for clients with cancer, Schwartz (2008) recommends that nurses advise clients to start exercising slowly and to progress in frequency and intensity in a slow step-by-step fashion. Referral to physical therapists or exercise professionals may also be warranted. There are, however, contraindications to exercise, and these include febrile neutropenia, platelet counts below 50,0000/mm, hemoglobin below 10 g/dL, and uncontrolled nausea, vomiting, or pain (Schwartz, 2008).

Some types of cancer require specific exercise rehabilitation (Franklin, 2007). For instance, in breast cancer after mastectomy and lymph node dissection, clients require progressive shoulder range of motion and upper extremity strengthening. Clients with head and neck cancer require instruction and support to undertake neck range of motion and strengthening exercises as well as rehabilitation interventions related to speaking and eating. Clients who require chemotherapy as part of the cancer treatment frequently experience fatigue and deconditioning, and they benefit from assistive devices for mobility and performance of activities of daily living.

Client–Family Teaching

Nurses provide support to clients and their family through the different stages of prevention, detection, and treatment of cancer. Clients often have to deal with issues related to adjustments after treatment that affect social enjoyment, relationships, and employment. Relationships may have suffered from the strain of the illness. Education involves a series of structured or nonstructured experiences designed to assist the clients to develop coping strategies to assist with the diagnosis, adjustments to the disease and its treatment, and development of self-care skills and attitudes. Teaching also involves the coaching aspects associated with rehabilitation and the adjustments required when function is limited. Self-help groups are also often available in many communities, and these groups assist other cancer survivors.

Evaluation of Outcomes

Evaluation of outcomes for clients with cancer involves acceptance of health status, the recognition of reality, the ability to make decisions about health matters, and increased psychological coping. Clients will also be able to discuss their anxiety and concerns about their disease and its treatment and have developed coping strategies.

Ethical Considerations

Rehabilitation ethical considerations for clients with cancer are associated with the principles of autonomy and beneficence. Clients have the right to choose to participate in treatment including rehabilitation after the diagnosis of cancer, and the rehabilitation team should maximize therapy options with the intention of doing no harm.

TERMINAL ILLNESS

Background, Statistics, and Significance of Problem

Modern health care enables clients to survive longer in the advanced stages of many complex and chronic diseases, and although life may be extended, clients do experience functional decline (Cheville, 2005). Terminal illness necessitates a comprehensive approach to symptom management that is often provided by the palliative care interdisciplinary healthcare team. Terminal illnesses are not only associated with cancer but other chronic diseases that result in end-stage organ failure.

The World Health Organization's (2007b) objectives for terminal illness and the provision of palliative care are to

- Palliate physical symptoms
- Alleviate disease and maintain independence for as long and as comfortably as possible
- Alleviate isolation, anxiety, and fear associated with advanced disease
- Provide as dignified a death as possible
- Support those who are bereaved

Terminal illnesses can last for months, if not years, during which fluctuations in health may occur, and it is highly likely that rehabilitation is an appropriate aim of care at one or more points throughout the course of a terminal illness (Schleinich, Wareen, Nekolaichuk, Kaasa & Watanabe, 2008). Unfortunately, rehabilitation possibilities are widely overlooked in the distribution of palliative care resources (Hopkins & Tookman, 2000) and that terminally ill clients report having unmet needs related to occupational functioning and symptom control (Morasso et al., 1999). Both palliative care and rehabilitation nursing have similar goals: to maximize function, reduce caregiver burden, and maintain psychological and spiritual well-being (Smith & Vargo, 2007).

Pathophysiology Review

Pathophysiological changes associated with end-stage cardiac and respiratory failure were dealt with in Chapter 21. Also see earlier in this chapter for reviews of CKD and cancer pathophysiology.

Physiological changes do occur during the terminal phases of all illnesses and are also part of the normal dying process. These changes result in the following side effects:

- Weakness and fatigue
- Difficulty talking or swallowing
- Nausea, abdominal distention
- Urinary and/or bowel incontinence, constipation
- Decreased urine output
- Decreased sensation, taste, and smell
- Weak, slow, and/or irregular pulse
- Decreasing blood pressure
- Changes in level of consciousness
- Restlessness, agitation, delirium
- Coolness, mottling, and cyanosis of extremities

Prevention

Although terminal illness cannot be prevented, planning for a dignified death and end-of-life care is appropriate. Advanced care directives, living wills, and do-not-resuscitate instructions can be prepared and documented in a client's records.

Assessment and Use of Screening Tools

In terminal illness assessment focuses on symptoms. Symptoms are continuously changing in intensity, quality, frequency, and level of associated distress (Cheville, 2005). There are numerous valid and reliable assessment tools for quality of life, pain, symptom distress, cognition, depression, anxiety, delirium, fatigue, and nutritional status. A client's subjective reports of experience and comfort play a greater role in palliative care. It is more important, therefore, for nurses to be alert to what the client is saying about the presence and severity of symptoms.

Nursing Diagnoses

Clients who are in the final stages of cancer or organ failure benefit from rehabilitation goals that focus on maximizing independence in the performance of activities of daily living. These clients are often quite concerned about becoming a burden to their family members. **Terminally ill** clients report that what they most need from the rehabilitation team are assistance with mobility, exercise, and activity (Schleinich et al., 2008). Often, simple rehabilitative strategies are used in combination with good symptom control and psychological support by palliative care nurses. The use of assistive devices and mobility aids maximize functional independence and quality of life. Engaging clients in constructive goals to maximize function may avoid engendering helplessness. Table 23.5 identifies rehabilitation nursing diagnoses for terminally ill clients.

Interventions

The palliative care nurse plays an important role in providing support and coping strategies for clients who are in the terminal stages of their illness. Interventions such as listening to expressions of grief convey a caring attitude and assist the nurse in determining how a client is coping with the situation (Haley & Daley, 2008). Using a constructive manner to help clients solve problems and encouraging family involvement also facilitate the grieving process.

As a client's physical condition deteriorates there is a diminishing sense of control over his or her life. A client-centered care approach aims to encourage greater choice and to treat clients as people rather than conditions (Becker, 2009). Although many clients, when asked, express a wish to die at home, the reality of care today is that few currently achieve that desire. With most of the population dying in some form of institution, careful attention to the environment can provide good psychological, emotional, and spiritual support by creating a milieu with which clients are comfortable. Some may prefer peace and quiet and wish to be in a side room. Others, however, like to be part of life on a ward and feel less iso-

---

TABLE 23.5   Rehabilitation Nursing Diagnoses for Terminally Ill Clients

- Acute/chronic pain related to direct tumor involvement
- Grieving related to loss of normal function as evidenced by expression of feelings of sadness, anger, inadequacy, hopelessness
- Imbalanced nutrition: Less than body requirements related to anorexia, nausea, vomiting and loss of taste or smell, and stomatitis
- Activity intolerance related to fatigue

lated in a bay environment. Although difficult to achieve in some clinical areas, the sense of continuity of care by assigning the same nurses to a client is often highly valued by both clients and relatives (Becker, 2009).

Nurses should avoid building a set of beliefs and values that unconsciously communicate to clients and families that their relative's death should represent an ideal (Becker, 2009). A key component in caring for the terminally ill is the maturity as a nurse to address the challenging intrapersonal issues intrinsic in caring for dying people and their families. There is a need for nurses to recognize and attempt to understand their own personal reactions that occur as a natural consequence of working with dying and bereaved people and to be able to reflect on how this affects care given in sensitive situations.

Interventions for pain, activity, and fatigue in terminal illness have many similarities to those described earlier in this chapter (see Cancer, above). Specific interventions for impaired nutrition due to anorexia and cachexia are discussed.

Anorexia and cachexia are common symptoms in the end stages of many chronic conditions such as cancer, AIDS, stage 5 CKD, chronic obstructive pulmonary disease and advanced cardiac disease. **Anorexia** is a lack or loss of appetite resulting in weight loss. **Cachexia** is a progressive wasting of fat and muscle even in the presence of a satisfactory intake of food and fluids due to

severe metabolic dysfunction (Cheville, 2005). Several treatments can be tried to reverse the cachexia such as nutritional supplements, parenteral nutrition, appetite stimulants (cyproheptadine, dexamethasone, prednisolone), or prokinetic agents (metoclopramide), which may provide temporary relief of these symptoms.

Client–Family Teaching

Palliative care nurses teach clients and others how to use assistive devices (see Chapter 10 for further details) and about environmental modifications that can be made to their home. One of the major challenges of providing palliative nursing care, particularly in nonspecialist environments, is reaching a collaborative decision regarding clients' care orientation that is focused on curative, life-preserving measures or toward more palliative, quality-of-life measures. Ideally, this should be done in conjunction with clients, relatives, and all team members (Becker, 2009). It is also important to assess which family and friends are available, how they wish to be involved in care, and what, if any, special needs they may. Table 23.6 provides recommended readings.

Evaluation of Outcomes

In terminal illness evaluation of client outcomes involves acceptance of health status, the recognition of reality, and the ability to make decisions about end-of-life matters. For the terminally person participating in rehabilitation, improved quality at end of life or the ability to return

TABLE 23.6   Recommended Readings

Bennett, P. N., Breugelmans, L., Barnard, R., Agius, M., Chan, D., Fraser, D., McNeill, L., & Potter, L. (2010). Sustaining a haemodialysis exercise program: A review. *Seminars in Dialysis, 23*(1), 62–73.

Hill, K. K., & Hacker, E. (2010). Helping patients with cancer prepare for hospice. *Clinical Journal of Oncology Nursing, 14*(2), 180–188.

Kutner, N. G. (2008). Promoting functioning and wellbeing in older CKD patients: Review of the literature. *International Journal of Urology and Nephrology, 40*, 1151–1158.

Qaseem, A., Snow, V., Shekelle, P., Casey D. E., Cross J. T., & Owens, D. K. (2008). Evidence-based interventions to improve the palliative care of pain, dyspnea, and depression at the end of life: A clinical practice guideline from the American college of physicians. *Annals of Internal Medicine, 148*(2), 141–146.

home to die with loved ones present may be the best possible outcome.

Ethical Considerations

The following are important ethical points for the nurse to consider when providing care to the terminally ill client:

- Quality of life is an important consideration for clients when weighing whether to begin or discontinue treatment.
- Client autonomy, or the client's right to self-determination regarding treatment decisions, applies both to initiating and discontinuing treatment.
- Assessing a client's capacity to make healthcare decisions, especially related to end-of-life issues, is a complex process involving physical, psychological, social, spiritual, and quality of life factors.
- If a decision is made to withdraw treatment, the healthcare team, client, and family should develop an appropriate follow-up plan that includes palliative care and hospice support.
- For the client with a terminal illness who chooses to participate in acute rehabilitation, staff members may need additional education and counseling to understand the client's perspective about this choice.

CRITICAL THINKING

Effective pain management is crucial for clients, particularly those with cancer, to actively participate in their rehabilitation. Explore the Oncology Nurses' Society Clinical Practice Resources available for pain management at www.ons.org/ClinicalResources/Symptom/Pain.

1. Does the nursing practice in your rehabilitation unit reflect best practice for pain management for clients with cancer?
2. Discuss your findings with the rehabilitation nursing team.

PERSONAL REFLECTION

Often, the goal of a rehabilitation nurse is to restore function or to have a client achieve the best functional outcome. At times, the rehabilitation nurse may provide nursing care to clients who are also terminally ill.

- What are your feelings about providing rehabilitation to a terminally ill client?
- How did you feel about that experience?

- What was your interaction with the client and his or her family?
- How were they coping with the changes brought about by the terminal illness?

REFERENCES

American Cancer Society. (2009). *Cancer Facts & Figures 2009.* Atlanta: American Cancer Society.

Axelsson, B., & Sjoden, P. (1998). Quality of life of cancer patients and their spouses in palliative home care. *Palliative Medicine, 12*(1), 29–39.

Becker, R. (2009). Palliative care 3: Using palliative nursing skills in clinical practice. *Nursing Times, 105*(15), 18–21.

Bennett, P. N., Agius, M., Simpson-Gore, K., & Barnard, B. (2007). A haemodialysis exercise programme using novel exercise equipment: A pilot study. *Journal of Renal Care, 33*(4), 153–158.

Bonner, A., & Douglas, B. (2008). Chronic kidney disease. In E. Chang & A. Johnson (Eds.), *Chronic illness and disability: Principles for nursing practice* (pp. 333–350). Sydney: Elsevier.

Bonner, A., Wellard, S., & Caltabiano, M. (2008). Levels of fatigue in people with ESRD living in far north Queensland. *Journal of Clinical Nursing, 17*(1), 90–98.

Bonner, A., Wellard, S., & Caltabiano, M. (2009). Determining patient activity levels in chronic and end stage kidney disease. *Journal of Nursing & Healthcare of Chronic Illness, 1,* 39–48.

Braun, I., Greenberg, D., & Pirl, W. (2007). Evidence-based report on the occurrence of fatigue in long term cancer survivors. *Journal of the National Comprehensive Cancer Network, 5*(1), 347–354.

Brick. N., & Ellis, P. (2009). The significance of the timing of referral for renal care. *Journal of Renal Care, 35*(1), 33–41.

Cheville, A. L. (2005). Palliative care. In J. A. DeLisa, B. M. Gans, N. E. Walsh, W. L. Bockenek, W. R Frontera, S. R. Geiringer, . . . R. O. Zafonte (Eds.), *Physical medicine & rehabilitation: Principles and practice* (4th ed., pp.531–551). Philadelphia: Lippincott Williams & Wilkins.

Corner, J., & Bailey, C. D. (2009). *Cancer nursing: Care in context.* Oxford: Wiley-Blackwell.

Cromes, G. J. (1978). Implementation of interdisciplinary cancer rehabilitation. *Rehabilitation Counselling Bulletin, 21,* 230–278.

Dietz, J. H. (1969). Rehabilitation of the cancer patient. *Medical Clinics of North America, 53,* 607–624.

Eades, M., Chasen, M., & Bhargava, R. (2009). Rehabilitation: Long-term physical functional changes following treatment. *Seminars in Oncology Nursing, 25*(3), 222–230.

Franklin, D. J. (2007). Cancer rehabilitation: Challenges, approaches and new directions. *Physical Medicine and Rehabilitation Clinics of North America, 18,* 899–924.

Grover, G., Gadpayle, A. K., & Sabharwal, A. (2010). Identifying patients with diabetic nephropathy based on serum creatinine under zero truncated model. *Electronic Journal of Applied Statistical Analysis, 3*(1), 28–43.

Guo, Y., & Shin, K. Y. (2005). Rehabilitation needs of cancer patients. *Critical Review in Physical and Rehabilitation Medicine, 17*(2), 83–99.

Haley, C., & Daley, J. (2008). Palliation in chronic illness. In E. Chang & A. Johnson (Eds.), *Chronic illness and disability: Principles for nursing practice* (pp. 168–184). Sydney: Elsevier.

Jhamb, M., Weisbord, S. D., Steel, J. L., & Unruh, M. (2008). Fatigue in patients receiving maintenance dialysis: A review of definitions, measures, and contributing factors. *American Journal of Kidney Disease, 52*(2), 353–365.

Karnofsky, D. A., & Burchenal, J. H. (1949). The clinical evaluation of chemotherapeutic agents in cancer. In C. M. MacLeod (Ed.), *Evaluation of chemotherapeutic agents in cancer* (pp. 191–205). New York: Columbia University Press.

Kilstoff, K., & Bonner, A. (2006). Renal health breakdown. In E. Chang, J. Daly, & D. Elliott (Eds.), *Pathophysiology applied to nursing practice* (pp. 169–199). Sydney: Elsevier.

Klang, B., Bjorvell, H., & Clyne, N. (1999). Predialysis education helps patients choose dialysis modality and increases disease-specific knowledge. *Journal of Advanced Nursing, 29*, 869–876.

Korstjens, I., Mesters, I., & Gijsen, B. (2007). Cancer patients' view on rehabilitation and quality of life: A programme audit. *European Journal of Cancer Care, 17*, 290–297.

Kutner, N. G. (2010). Rehabilitation in the renal population: Barriers to access. *Seminars in Nephrology, 30*(1), 59–65.

Lee, B. O., Lin, C. C., Chaboyer, W., Chiang, C. L., & Hung, C. C. (2007). The fatigue experience of haemodialysis patients in Taiwan. *Journal of Clinical Nursing, 16*, 407–413.

Levey, A. S., Atkins, R., Coresh, J., Cohen, E. P., Collins, A. J., Eckardt, K-U., . . . Eknoyan, G. (2007). Chronic kidney disease as a global public health problem: Approaches and initiatives—a position statement from Kidney Disease Improving Global Outcomes. *Kidney International, 72*, 247–259.

Mikkelsen, T. H., Sondergaard, J., Jensen, A. B., & Olesen, F. (2008). Cancer rehabilitation: Psychosocial rehabilitation needs after discharge from hospital? *Scandinavian Journal of Primary Health Care, 26*, 216–221.

Mobley, A. M. (2009). Slowly the progression of chronic kidney disease. *Journal for Nurse Practitioners, 5*(3), 188–194.

Morasso, G., Capelli, M., Viterori, P., DiLeo, S., Alberisio, A., Costantini, M., . . . Henriquet, F. (1999). Psychological and symptom distress in terminal cancer patients with met and unmet needs. *Journal of Pain Symptom Management, 17*, 402–409.

National Institutes of Health. (1994). Morbidity and mortality of renal dialysis: an NIH consensus conference statement. *Annals of Internal Medicine, 121*(1), 62–70.

National Kidney Foundation. (2002). KDOQI clinical practice guidelines for chronic kidney disease: Evaluation, classification and stratification. *American Journal of Kidney Disease, 39*(Suppl 1), S1–S000.

National Kidney Foundation. (2009). 2009 annual report. Retrieved from www.kidney.org

Oken, M. M., Creech, R. H., Tormey, D. C., Horton, J., Davis, T. E., McFadden, E. T., & Carbone, P. P. (1982). Toxicity and response criteria of the Eastern Cooperative Oncology Group. *American Journal of Clinical Oncology, 5*, 649–655.

Ouzouni, K., Kouidi, E., Sioulis, A., Grekas, D., & Deligiannis, A. (2009). Effects of intradialytic exercise training on health-related quality of life indices in haemodialysis patients. *Clinical Rehabilitation, 23*, 53–63.

Painter, P., Carlson, L., Carey, S., Paul, S., & Myll, J. (2000). Physical functioning and health-related quality-of-life changes with exercise training in hemodialysis patients. *American Journal of Kidney Diseases, 35*(3), 482–492.

Periman, R. L., Finkelstein, F. O., Liu, L., Roys, E., Kiser, M., Eisele, G., . . . Saran, R. (2005). Quality of life in chronic kidney disease (CKD): a cross-sectional analysis in the Renal Research Institute-CKD study. *American Journal of Kidney Diseases, 45*, 658–666.

Pryor, J., Stewart, G., & Bonner, A. (2005). Is rehabilitation a function of nephrology nursing? *Collegian, 12*(3), 20–26.

Saarik, J., & Hartley, J. (2010). Living with cancer-related fatigue: Developing an effective management programme. *International Journal of Palliative Nursing, 16*(1), 6, 8–12.

Salzberg, D. J. (2009). Quality of life and rehabilitation in dialysis patients. In W. L. Henrich (Ed.), *Principles and practice of dialysis* (4th ed., pp. 570–584). Philadelphia: Wolters Kluwer.

Schleinich, M. A., Wareen, S., Nekolaichuk, C., Kaasa, T., & Watanabe, S. (2008). Palliative care in rehabilitation survey: A pilot study of patients' priorities for rehabilitation goals. *Palliative Medicine, 22*, 822–830.

Schwartz, A. L. (2008). Physical activity. *Seminars in Oncology Nursing, 24*(3), 164–170.

Smith, R. G., & Vargo, M. M. (2007). Rehabilitative medicine. In A. M. Berger, J. L. Shuster, & J. H. Von Roenn (Eds.), *Principles and practice of palliative care and supportive oncology* (3rd ed., pp. 765–776). Philadelphia: Lippincott Williams & Wilkins.

Spence, R. R., Heesch, K. C., & Brown, W. J. (2010). Exercise and cancer rehabilitation: A systematic review. *Cancer Treatment Review, 36*(2), 185–194.

Tawney, K. W., Tawney, P. J. W., & Kovach, J. (2003). Disablement and rehabilitation in end-stage renal disease. *Seminars in Dialysis, 16*(6), 447–452.

Thomas-Hawkins, C. (2000). Symptom distress and day-to-day changes in functional status in chronic hemodialysis patients. *Nephrology Nursing Journal, 27*(4), 369–379.

Unruh, M. L., Weisbord, S. D., & Kimmel, P. L. (2005). Health-related quality of life in nephrology research and clinical practice. *Seminars in Dialysis, 18*, 82–90.

Vargo, M. M., & Gerber, L. H. (2005). Rehabilitation for patients with cancer diagnoses. In J. A. DeLisa, B. M. Gans, N. E. Walsh, W. L. Bockenek, W. R. Frontera, S. R. Geiringer, . . . R. O. Zafonte (Eds.), *Physical medicine and rehabilitation: Principles and practice* (4th ed., pp. 1771–1794). Philadelphia: Lippincott Williams & Wilkins.

Vassalotti, J. A., Stevens, L. A., & Levey A. S. (2007). Testing for chronic kidney disease: a position statement from the National Kidney Foundation. *American Journal of Kidney Disease, 50*(2), 169–180.

William, J., Hogan, D., & Battle, D. (2005). Predicting the development of diabetic nephropathy and its progression. *Advances in Chronic Kidney Disease, 12*(2), 202–211.

Williams, M. (2010). Improving outcomes for diabetic patients on dialysis: An introduction. *Seminars in Dialysis, 23*(2), 127–128.

World Health Organization. (2007a). *Cancer control: Knowledge into action. WHO guide for effective programs: Prevention.* Geneva: World Health Organization.

World Health Organization. (2007b). *Cancer control: Knowledge into action. WHO guide for effective programs: Palliative care.* Geneva: World Health Organization.

Zimmermann, C., Burman, D., Bandukwala, S, Seccareccia, D., Kaya, E., Bryson, J., . . . Lo, C. (2010). Nurse and physician inter-rater agreement of three performance status measures in palliative care outpatients. *Supportive Care in Cancer, 18*(5), 609–616.

CHAPTER 24

Cultural Perspectives Within Rehabilitation Nursing

Margaret M. Andrews
Teresa L. Cervantez Thompson

LEARNING OBJECTIVES

At the end of this chapter, the reader will be able to

- Describe the impact of cultural attitudes, beliefs, and practices as it relates to disability and rehabilitation.
- Discuss key models in the provision of culturally congruent with people with disabilities.
- Apply Leininger's three action modes for transcultural nursing decisions and actions in rehabilitation.
- Identify the potential impact for folk and complementary interventions on the provision of care in rehabilitation nursing.
- Critically analyze cultural influences on the nurse–patient interaction in rehabilitation nursing.

KEY CONCEPTS AND TERMS

Activism	Disability	Minority cultures
Americans with Disabilities Act of 1990	Disability culture	Nurse–patient communication
	Environmental context	Nursing culture
Caregiver roles	Ethnic culture	Nursing intervention
Caregiving experience	Ethnic minority groups	Paralympic
Communication	Ethnohistory	Peer groups
Complementary and alternative medicine (CAM)	Goals of independence	Professional Professional subculture
	Handicap	
Conflicts of interpretation	Health disparities	Rehabilitation delivery system
Cultural diversity	Illness mode	Resilience
Cultural expressions of care	Impairment	Self-care
Cultural imperialism	Incongruence	Shared primary language
Culturally competent care	Individualism	Societal changes
Culturally congruent care	Language	Spiritual blessing
Culture	Language barriers	Subculture
Culture care accommodation/ negotiation	Legislative action	Thompson Model of Care Congruence
	Leininger's Culture Care Theory	
Culture care preservation/ maintenance	Leininger's Sunrise Enabler	Transcultural care decisions and actions
	Life span	
Culture care repatterning/ restructuring	Lived experience	Wheelchair sports teams
	Mainstreaming	

CULTURAL DIVERSITY IN THE UNITED STATES

With a population that exceeds 310 million, the United States is a nation rich in **cultural diversity**, a term that is sometimes used interchangeably with multiculturalism or cultural pluralism. Cultural diversity refers to the differences that occur between human societies and cultures. Although recognizing that diversity includes a wide variety of characteristics including religion, gender, sexual orientation, age, and related factors, the federal census data report only an overview of the types of racial and ethnic diversity found in contemporary U.S. society. More than 100 million, or one in three people, self-identify with one or more of the federally recognized racial or **ethnic minority groups**.[1] Recent census data reveal that there are more minorities in this country today than there were people in the United States in 1910. To put this into a broader context, the U.S. minority population is larger than the total population of all but 11 countries in the world (U.S. Census Bureau, 2009).

Health Disparities

Racial and ethnic disparities in health care have been well documented in the professional healthcare and rehabilitation literature (National Institutes of Health, 2010b). **Health disparities** refer to differences between groups of people that affect how frequently a disease occurs in a group, how many people become sick, and how often the disease causes death. The Institute of Medicine of the National Academies (2010) identified more than 175 studies demonstrating racial and ethnic disparities in the diagnosis and treatment of key health conditions such as cardiovascular disease, diabetes mellitus, low birth weight, asthma, cancer, and other problems that frequently lead to chronic illness, disability, and the need for rehabilitation. Disability is reported at higher rates in **minority cultures** overall, with the African American population the highest (Nathenson, 2009). Although the causes of the disparities are complex, social factors external to the healthcare delivery system contribute

---

[1]Refers to the following major categories used during the most recent census conducted in 2010: Black/African American, Hispanic, Asian, Native Hawaiian or Other Pacific Populations, and American Indian/Alaska Natives. The option to self-identify with two or more categories also is provided. Some view the term "minority" as offensive because it sets certain individuals or groups apart from the rest of society and focuses on differences rather than similarities among people.

significantly. Although minorities should play a key role in solving the health disparities problem, this important challenge cannot be fully addressed until every healthcare professional is prepared to deal with any patient regardless of race, gender, ethnicity, culture, or socioeconomic status in a respectful, culturally competent manner. Fewer than 40% of nurses and 25% of nursing faculty have formal academic preparation relative to the provision of culturally congruent and competent nursing care (Leininger & McFarland, 2006).

Although health indicators such as life expectancy and infant mortality have improved for most Americans, people from some cultures experience a disproportionate burden of preventable disease, death, and disability. Patients from traditionally under-represented populations tend to be more socioeconomically disadvantaged, less educated, work in jobs having higher rates of occupational hazards, and live in neighborhoods with greater environmental pollution and threats to personal safety than members of the general population. With the exception of some Asian cultures, people who self-identify as members of one or more of the federally identified racial and ethnic minority groups are likely to be uninsured or underinsured. For example, Hispanics represent 15.8% of the total U.S. population but account for 33% of those without health insurance (Centers for Disease Control and Prevention, 2009). Lack of insurance translates into less access to preventive services, higher rates of emergency department use and avoidable hospitalizations, and lower adherence to prophylactic measures and inability to obtain prescription medications.

Similarly, the impact of racism has been studied and linked to poor health outcomes among African Americans. Even when studies control for socioeconomic status, insurance, location of care delivery, stage of disease, age, gender, and comorbidities, racial and ethnic disparities are prevalent. Reasons for the disparities include variations in patients' health-related values, beliefs, and practices; personal preferences; genetic makeup; and behaviors. These include variability in patients' recognition of symptoms, decision making related to the timing for seeking care, choice of healers and healing systems, ability to effectively communicate symptoms to nurses and other care providers, and decreased ability to understand the management and/or treatment plans developed by professional healthcare providers. As a result of these and related factors, the emphasis on cultural competence in health care has emerged.

Defining Cultural Competence

Culture refers to integrated patterns of human behavior that include the language, thoughts, actions, customs, beliefs, and institutions of racial, ethnic, social, or religious groups. Cultural competence refers to the ability to respect the beliefs, language, interpersonal styles, and behaviors of individuals, families, and communities receiving services as well as the healthcare professionals who are providing those services. Cultural competence requires a willingness and ability to draw on community-based values, traditions, and customs and to work with knowledgeable persons of and from the community in developing targeted interventions, communication, and other supports (U.S. Department of Health and Human Services, 2009).

Striving to achieve cultural competence is a dynamic, ongoing, sustained developmental process that requires a long-term commitment to mastery of specific knowledge and skills and constructively critical self-reflection on feelings, values, attitudes, beliefs, and motivations, including those related to prejudice, bigotry, discrimination, and racism. In rehabilitation nursing this means feelings and attitudes toward people with mobility, visual, and/or hearing impairments and those with genetic and/or acquired developmental disabilities. In some cultures, for example, the birth of an infant with one or more impairments is viewed as a burden or may be perceived as parental punishment by God or gods(s) for past family or personal transgressions (e.g., marital infidelity, past decision to have an abortion, or related actions). In other cultures the infant is viewed as a sign of favor by a supreme being who has entrusted the parents with a "special" baby.

Types and Levels of Cultural Competence

The movement toward cultural competence in health care has gained national and international attention, with cultural barriers being identified at two levels: (1) organizational or leadership level and (2) clinical or individual patient–provider level.

Organizational Cultural Competence

Organizational cultural competence refers to the activities to ensure that the key leadership and workforce of a healthcare delivery system are diverse and representative of its patient population (Sullivan Commission, 2005). Ludwig-Beymer (2008) states that organizational cultural competence includes the presence of an infrastructure for communicating effectively with patients and helping nurses and other members of the rehabilitation team to provide the best possible care. For communication to be effective, the information provided must be complete, accurate, timely, unambiguous, and understood by the patient. Some patients require alternative communication methods. Examples of this include patients who speak and/or read languages other than English, patients who have limited literacy in any language, patients who have visual or hearing impairments, patients on ventilators, patients with cognitive impairments, and children. There are many options available to assist in **communication** with these individuals, such as interpreters, translated written materials, pen and paper, communication boards, and speech therapy. Various laws, regulations, and guidelines are relevant to the use of interpreters. In addition, the Joint Commission has set standards to ensure patients receive care that respects their cultural, psychosocial, and spiritual values (Joint Commission, 2002–2010). Similarly, the American Nurses Credentialing Center (2010), the American Association of Colleges of Nursing (2008), and the American Nurses Association (2010) also have addressed the need for culturally competent care.

Individual or Clinical Cultural Competence

Individual or clinical cultural competence refers to efforts that enhance or expand the rehabilitation nurse's knowledge of the relationship between sociocultural factors and patients' health beliefs and practices or behaviors. Individual cultural competence also refers to a complex integration of knowledge, attitudes, beliefs, skills, and encounters with those from cultures different from one's own that fosters effective interactions in cross-cultural situations. It allows nurses and other healthcare professionals to "increase their understanding and appreciation of cultural differences and similarities within, among, and between groups" (U.S. Department of Health and Human Services, 2006, p. 99). For a comprehensive overview of definitions and references on cultural competence, visit Cultural Competence at www.nccc.georgetown.edu/foundations/need.htmlt

FRAMEWORK FOR CULTURAL COMPETENCE IN REHABILITATION

It is useful for nurses working with individuals with disabilities and groups or communities from diverse backgrounds to have an organizing or theoretical framework as they engage in the process of assessing, planning, implementing, and evaluating nursing and rehabilitation care.

Leininger's Culture Care Theory

Dr. Madeleine Leininger is a nurse-anthropologist who established the nursing specialty called transcultural nursing. She developed the Theory of Culture Care Diversity and Universality that focuses on describing, explaining, and predicting nursing similarities and differences in human care and caring. The theory is intended to guide nurses in providing care that is culturally congruent and competent. To provide a comprehensive, holistic view of culture care Leininger uses concepts such as world view, social and cultural structure dimensions, **language**, **ethnohistory**, environment, generic, indigenous or folk health systems, and professional health systems. The social and cultural structure dimensions include people's beliefs and practices concerning technology, religion, kinship, cultural values, beliefs and lifeways, politics, law, economics, and education. Culturally based care factors are recognized as major influences on human expressions and experiences related to health, illness, and well-being or on facing chronic illness, disability or death.

Finally, **Leininger's Culture Care Theory** includes three action modes to guide nurses when making transcultural care decisions or taking actions. The action modes are intended to assist in the provision of **culturally congruent care**, that is, care consistent or congruent with the patient's cultural beliefs and practices. The three action modes are (1) **culture care preservation and/or maintenance**, (2) **culture care accommodation and/or negotiation**, and (3) **culture care repatterning and/or restructuring** (Leininger & McFarland, 2002, 2006).

Box 24.1 applies Leininger's Culture Care Theory to a case involving an Amish infant with spina bifida and apnea. Using knowledge of Amish ethnohistory and beliefs about technology, the process followed by the nurses in **transcultural care decisions and actions** is described in the case. In addition to technological factors, the nurses also applied knowledge about Amish kinship and social structures, lifeways, care expressions, **environmental context**, and related factors they considered in developing a culturally congruent discharge plan.

The pediatrician has written a discharge order for an apnea monitor for Jonas Yoder, an Amish infant with spina bifida and life-threatening episodes of apnea. Jonas was born to parents who belong to a rural ethnoreligious group called the Old Order Amish. Ethnoreligious practices among members of this community dictate that families refrain from using electricity in their homes. Instead, it is common for the Old Order Amish to rely on candles, wood-burning fireplaces, and similar items for light and warmth. In assessing the cultural and social structure dimensions of the Yoder family, the nurse identifies technological factors as an area in which there is a lack of congruence between the cultural beliefs and practices of the pediatrician, nurses, and others who embrace the highly technological biomedical practices and the Yoder's.

Using Leininger's Culture Care Theory the nurse considers the closely knit extended family kinship and other social factors; Amish lifeways, religious, and philosophical factors; environmental context; and Amish care expressions, patterns, and practices such as the high level of community interdependency in supporting sick, disabled, or handicapped members. Amish expressions of care include being kind to others; doing for others and less for oneself; knowing, trusting, and relying on friends within the Amish community; and accepting help from kin. The nurse critically analyzed the three action modes in providing culturally congruent or culturally competent care for Jonas and decided that the most culturally congruent action would be culture care preservation and/or maintenance. The nurse encouraged the Yoder parents to garner the support of their interdependent, extended Amish community to provide direct observation of Jonas' breathing around the clock rather than rely on an apnea monitor. The nurse also considered the second action mode, culture care negotiation and/or accommodation. If the Yoder's could be convinced to attach the apnea monitor to a battery, the nurse reasoned that the lack of congruence concerning technological factors might be resolved. The nurse quickly dismissed the third action mode, culture care restructuring and/or repatterning, because this would require the Yoder's to allow electricity to be wired into their house, a decision that would violate their ethnoreligious beliefs and alienate them from long-standing friends in their extended Amish community.

BOX 24.3   Web Exploration

Visit Mobility International, USA ©2010. CEO Susan Sygall states, "**I believe that all people with disabilities are members of a global family. Working together across borders is our most powerful way of effecting changes.**" Surf this website in search of the advocacy efforts undertaken to make this happen: http://www.miusa.org.

Among the strengths of Leininger's theory is its flexibility for use with individuals, families, groups, communities, and institutions in diverse health systems. **Leininger's Sunrise Enabler** to Discover Culture Care (Figure 24.1) depicts components of the Theory of Culture Care Diversity and Universality. The figure illustrates the key components of the theory and the interrelationships among its parts. As the world of nursing, health care, and rehabilitation have become increasingly diverse, the theory's relevance has increased as well. For further information about Dr. Leininger and her Theory of Culture Care Diversity and Universality, visit either Dr. Leininger's website at www.madeleine-leininger.com or the Transcultural Nursing Society's website at www.tcns.org.

Using key components of Leininger's Culture Care Theory, we identified cultural influences on the nurse–patient interaction in rehabilitation settings. The goal of the model is the delivery of culturally appropriate, meaningful, helpful, and relevant nursing and rehabilitation care that is congruent with the patient's cultural beliefs and practices (Figure 24.2).

Throughout this chapter we expand on selected concepts presented in Figure 24.2 as they relate to culturally

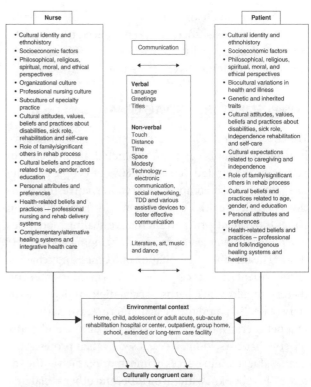

FIGURE 24.2   Andrews/Thompson conceptual model for understanding cultural influences on the nurse-patient interaction in rehabilitation settings.

Source: © Margaret Andrews & Teresa Cervantez Thompson

congruent and **culturally competent care** in rehabilitation nursing. We discuss the importance of cultural identity, religious and philosophical factors, and cultural attitudes, values, beliefs, and practices about disabilities, sick role, rehabilitation, self-care, the role of family/significant others in the rehabilitation process, cultural expectations related to caregiving and independence, professional nursing and rehabilitation systems, folk/indigenous healing systems, complementary/alternative healing medicine/healing systems, integrative health care, and **nurse–patient communication**. The model for understanding cultural influences on the nurse–patient interaction is intended for use within environmental contexts associated with rehabilitation nursing such as the patient's home; acute and subacute settings for children, adolescents, and adults; rehabilitation center or hospital; outpatient setting; group home; school; and extended or long-term facility.

It is assumed that cultural diversity exists in many environmental contexts and requires rehabilitation nurses to consider cultural influences on themselves, patients and their families/significant others, and all members of

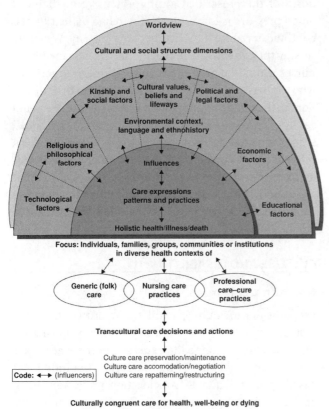

FIGURE 24.1   Leininger's Sunrise Enabler to discover culture care.

Source: Used with permission of Dr. Madeleine M. Leininger

the rehabilitation team—physicians, physical and occupational therapists, social workers, speech pathologists, psychologists, disability counselors, and professionals in the **rehabilitation delivery system**.

COMPLEMENTARY AND ALTERNATIVE MEDICINE

We chose to emphasize complementary and alternative healing systems because an estimated 40% to 60% of people in the United States and 80% of people globally use one or more complementary/alternative interventions (World Health Organization, 2010); rehabilitation patients frequently turn to alternative healing modalities when biomedicine is ineffective in bringing about their desired health and rehabilitation outcomes; and rehabilitation patients have access to a plethora of information on dietary supplements, herbs, special diets, and a wide variety of healing modalities (acupuncture, aromatherapy, magnet therapy, mental imaging, relaxation, and many others) that are seldom, if ever, used by their professional healers. Electronic sources of information such as the Internet, Facebook, Twitter, YouTube, and other social networks provide rehabilitation patients and their families/significant others with fast, easily accessible information on complementary and alternative healing.

Complementary and alternative medicine (CAM) is a group of diverse medical and healthcare systems, practices, and products that are not generally considered part of conventional medicine as practiced by those who have earned M.D. (medical doctor) and D.O. (doctor of osteopathy) degrees and by health professionals, such as registered nurses, nurse practitioners, physical therapists, psychologists, and physician assistants. The boundaries between CAM and conventional medicine are not absolute, and specific CAM practices may, over time, become widely accepted (National Institutes of Health, 2010a). Folk, traditional, integrative, and non-Western medicine are other terms used to describe healing and care not generally considered part of the allopathic, biomedical, conventional mainstream.

Since prehistoric times people have attempted to identify plants, marine organisms, arthropods, animals, and minerals with healing properties. According the World Health Organization (2010) 80% of people residing in less developed countries use traditional or folk medicine, including medicinal plants, for their major primary healthcare needs. Although the exact number of plants being used medicinally worldwide is unknown, approximately 5% of the 250,000 known species of plants

have ever been studied for bioactive compounds that might have healing effects.

Many of the active ingredients in plant-derived drugs or herbs are unknown and remain largely unregulated by government agencies, except for customs officials who make efforts to control the flow of illegal drugs. Fresh or dried herbs are usually brewed into a tea, with the dosage adjusted according to the chronicity or acuteness of the illness and the age and size of the patient. Traditional Chinese medicine typically is used only as long as symptoms persist. Some patients extend the same logic to Western biomedicine. For example, they might stop taking an antibiotic as soon as the symptoms subside instead of completing the course of treatment for the prescribed length of time.

It is important to consider the potential interaction of herbs with Western biomedicines. The root of the shrub ginseng, for example, is widely used for the treatment of arthritis, back and leg pains, and sores. Because ginseng is known to potentiate the action of some antihypertensive drugs, nurses must ask the patient whether he or she is experiencing side effects or toxicity and monitor blood pressure frequently. It might be necessary to withhold doses of the prescribed antihypertensive medicine if blood pressure is low or to ask the rehab patient to discontinue or reduce the strength of the ginseng. When assessing the patient's use of traditional Chinese medicine, nurses should be aware that some Chinese Americans who use herbs topically do not consider them to be drugs. For further information about herbs, the nurse should ask the patient and family, consult with an herbalist, search for reputable sources on the Internet, or check reference books on herbal remedies. Table 24.1 provides an overview of selected conditions, types of CAM that are used by some people for prevention or treatment of conditions, and current research to guide evidence-based and best practices.

CULTURE AND DISABILITY

Nonethnic Cultures

People belong to a number of different cultures; the ethnic culture is the one to which an individual is born and/or lives. Through one's life experiences there are other cultures and subcultures that influence the individual based on the individual's work location, profession, living environment, education, or experiences in common with others. Individuals may consciously or unconsciously adopt values, beliefs, attitudes, or actions based on close

TABLE 24.1 Complementary and Alternative Healing for Selected Conditions Associated with Disability and Rehabilitation

Condition	Healing Modality	Evidence-based Practice
Arthritis (osteoarthritis)	Dietary supplements (such as glucosamine, chondroitin)	Research demonstrates that glucosamine and chondroitin sulphate alone or in combination did not reduce pain effectively overall for people with osteoarthritis of the knee but may be effective in a subgroup of those with moderate-to-severe knee pain.
Arthritis (rheumatoid)	Mind–body techniques such as relaxation, mental imaging, biofeedback, mindfulness-based stress reduction	When added to conventional medical treatment, research demonstrates beneficial effects on pain, physical function, psychological state, and ability to cope.
	Dietary supplements such as fish oil, gamma linoleic acid (GLA)	No supplement has shown clear treatment benefits, but preliminary studies show GLA may relieve symptoms such as joint pain, stiffness, and tenderness and reduce need for NSAIDs.
	Thunder god vine (*Tripterygium wilfordii*)	Research shows some anti-inflammatory and immunosuppression effects. Caution: May cause serious side effects such as hair loss, diarrhea, and skin rash.
	Acupuncture	No evidence to determine effectiveness.
	Special diets (vegetarian, Mediterranean), periods of fasting	No evidence to determine effectiveness.
Back pain	Chiropractic/manipulation, massage	Mixed evidence on effectiveness. Further research in progress.
	Acupuncture	Research demonstrates decreased low back pain; use of acupuncture needles may stimulate production of body's natural pain-reducing chemicals such as endorphins, serotonin, and acetylcholine.
Cardiovascular disease	Aspirin (325 mg daily prophylactic dose)	Research demonstrates gender differences: Lowers risk of heart attack in men and stroke in women.
	Fish oil	Some research shows it reduces cholesterol and cardiovascular disease, but not recommended for high-risk populations such as those with diabetes or severe congestive heart failure.
	Garlic	No evidence to determine effectiveness in lowering blood pressure.
	Hawthorn	Safe and effective for mild forms of heart failure.
	Other dietary supplements (antioxidant supplements, vitamin C, vitamin D, calcium, coenzyme Q10, or combinations of these)	Mixed research findings in efficacy for the prevention or treatment of cardiovascular disease.
Diabetes mellitus noninsulin dependent	Dietary supplements Green tea Magnesium	May have a beneficial effect on insulin activity and glucose control by lowering blood levels. Caution: Green tea is caffeinated, which may cause in some people insomnia, anxiety, or irritability. Also contains small amounts of vitamin K, which can make anticoagulants (e.g., warfarin) less effective.
	Other dietary supplements (aloe vera, bitter melon, cactus pear, coenzyme Q10, garlic, fenugreek, ginseng)	Eating a diet high in magnesium may prevent diabetes, but studies on magnesium supplementation to lower blood glucose for people already diagnosed with diabetes have been mixed. Inconsistent research findings on control of glucose levels.

NSAIDs, nonsteroidal anti-inflammatory drugs.

Source: Data from National Center for Complementary and Alternative Medicine, retrieved from http://www.nccam.nih.gov; Agency for Healthcare Research and Quality, retrieved from ahrq.gov/consumer; National Institute of Arthritis and Musculoskeletal and Skin Diseases, retrieved from http://www.niams.nih.gov/Health_info/back_pain; National Institute of Diabetes and Digestive and Kidney Diseases, retrieved from htpp://www.diabetes.niddkd.nih.gov/dm/pubs/alternativetherapies.

association with others. The latter influences are usually considered nonethnic cultures because they often relate more to experiences in which a person is immersed. The individual then has an overlay of values, beliefs, attitudes, and actions that influence or mediate his or her lifeways or ways of perceiving situations (Andrews & Boyle, 2008.) Examples of nonethnic cultures are individuals in the military adopting a clear set of values, beliefs, attitudes, and actions specific to that role or an individual who lives in an institutional setting such as a long-term care facility where there are values, beliefs, attitudes, and norms that provide an overlay of expectations for those residents. Finally, within a profession one takes on cultural expectations.

Disability

For consistency in word use, although the term "disability" is used in most of this discussion, the distinction between "impairment," "disability," and "handicap" is shared to ensure understanding. **Impairment** relates to the part that is affected. For example, eyes, ears, legs, or speech may be impaired. The degree to which the impairment affects an individual's function defines the perception of **disability** experienced by the individual. **Handicap** has to do with the external or societal limitation on the individual who has the disability. The World Health Organization (2010) has an international classification system that addresses this distinction through three domains of the body, person, and society. The person who is limited in sight (impairment or body) may be able to compensate for it with glasses and thus only without glasses does the individual experience distinguishable disability and handicap. On the other hand, if a person has a visual impairment for which there is no treatment or remediation, the person may experience a disability (person), and if there are not resources such as audible announcements for each floor exit on an elevator, the person may also be handicapped by the environment/society.

The values, beliefs, and attitudes within a particular **ethnic culture** related to disability are not universal. To begin to understand the concept of disability within a culture, one must fully understand definitions of roles and attitudes related to independence, dependence, and productivity, along with expectations about caregiving in general and then as it relates to individuals who have disabilities. Some specific culture studies related to disability describe within a group experiences and attitudes that impact how individuals or their cultural group view a disability (Thomas, 2009; Wiley, 2009). For example,

does a culture value independence, not being a burden, or have expectations about privacy, especially within the family, if there is a member with a disability? Just as one works to identify the cultural background and expectations of the individual for any **caregiving experience**, another level of inquiry needs to be considered to understand the underpinnings of the cultures attitude toward disability.

As we consider cultural values, beliefs, attitudes, and actions as they relate to individuals with a disability, the Leininger Sunrise Enabler to Discover Culture Care (Figure 24.1) serves as a guide to identify all areas that influence and the ways in which a culture comes to develop its attitudes related to disability. Unfortunately, through the ages individuals who were considered different or less able were not always seen as a part of a culture. From Biblical times, the blind, lame, and lepers were ostracized or set apart. Those seen as unproductive or considered to be other than "normal" have often been put aside and, in the most severe circumstances, abandoned or left to die. Some cultures do not expect individuals with disabilities to be seen: It is considered abnormal or offensive. The person with the disability in these cultures avoids being seen in by others. Through the ages disabilities have been viewed as a curse for wrong doings by the individual or their family. Others cultures attached shame to having a child with a developmental disability, and still others view certain impairments as a **spiritual blessing** or god-like characteristic, as is the case of epilepsy. This was true of Julius Caesar and Augustine the Great.

Cultural beliefs can also impact the interpretation of illness, as discussed in Fadiman's (1997) book, *The Spirit Catches You and You Fall Down: A Hmong Child, Her American Doctors, and the Collision of Two Cultures.* In this case the seizures experienced by their child were deemed by the family to be spiritual; this was coupled with a **language barrier** that delayed diagnosis and resulted in **conflicts of interpretation** for the family and healthcare providers. Finally, some attach meaning to how the disability came about as part of their beliefs and attitudes. For example, a childhood accident may be seen as unfortunate, whereas a careless or violent activity of an adult that resulted in a disability may be viewed with differing attitudes.

In the United States it was rare to see individuals in wheelchairs or with a disability in public before the 1960s and 1970s. After the polio epidemic and the return of Vietnam veterans there were numbers of young people with disabilities who were looking for the same rights and opportunities as others. There were active demonstrations to be a part of society. This lack of visibility in the United States existed despite having had a president, Franklin Delano Roosevelt, with impaired mobility due to polio. He was rarely seen standing or in pictures; more commonly he was portrayed sitting with world leaders. Few were aware that in reality his major mode of mobility was a wheelchair. In fact, there was great debate about whether a memorial statue should portray him sitting in a wheelchair. Today, that would be impossible to control or hide. **Activism** and **legislative action** undertaken by the disability and rehabilitation community pushed for the passage of the **Americans with Disabilities Act of 1990**. From that time **mainstreaming** of individuals with disabilities in the education system, accessibility requirements, and equal opportunity hiring requirements brought about raising of consciousness resulting in **societal changes**.

Media has in the last 20 years begun to include individuals with disabilities into movies, television, and advertisements. Today, accessibility efforts, society's way of limiting the handicapping impact of disability, are seen in all aspects of American life. Understanding this relatively recent change in the United States helps one recognize the realities that this took legislation and a conscious effort to influence a cultural change within this country. Even so, this does not mean all people who live in this country have the same attitude or value of individuals with disabilities. Data show that individuals with disability have significantly lower employment rates than any other group (Nathenson, 2009). In addition, recognition of individuals with disabilities as valued members of a cultural group may or may not reflect this societal movement. There are the other restraining factors of values, beliefs, and attitudes that change much more slowly if at all. In summary, knowing what the **cultural role** and view of disability is for the individual and family is important as a foundation for assessment and required to assist the individual to set personal goals.

Along with a culture's expectations related to disability is the culture's attitude about **individualism** and caregiving. An individualist perspective holds high the expectation of **self-care** and independence. Other cultures hold an expectation of taking care of the less able and have **caregiver roles** even designated within the hierarchy of the family. These two different attitudes about roles and expectations impact how the individual and family view the expectations related to a disability. It may counter rehabilitation philosophy and undermine expectations if not addressed.

Disability Culture

The discussion of disability culture is not a simple one. Just as with all ethnic cultures there are differences within cultures, so too are disabilities far from being the same, in some cases not even similar. One would not expect all groups included in Hispanic designation to have the same cultural norms; likewise, individuals with disabilities cannot be put together into one group. Disabilities occur in a variety of forms and can occur at different times during a **life span**. Some individuals are born with a congenital impairment, others have accidents, and still others have chronic disease that results in impairment. So, the **lived experiences** of individuals with disabilities have a wide variety across the life span as well as to the type of disability. There are impairments of vision, speech, hearing, cognition, and mobility, to name a few. Combining all these into one culture implies that all had similar life experiences and developed the same values, beliefs, and attitudes about their lived experiences. Nonetheless, there is extensive literature that speaks to a culture of disability or a **disability culture** (Ingstad & Whyte, 1995; Lipson & Rogers, 2000; McDermott & Varenne, 1994; Nathenson, 2009). The positions taken relate to common experiences of cognitive, mobility, visual, or hearing impairments that result in a shared sense of devaluation or oppression. **Resilience** is also seen as a shared experience as individuals with disabilities confront a world that is not adapted to meeting the needs of all.

Finally, poverty and marginalization are other common characteristics (Lipson & Rogers, 2000). Although we do not deny shared experiences and values may exist, in reality there are also major differences within as well as between individuals with different disabilities. Thus, there are likely **subcultures** within the disability culture. As an example, a group that may be seen to have very similar experiences is the deaf community. Those born without hearing and in a deaf family may have a very specific upbringing and experience, including a **shared primary language** (American Sign Language), that tie them with a common nonethnic cultural experience (Luey, Glass, and Elliot, 1995). However, within the hearing-impaired community, although some individuals born deaf may be born into hearing families, others are not. Still others may lose hearing for various reasons in childhood and have both hearing and nonhearing experiences, and others may lose hearing over time and have varying hearing loss as they age. Luey, Glass, and Elliot (1995) describe these differences and share the realities that the experiences of individuals with hearing loss or deafness are variable and require a full understanding of the individual's experience. Aguayo and Coady (2001) note that three of four individuals who are deaf have an onset after 19 years of age. Thus, each would have different experiences and attitudes about being hearing impaired and may not share similar values and beliefs.

Other disabilities, such as cerebral palsy, have childhood onsets, but the degree of impairment may or may not result in the child interacting or knowing other children with similar impairments. So the child's experiences may relate more to their work with disability/rehabilitation specialists or to the educational experiences for them to begin to formulate what the values and beliefs are related to disability. Finally, when a disability occurs in adulthood, values, beliefs, and attitudes are well formulated and the adult is suddenly confronted by change in what he or she is able to do.

The formation of values, beliefs, attitudes, and actions come with time and exposure to this new nonethnic culture into which a person with a new impairment is immersed. Time is a major factor, as is experience. Depending on type of disability, the time and intensity of rehabilitation may provide a shared experience of what it is like to live with a particular disability. **Peer groups** of spinal cord–injured individuals and support groups for individuals with stroke and their caregivers provide another way to learn about the disability but may or may not result in creating an affinity within group or a shared experience per se. One group that traverses across different types of disabilities is athletics. The **paralym-**

pic, **wheelchair sports teams** and other sports-related experiences can serve to create a subculture of its own. In general, there is a variability in related experience within the disability culture that includes dimensions of extent and type of disability, duration, and commonality of shared experiences.

NURSING CULTURE

Nursing has its own culture formalized through standards, codes, and regulations or through the lived experiences within the educational and professional experience. Indeed, within nursing there are many subcultures that tend to center around area of specialty practice. Thus, the nurse identifies her- or himself as a rehabilitation nurse, an intensive care unit nurse, or a maternal child and the nurse can articulate what that means and how it differs from other specialties. It is more than a place of work. There are subcultural values, beliefs, attitudes, and actions that inform the nurse and impact how one interacts with patients and families and sets expectations for one's peers.

Rehabilitation nurses were identified in the research by Thompson (1990) as taking on roles that included being the patient's coach, fan, and cheerleader. As a coach the nurse taught and reinforced compensatory and strengthening techniques, worked to increase function, and attended to physical needs. As a fan the nurse developed trust and relationships and undertook advocacy for the patient. As the cheerleader the nurse encouraged, praised, and acknowledged progress. At the same time the nurse valued progression, the hard work it took to learn or relearn skills, and looked for ways to work with the team to reach **goals of independence**. A conflicting theme was expecting patients to work on doing for themselves while conforming with the system expectations related to safety. Rehabilitation nurses are clear that patients new to disability have no idea what rehabilitation is about and likely view themselves in the **illness mode**. Helping the individual adjust to rehabilitation and its expectations are foremost in the nurses mind to support the patient's success and continuation in rehabilitation.

Nursing Interventions

Melding the ethnic culture, the nonethnic cultures, the new culture of disability, and rehabilitation nursing is central to culturally relevant care in this specialty. The practice of **cultural imperialism** (Bickenbach, 2009) is seen as applying the provider's culture on the client. This

---

BOX 24.5   Web Exploration

Search the web by entering "disability etiquette." There are numerous items available, including Youtube videos; choose one or two to view. An example can be found at http://www.youtube.com/watch?v=mVqz0LKphws, but you may find others of interest. How would you use this information?

can be particularly true when the values of the services to be provided are strongly viewed as being more informed than that of the patient and family. This may not be done consciously or maliciously but as a means to a known end. Thus, it is key for professionals to know first their own cultural beliefs and those of their **professional subculture** to better understand their own actions and attitudes. That is the first step in understanding one's actions. Then, a true assessment of the individual and family perspectives need to be identified to discover how and where there may be **incongruence**.

Figure 24.2 illustrates potential components of that assessment as it relates to rehabilitation. Only from that point can patient-centered plans be developed. The **Thompson Model of Care Congruence** (Figure 24.3) illustrates how the care process should proceed and, using the Leininger enablers, allows for a mechanism to work through differences. Cultural beliefs that counter the rehabilitations process need to be discussed. When possible, preservation or accommodation is done. When that is not possible, education, negotiation, and identification where restructuring is understood and possible will be the only way to move forward with congruent care. Open discussion about where each is coming from is the way to lay a trusting foundation for care.

When a family's culture is to care for and do for their loved one, and indeed there are expectations of roles within family to do this, the rehabilitation of a stroke patient may be limited without an open discussion. The rehabilitation team may know from experience that the level of impairment would result in the patient being able to feed and dress him- or herself but find the family doing this for them or the patient might identify who would be doing this for them. Without a full team meeting to discuss this and define what can be and what is desired,

the rehabilitation process may be thrown into conflict. Instead, a restructuring of expectations on both sides needs to be identified for true patient goal setting.

SUMMARY

This chapter has shared the basic culture within the United States, cultural competence, related Leininger's Culture Care Theory, and provided insights into related CAM that may be encountered. Two models to illustrate nurse–patient in rehabilitation and a model for culture care congruence were shared. Understanding of various cultures and the overlay of experiential and nonethnic cultures and subcultures of both the individual and the provider is key to truly culturally competent care. However, no one person will know all possible cultures or nonethnic cultures because this is not just a listing to be found in a book. Each person and family has their own experience, history, and understanding of their culture. Thus, professionals need to have an awareness of their own values beliefs, attitudes, and actions from both a cultural and professional standpoint. This is the foundation point on which to build. Knowing the lens ones looks through helps to understand when one is practicing cultural imposition.

CRITICAL THINKING

1. Go to the web and search for culture + disability + (enter your own culture.) If nothing is found, enter another culture. What kind of information did you find? See if there are any evidence-based reports.
2. Cultural competence has been linked to safety in health care. How do you see the interconnection between safety and cultural competence in rehabilitation nursing? Describe a situation that could lead to safety concerns in caring for an individual with disability due to cultural values, beliefs, attitudes, or actions. How might the nurse intervene?
3. Identify if there is a wheelchair team (basketball, rugby, or other) in your area. Go to a game. What surprised you about this event? How might this impact your or a newly spinal cord–injured patient's attitudes about disabilities?
4. Visit Family Village: A Global Community of Disability Resources (www.familyvillage.wisc.edu). Applying the Leininger Culture Care Model view the various components and see if there are links you can identify that would fit from this site.

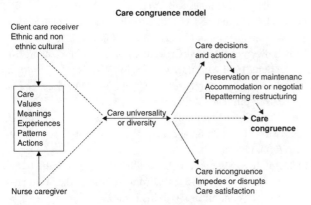

FIGURE 24.3   Thompson Care Congruence Model.

Source: © Teresa Cervantez Thompson (2010)

PERSONAL REFLECTION

- Consider your own culture, society, and family. Have you had direct experience with individuals with disabilities? How did that relationship impact your beliefs, values, and attitude about individuals with disabilities?

- Imagine you are at the mall with your friend or family member who has a disability. The clerk addresses you instead of the individual with disability. Why do you believe they might do that? How would you handle this?

- A young mother has a child with cerebral palsy. She is wondering what she has done wrong in her life to be punished in this way. What might lead a person to come to that concern? What information would you need to gather to begin to assist this mother and family?

ADDITIONAL RESOURCES

Transcultural Nursing Society (TCNS)

www.tcns.org

The mission of TCNS is to enhance the quality of culturally congruent, competent, and equitable care that results in improved health and well-being for people worldwide.

Cultural Competence Project Health Resources and Service Administration

http://www.cultural-competence-project.org/en/index.html or you can get there via Facebook http://af-za.facebook.com/pages/Cultural-Competence-Project/260484419764?v=info

This project is funded by grant number D11HP09759, U.S. Department of Health and Human Services

National Center for Cultural Competence

http://www11.georgetown.edu/research/gucchd/nccc/foundations/frameworks.html

This site has a number of excellent resources and a link for a self-assessment.

REFERENCES

Aguyao, M. O., & Coady, N. F. (2001). The experience of deafened adults: Implications for rehabilitative services. *Health and Social Work, 24*(4), 269–276.

American Association of Colleges of Nursing. (2008). Cultural competency in baccalaureate nursing education. Retrieved August, 24, 2010, from http://www.aacn.nche.edu/Education/pdf/competency.pdf

American Nurses Association. (2010). ANA receives grant to support nurses' cultural competency. Retrieved August, 24, 2010, from http://www.nursingworld.org/ANA-What-Is-New/ANA-Receives-Cultural-Competency-Grant.

American Nurses Credentialing Center. (2010). An action plan for cultural competence. Retrieved August 24, 2010, from http://ce.nurse.com/CE255-60/An-Action-Plan-for-Cultural-Competence.

Andrews, M.M., & Boyle, J. S. (2008). *Transcultural concepts in nursing care.* Philadelphia: Lippincott Williams & Wilkins.

Bickenbach, J. E. (2009). Disability, culture and the UN convention. *Disability and Rehabilitation, 31*(14), 1111–1124.

Centers for Disease Control ad Prevention. (2009). National Center for Health Statistics. Retrieved August 24, 2010, from http://cdc.gov/nchs/faststas/hispanic_health.htm.

Fadiman, A. (1997). *The spirit catches you and you fall down: A Hmong child, her American doctors, and the collision of two cultures.* New York: Farrar, Straus, and Giroux.

Ingstad, B., & Whyte, S. R. (1995). *Disability culture.* Berkley, CA: University of California Press.

Institute of Medicine of the National Academies. (2010). Future directions for the national healthcare quality and disparities reports. Released April 4, 2010. Retrieved July 1, 2010, from http://www.iom.edu/Reports/2010/Future-Directions-for-the-National-Healthcare-Quality-and-Disparities-Reports.aspx.

Joint Commission. (2002–2010). WBT cultural competence in healthcare. Retrieved August 24, 2010, from http://www.jcrinc.com/WBT-Course-Cultural-Competence-in-Healthcare.

Leininger, M., & McFarland, M. (2002). *Transcultural nursing: Concepts, theories, research and practice.* New York: McGraw-Hill.

Leininger, M.M., & McFarland, M.R. (2006). *Culture care diversity and universality: A worldwide nursing theory* (2nd ed). Sudbury, MA: Jones & Bartlett.

Lipson, J. G., & Rogers, J. G. (2000). Cultural aspects of disability. *Journal of Transcultural Nursing, 11*(3), 212–219.

Ludwig-Beymer, P. (2008). Creating culturally competent organizations. In M. M. Andrews & J.S. Boyle, (Eds.), *Transcultural concepts in nursing care* (5th ed., pp. 197–225). Philadelphia, PA: Lippinncott, Williams and Wilkins.

Luey, H. S., Glass, L. & Elliot, H. (1995). Hard-of-hearing or deaf: Issues of ears, language, culture, and identity. *Social Work, 40*(2), 177–182.

McDermott, R.& Varenn, H. (1994–2010). Culture as disability. Retrieved December 13, 2010, from http://serendip.brynmawr.edu/sci_cult/culturedisability.html

Nathenson, P. (2009). Culturally competent care complements interactions with people with disabilities. *Rehabilitation Nursing, 34*(3), 91–95, 109.

National Institutes of Health. (2010a). National Center for Complementary and Alternative Medicine. Retrieved August 24, 2010, from http://www.nccam.nih.gov

National Institutes of Health. (2010b). Progress report on Healthy People 2010: Health disparities. Retrieved August 24, 2010, from http://www.nlm.nih.gov.

Sullivan Commission. (2005). Missing persons: Minorities in the health professions. Retrieved August 24, 2010, from http://www.aacn.nche.edu/media/pdf/sullivanreport.pdf

Thomas, D. M. (2009). Culture and disability: A Cape Verdean Perspective. *Journal of Cultural Diversity, 16*(4), 178–186.

Thompson, T. C. (1990). A qualitative investigation of rehabilitation nursing care in an inpatient unit using Leininger's theory. Doctoral dissertation. Wayne State University. Retrieved December 1, 2010, from http://digitalcommons.wayne.edu/dissertation/AA1918944.

U.S. Census Bureau. (2009). International census projections, 2009. Retrieved July 1, 2010, from http://www.census.gov/population/www/projections/2009comparisonfiles.html

U.S. Department of Health and Human Services. (2006). *Nurse education practice and retention program guidance.* Rockville, MD: Author.

Wiley, A. (2009). At a cultural crossroads: Lessons on culture and policy from the New Zealand disability strategy. *Disability and Rehabilitation, 31*(14), 1205–1214.

World Health Organization. (2010). International classification of functioning, disability and health (ICF). Retrieved August 10, 2010, from http://www.who.int/classifications/icf/en

CHAPTER 25

Ethical and Legal Issues

Ryan Bratcher
James J. Farrell
Kathleen A. Stevens
Kevin W. Vanderground

LEARNING OBJECTIVES

At the end of this chapter, the reader will be able to

- Use the American Nurses Association Code of Ethics and Interpretive Statements as a guide for practice.
- Discuss how nurses apply ethical concepts to decision making in rehabilitation.
- Describe why guardianship is important and when it should be considered in rehabilitation.
- Recognize different types of advance directives and relevance in rehabilitation. Explain key protections within the Americans with Disabilities Act.

KEY CONCEPT AND TERMS

Advance directive	Capacity	Living will
American Nurses Association Code of Ethics	Do not resuscitate (DNR)	Medical power of attorney
	Guardian ad litem	Nonmaleficence
Americans with Disabilities Act (ADA)	Guardian	Patient Self-Determination Act
	Guardianship	Psychiatric advance directive
Autonomy	Individuals with Disabilities Act	Reasonable accommodations
Beneficence	Informed consent	Veracity
Bioethics	Justice	

Ethical issues have been known to cause distress among nurses, resulting in decreased job satisfaction and increased turnover intention (Hart, 2005). This is especially problematic when the ethical concern has some legal consequences. In some cases new laws have been created to provide guidance in response to ethical dilemmas. The two offer different ways of thinking about common problems related to rights of individuals with a disability within our society. For this reason we address both ethical and legal issues in this chapter. The intent is for the reader to appreciate the basis for ethical decision making and utilize resources that can provide guidance in decision making. For more details on ethics and models of ethical decision making for nurses, please see texts on these specific topics.

DEFINING ETHICS

In the course of daily life we make decisions as to the best or morally right action to take. How we make decisions is based on our values and beliefs as well as laws or rules of society. Ethics is the branch of philosophy that deals with the values relating to human conduct and with respect to the rightness or wrongness of certain actions and to the goodness and badness of motives and ends of such actions. These values of human conduct are based on shared beliefs within a society or culture. Ethics most commonly refers to the reasons for decisions about how one should act based on the shared values and beliefs of the group. Ethics refers not to a specific set of principles or rules but rather presents a way of guided thinking.

In our society there are values outlined in the U.S. constitution that provide the foundation for our society. The guiding principles of ethical decision making are autonomy, beneficence, justice, nonmaleficence and veracity (Masters-Farrell, 2007). **Autonomy** is the duty to allow the individual the right to make his or her own decision. Conflicts arise when individuals or persons served make a decision that conflicts with that of the healthcare team, such as refusing treatment or pursuing a discharge plan the team believes is unsafe. The individual's decision may not be what the healthcare team prefers or recommends; however, the principle of autonomy says that professionals must respect the decision made by the person served. Decision making can be problematic when the individual is unable due to illness, functional level, cognition, language, or age to participate in the decision-making process, so a surrogate is used to execute decision making. This has been an important principle in several prominent court decisions and is discussed later in this chapter.

> The value of human life and our responsibility as nurses to do good, promote health, and serve as a patient advocate should be the foundation for our practice.

The second principle is **beneficence**, which is the duty to do good. It frequently is paired with **nonmaleficence**, which is the duty to do no harm. So when presented with a choice of treatment options, the nurse is expected to elect to choose the option will do good and cause no harm. A conflict arises when a treatment with a high likelihood for success comes with exceptional risk. Should a nurse recommend a patient take a medication that poses significant health hazards to affect a cure and yet could be potentially lethal for the person? In this case the conflict for the nurse occurs in deciding between the potential for doing good and doing no harm.

The principle of **veracity** refers to the duty to be truthful and provide the person served with adequate information necessary to make an informed decision. This principle is the foundation for **informed consent** in patient care and research studies. In the case of the medication that is beneficial but carries significant risk, the importance of truth telling is key. The clinician would be expected to disclose the risks and benefits to the person in a manner that is understandable and in a language the person can understand. Upon disclosing full information, if the person freely elects to take the medication, then no moral or ethical issue results. In this case the clinician has provided full disclosure, verified understanding, and allowed the individual to make a choice, supporting the competent person's autonomy. Conflicts arise when before administering a medication the nurse assesses the patient does not have full or adequate knowledge to make a decision or is incompetent to do so.

The last ethical principle is **justice**. Justice is the duty to treat all fairly or act in a manner such that risks and benefits are distributed equally. When healthcare services depend on payer, decisions about type, frequency, and duration of treatment occur. Some clinicians question whether justice is being served. Some have argued that having paid more dollars to an insurance carrier that negotiates a more comprehensive benefits package than the public payer is fair, whereas others see this as preferred treatment. When confronted with an ethical dilemma, rarely does one principle alone provide adequate guidance for decision making. The best decisions occur when all the principles are considered and applied to the thought process.

MODELS FOR ETHICAL DECISION MAKING

Several models for ethical and moral decision making have been developed by nurses. These include the three-step ACT model by Graham-Eason (1996) and the Savage Model for Facilitating Ethical Decision Making (Savage, & Michalak, 1999). These models have several commonalities. First, it is important to gather the facts and engage all stakeholders, including family, healthcare providers, and the healthcare organization early on. Second, identify the ethical principles that are the source of conflict, and, finally, discuss options with key stakeholders. Often, it is helpful to engage the assistance of the organization's ethics committee to serve as a neutral facilitator in these discussions. The cases mentioned here have all led to legal precedents or legislation designed to help guide future decision making, especially in cases when an individual is not able to express their own healthcare wishes.

PROFESSIONAL CODE OF CONDUCT

To provide guidance, many societies or professions have formal written codes of conduct that outline the values of the group and expectations of those that belong to the group. The **American Nurses Association Code of Ethics** (2001) is the code of conduct that guides nursing practice within the United States. In essence, the Code of Ethics (American Nurses Association, 2001) defines the ethical obligations and duties of individuals who have entered into and practice within the profession of nursing. The Code is based on the shared belief that "nursing encompasses the prevention of illness, the alleviation of suffering, and the protection, promotion, and restoration of health in the care of individuals, families, groups and communities" (American Nurses Association, 2001, p. 5). All nurses are expected to be familiar with the Code and act in accordance with the beliefs and values set forth in the Code.

In the rehabilitation setting, nurses work with colleagues from a variety of different disciplines as a member of the rehabilitation team. Each discipline has a unique set of beliefs and values that underscore the philosophy of the discipline. Each profession also has a code of ethics that serves to guide professionals within the discipline. Although many disciplines share some common values and beliefs related to the value of human life, respect for the humanness, and desires of the person seeking services of the professional, there are also differences in relation to delivery of services that can be a source of conflict (Savage, Parson, Zollman, & Kirschner 2009). For example, a nurse may believe it is important for a physical therapist to treat a patient. If the therapist determines there are no active goals that can be achieved with therapy services, then according to the profession's code of ethics it would be unethical for the therapist to treat the patient and charge for services delivered. Team members should be

knowledgeable of their code of ethics as well as those of other disciplines (Table 25.1).

Another potential source of conflict in the rehabilitation setting is consumer expectations and beliefs as set forth in regulatory requirements. In particular, the Commission on Accreditation of Rehabilitation Facilities, a regulatory body for rehabilitation, expects the team to include and respect the decisions of the person served throughout the rehabilitation process. When patients and/or family members refuse healthcare provider recommendations or treatments, this can pose a moral dilemma for staff. A moral dilemma occurs when two or more clear moral principles apply but they support mutually inconsistent sources of action (Redman & Fry, 1998). Case Study 25.1 describes how nurses at one facility addressed a conflict with a parent over unsafe oral feeding of a child.

Ethical conflicts can arise when two or more individuals on the rehabilitation team have different expectations of what is right or morally appropriate action. Savage et al. (2009) suggests guidelines for resolving team disagreements regarding patient care during nonemergent situations (Box 25.1).

Although many of these conflicts can be resolved through respectful communication and guidance provided by the discipline's code of conduct, some require more in-depth discussion to discern appropriate action to be taken. It may be helpful to seek consultation from

TABLE 25.1 Rehabilitation Disciplines' Web Links to Code of Ethics	
Profession	**Web Link**
Physiatrist	http://www.ama-assn.org/ama/pub/physician-resources/medical-ethics/code-medical-ethics/principles-medical-ethics.shtml
Rehabilitation nurse	http://nursingworld.org/ethics/code/protected_nwcoe629.htm
Physical therapy	http://www.apta.org/AM/Template.cfm?Section=Policies_and_Bylaws1&TEMPLATE=/CM/ContentDisplay.cfm&CONTENTID=73012
Occupational therapy	http://www.aota.org/Consumers/Ethics/39880.aspx
Speech-language pathology	http://www.asha.org/docs/html/ET2010-00309.html
Psychology	http://www.apa.org/ethics/code/index.aspx
Respiratory therapy	http://www.aarc.org/resources/position_statements/ethics.html
Pharmacy	http://www.uspharmd.com/pharmacist/pharmacist_oath_and_code_of_ethics
Therapeutic recreation	http://www.atra-online.com/displaycommon.cfm?an=1&subarticlenbr=41
Social work	http://www.naswdc.org/pubs/code/code.asp

CASE STUDY 25.1

The following case study is excerpted from Savage (2005).

An 11-year old girl who is several years post–traumatic brain injured is admitted to the rehabilitation unit after hip surgery. She is nonambulatory, nonverbal, and cortically blind. She has a gastrostomy tube in place; however, at home her mother feeds her pureed foods with a spoon or eye-dropper. It usually takes the mother an hour to feed her daughter about 8 ounces of food. The mother believes her daughter has few pleasures in life and that oral feeding, while risky, provides some degree of pleasure for her daughter. The mother has asked that her daughter be fed by mouth during her hospitalization. Staff members on the unit were uncomfortable with oral feeding and feared potential harm would occur with feeding.

The ethics consultant recommended several actions to the staff. First, approach the mother acknowledging the love and concern she has for her daughter and her willingness to go to great lengths to provide oral feeding in the home. Second, express the shared concern of staff about the safety of oral feedings and concern that they may not be adequately prepared to feed the child safely and in a manner consistent with what the mother has done at home. Third, seek a compromise or common ground. Perhaps offer that for the child's safety staff

provide nourishment via gastrostomy feedings during hospitalization; however, if the mother is present staff would be able to secure a pureed meal so the mother can feed the child. Seek consultation from experts in pediatric feeding who can provide strategies to provide adequate nourishment as the child's needs change as the child matures. Finally, suggest other interventions such as gentle rocking, skin massages, warm showers, or play that offer pleasure to the child but are safer than oral feeding. The ultimate goal according to the consultant is to provide nourishment while maintaining the mother–child bond, respecting the integrity of the nursing staff, and forging an alliance between the mother and the rehabilitation team.

Questions

1. What would the next step be in this process if the mother refuses to heed the advice of the consultant?
2. If this case came before the ethics board of the facility, how would you respond to this dilemma as a rehabilitation nurse? As an ethics board member? As the nurse manager on the unit?
3. What risks are inherent in this situation to the hospital? To the unit? To the patient? To the mother?

BOX 25.1   Suggested Guidelines for Resolving Team Disagreements

1. Clarify the plan of care with other members of the healthcare team.
2. Identify the specific issue that is the source of conflict.
3. State the source of the disagreement and rationale.
4. Propose an alternative action or plan.
5. Determine whether there is agreement, consensus, or acceptance of the new plan that is acceptable for all.
6. Implement the plan of care.

Adapted from Savage et al. (2009).

a hospital ethics committee or ethics consultant in these cases. The latter can serve as objective reviewers and offer alternatives to help the team reach a mutually acceptable decision.

DILEMMAS IN REHABILITATION: WHERE ETHICS AND LEGAL ISSUES COME TOGETHER

Advances in technology and knowledge since the turn of the 20th century allow modern medicine to accomplish feats of supporting birth, sustaining life, and promoting longevity for individuals with chronic illness or disability. Concurrently, the Internet has increased public awareness of healthcare options while creating a forum for dialogue on ideological issues. **Bioethics** is the branch of ethics concerned with issues surrounding health care and the biological sciences. Bioethical issues may occur from before birth, in the case of in vitro fertilization and abortion, to end-of-life decision making and euthanasia. The 20th century began with bioethicists asking how far modern medicine could go in prolonging life, and now the debate has shifted to how far should modern medicine go and how should end-of-life decisions be made.

Some of the most notable cases in bioethics are related to end-of-life decision making and the subsequent legal decisions that have significant relevance for rehabilitation nursing.

DECISION MAKING FOR THE INCOMPETENT AND DYING

Perhaps the most commonly debated ethical and legal dilemma has been when an individual is incapacitated and unable to make healthcare decisions on his or her behalf. How far can a surrogate decision maker go in terms of removing life support devices? In the current era, when modern medicine appears to be at the point of being capable of supporting vital organs almost indefinitely, serious ethical issues have arisen. Should individuals be able to terminate their own existence where no hope of quality or cure exists? Or should the family, acting on behalf of the individual, be permitted to withdraw life-prolonging medical procedures, even when withdrawing life-prolonging procedures will almost certainly cause death? How far can the individual and/or family go in deciding to terminate life? At what point does terminating life become homicide and prohibited by the law? Furthermore, what can be done to prevent some mistakes of the past from being repeated? Three cases, Quinlan, Cruzan, and Schiavo, stand at the crossroads of ethical and legal issues in medical practice. These cases, which started as ethical issues, evolved into legal cases that ultimately set the precedent for the national use of living wills and future advance directive laws. These cases are examined as examples in the following sections.

Quinlan and Advance Directives

The Quinlan case is the landmark case in the patient's right of self-determination. On the night of April 15, 1975, Quinlan ceased breathing for two 15-minute intervals and was transported to the hospital, where it was determined her pupils were unreactive and she failed to respond to deep pain (Karen Ann Quinlan Memorial Foundation, 2010). She was placed on a ventilator at the hospital and received a tracheotomy. In the ensuing days after her respiratory arrest, her parents watched the condition of their daughter further deteriorate. After much discussion and counseling, the family determined that it was in her best interest to remove the ventilator. Whereas the hospital initially consented to authorize removing the ventilator and life support, the hospital would later disagree with the decision and took the case to court (Karen Ann Quinlan Memorial Foundation, 2010).

The case went to the Supreme Court of New Jersey where it was acknowledged that Karen was in a "persistent vegetative state." Her condition was clearly determined to be incurable, and the court was confronted with determining if a person in her position possessed the right of choice regarding the disruption or continuance of life-prolonging medical procedures. The court concluded that the family could, after consultation with the hospital ethics committee, withdraw life-sustaining equipment. The court only required that a responsible physician first determine that there was no possibility of Karen ever coming out of her present condition to a cognitive, functional state (Karen Ann Quinlan Memorial Foundation, 2010).

In the aftermath of this case, several interesting things occurred. Most importantly, living wills evolved from this case as a means of communicating to family members and medical staff the wishes of the competent patients in the event they are unable to make their wishes known.

Cruzan and Schiavo and the Patient Self-Determination Act of 1990

The cases of Nancy Cruzan and Theresa Schiavo are unmistakably linked with the Quinlan case in the public debate over honoring an individual's wishes. Although removing someone from a ventilator in current society appears to a socially acceptable and even a benevolent act, the removal of a feeding tube, as in these cases, raised concern for many individuals, including some healthcare workers. Some even argued that it was cruel and inhuman punishment, because no one would voluntarily choose to "die of starvation."

Nancy Cruzan was born in Missouri and on the night of January 11, 1983 she lost control of her car and crashed into a ditch with the injury resulting in anoxia to the brain (FindLaw, 2010). After determining that her condition was irreversible, the family asked the hospital to cease nutrition and hydration. The hospital refused to grant the family's wishes without a court order requiring them do so. The family then appealed to a trial court who agreed that Nancy's wishes, as declared in a conversation with a housemate, should be upheld. The decision was appealed to the Supreme Court of Missouri, who reversed the decision, stating they found insufficient grounds for removing the feeding tube.

The case made its way to the Supreme Court, who supported the right of Nancy to have a feeding tube removed once sufficient evidence was found stating this was Nancy's wish. In the aftermath of the Supreme Court decision, the family found additional witnesses who testified on Nancy's behalf regarding her desires about life-sustaining medical treatment and ultimately the feeding tube was removed. As a follow-up to this case, the **Patient Self-Determination Act** was enacted in 1990 requiring all medical facilities that accept Medicare or Medicaid funding to provide counseling for patients on advance directives.

Most recently, the case of Theresa Marie Schiavo (Cerminara & Goodman, 2010) may have started as an ethical concern about the right to remove a feeding tube, but it would become a legal quagmire and a highly political battle. In this case disagreement among family members would lead to a protracted court battle. Terri Schiavo suffered a cardiac arrest in February 1990. Although her husband sought medical intervention and rehabilitation therapy with the hope of Terri regaining some level of consciousness, he would eventually lose hope and request to have the feeding tube removed.

The legal battles over Terri began in 1998 when her husband asked the court for permission to have her feeding tube removed. Her parents opposed the motion. In February 2000 Judge Greer ruled for the first time that sufficient evidence existed to demonstrate that Terri would want the feeding tube removed.

Ultimately, due to the parents' public statements and widespread discussion in the public media and on the Internet, politicians stepped into the fray over Terri's right to die. Now for the first time the legal debate extended beyond the courts into the political and legislative arena. In October 2003 the Florida House and Senate passed the bill into law, informally known as "Terri's Law," which prohibited the removal of Schiavo's feeding tube. Judge Baird and the Florida Supreme Court declared this law unconstitutional in September 2004. In December 2004 the Governor of Florida asked the U.S. Supreme Court to overturn the Florida Supreme Court's decision, repealing Terri's Law. The Supreme Court rejected this motion (Cerminara & Goodman, 2010).

In 2005 the federal government got involved when a congressional committee subpoenaed Terri's family. The congressional committee asked for a stay on the removal of the feeding tube. The stay was denied, and Terri's feeding tube was removed for the last time on March 18, 2005 (Cerminara & Goodman, 2010). She passed away 2 weeks later on March 31.

The pivotal person in this case was the Circuit Judge, George W. Greer. He presided over this case and made his decision to allow the feeding tube to be removed on 11 February 2000. In his ruling he cited the case of Guardianship of Estelle M. Browning in which it was determined that every person has the "fundamental right to the sole control of his or her person" (*In Re: The Guardianship of Theresa Marie Schiavo* from the Circuit Court for Pinellas County, Florida Probate Division File No. 90-2988GD-003). Furthermore, he stated the Browning case established this right to reject medical treatment was not "diminished by virtue of physical or mental incapacity or incompetence" (*In Re: The Guardianship of Theresa Marie Schiavo* from the Circuit Court for Pinellas County, Florida Probate Division File No. 90-2988GD-003). To invoke the patient's rights of self-determination, the surrogate or guardian must meet three criteria: (1) the surrogate must be satisfied that evidence in regards to the patient's wishes is uncoerced and reliable, (2) the surrogate must have reasonable assurance that the patient does not have probability of recovering competence, and (3) the surrogate must ensure that any written or oral statements are considered and honored.

The laws regarding end-of-life decisions are not unclear. It is without question that decisions like this one and others related to intensity and use of healthcare interventions are made in hospitals across the nation. When family members disagree, authority for decision making is by state law assigned to the closest next of kin unless the individual has created an advance directive assigning a surrogate to act on his or her behalf. The importance of communication between healthcare providers and family members is often key to resolving ethical dilemmas.

ADVANCE DIRECTIVES

It is important for individuals to make their wishes known before an event occurs. The Quinlan case encouraged individuals and families to have discussions about end-of-life care and encouraged the use of advance directives, such as a living will. After the Cruzan case, the Patient Self-Determination Act of 1990 institutionalized this decision making by mandating that all patients upon entry into a healthcare facility be queried about the existence of an advance directive and if none exists it was the duty of the healthcare facility to offer education and assistance should an individual wish to create an advance directive. There are several types of advance directives, and nurses should be aware of the different types and limitations associated with each type of advance directive.

Advance directives are legal documents that convey an individual's decisions regarding end-of-life care and treatment. These documents are used to direct family members, friends, and healthcare providers' decisions regarding health care and treatment in the event the patient is unable to make or convey these decisions on his or her own due to some incapacity, such as a coma. In theory, by preparing an advance directive the patient can maintain some control over his or her medical treatment while at the same time relieving family, friends, and doctors of making difficult decisions on behalf of the patient when the patient is unable to express his or her intentions. Often, an advance directive will set forth the patient's wishes depending on the extent of his or her ailment or incapacity. For example, an advance directive could describe what treatment, if any, the patient desires in the event he or she is unlikely to recover or is permanently unconscious. The advance directive can also direct healthcare providers to provide treatment regardless of the severity of the patient's ailment or condition.

Living Will

Generally speaking, there are three types of advance directives: a living will, a power of attorney for healthcare decision making, and a do not resuscitate (DNR) order. A **living will**, otherwise known as a healthcare declaration or healthcare directive, is a written document that sets forth the types of medical treatments or life-sustaining measures the patient wants or does not want in the event the person has a terminal illness and is unable to communicate. This document goes into effect once the patient has been deemed terminal by a duly authorized physician and is unable to articulate his or her own desires regarding treatment. When preparing a living will, a patient can choose the treatments he or she would like to receive if unable to articulate these on his or her own due to an incapacity. Typically, a living will sets forth whether or not the patient would like to receive treatments as described in Box 25.2.

A living will can convey the patient's decision regarding organ donation as well.

It should be noted that a living will does not necessarily convey the patient's decision to obtain or refrain from certain treatments. In some cases the patient, by his or her living will, may expressly state that he or she is intentionally making no decision regarding what treatment to receive. In doing so, the patient is purposely leaving such decisions to family members and doctors. Regardless of the patient's decisions set forth in a living will, it is advisable for healthcare providers to discuss the treatments available. In doing so, the patient can make informed decisions regarding prospective treatments and possible outcomes of those treatments.

> **BOX 25.2   Sample of Items Addressed by a Living Will**
>
> - **Resuscitation.** Resuscitation is the attempt to restart the heart when it has stopped beating. Common forms of resuscitation are by cardiopulmonary resuscitation (CPR) or a defibrillator device that administers an electric shock in an effort to stimulate the heart.
> - **Artificial nutrition and hydration.** The patient can express whether or not he or she desires nutritional and hydration assistance via a tube or intravenously. In his or her living will, the patient can express the duration of time he or she would desire life to be sustained by these methods.
> - **Mechanical ventilation.** Mechanical ventilation refers to devices that substitute or assist spontaneous breathing. Again, the patient can express the duration of time he or she would desire life to be sustained by mechanical ventilation.
> - **Dialysis.** Dialysis refers to artificial replacement for diminished or lost kidney function. In receiving this treatment, machinery will assist the body by removing waste from the patient's blood. In a living will, the patient can determine the duration of time he or she is desirous of this treatment.

Medical or Durable Power of Attorney for Healthcare

A second type of advance directive is a **medical power of attorney**, also known as a durable power of attorney with healthcare powers. The medical power of attorney has broader powers than a living will. A medical power of attorney allows the patient to choose an individual to make medical decisions on his or her behalf when the patient is unable to do it him or herself. This allows the patient to give decision-making powers to a trusted individual in the event the patient's living will does not address a particular situation. This appointed individual acts as the patient's healthcare agent (or proxy) and may make a broad range of healthcare decisions on the patient's behalf. This person is entrusted to make decisions on behalf of the patient that are consistent with the patient's living will or discussed wishes related to healthcare decisions.

For obvious reasons an individual should select a healthcare agent they trust and who is not opposed to the individual's healthcare or end-of-life wishes and desires. In fact, choosing a healthcare agent is perhaps one of the most important decisions in advance directive planning. This person should have the individual's best interests at heart, and most importantly should understand the individual's wishes. The individual should discuss the issue with the potential healthcare agent to ensure they are willing to serve in this capacity. When choosing a healthcare proxy or surrogate, the individual should choose a person who is mature and capable of making difficult decisions. The person selected need not be a family member, and at times the patient's best interests may best be served by choosing an agent who is not family. In any event the patient should not choose an agent out of a sense of obligation or feelings of guilt. It is also a good idea, for practical reasons, that the agent live near the patient. This allows the agent to more readily consult with the patient's healthcare providers and to make better-informed decisions regarding care. Selecting an alternate power of attorney is also recommended in the event the primary power of attorney is unable or unwilling to serve if the time to do so arises.

It is important to understand the distinction between a power of attorney and a medical power of attorney. With the former, the authority conveyed typically allows the agent to conduct business or financial transactions on behalf of the person who has granted the authority to act in this way. A medical power of attorney conveys specific authority to an agent for the express purpose of making medical decisions on behalf of the grantor. Given this distinction, it is important that the healthcare provider be aware of the extent to which the agent has authority to make decisions on behalf of a patient. A doctor should not look to a patient's agent for medical treatment decisions if the only authority conveyed to the agent by the patient is to sign checks on his or her behalf.

DNR Order

A third common advance directive is a **DNR** order. This is a request by the patient to not receive cardiopulmonary resuscitation in the event his or her heart stops or he or she stops breathing while at the hospital. A DNR order can typically be placed in the patient's chart by the request of the patient. Hospital policy defines the organization's responsibilities for who can request a DNR order and the organization's responsibility for honoring the DNR order.

Typically, the DNR applies only when the individual is undergoing care and treatment at the hospital, but nursing home residents may have a standing DNR on the medical record after going through the proper channels to have this implemented. Within the past few years a select number of states have created a universal or uniform DNR order request that is initiated by the individual

and is carried by them from one healthcare setting to the next (Illinois Department of Public Health, 2005). This order spells out what the individual wants in terms of resuscitation while they are being transported from one facility to another or in the case of some patients in rehabilitation when they are being seen as an outpatient at another hospital or physician office. The nurse should be aware of their hospital policy and state rules and regulations on DNR orders. In addition, residents in long-term care facilities are now urged to place their living wills and DNR orders on their refrigerators so that in the event of an emergency, rescue personnel have ready access to these legal documents that can aid in upholding the person's wishes.

PSYCHIATRIC ADVANCE DIRECTIVE

A relatively new way to deal with mental health decisions in advance is through a **psychiatric advance directive**, sometimes called a declaration for mental health treatment. As the name implies, this legal document can be used to declare in advance one's desires regarding the psychiatric or mental health treatment they wish to receive. A psychiatric advance directive may be used to document a competent person's specific instructions or preferences regarding future mental health treatment. This is done in preparation for the possibility that the person may lose capacity to give or withhold informed consent to treatment during acute episodes of psychiatric illness.

Advance directives can be prepared in a variety of ways. Many times, healthcare professionals have a form a patient can fill out to make known his or her desires. A patient can also write his or her own desires. Another potential resource is also a local health department or other local or state agency that can provide a form. Finally, and perhaps the best resource for preparation of an advance directive, is an experienced, licensed attorney. Although this may be slightly more expensive for the patient, the cost for this type of legal work is relatively small, and counseling offered by the attorney can go a long way in avoiding future complications. The legal requirements for advance directives vary from state to state, and the individual creating the documents should keep this in mind.

Regardless of the source for the advance directive, the preparer should keep in mind that the document need not be long and complicated. A short, simple statement of the patient's desires regarding treatment should suffice. Once an advance directive is prepared, it is advisable to have the patient review the document with his or her doctor. This will assist the healthcare provider to understand exactly what the patient's intentions are regarding treatment. Any advance directive should be notarized and a copy given to the patient's doctor and any agent appointed in the medical power of attorney document.

The patient should also be aware that an advance directive can be changed at any time as long as the patient is of sound mind. To be of sound mind means that the patient can think rationally and can communicate his or her wishes clearly (i.e., is deemed competent). It is also recommended that the patient periodically review his or her advance directives to ensure the documents still accurately reflect his or her intentions. Any changes should be made known to the patient's doctor and any individuals appointed as a healthcare agent. In the absence of an advanced directive, family members and physicians are left with the unfortunate task of making difficult decisions without the benefit of knowing the patient's wishes and desires. State law dictates the legal order of decision making within the state. The typical order is spouse, parent, child, and sibling. Only a few states have a provision allowing domestic partners to serve as decision makers. At times the order of decision making can be a source of conflict, as in the case of a woman with a traumatic brain injury sustained as a result of domestic abuse. If criminal charges are not filed against the spouse, the spouse will in most states be primary decision maker (see Case Study 25.2). Dealing with such situations is stressful enough, but often the absence of an advance directive can lead to conflict among family members, friends, and healthcare providers. Nurses as patient advocates should encourage individuals to consider preparing an advance directive long before it is actually needed.

GUARDIANSHIP

Safe decision making is part of every day life, yet some patients in rehabilitation are unable to make decisions without jeopardizing their welfare. One of the most common ethical and legal dilemmas in rehabilitation is how to care for those who may not be able to make decisions in a cogent manner. As a result the law has developed a tool called "**guardianship.**" The number of guardianships is increasing, and as the so-called baby boomer generation ages, the number of guardianships in the United States is projected to continue to grow.

Rehabilitation nurses should have an understanding of the general principles surrounding guardianship and the specific rules applicable in the jurisdiction you

---

CASE STUDY 25.2

You are working with a female patient who has sustained a C-5 complete ASIA A spinal cord injury. The patient is dependent for all activities of daily living and has a tracheostomy in place. The patient tells you she wants to die rather than live with this disability. She has been eating poorly and refusing turns and therapy. At team conference several team members are recommending discharge to a skilled nursing facility because the patient has no rehabilitation goals. You and other team members are concerned about her well-being and not comfortable with the discharge plan.

Questions

1. How can this dilemma be resolved?
2. What factors should be considered?
3. What role might the ethics board play in a situation such as this?
4. What legal and ethical factors/principles should be considered?

---

are working in. Generally, once an individual has been determined to be incapacitated, the court can appoint a guardian to make some or all decisions for that individual.

Identifying a Guardian

A "**guardian**" is a person who has the legal authority and duty to care for another's person or property (Garner, 1999). A guardian or conservator may be appointed for all purposes, for a specific purpose, or a specific period of time. The term includes a temporary guardian, a limited guardian, and a successor guardian but excludes one who is only a guardian ad litem (a **guardian ad litem** usually only appears in court for the incapacitated individual). The guiding principle in all guardianship is that of least intrusive measures to ensure as much autonomy as possible. The guardian's authority is defined by the court, and the guardian may not operate outside that authority. However, guardianship duties are often not clearly defined. A good guardian takes into account the wishes and desires of the incapacitated person, often called a "ward," when making decisions about residence, medical treatments, and end-of-life issues. The courts will remove only those rights that the proposed ward is incapable of handling.

When the courts appoint a guardian, certain rights of the ward are removed. Table 25.2 lists the rights of the

TABLE 25.2 Rights of the Ward Removed During Guardianship	
Consent to medical treatment	Make end-of-life decisions, such as the withdrawal of life support or withholding of medical care
Determine place of residence	Possess a driver's license
Manage, buy, or sell property	Own or possess a firearm or weapon
Enter into a contract	Marry
Vote	

ward that are removed during guardianship. These rights are rights typically guaranteed by federal or state law to citizens so any removal of these rights can significantly limit an individual's role within society and thus the process of guardianship is highly regulated.

Capacity Determination

The first step in the guardianship process is to determine "incapacitation." An incapacitated person is a person who is impaired, for any of a variety of reasons, to the extent that personal decision making is impossible (Garner, 1999). Each state has an official legal definition of an incapacitated person. The legal definition is not the same as a medical definition of incapacitation. The legal definition often is based on a determination of an individual's inability to manage his or her own property and/or provide self-care (Indiana Code § 29-3-1-7.5). Several states have very detailed explanations of what a determination of incapacity involves. For example, Virginia defines an incapacitated person as follows (Virginia Code § 37.2-1000):

> An adult who has been found by a court to be incapable of receiving and evaluating information effectively or responding to people, events, or environments to such an extent that the individual lacks the capacity to (i) meet the essential requirements for his health, care, safety, or therapeutic needs without the assistance or protection of a guardian or (ii) manage property or financial affairs or provide for his support or for the support of his legal dependents without the assistance or protection of a conservator.

It is important for rehabilitation nurses to know the official definition for their state to articulate the standard by which the capacity of patients will be judged.

Poor judgment does not constitute incapacity. For relatives of elderly individuals, there is a temptation to have the relative declared to be an incapacitated person when family members perceive the individual is exercising poor judgment. When an elderly person has assets that are desired by his or her heirs, many times the family members attempt to have the individual declared to be an incapacitated person so they can establish a guardianship and control the assets of the individual. As a result, family members will try to attribute what they perceive to be a bad decision to incapacity.

Another common cause for guardianship requests is dementia. Many times the one suffering from dementia is unaware of the seeming absurdity of his or her decisions and will thus fight the guardianship proceedings. In this situation it is often difficult for the court and medical personnel to tell the difference between family and friends of the patient who are acting with the well-being of the patient in mind and those acting in their own self-interest. Some research has indicated that persons with dementia may fluctuate in their decision-making abilities (Menne & Whitlatch, 2007), further complicating the issue. How then should courts and practitioners examine whether an individual is incapacitated? Many courts use some or all of the following criteria in assessing the capacity of an individual:

- What is the current cognitive ability of the patient?
- What is the medical condition that caused the current condition?
- Is it temporary or reversible?
- Can the person perform the activities of everyday living (e.g., grooming, toileting, eating, dressing)?
- What is the risk of harm associated with the least restrictive means available?

Some courts attempt to understand the values or preferences of the incapacitated person. Of course, if the incapacity is mental or psychological, such as dementia, understanding the person's preferences can become rather complicated.

Establishing guardianship is a legal process that involves the removal of an individual's rights. There are several due process hurdles one seeking a guardianship of another must overcome:

- The individual must be notified of all court proceedings.
- The individual is entitled to representation by an attorney.
- The individual can and may be compelled to attend hearings regarding his or her capacity/guardianship unless excused due to physical impossibility.

- The individual is entitled to compel, confront, and cross-examine all witnesses and present his or her own evidence.
- The individual may appeal the determination of the lower court.
- The individual has the right to a jury trial.

The due process required for the removal of an individual's rights may vary from state to state, and as such the state's statutes and case law will be the final authority.

Anyone can act as a guardian. The court will decide who should be the guardian of an incapacitated individual. There may be different types of guardians specified, depending on the patient's condition and needs. For example, a patient with complex needs and a large estate may have a guardian of person (who handles daily affairs including health and home maintenance), a guardian of his or her estate (who handles all financial aspects), and a guardian ad litem (for legal counsel).

As a general rule, courts prefer close relatives to be the guardian (of person) because they are often best prepared to understand the individual's needs and desires. Many community organizations, and some state and national organizations, can connect individuals with volunteer advocates who will act on behalf of the incapacitated individual. When the court appoints a guardian of the person, the responsibilities of the guardian are as follows:

- Determine and monitor the residence of the incapacitated individual
- Consent to and monitor medical treatment
- Consent to and monitor services such as education and counseling
- Consent to and release of confidential information (i.e., healthcare records)
- Make end-of-life decisions
- Act as representative payee
- Report to the court about the guardianship status at least annually

Often, a guardian will have to right to make financial decisions on behalf of the incapacitated person. Practitioners need to be careful as well when deciding for themselves as to the capacity of an individual. Often, physicians and other medical personnel can be called to testify in court as to what they observed and the functionality of an individual. Because so much is at stake for the supposedly incapacitated person and there is so much risk of wrongdoing and potential loss, some laws create a duty to maximize the independence of the individual.

At the very least one could argue for an ethical obligation to entrust as much of his or her own affairs as possible to the individual.

One tool that has been increasing in popularity is the limited guardianship. A limited guardian has only those powers specifically stated in the court order making him or her a guardian. In other words, the court can decide the guardian can only do certain things on behalf of the incapacitated person. For example, an incapacitated individual may be perfectly capable of determining living arrangements or his or her degree of participation in family or religious events, but a court may decide he or she are not currently capable of understanding a new lease agreement on an apartment or making a major purchase. The decision to pursue guardianship is not to be taken lightly. Yet when used properly guardianship can be a valuable resource, allowing the individual to live with a high quality of life.

INDIVIDUALS WITH DISABILITY AND RIGHT TO LIFE ISSUES

A second area where ethical and legal issues merge is related to rights of individuals with disability within society. For many years individuals with disability where denied either by law or societal handicap basic rights as citizens, such as right to a public education or the right to vote. As recently as 1979 it was legal for some state governments to sterilize disabled individuals against their will or prohibit people with certain disabilities from marrying (Regents of the University of California, 2004). In the early 1970s the disability rights movement started at the University of California at Berkley. The disability rights movement asserts that people with disabilities are human beings with rights equal to any American citizen. The movement sought to secure these rights through political action. As a result of their efforts a number of legislative victories have occurred within our society. Table 25.3 outlines 20 years of legislation to secure rights for individuals with disabilities.

One of the first successes was the passage of the Rehabilitation Act of 1973. This federal law for the first time protects individuals with disabilities from discrimination based on their disability. The Act defined qualified individuals with disabilities as persons with a physical or mental impairment that substantially limits one or more major life activities as well as persons who have a history of or are regarded as having a physical or mental disability. According to the Act, major life activities

TABLE 25.3 Federal Disability Rights Laws and Court Decisions		
Law	**Date**	**Summary**
Architectural Barriers Act (ABA)	1968	Requires that buildings and facilities that are designed, constructed, or altered with Federal funds, or leased by a Federal agency, comply with Federal standards for physical accessibility. Facilities of the U.S. Postal Service are not covered by this Act.
Rehabilitation Act	1973	Prohibits discrimination on the basis of disability in programs conducted by Federal agencies, in programs receiving Federal financial assistance, in Federal employment and in the employment of Federal contractors.
Individuals with Disabilities Education Act (IDEA)	1975	This Act requires public schools to make a free appropriate public education in the least restrictive environment available to all eligible children. It also requires public school systems to develop appropriate individualized education programs (IEPs) for each child. The IEP must be developed by a team of knowledgeable persons and must be reviewed at least annually.
Voting Accessibility for the Elderly and Handicapped Act	1984	This Act requires polling places across the U.S. to be physically accessible to people with disabilities for federal elections. If no accessible location is available, an alternate means of casting a ballot must be offered. States must make registration and voting aids available for disabled and elderly voters.
Fair Housing Act	1988	Prohibits housing discrimination on the basis of race, color, religion, gender, disability, familial status, and national origin. Amendments are applicable to government housing as well as private housing that receives federal assistance. It also requires landlords to allow tenants with disabilities to make reasonable access-related modifications to their private living space, as well as common areas. Any new multifamily unit with four or more units be designed and built to allow access for persons with disabilities.
Americans With Disabilities Act (ADA)	1990	The ADA prohibits discrimination on the basis of disability in employment, state and local government, public accommodations, commercial facilities, transportation and telecommunications. It also applies to the U.S. Congress.
Air Carrier Access Act	1990	Prohibits discrimination in air transportation by domestic and international carriers against qualified individuals with physical or mental impairments. It applies only to air carriers that provide regularly scheduled services for hire to the public.
National Voter Registration Act "Motor Voter Act"	1993	This Act requires all offices of state-funded programs that are primarily engaged in providing services to persons with disabilities to provide all program applicants with voter registration forms, to assist them in completing the forms, and transmitting the completed forms to the appropriate state official.
Telecommunications Act	1996	Requires manufacturers of telecommunications equipment and providers of telecommunications services to ensure that such equipment and services are accessible and usable by persons with disabilities, if readily achievable. The amendments ensure that people with disabilities have access to a broad range of products and services such as telephones, cell phones, pagers, call waiting, and operator services that previously were inaccessible to persons with disabilities.
Civil Rights of Institutionalized Persons Act	1997	This Act authorizes the U.S. Attorney General to investigate conditions of confinement at state and local institutions such as prisons, jails, pretrial detention centers, juvenile correctional centers, publicly operated nursing homes, and institutions for persons with psychiatric or developmental disabilities. The purpose is to all the Attorney General to uncover and correct any widespread deficiencies that would jeopardize the health and safety of the residents.
Olmstead Decision	1999	U.S. Supreme Court affirmed that unjustified institutionalization of people with disabilities is discrimination and violation of the ADA. States are required to provide community-based services for persons with disabilities otherwise entitled to institutional services when the state's treatment professionals reasonably determined that community placement is appropriate; the person does not oppose such placement; and the placement can reasonably be accommodated, taking into account resources available to the state and the needs of others receiving state-supported disability resources.

Source: Adapted from U.S. Department of Justice (2005).

include caring for one's self, walking, seeing, hearing, speaking, breathing, working, performing manual tasks, and learning (U.S. Department of Justice, 2005). Under the Act employers may not deny qualified individuals the opportunity to participate in or benefit from federally funded programs, services, or other benefits. Qualified individuals with a disability could not be denied access to programs, services, benefits, or opportunities to participate as a result of physical barriers and, finally, could not be denied employment on grounds of their disability. The law applied to employers or organizations receiving federal funding, so there were still a number of private entities exempt from the Act. The Act for the first time provided a legal definition of individuals with disability and clearly prohibited discrimination on these grounds.

A second major piece of legislation provided individuals with a disability access to public schooling. The **Individuals with Disabilities Act**, commonly referred to as IDEA, provides eligible children with disabilities a free appropriate public education in the least restrictive environment. Previously, many children with disabilities were segregated in schools dedicated to children with disabilities. Children with disabilities were now accorded public education opportunities equivalent to able bodied children.

Over the next 10 years federal legislation eliminated barriers in voting and housing with federal funding. Although the federal government was moving to eliminate barriers, a number of barriers continued to exist in the private sector. In 1990 President George H. Bush signed the **Americans with Disabilities Act (ADA)**, a landmark piece of legislation often considered the civil rights bill for individuals with disabilities. The ADA is a federal civil rights law that prohibits discrimination in employment, public services, and public accommodations against a person with a disability. According to the Act, a disability, consistent with the Rehabilitation Act of 1973, is a physical or mental impairment that substantially alters one or more major life activities.

Unlike the Rehabilitation Act of 1973, the ADA applies to both governmental and private entities (U.S. Department of Justice, 2005). However, the discrimination is not barred everywhere, only in employment, public services, ad public accommodations. In employment, employers are required to make **reasonable accommodations** for a disabled employee. The word "reasonable" has sparked a lot of litigation. Also, the government is not allowed to discriminate against the disabled in the provision of public services. Of particular importance for

healthcare professionals is the prohibition of discrimination against those with disabilities within the realm of public accommodations.

Private hospitals or medical offices are covered by Title III of the ADA as places of public accommodation. Public hospitals and clinics and medical offices operated by state and local governments are covered as programs of public entities. Section 504 covers any of these that receive federal financial assistance, which can include Medicare and Medicaid reimbursements. In other words, if you provide medical care, it is highly likely that you are required to abide by the ADA. The ADA requires that medical care providers provide individuals with disabilities

- Full and equal access to their health care services and facilities; and
- Reasonable modifications to policies, practices, and procedures when necessary to make healthcare services fully available to individuals with disabilities, unless the modifications would fundamentally alter the nature of the services (i.e., alter the essential nature of the services).

Equal treatment for individuals with disabilities can mean an adjustment to the normal practices of healthcare providers. For instance, generally it is not acceptable to examine an individual in his or her wheelchair because the exam would not be as thorough as an exam on an exam table. Thus, accommodations may be necessary to get the patient from the wheelchair to the exam table. Accessible room design, training in proper techniques, and certain equipment (such as adjustable exam tables and medical testing equipment) are likely necessary to ensure equal treatment. For nurses in particular, training regarding the proper techniques for lifting and moving patients is becoming increasingly valuable. Because most medical service personnel are not in control of the equipment or facilities available to them, the most they can do is be sure they are using proper techniques. Because employers have a legal obligation to provide equal treatment, this training often readily available.

OLMSTEAD DECISION: INSTITUTIONALIZATION OR COMMUNITY-BASED SERVICES

In the late 1990s two women in Georgia whose disabilities included mental retardation and mental illness filed suit stating that their institutionalization was discriminatory and in violation of the ADA (U.S. Department of Health and Human Services, 2000). At the time the women were covered by the state Medicaid program that restricted payments for ongoing health services to payment for services provided during an inpatient stay at healthcare institution. According to the suit, local health professionals involved in the care of the women had determined that appropriate mental health services could be provided in a community setting, yet at the time Medicare and Medicaid funding was not available to provide the support needed for community care. As a result of the court decision the Department of Health and Human Services committed to working with state Medicaid directors to craft fiscally responsible solutions that support compliance with the ADA, including making funding available for individuals with disability to live in the community with the right support (U.S. Department of Health and Human Services, 2000).

INDIVIDUALS WITH DISABILITIES: A GROWING VOICE

Individuals with disabilities were vocal not only about legal issues but also ethical matters related to the value and quality of life associated with disability. One specific concern was the case of Ashley X (Kirschner, Brashler, & Savage, 2007), a young disabled girl diagnosed with static encephalopathy. As a result of the disability she was dependent in all activities of daily living, nonverbal, and received all nutrition through a feeding tube. As Ashley approached puberty her parents were concerned that her physical growth would make it difficult for them to care for Ashley at home. After discussion with her physician, a plan was devised to provide high-dose estrogen to attenuate her growth. Concurrently, Ashley underwent a hysterectomy and breast bud removal. The combination of medication regimen and the surgery was referred to as the "Ashley treatment" (Kirschner et al., 2007). This treatment raised significant concern among individuals with disabilities who viewed the parents' decision as evidence of an ongoing stigma against individuals with disabilities in society. Did the parents' decision to have the hysterectomy performed in the absence of disease violate the rights of Ashley as a person? Do cases such as this further the image of life with disability as less than adequate?

Similar concerns have been voiced related to decisions on euthanasia and genetic testing. In the case of genetic testing, if testing reveals gene for one of several diseases that result in severe disability, is it ethical to then proceed with a therapeutic abortion? Is manipulation of genes in utero a violation of the embryo? Does genetic

---

testing reinforce the belief that life is only valued for able bodied children and that children with disability should not be allowed to live?

The therapeutic use of stem cells is a potential ethical concern for many. Scientists postulate that stem cell therapy may be of benefit to patients with a number of chronic illnesses, such as diabetes and Alzheimer's disease, as well as individuals with disabilities such as spinal cord injury (Chapman, Frankel, & Garfinkel, 1999; National Institutes of Health, n.d.). Currently, there is a limited supply of available stem cells, and it is anticipated that new sources of live stem cells will be needed in the future. Under the Bush administration federal funding for human embryonic stem cell research was limited by presidential order. In March 2009 President Obama revoked this order and removed the limitation on scientific exploration of the use of stem cell therapy to reduce disease and disability (National Institutes of Health, www.stemcells.nih.gov/policy/defaultpage.asp). For some individuals the use of stem cells presents a moral and ethical challenge to their values.

SUMMARY

Perhaps it was inevitable that with the advances in modern medicine since the turn of the 20th century that ethical issues would arise. Where the life expectancy once was in the 40s, modern medicine has increased it to 78 years old. With increased life expectancy came the increase of chronic disease and associative suffering. Also, modern medicine found a way to sustain people on life support nearly indefinitely. Consequently, we began the 20th century asking how far modern medicine *could* go. We ended the 20th century asking how far modern medicine *should* go.

The collision between personal rights and modern medicine continues today. The battle between rights and medicine will likely continue throughout the 21st century. Rehabilitation nurses will encounter some of the difficult decisions in their practice or work settings. Yet, certain foundational beliefs such as the belief in our society that all life has value and meaning will hopefully underscore ethical decision making in the future. Second, the rights of the individual cannot be infringed upon except when such exercise of those rights endanger others. Third, medical treatment and procedures must be received voluntarily and the medical community must honor all stated wishes except where those wishes violate personal ethical responsibility to do no harm. The value of human life and our responsibility as nurses to do good, promote health, and serve as a patient advocate should be the foundation for our practice.

CRITICAL THINKING

1. Describe how you respect a patient's autonomy in your daily practice as a nurse.
2. Your patient today is a young woman who sustained a traumatic brain injury as a result of an assault. She has significant cognitive impairments and is dependent for most activities of daily living. She has a gastrostomy tube in place for nutrition. Her husband is the suspected assailant; however, criminal charges were never filed against him. The discharge plan is for the woman to return home with the husband as the primary caregiver. What should you consider when preparing this patient for discharge?
3. You are working in the outpatient clinic. Today your patient's family members report her memory is becoming more impaired and they are fearful of her living alone. The physician has recommended the family pursue obtaining guardianship. The family asks you about pros and cons of guardianship. What advice do you have for the family?
4. What are the critical factors to be considered when allowing a surrogate to make healthcare decisions on a patient's behalf?
5. You are a nurse manager. A qualified applicant just accepted a position on your unit. The human resources representative notifies the nurse has a lower extremity amputation and uses a prosthesis. What should you consider when planning the nurse's orientation?
6. Your patient has a medication ordered that is derived from human embryonic stem cells. You believe the use of stem cells is morally wrong. What options are available to you and how will do decide what option to pursue?

PERSONAL REFLECTION

- Do you have an advance directive? If so, why? If not, why not?
- Think about three or four individuals with whom you have had conversations about your end-of-life wishes. How would they represent your decisions when questioned by the court?
- Do you know someone with a disability? When you initially learned about the disability how did you react? How does this person describe his or her life since the onset of the disability? Has this changed your initial perception about the person's life with a disability?
- Can you describe a scenario in a clinical setting when you had a hard time deciding on the right action to take? Think about how you made the decision. What factors did you take into account when deciding?

RECOMMENDED BOOKS ON ETHICS AND NURSING

American Nurses Association. (2001). *Code of ethics for nurses with interpretive statements.* Washington, DC: Author.

Bandman, E., & Bandman, B. (2002). *Nursing ethics through the life span* (4th ed.). New York: Prentice Hall.

Bartter, K. (2001). *Ethical issues in advanced nursing practice.* Philadelphia: Elsevier.

Beauchamp, T. L., & Childress, J. F. (2001). *Principles of biomedical ethics* (5th ed.). New York: Oxford University Press.

Bosek, M. S. D., & Savage, T. A. (2007). *The ethical component of nursing education: Integrating ethics into clinical experience.* Philadelphia: Lippincott Williams & Wilkins.

Danis, M., Clancy, C., & Churchill, L. R. (2005). *Ethical dimensions of health policy.* New York: Oxford University Press.

Jecker, N. S., Jonsen, A. R., & Pearlman, R. A. (2007). *Bioethics: An introduction to the history, methods, and practice* (2nd ed.). Sudbury, MA: Jones & Bartlett.

Macrina, F. (2005). *Scientific integrity: An introductory text with cases* (3rd ed.). Washington, DC: American Society for Microbiology Press.

Morrision, E. E. (2006). *Ethics in health administration: A practical approach for decision makers.* Sudbury, MA: Jones & Bartlett.

REFERENCES

American Nurses Association. (2001). *Code of ethics for nurses with interpretive statements.* Washington, DC: Author.

Cerminara, K. A., & Goodman, K. (2010). Schiavo case resources: Key events in the case of Theresa Maria Schiavo. Retrieved May 20, 2010, from http://www6.miami.edu/ethics/schiavo/schiavo_timeline.html

Chapman, A. R., Frankel, M.S., & Garfinkel, M.S. (1999). *Stem cell research and applications, monitoring the frontiers of biomedical research*. American Association for the Advancement of Science and the Institute for Civil Society. Retrieved September 1, 2010, from http://stemcells.nih.gov/info/ethics

FindLaw. (2010). *Cruzan v. Director*, Missouri Department of Health. Retrieved August 1, 2010, from http://caselaw.lp.findlaw.com/scripts/getcase.pl?court=us&vol=497&invol=261

Garner, B. A. (1999). *Black's law dictionary* (7th ed.). St. Paul, MN: West Group.

Graham-Eason, C. (1996). Ethical considerations for rehabilitation nursing. In S. Hoeman (Ed.), *Rehabilitation nursing: Process and application* (2nd ed., pp. 34–46). St. Louis, MO: Mosby.

Hart, S. E. (2005). Hospital ethical climates and registered nurses' turnover intentions. *Journal of Nursing Scholarship, 37*, 173–177.

Illinois Department of Public Health. (2005). Illinois Department of Public Health announces new uniform do-not-resuscitate order form. Press release June 1, 2005. Retrieved April 15, 2010, from http://www.idph.state.il.us/public/press05/6.1.05.htm

In Re: The Guardianship of Theresa Marie Schiavo from the Circuit Court for Pinellas County, Florida Probate Division File No. 90-2988GD-003.

Karen Ann Quinlan Memorial Foundation. (2010). Karen Ann Quinlan: She changed the way people looked at life and death. Retrieved July 1, 2010, from http://www.karenannquinlanhospice.org/history.htm

Kirschner, K., Brashler, R., & Savage, T. A. (2007). Ashley X. *American Journal of Physical Medicine and Rehabilitation, 86*, 1023–1029.

Masters-Farrell, P. A. (2007). Ethical, moral and legal considerations. In K. Mauk (Ed.), *The specialty practice of rehabilitation nursing: A core curriculum* (5th ed., pp. 27–34). Glenview, IL: Association of Rehabilitation Nurses.

Menne, H. L., & Whitlatch, C. J. (2007). Decision-making involvement of individuals with dementia. *The Gerontologist, 47*(6), 810–819.

National Institutes of Health. (n.d.) Stem cell information—federal policy. Retrieved September 10, 2010, from http://stemcells.nih.gov/policy/defaultpage.asp

Redman, B. K., & Fry, S. T. (1998). Ethical conflicts reported by certified rehabilitation registered nurses. *Rehabilitation Nursing, 23*(4), 179–184.

Regents of the University of California. (2004). The disability rights and independent living movement: Introduction. Retrieved from http://bancroft.berkeley.edu/collections/drilm/introduction.html

Savage, T. A. (2005). Clinical consultations: How do we handle conflicts with parents over unsafe oral feedings? *Rehabilitation Nursing Journal, 30*(1), 7–8.

Savage, T. A., & Michalak, D. R. (1999). Ethical, legal and moral issues in pediatric nursing. In P. A. Savage, T. A., Parson, J., Zollman, F., & Kirschner, K. L. (2009). Rehabilitation team disagreement: Guidelines for resolution. *Physical Medicine and Rehabilitation, 1*, 1091–1097.

U.S. Department of Health and Human Services. (2000). The Olmstead decision fact sheet. Retrieved December 1, 2010, from http://www.acf.hhs.gov/programs/add/otherpublications/olmstead.html

U.S. Department of Justice. (2005). A guide to disability rights laws. Retrieved December 10, 2010, from http://www/ada.gov/cguide.htm

CHAPTER 26

Health Policy and Healthcare Financing

Anne F. Deutsch
James J. Farrell

LEARNING OBJECTIVES

At the end of this chapter, the reader will be able to

- Describe the most common types of healthcare insurance.
- Distinguish between Medicare and Medicaid coverage.
- Discuss three trends that have impacted financing of rehabilitation services and what this has meant for healthcare consumers.
- Differentiate between structure, process, and outcome quality measures.
- Identify categories of quality measures used in rehabilitation.
- Recognize how nurses can participate in the healthcare policymaking process.

KEY CONCEPTS AND TERMS

75% rule	Managed care	Quality measures
Consolidated Omnibus Budget Reconciliation Act (COBRA)	Medicaid	Resource utilization groups
	Medicare	Safe care
Diagnosis-related group (DRG)	Medigap	State children's health insurance program (SCHIP)
Effective care	Outcome measure	
Efficient care	Point of service	Structure measures
Fee for service (FFS)	Preferred provider organization	Tax Equity and Fiscal Responsibility Act (TEFRA)
Health maintenance organizations (HMOs)	Process measures	
	Prospective payment system (PPS)	
Inpatient rehabilitation facility		

Changes in health policies can significantly alter access to and delivery of healthcare services. Health professionals are increasingly expected to have an understanding of key health policy issues and the policy development process, and this knowledge is essential for those professionals who seek to influence the policymaking process (Leavitt, Chaffee, & Vance, 2002). This chapter provides an introduction to healthcare policy with a special emphasis on healthcare financing. We begin the chapter with an overview of how the American healthcare system has been shaped by public and private health policies, with some major shifts in the focus over time.

HEALTH POLICY

Health policy can be defined as the authoritative decisions made within government that pertain to health and the pursuit of health (Longest, 2006). Authoritative decisions refers to decisions that are made within any of the three branches of government—the executive, legislative, and judicial branches—and at any level of government—federal, state, or local (Longest, 2006). Health policy's role in health spans many aspects of our lives, because health is determined by many factors: our genetic makeup, our physical environment, our work and home situations, our social environment, our behavioral and access to healthcare services, and the delivery of healthcare services.

The focus of this chapter is health policy related to the access to and delivery of healthcare services; we do not address policies not focused primarily on health delivery, such as environmental or employment policies. It is also important to note that the American healthcare delivery system is affected by a complex mix of both public and private-sector policies. The private-sector policies are the result of authoritative decisions made by executives of the organization (e.g., insurance company, pharmaceutical manufacturer).

GROWTH AND DEVELOPMENT

Between 1965 and 1980 the healthcare industry can best be described in terms of growth and development of the healthcare delivery system. During this time the delivery system included small independent physician group practices; larger multispecialty clinics were developing but were uncommon. Hospitals provided secondary and tertiary care. The supply of and demand for healthcare services expanded in response to the introduction of **Medicare** and **Medicaid** programs in 1965; an increased need for the capacity, capabilities, and number and types of healthcare providers; an increased number of people accessing the delivery system; an increased amount of care provided; and new and improved treatments and technology (Nosse, Friberg, & Kovacek, 1999).

COST CONTAINMENT

Between 1981 and 1991 the focus for health care was on cost containment. It was a concern for physicians, hospitals, the public, and private insurers. The acute care inpatient prospective payment system began in 1983 and reduced costs of inpatient hospital care by decreasing the average length of stay, decreasing the use of routine diagnostic tests during inpatient hospitalizations, shifting care to outpatient settings, and increasing the use of post–acute care services (e.g., home care, rehabilitation hospitals and units, skilled nursing facilities). The decrease in inpatient hospital use resulted in excess acute care bed capacity, decreased profits for hospitals and physicians, and imposed financial limits on purchasing new technologies and upgrading facilities. As a result, providers took several measures, including reducing costs through reorganization and staff layoffs, developing and

modifying alternative care options (e.g., rehabilitation services, home care, ambulatory care, long-term care), restructuring the organization through vertical and horizontal integration with other providers so that hospital networks cover larger geographic areas, and providing a full continuum of services. New attention was also focused on marketing of provider services (Nosse et al., 1999).

ASSESSMENT AND ACCOUNTABILITY

In 1988 Relman reported the beginning of the next era of health care as a time for "assessment and accountability." He highlighted the need to learn more about the variations in the performance of healthcare practitioners and the need to link medical care and outcomes data. These data would provide a better understanding of the costs, safety, and effectiveness of the care being provided. Roper, Winkenwerder, Hackbarth, and Krakauer (1988) described the benefits as "better information for physicians and patients to use in making decisions, improved guidelines for medical practice . . . and wiser decisions by health care purchasers." (p. 866). The Patient Protection and Health Care Affordability Act of 2010 and the Healthcare and Education and Health Care Reconciliation Act of 2010 will likely mean shifts with its plans of increasing health insurance coverage, expansion of public reporting of quality measures, and further payment reform efforts in the areas of value-based purchasing, including pay-for-performance and several pilot studies that test the concept of paying for bundled of services and the chronic care hospital pilot.

OVERVIEW OF HEALTHCARE FINANCING

Health care in the United States costs approximately 2 trillion dollars each year. When compared with the total gross domestic product of all other countries, the United States spends more on health care than the total gross domestic product of all other countries except France, the United Kingdom, China, and Japan. The United States is the only industrialized nation in the world without a form of national health care or healthcare insurance. The primary sources of financing for health care in the United States include both public and private funding. Private funding in the United States makes up over half of the dollars spent on health care and comes from private insurances, the Consolidated Omnibus Budget Reconciliation Act (COBRA), and out-of-pocket expenditures (Figure 26.1).

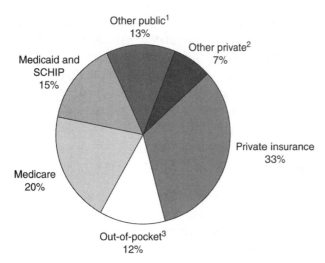

FIGURE 26.1   Healthcare funding in the United States

Centers for Medicare and Medicaid Services, Office of the Actuary, National Health Statistics Group

Nevertheless, public financing is a significant source of healthcare financing and plays an increasingly even greater role in decisions made by payers and providers. The public sources for healthcare financing include Medicare, Medicaid, **state children's health insurance program (SCHIP)**, Veterans Administration (VA), and Tri-Care. Many of these public sources for healthcare financing are the result of recent legislation. Although some forms of public financing have increased access to groups who could otherwise not afford it, it has been suggested that public financing is partly to blame for increasing costs. As noted above, discussion on cost containment and accessibility for the under- and uninsured has become a major focus in the political arena.

HISTORY OF HEALTHCARE FUNDING BEFORE THE 20TH CENTURY

Healthcare financing before the 20th century was fairly uncomplicated, with the primary source of funding coming from private payment. The healthcare industry in the 19th century is best described as a cottage industry with limited resources and consequently poor outcomes. Hospitals were more designed to protect the well from the sick rather than cure diseases, leading to the nomenclature "pest houses" for these rudimentary places. Both financing and healthcare delivery changed significantly in the 20th century.

PRIVATE FINANCING

In the 20th century most private funding for health care was derived from healthcare insurance. Healthcare insurance is a means of sharing risk. From the insured or subscribers' perspective, insurance is a means of protecting themselves from catastrophic financial loss. Grouped together, they share the risk with other subscribers. From the insurance perspective, it is a means of pooling resources (premiums) from multiple subscribers and sharing the risk of financial loss from a possible large claim against them.

Healthcare insurance companies inherently face risks unique to their industry. These risks include adverse selection, subscriber expectations for services, and information asymmetry. One risk for insurance companies is adverse selection. In an ideal case insurance would be purchased by individuals with varying degree of risk so that claims would be infrequent and random. But with adverse selection, insurance is purchased for nonrandom, predictable losses, and insurances are paying for claims that occur regularly.

The second problem is subscriber expectations and use of services. Generally, before individuals use money from their discretionary spending they evaluate where they can get the best "bang for the buck." But in healthcare spending, individuals and families are more likely to spend dollars on more expensive tests or costlier hospitals because they have coverage without regard to costs and benefits. This is primarily because it is a "covered expense" and does not directly come out of their own pockets. This has the potential to relieve the individual of self-responsibility for their own health and increase the costs of health care to all.

Finally, healthcare insurances face information asymmetry. There are facts known to the individuals that may affect the risk faced by the insurance company that are withheld from the insurance company until a claim is made. The information that is needed to evaluate the proper premium is held by the subscriber, not by the policy writer. Examples of this include untreated conditions like elevated blood pressure or chronic back pain. After an individual signs for a healthcare insurance policy there may be financial costs associated with treating those conditions that will have to be paid by the insurer. Consequently, the insured has more information than the policy writer, or there is an asymmetrical relationship regarding information.

DEVELOPMENT OF BLUE CROSS AND BLUE SHIELD

In the first part of the 20th century the primary "costs" incurred from sickness were not medical costs but lost wages. Insurance in the early 20th century continued to focus more on income reimbursement than on medical expenses. With advances in medicine in the first part of the 20th century, the costs of health care began to rise. Three factors, increasing costs of health care, decreasing occupancy rates, and the loss of philanthropic support, put hospitals in a financially dire situation. As a result, hospitals sought to reclaim reimbursement for expenses to a greater degree from their patients to make up for economic shortfalls. This placed fiscal pressure on patients during a period when income was scarce. With both forces in play, financial stresses on hospitals and financial distress on patients, the idea of healthcare insurance was revived. Starting in Dallas, a group of teachers and a former school superintendent created the first healthcare insurance company, which would later evolve into Blue Cross. In 1929 J. F Kimball, a hospital administrator and former school superintendent, enrolled 1,200 teachers into the nation's first true healthcare plan at Baylor University Hospital at the cost of $0.50 per month (Health Care Service Corporation). This eventually became the genesis for Blue Cross Hospital Insurance, and the "blues" were born. By 1946 Blue Cross had over 20 million members in 43 states. Blue Shield, which was created to pay for physician services came along a decade later and merged with Blue Cross to become the Blue Cross Blue Shield Association.

Two key events in the mid-20th century contributed to that rapid growth of healthcare insurance. First, wages were frozen during World War II, but healthcare insurance was excluded from the wage freeze. In 1947 the Taft-Hartley Act made health benefits a "condition of employment" that could be negotiated by employees with employers (Stahl, 2004). To attract good workers, employers could negotiate with employees over covered benefits within healthcare insurance or increase the amount employers paid into healthcare insurance. In addition, the government made prepaid healthcare insurances tax exempt (Emanuel, 2008). Employer-provided healthcare insurance became an attractive benefit from both the employee and employer perspective.

WORKERS' COMPENSATION

Although workers' compensation is more directly tied to reimbursement of lost wages, a discussion on healthcare financing, especially rehabilitation medicine, must include workers' compensation. Workers' compensation has roots as far back as 2050 B.C. In the Code of Hammurabi, each body part had a "price tag" on it that made certain parts more valuable and costly to an employer. This idea was carried on during feudal times and instilled into Prussia by Chancellor Otto Von Bismarck. In the United States in 1911 the Workers' Compensation Act was enacted into law. Wisconsin was the first state to enact a workers' compensation law. Other states gradually followed, and the last state to sign workers' compensation into law was Mississippi in 1948 (Guyton, 1999).

Unlike other forms of health insurance, workers' compensation often has a special rehabilitative focus. Because workers' compensation involves a replacement of wages, employers have an earnest interest in getting workers back to work through rehabilitation and work hardening programs. Consequently, employers are willing to pay for rehabilitation through workers' compensation, even when it is not required by law.

GROWTH OF HEALTH MAINTENANCE ORGANIZATIONS

From the onset of third-party payers for health care, costs for health care have risen at alarming rates. This is especially noted during the 1970s and early 1980s when healthcare costs rose faster than the economy and the costs of premiums grew at four times the rate of inflation (Figure 26.2). Healthcare insurance companies in the late 1980s created a series of initiatives to slow down the growth of healthcare costs. Under the auspices of **health maintenance organizations (HMOs)**, insurance companies implemented some control on costs. These controls included a gatekeeper process, a network of preferred providers, and a capitated payment system. The "gatekeeper," typically the patient's family physician, would screen patients at lower costs and reduce the overuse of specialists prevalent in the 1980s. Second, HMOs created a network of providers who were chosen based on their willingness to accept the payment rates set by the insurance company. The patient was restricted to the network of providers, except in the case of emergencies or where services were unavailable in the network. Third, HMOs

The Nation's Health Dollar, Calendar Year 2009: Where It Went

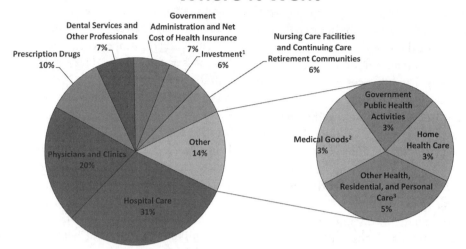

¹ Includes Research (2%) and Structures and Equipment (4%).
² Includes Durable (1%) and Nondurable (2%) goods.
³ Includes expenditures for residential care facilities, ambulance providers, medical care delivered in nontraditional settings (such as community centers, senior citizens centers, schools, and military field stations), and expenditures for Home and Community Waiver programs under Medicaid.
Note: Sum of pieces may not equal 100% due to rounding.

SOURCE: Centers for Medicare & Medicaid Services, Office of the Actuary, National Health Statistics Group.

FIGURE 26.2   National Health Expenditures Trends

Source: Centers for Medicare and Medicaid Services, Office of the Actuary, National Health Statistics Group, at http://www.cms.hhs.gov/ NationalHealthExpendData/ (Historical data from NHE summary including share of GDP, CY 1960–2007, file nhegdp07.zip; Projected data from NHE Projections 2008–2018, Forecast summary and selected tables, file proj2008.pdf)

changed the way providers would be paid. The primary method of payment before HMO was **fee for service (FFS)**. Under FFS, a provider would bill an insurance company for services provided and negotiate payment after the services were provided. The problem with FFS is that this payment structure incentivized providers to maximize utilization of services to maximize profits. With the advent of HMOs, insurance companies paid providers a "capitated rate." Under capitation providers received a set payment for each subscriber in their community who carried their insurance (Gapenski, 2007). As a result of capitation the provider's financial goal refocused to reduce utilization of services by patients. The means of controlling costs and improving profits is to provide more preventative services and less unnecessary tests or procedures. The hope, for both the insurance company and the provider, is that patients would be kept healthier by early proactive measures.

> *Regarding HMOs: The hope, for both the insurance company and the provider, is that patients would be kept healthier by early proactive measures.*

MANAGED CARE

Closely aligned with HMOs and often confused is the concept of **managed care**. Although HMO is a form of managed care, it is incorrect to assume that all managed care is a form of HMOs. Managed care is a system "that influences or controls utilization of services and costs of services" (Kovner & Knickman, 2008, p. 535). Several steps are taken to ensure payment rendered does not exceed what is deemed reasonable and necessary. The first measure is setting a capped rate based on clinical criteria and average costs expected. If the hospital can more efficiently manage the patient, then the extra payment received is retained by the hospital's profit margin. If the patient becomes sicker during their stay (without legitimate upcoding) or the provider does not manage costs effectively, then the costs incurred negatively affect their bottom line.

The second measure is a prospective review and approval process. In this case, before a medical procedure is undertaken, when possible, the insurer must review the services and decide whether they are medically necessary.

The goal in this measure is to filter out unnecessary tests, procedures, and so on that may be provided or ordered by a healthcare provider.

The third measure taken under managed care is the concurrent review process. Most often associated with inpatient hospital stay, a concurrent review is done by a clinician working for an insurer to determine whether or not a continued inpatient stay is deemed necessary. In the case of concurrent review, the insurer reviews information provided by the hospital to support the need for continued inpatient hospitalization. If it is deemed unnecessary, the insurer will deny further payment for services. The provider can either concur with the decision by the insurer and discharge the patient to another setting or appeal the decision. Typically, the appeal for ongoing inpatient services proceeds to a physician within the insurance company who reviews the case and either overturns or affirms the denial.

Finally, the last measure taken under managed care is the retroactive review. Under the retroactive review all care provided is reviewed for medical necessity. Whereas the concurrent review involves selective information given by the provider to the insurance either by phone, electronic mail, or fax, a retroactive review is a more thorough review that ensures information that may have caused the case to be denied was not excluded or overlooked in the concurrent review process. Much like the concurrent review process, payment can be denied because of lack of necessity, but the provider is permitted to appeal the denial to receive part or all payment for services rendered.

Managed care is often credited with reducing the rising costs of health care. Unfortunately, some of the controls were repealed as a result of complaints by patients and providers and much of the reduction in rising healthcare costs was lost.

EMPLOYER-FUNDED INSURANCE

Employer-funded insurance in its truest form is primarily an invention of the 20th century. Since the inception of employer-funded insurance many variations of the original model have arisen. The original model was FFS, but because of rising costs, other means of healthcare payments and cost containment were necessitated. The first one developed after HMO was the **point of service** insurance plan. As a compromise, or regression from the strictest provision of healthcare services, point of service allowed the insured to receive health care at providers outside the network, albeit with higher copays and deductibles. Like the HMO, a gatekeeper screens

referrals and consequently offers low or no deductibles when patients receive care within the network. A second form of employer-funded insurance is **preferred provider organizations**. The most liberal form of healthcare insurance, it allows individuals to freely choose their providers. Financial incentives and lower deductibles and copays to receive care within a selected network of providers still remain. Preferred provider organizations make up the majority of employer-funded healthcare insurance in the United States today

> *Point of service allowed the insured to receive health care from providers outside of the network, albeit with higher copays and deductibles.*

COBRA

An extension of employee-provided insurance is insurance provided under the **Consolidated Omnibus Budget Reconciliation Act (COBRA)**. Signed into law in 1986, under COBRA any employee who works for an employer with 20 or more employees for 50 days of the year or more is qualified to continue temporary insurance coverage at group rates. This coverage is provided in the event the employee becomes unemployed or has a reduction in hours. In most cases the beneficiary is fully responsible for the cost of the premium. Although the cost of COBRA insurance is higher than employer-provided insurance, in many cases it is more affordable than private insurance.

MEDICARE SUPPLEMENTAL INSURANCE

Medicare supplemental insurance, or Medigap, is very much like a public version of COBRA. **Medigap** is private insurance that picks up where Medicare drops off. Without spending a great deal of time in this section describing Medicare, it is important to note that Medicare pays up to 80% of most costs. For many Medicare recipients, 20% of the incurred expenses can represent a significant portion of their income and may surpass the amount an individual can afford. As a result, many obtain a second insurance to pick up the additional costs. Consequently, 90% of seniors in the United States who have Medicare also have a second insurance plan to help pay the copays and deductibles left by Medicare (2002).

PUBLIC FINANCING

Public financing makes up less than half of the revenue for healthcare costs. Despite its role as a minority player, public financing has a significant role in the provision of healthcare services. In fact, decisions made at the federal or state level affect the private financing sector, which will follow similar guidelines for reimbursement. Public financing for health care in the United States began with introduction of the Social Security Act.

EARLY ATTEMPTS AT HEALTHCARE REFORM

The original Social Security Act was passed in 1935, during the Roosevelt administration under the New Deal plan. Although the idea of putting in a system to pay for health care as part of Social Security was considered at the time, Franklin D. Roosevelt and, later, Harry Truman were not able to accomplish this goal. At the signing of the Social Security Act of 1965, Lyndon Johnson partially credited Harry Truman with the passage of Medicare and Medicaid, and the first Medicare cards were issued to Harry and Bessie Truman. After Truman left office, healthcare reform was part of the political agenda for congressional democrats in the 1950s. Without a sweeping majority or a president willing to push for reform, healthcare reform attempts were futile. Meanwhile, public pressure mounted to pass a bill that would provide healthcare coverage for the poor and elderly.

MEDICARE AND MEDICAID

Under President Lyndon Johnson's leadership, with the assistance of democratic majorities in both sides of the House, and with continued public pressure, the Social Security Amendment Act of 1965 was passed and signed into law. It included three main "layers" that included hospital coverage for seniors (Medicare Part A), physician coverage for seniors (Medicare Part B), and healthcare coverage for the poor (Medicaid) (Blumenthal & Morone, 2008). Although it is accurate to say that private health insurance pays a greater portion of the costs for health care in the United States than Medicare, Medicare is the single largest payer of health care. Although it was originally run by the Social Security Administration in 1965, oversight was transferred to the Health Care Financing Administration in 1977, until it passed hands to the Centers for Medicare & Medicaid Services (CMS) in 2001.

There are several key differences between Medicare and Medicaid. Fist, Medicare is administered by the federal government with revenue obtained from payroll taxes and premiums received from enrollees. To be eligible for Medicare you must be over 65 years old and have contributed to the system for 10 years. There are two exceptions

to the age requirement: individuals who are disabled or have end-stage renal disease (CMS, n.d.)

Another key difference between Medicare and Medicaid is that the original Medicare plan does not contain prescription drug coverage. In addition, Medicare has strict limitations on coverage for nursing home care. For an enrollee to receive care in a nursing home, they must qualify for skilled care, which is care provided by a nurse or a trained therapist. Much of the care provided in nursing homes is described as custodial care (e.g., assistance with bathing, grooming, feeding) and therefore does not qualify for Medicare coverage.

There are two parts to Medicare. Part A coverage pays for 100% of inpatient care for days 1 through 60 of an episode of care and approximately 80% for days 61 through 90. In addition, Medicare Part A covers 100% of care in a skilled facility for days 1 to 20 and everything but a set uncovered per day amount for days 21 to 100. Medicare Part A carries no monthly premium but does have an annual deductible of $992. Medicare Part B also covers home health care, durable medical equipment, and preventative care. Medicare B covers physician and outpatient services and carries a monthly premium of around $100 per month.

Health policy initiatives set in motion by stakeholders have resulted in some significant changes in Medicare since its original enactment. When Medicare was originally enacted, it was designed to cover only those eligible enrollees who were over 65 years old. In 1972 President Nixon expanded Medicare coverage to include patients with end-stage renal disease. Second, initially Medicare started out paying under FFS, but it became readily apparent that cost containment was necessary. Even at its inception, enrollees were permitted to take an HMO alternative instead of traditional Medicare, but the lack of enrollment made the measure ineffective. From 1975 to 1980 Medicare spending more than doubled, from $14.8 billion to $35 billion (Tieman, 2003). In response to rising costs, in 1983, Medicare revised payment provisions for inpatient hospitalization from FFS to a prospective payment system (PPS) based on **diagnosis-related groups (DRGs)**. There are approximately 500 DRGs in the current CMS classification system. In a hospital setting, patients' charts are reviewed by a coder who submits a claim after applying strict criteria in a manual called the International Classification of Disease and Related Health Related Problems version 9, which leads to a DRG. The most recent change in Medicare was the addition of prescription coverage, under Medicare D. Although intended to help cover cost of prescription drugs, significant gaps in coverage have limited its usefulness.

Despite early fears of hospitals discharging patients "quicker and sicker," the Medicare PPS system has led to a system that provides satisfactory healthcare coverage for many senior citizens in the United States (Tieman, 2004). Average life expectancy in the United States is 77 years old, which ranks 40th in the world. In contrast, for citizens in the United States who live to be 65 years old and subsequently become eligible for Medicare, the life expectancy is 83 years old, which is similar to most industrialized nations. Additionally, it has proven to be profitable for hospitals and led to cost containment on Medicare's side. In fact, it has been such a successful system that the governments of other countries, including Australia, France, and Germany, have taken note and copied the PPS system in their respective countries (Tieman, 2004).

In contrast to Medicare, Medicaid is administered by state governments. Although Medicaid in each state may have general federal guidelines it must follow, Medicaid is managed in a variety of ways at each state level. For example, to qualify for Medicaid the applicant must meet income criteria that can vary from 11% to 200% of the poverty level depending on his or her state of residence (Kaiser Family Foundation, 2011). Thirty-five of the 50 states charge a premium for enrollees. Similarly, 35 have waiting periods for children enrolling in their state Medicaid program. Also, 44 of the states' Medicaid programs cover tobacco cessation products (Kaiser Family Foundation, 2011). Most notably for rehabilitation nurses, Medicaid coverage for rehabilitation and most particularly for brain injury care varies greatly. Some states require preauthorization under Medicaid before a patient receives inpatient rehabilitation, whereas others do not. Some states' Medicaid programs cover subacute brain injury programs, whereas other states have no such coverage.

Despite the uniqueness of each state's Medicaid plan, there are some general similarities. First, to qualify you must meet an income threshold. Second, Medicaid coverage is more comprehensive than Medicare in that it provides coverage for dental and prescription drug needs. Finally, as a result of recent court decisions, Medicaid programs provide for home and community-based waiver programs that subsidize additional services to help recipients remain in their home environment. Some examples of these subsidies include payment for wheelchair ramps, payment for at-home caregivers, and adult day care services while family members are at work. The extent and type of coverage for home and community-based services varies from state to state, but each state offers some kind of "waiver" services.

TAX EQUITY AND FISCAL RESPONSIBILITY ACT (TEFRA)

With the advent of PPS in the inpatient hospitals in 1983, a system for payment for acute inpatient rehabilitation was needed. Under the **Tax Equity and Fiscal Responsibility Act (TEFRA)**, inpatient rehabilitation units and hospitals were excluded from the DRG system and paid at a per diem rate with a maximum ceiling. Each **inpatient rehabilitation facility** was given a maximum TEFRA threshold based on historic billing patterns. If the inpatient rehabilitation facility billed Medicare for less than the TEFRA limit, a bonus was given as an incentive to keep costs lower than the TEFRA limit. Consequently, this was a financial win for acute hospitals that also had inpatient rehabilitation units because they received payment for both the acute care and inpatient rehabilitation (Braddon, 2005). Shortly after the introduction of DRGs there was a sudden increase in the number of hospital-based rehabilitation units, as hospitals without rehabilitation units sought to open them to share in the financial profit to be gained.

75% RULE

Along with the initiation of TEFRA payments in 1983 was the creation of the so-called **75% rule**. Devised to separate inpatient rehabilitation from acute care, Medicare devised a list of eight diagnoses to determine which patients would most likely qualify for acute inpatient rehabilitation. A rehabilitation hospital or unit, to bill for TEFRA payments, had to demonstrate that 75% of the patients admitted were diagnosed with one of those eight diagnoses. In 1984 Health Care Financing Administration was asked to lower the threshold to 60% but refused to amend the 75% requirement. Instead, Health Care Financing Administration added two more diagnosis, neurological disorders and burns (Box 26.1).

The 75% rule was intended to deter hospitals from sending patients to rehabilitation hospitals or units merely to avoid incurring costs. Unfortunately, fiscal intermediaries working for Medicare were inconsistent in applying the rule. In 1995 only 13% of rehabilitation units or hospitals were in compliance with the 75% rule (Braddon, 2005). The 75% rule became more of an issue when facilities in New Jersey and Tennessee received letters of noncompliance, threatening their revenue and

---

BOX 26.1 75% Rule Classifications

Currently, there are 13 diagnostic categories:

- Stroke
- Spinal cord injury
- Congenital deformity
- Amputation
- Major multiple trauma
- Hip fracture
- Brain injury
- Neurological disorders
- Burns
- Polyarthritis (split into four subcategories of arthritic-related conditions)

Source: Adapted from American Academy of Physical Medicine and Rehabilitation (2010).

---

status as rehabilitation facilities. In 2002 the rehabilitation industry became alarmed with both the difficulty in meeting the 75% and the risk of being declassified by CMS. After several suspensions of the rule, a decision was made in 2000 to revise the listed diagnoses that fit the criteria for admission to an inpatient rehabilitation unit and reduce the requirement to 60%.

PROSPECTIVE PAYMENT SYSTEM

A PPS is a method of paying based on foreseen costs rather than billed costs. The implementation of the Medicare PPS system has taken on various forms, based on the setting. In the acute side, PPS was implemented in 1983 with the advent of DRGs. After the creation of the Balanced Budget Amendment of 1997, post–acute settings were included in the PPS structure. In nursing home settings payment was based on **resource utilization groups**, which provided a fixed payment based on anticipated costs for skilled services. During the late 1990s, as a result of this restructure, the nursing home industry lost billions of dollars in the first years after its implementation. Eight of the top 10 owners of nursing homes declared bankruptcy within the first couple of years. Among them were Sun Healthcare, Vencor, Mariner, and Integrated Health Services.

PPS also impacted home health with the implementation of the home health resource groups. After the implementation of PPS, home health services were no longer able to bill for each visit; instead, they received capped payments for a 60-day episode of care. When first implemented provider-based and for-profit home health agencies received a decrease in reimbursement from CMS. Nonprofit and government-run home health agencies received a net increase.

Increased public reporting was not associated with higher use of quality information for selecting health providers, but public reporting did stimulate hospitals to engage in quality improvement activities (Fung, Lim, Mattke, Damberg, & Shekelle, 2008).

Implementation of PPS in the acute rehabilitation industry was not without its own corresponding backlash. Fearful that PPS would result in bankruptcies like the ones seen in the nursing home industry or severely capped payments like those seen in home health, the acute rehabilitation industry appealed for modifications in PPS reimbursement and the 75% rule. As previously stated, CMS refused to eliminate the 75% rule but did reduce the requirement to 60% and added three diagnoses. In addition to Medicare and Medicaid, there are several publicly funded programs for special groups.

PROGRAMS FOR SPECIAL GROUPS

There are healthcare payment programs for groups who meet certain eligibility criteria. These programs include VA, Tri-Care, Indian Health Service (IHS), and SCHIP.

Veterans Administration

Veterans of the armed forces in the United States may qualify for care at a VA facility. Disabled veterans, former prisoners of war, and Purple Heart recipients are able to access health care at a VA facility at no or little charge. Eligible veterans receive inpatient hospital care, medicines, and access to many of the clinics available at a VA hospital. As an incentive to provide high-quality care to World War II veterans, subsidies were provided to academic medical centers affiliated with a VA facility. This public–private partnership was quite successful and advantageous to both groups for a number of years.

Indian Health Service

The IHS provides care for approximately 1.9 million Native Americans and Alaska Natives. To receive coverage, a person must either reside on an Indian reservation or be a descendent of someone who resided on a federal Indian reservation as of 1934 or be one-half or more Native American from tribes indigenous to the United States (http://www.ihs.gov). The IHS manages 38 hospitals and 56 health centers in the United States (Sultz & Young, 2009). The IHS receives money as part of the federal budget. The annual budget for IHS for fiscal year 2010 is over $4 billion. Alcohol-related deaths are six times more frequent among Native Americans and Alaska Natives; consequently, of the total budget for

IHS, over $250 million is spent to cover care for alcohol and substance abuse (http://info.ihs.gov/Budget10.asp). Funding is also available under IHS for dental care as well as diabetes prevention and treatment (http://info.ihs .gov/Budget10.asp).

State Children's Health Insurance Program

As a means of helping families who did not qualify for Medicaid but could not afford health insurance for their children, in 1997 the Clinton administration signed SCHIP into law. The program provided $24 billion to be spent over 10 years to assist families with healthcare costs. SCHIP was underused for many years, in large part because very little was done to publicize the program. It has been estimated that one-third of eligible children remain uncovered despite the fact that SCHIP has shown to provide needed preventative care. One study showed that children enrolled in SCHIP suffered fewer asthma-related attacks than children without insurance (Lambrew, 2007). SCHIP is funded by a matching contribution, with 70% coming from the federal government and 30% coming from the states.

UNINSURED

Americans without healthcare insurance comprise 15% of all Americans, with numbers estimated at 46 million. Equally problematic is the number of underinsured, those with limited insurance coverage. Consequently, the health care of uninsured and underinsured Americans is appreciably worse than insured Americans (The Associated Press, 2009). The uninsured and underinsured are less likely to see a family doctor or receive preventative care, which can reduce the risk of major illness and costlier healthcare needs (Pifer-Bixley, 2009). As a result of the Emergency Medical Treatment and Active Labor Act (EMTALA), the main source of medical treatment for these individuals is the emergency room. According to EMTALA, any patient who shows up in an emergency room must be properly triaged and stabilized before they can be discharged or transferred. The law is reinforced by the ominous threat from the federal government to withdraw Medicare dollars for hospitals that fail to comply. In addition to requiring emergency triage and treatment of patients presenting to the emergency room, hospitals must also adhere to the "250 yard rule." According to the 250 yard rule, any patient who is within 250 yards of the hospital campus and is perceived by a lay person as needing medical treatment must receive treatment from hospital medical personnel (Schecter, 2010).

PROCESS OF MAKING HEALTH POLICY

Phases of Health Policymaking

Health policymaking can be divided in three phases: policy formulation, policy implementation, and policy modification (Longest, 1996). At each phase stakeholders can play an important role in policy design, which can have a significant impact on healthcare delivery. Policy formulation begins with agenda setting and refers to the identification of problems and possible solutions proposed by stakeholder with diverse interests. For example, concerns about the rising costs of Medicare, the growing number of uninsured and under-insured individuals, and gaps in the quality of healthcare delivery led to the health reform law passed in 2010. Once an issue becomes prominent in the political agenda, it can proceed to the next stage of policy formulation: the development of legislation. However, only a small percentage of issues reach that point. See Figure 26.3.

The legislative process begins with proposals (e.g., bills) that may be drafted by senators or representatives and their staff members, by members of the executive branch, by political or special interest groups, or by individual citizens. Only members of Congress can officially sponsor a bill. Occasionally, identical bills are simultaneously introduced in the Senate and the House of Representatives for consideration. Each bill is assigned to the appropriate committee(s) based on its content and the jurisdiction of the committees and subcommittees. Hearings are held, and the bill is marked up.

Once it is approved by the full committee, the House or Senate receives the bill and places it on the legislative calendar for floor action. The bill may be further amended during debate on the floor. If the bill passes either the House or the Senate, it is sent to the other chamber of Congress, where the process is repeated. If the second chamber passes the bill, any differences between the House and Senate versions must be resolved before the bill is sent to the White House for presidential action. The president then has the option to sign the bill to make it a law or to veto the bill and return it to Congress with an explanation for the rejection. A presidential veto may be overridden by a two-thirds vote in both houses of Congress. If the president does not sign or veto the bill after 10 days, the bill automatically becomes law.

After a law is enacted, policy implementation, which includes rule making and policy operation, becomes the responsibility of the executive branch of the government. Cabinet departments such as the Department of Health and Human Services and its agencies, such as the CMS

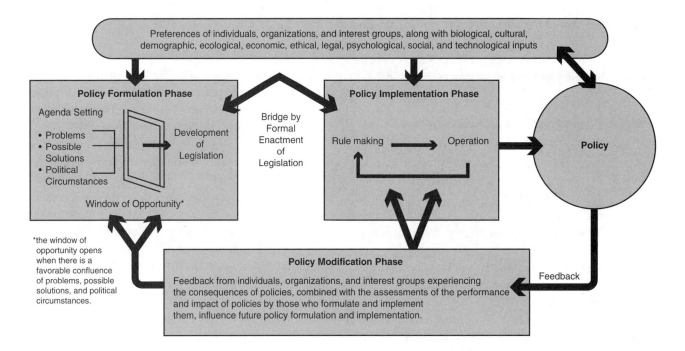

and the Centers for Disease Control and Prevention, oversee the implementation. Oversight of the implementation is the responsibility of agencies such as the Government Accountability Office, the Congressional Budget Office, the Congressional Research Office, and the Office of Technology and Assessment. Laws frequently are vague on implementation details, so the organization responsible for implementing the law publishes a "Notice of Proposed Rule Making" and "Final Rule" in the *Federal Register*. Any person may comment on the proposed rules/regulators, and the final rule serves as a notice to those individuals affected by the rules/regulations regarding the details of the policy implementation and operation of the enacted legislation. This is an important and often powerful vehicle for stakeholder to influence the regulations that govern implementation of policy.

Policy modification occurs when prior decisions are modified once the outcomes, perceptions, and consequences of existing policies are discovered. Modifications to any legislation begin with at the agenda-setting stage.

Rehabilitation nurses can influence the health policy-making process at any stage of the process. For example, within the policy formulation phase, the nurse can help with agenda setting by defining and documenting problems, developing and evaluating solutions to problems, and shaping political circumstances through lobbying or working through the legal system. Within the legislation development phase, the nurse can participate in drafting legislation or testify at legislative hearings. During the policy implementation (e.g., rule making) phase, nurses can provide formal comments on proposed rules published in the *Federal Register* or serve on and provide input to rule-making advisory bodies. Nurse can influence policy modification by documenting the rationale for modification through operational experience and formal evaluations, such as research.

MAJOR STAKEHOLDERS IN THE U.S. HEALTHCARE INDUSTRY

The American healthcare system has a large and diverse group of stakeholders (Kovner & Knickman, 2008; Sultz & Young, 2009). In general, health policies affect or influence groups or classes of individuals (e.g., nurses, the elderly, the disabled, the poor) or certain types of organizations (e.g., hospitals, skilled nursing facilities, health plans, biotech entities, or employers). Thus, support or opposition to healthcare reform efforts often vary by stakeholder groups. In addition, stakeholder groups' level of interest and their support or concern about a given policy may be shared or conflicting (Kovner & Knickman, 2008; Sultz & Young, 2009). Table 26.1 describes key stakeholder groups for the healthcare industry.

KEY ISSUES IN HEALTH POLICY

Many health policy issues affect access to and delivery of healthcare services. Some of the key issues include quality measures, healthcare costs, access to care, health disparities, stem cell research, and technology.

TABLE 26.1	Key Stakeholders in the Healthcare Industry	
Stakeholder Group	**Tend to Favor**	**Tend to Oppose**
Patients: Users of healthcare services.	Comprehensive coverage, high-quality health care, and low out-of-pocket expenses	Limited access to care and increased patient payments
Taxpayers: Public pays taxes to the government, which are used to fund healthcare services.	Limits on provider payments	Higher taxes
Consumer organizations: Organizations such as the American Stroke Association and the Paralyzed Veterans' Association are politically active.	Securing funding for research and public education	
Employers: An important stakeholder, because they are paying for a high percentage of healthcare costs and are involved in negotiating insurance coverage for their employees, including coverage and copayments.	Cost containment, administrative simplification, and elimination of cost shifting	Government regulation
Healthcare professionals: Include nurses, physicians, physical therapists, occupational therapists, speech language pathologists, social workers, case managers, dietitians, pharmacists, and dentists, who deliver and supervise health care provided to patients.	Income maintenance, autonomy, and comprehensive coverage	Limits on payments
Hospitals, facilities, home health agencies, and nursing homes.	Autonomy and comprehensive coverage	Limits on provider payments
Federal, state, and local governments: The federal and state governments are key given their role in oversight of the Medicare and Medicaid programs.	Disclosure and reporting by providers, cost containment, access to care, and high-quality health care	Provider autonomy
Pharmaceutical manufacturers, biotech, assistive technology vendors, and suppliers	Comprehensive coverage	Limits on provider payments
Private insurance companies: Insurance companies offer managed care or indemnity plans.	Business autonomy	

Quality and Quality Measures

The Institute of Medicine (IOM, 2006) defines quality as "degree to which health services for individuals and populations increase the likelihood of desired health outcomes and are consistent with current professional knowledge" (p. 468). The United States offers advanced healthcare services; however, the care is not always accessible, effective, safe, and efficient (IOM, 2004). In calling for a strong response to improve the quality of health care, the IOM noted that the only way to know if health care quality is improving is to document performance using standardized measures of quality. The term "**quality measure**" has been defined as the "quantification of the degree to which a desired health care process or outcome is achieved or the extent that a desirable structure to support health care delivery is in place" (IOM, 2006, p. 42).

Quality measures address several aspects of care, which have been defined by Donabedian (2005) as structure measures, process measures, and outcome measures. **Structure measures** track whether a particular mecha-

nism or system is in place, and **process measures** track performance of a particular action. **Outcome measures** consider the results of care, such as morbidity and mortality resulting from a disease.

The IOM identified the six aims of healthcare delivery as care that is safe, effective, patient-centered, timely, efficient, and equitable. **Safe care** refers to the avoidance of injuries to patients from the care that is intended to help. **Effective care** means that services are based on scientific knowledge and provided to all who could benefit and refraining from providing services to those not likely to benefit. *Patient-centered care* refers to care that is respectful of and responsive to individual patient preferences, needs, and values, and *timely care* is provided in a way that reduces wait times. **Efficient care** avoids waste, including waste of equipment, supplies, ideas, and energy, and *equitable care* refers to care that does not vary in quality because of personal characteristics (e.g., gender, ethnicity, geographic location, and socioeconomic status).

The IOM (2001) proposed rules for redesigning healthcare processes to improve care:

- *Care based on continuous healing relationships:* Care should be available 24 hours a day and 7 days a week, and access to care should occur over the Internet, by telephone, and by other means as well as face-to-face.
- *Customization based on patient needs and values:* The system should meet the most common types of needs and have the ability to respond to patient choices and preferences.
- *Patient as the source of control:* Patients should be given the necessary information and opportunity to be involved in shared decision making.
- *Shared knowledge and the free flow of information:* Patients should have access to their own medical information and clinical knowledge.
- *Evidence-based decision making:* Patients should receive care based on the best scientific knowledge.
- *Safety:* Patients should be safe from injury that is caused by the system.
- *Transparency:* The system should make information available to patients and their families that allow them to make informed decisions when selecting a health plan, hospital, or clinician.
- *Anticipation of needs:* The system should anticipate patients' needs.
- *Continuous decrease in waste:* The health system should not waste resources or patients' time.
- *Cooperation among clinicians:* Clinicians and institutions should actively collaborate and communicate to foster greater coordination of care and integration. Transition measures seek to reduce "hand-off" errors as patients move from one setting to another (e.g., acute care hospital to rehabilitation unit, rehabilitation unit to home) and reduce duplicative testing.

Quality measures (also known as performance measures, quality indicators, or performance indicators) evaluate healthcare performance in a manner that permits comparisons across facilities and across time. Three activities that use quality measures that have been shown to improve care are public reporting, quality improvement, and pay-for-performance activities (IOM, 2006). The CMS and private-sector payers have been leaders in using quality measures for public reporting and pay-for-performance. Public reporting of quality data from acute care hospitals is incorporated into federal law and many states have mandatory public reporting. Proponents of public reporting of quality information argue that it helps patients, referring physicians, and purchasers of healthcare make better, more-informed choices about which providers offer the best care. In a recent systematic review, Fung et al. (2007) found that increased public reporting was not associated with higher use of quality information for selecting health providers, but public reporting did stimulate hospitals to engage in quality improvement activities. Hibbard (2007) recommended more thoughtful public reporting aimed at consumers, because information meant for the public has thus far been incomplete, confusing, inaccurate, or distorted. Public reporting of rehabilitation quality information also found problems with the presentation of the material, including patients' limited comprehension of terms and their inability to link measures with quality of care (Taylor, 2010).

Another quality measure that has the potential to improve the delivery of health care is the use of incentives to reward providers that demonstrate better quality of care based on performance data (i.e., pay-for-performance programs). Research on managed care organizations demonstrates that this approach can lead to improved care. Medicare has linked payment incentives to reporting on measures for hospitals, home health agencies, and physicians; plans for incentive payments for performance, efficiency, and eventually value are underway.

Healthcare Costs

As previously noted, policymakers have struggled with controlling the increasing costs of healthcare delivery for several decades. In 1960 the national health expenditures represented 5.1% of the gross domestic product. By 2008 national health expenditures increased to 16% of the gross domestic product (Medicare Payment Advisory Committee, 2010). The rising costs have been attributed to many factors, including population growth, increased utilization of services, advances in healthcare technology, increasing labor costs, increases in the costs of pharmaceuticals, and malpractice insurance. With the rapidly rising costs of health care, less money is spent on other areas, such as education or housing. Although almost all agree rising healthcare costs are a problem, developing policies aimed at controlling costs are challenging, because one or more stakeholder group will receive less money and access to care may become more limited. Some economists argue that substantial cuts in spending could be made based on the following:

- Value of health delivery is related to care as well as cure.
- Benefit occurs as a result of medical science and public health rather than costly hospital stay and other healthcare delivery.
- Need to distinguish between average and marginal benefits.
- Issues that have been proposed to control costs include managed care, use of information technology, evidence-based care, management initiatives, controlling prescription drug costs, Medicare and Medicaid reform, using competition, fraud prevention and detection, and price controls.

Access to Care

Individuals do not have equal access to health care for a variety of reasons. The most common reason for limited access to necessary health services is the inability to pay for care (Sultz & Young, 2009). A growing number of people have no health insurance or are underinsured, an issue that is addressed in the health reform law passed in 2010. There are many other individuals with limited access to care, because healthcare personnel and facilities are not close to where they live, accessible by transportation, culturally acceptable, or capable of providing the type of needed care (Sultz & Young, 2009).

Technology

Healthcare technology includes clinical equipment/devices and information technology. Information technology has the potential to improve the storage and access of patient information, reduce errors, manage workflow, and lead to faster and more accurate billing (Kovner & Knickman, 2008). The American Recovery and Reinvestment Act of 2009 provided funding to increase the use of health information technology.

KEY FACTORS SHAPING THE FUTURE OF HEALTHCARE DELIVERY IN THE UNITED STATES

The changing demographic characteristics of the U.S. population are expected to affect how health care is organized and delivered (Kovner & Knickman, 2008; Sultz & Young, 2009). Americans older than 65 represent less than 15% of the population but account for almost half of the acute care hospital admissions and approximately 65% of patients treated in rehabilitation hospitals/units (Deutsch, Fiedler, Granger, & Russell, 2002). The number of individuals older than 65 is expected to double in the next 25 years, thus increasing utilization of healthcare services

and leading to an increase in costs. The U.S. population is also becoming more diverse in the areas of race and ethnicity. According to the U.S. Census Bureau, most Americans will be ethnic "minorities" by the year 2060, but the differences vary by geographic region (Kovner & Knickman, 2008; Sultz & Young, 2009). Disparities in the access to and outcomes of health care by race and ethnic groups when compared with the non-Hispanic White population have been demonstrated in many studies, with worse outcomes often occurring among minority populations. Many ethnic minorities prefer to receive care from providers who understand their culture. Creating a more racially and ethnically diverse healthcare workforce is a key goal for the upcoming years.

Medicare and Medicaid reform will affect the entire healthcare marketplace. These two programs combined account for 36% of personal health expenditures, 48% of hospital expenditures, 33% of physician and professional expenditures, 61% of nursing home care, and 26% of home health care (Kovner & Knickman, 2008; Shultz & Young, 2009).

There is increasing recognition that individuals and their families need to be more involved in their care decisions. For example, among the IOM's 10 rules for improving care (described previously), 6 refer to direct involvement of the patient and family in their care (IOM, 2001). Individuals are increasingly aware that their own behaviors affect their health, and efforts to help individuals become more informed consumers of health care have increased. There is increasing understanding that the determinants of health have little to do with the healthcare system and more to do with the way we lead our lives and the environment in which we live.

SUMMARY

Healthcare policies affect access to and delivery of healthcare services. A key healthcare policy issue in the United States is healthcare financing, which includes an array of private health insurance programs, dominated by managed care, and public health insurance programs, such as Medicare and Medicaid. The Medicare program covers the elderly, individuals who are disabled, and those with end-stage renal disease, whereas Medicaid provides health insurance coverage for individuals with a low income. Medicare, a major payer of health services, has moved from cost-based reimbursement systems to a PPS tied to patient complexity. High-quality health care, a second key policy issue, means that care delivery is safe, effective, patient-centered, timely, efficient, and equitable.

Measures of quality can be classified as structure measures, process measures, or outcome measures. Health reform plans include tying Medicare payments to the quality of care provided.

Nurses, one of the many diverse healthcare stakeholders, should be familiar with the health policymaking process. They can play an important role in policy design, which furthermore can have a significant impact on healthcare delivery.

CRITICAL THINKING

1. Describe three trends that are impacting healthcare reform. Which of these trends do you foresee as having the most significant impact on your career?

2. Identify two types of quality measures.

3. Go to two different hospital websites and review their quality information. Based on this information, which hospital would you choose and why?

4. Ask your parents or grandparents why they use a particular physician and hospital for their healthcare services. How do their responses compare with your perspective on the physician and hospital quality of care?

5. Describe three ways you can have a voice on healthcare reform.

PERSONAL REFLECTION

- What type of healthcare insurance do you have and why? Does your own insurance seem to adequately cover your healthcare needs? What is your prescription plan like? How much do you pay out of pocket for medications per year?

- What is your major concern about your or your family's healthcare insurance?

- Have you read the healthcare plans for candidates to federal elected positions?

- How involved are you in policymaking within your professional specialty? How could you become more active in this area?

- Could you name your congressmen and state senators? If not, look them up.

REFERENCES

American Academy of Physical Medicine and Rehabilitation. (2010). What is the so-called "75% rule"? Retrieved January 14, 2010, from http://www.aapmr.org/hpl/legislation/whats75.htm

American Association of Preferred Provider Organizations. (n.d.). PPO—a leading, proven, health care delivery model. Retrieved from http://www.aappo.org/index.cfm?pageid=10

Anna, Y. S. (2002). Legislative and regulatory processes. In D. J. Mason, J. K. Leavitt, & M. K. Chaffee (Eds.), *Policy & politics in nursing and health care* (pp. 451–461). St. Louis, MO: Saunders.

Blumenthal, D., & Morone, J. (2008). The lessons of success—revisiting the Medicare story. *New England Journal of Medicine, 359*, 2384–2389.

Braddon, R. L. (2005). Medicare funding for inpatient rehabilitation: how did we get to this point and what do we do now. *Archive of Physical Medicine and Rehabilitation, 86*, 1287–1992.

Centers for Medicare & Medicaid Services. (n.d.). History of Medicare. Retrieved April 1, 2010, from http://www.cms.gov/History

Centers for Medicare & Medicaid Services. (n.d.). President milestones. Retrieved from https://www.cms.gov/History/Downloads/PresidentCMSMilestones.pdf

Centers for Medicare & Medicaid Services. (2008). *Roadmap for quality measurement in the traditional fee-for-service program.* Centers for Medicare & Medicaid Services.

Deutsch, A., Fiedler, R. C., Granger, C.V., & Russell, C.F. (2002). The uniform data system for medical rehabilitation report of patients discharged from comprehensive medical rehabilitation programs in 1999. *American Journal of Physical Medicine and Rehabilitation, 81*, 133–142.

Donabedian, A. (2005). Evaluating the quality of medical care. *Milbank Q, 83*(4), 691–729.

Emanuel, E. (2008). The problem with tax-exempt health insurance. *The New York Times*, October 10. Retrieved from http://campaignstops.blogs.nytimes.com/2008/10/10/the-problem-with-tax-exempt-health-insurance/

Fung, C. H., Lim, Y. W., Mattke, S., Damberg, C., & Shekelle, P. G. (2008). Systematic review: The evidence that publishing patient care performance data improves quality of care. *Annals of Internal Medicine, 148*(2), 111–123.

Gapenski, L. C. (2007). The healthcare environment. In *Understanding healthcare financial management* (pp. 3–73). Chicago: Health Administration Press

Guyton, G. P. (1999). A brief history of worker's compensation. *The Iowa Orthopaedic Journal, 19*, 106–110. Retrieved from http://www.ncbi.nlm.nih.gov/pmc/articles/PMC1888620/

Health Care Service Corporation. (n.d.). History of the company. Retrieved from http://www.hcsc.com/about-hcsc/history.html

Hearing before subcommittee on health of the committee on ways and means House of Representatives one hundred seventh congress second session. (2002, March 14). Serial 107-60. In Medicare Supplemental Insurance. Retrieved June 8, 2010, from http://waysandmeans.house.gov/legacy/health/107cong/3-14-02/107-60final.htm

Hibbard, J. H. (2008). What can we say about the impact of public reporting? Inconsistent execution yields variable results. *Annals of Internal Medicine, 148*(2), 160–161.

Indian Health Services. (n.d.). Eligibility statement. Retrieved July 1, 2010, from http://www.ihs.gov/FacilitiesServices/areaOffices/California/Universal/PageMain.cfm?p=2

Institute of Medicine (IOM). (2001). *Crossing the quality chasm: A new health system for the 21st century.* Washington, DC: Institute of Medicine.

Institute of Medicine (IOM). (2006). *Performance measurement: Accelerating improvement.* Washington, DC: National Academies Press.

Kaiser Family Foundation. (2011). State health facts. Retrieved from www.statehealthfacts.com

Kovner, A. R., & Knickman, J. R. (Eds.). (2008). *Health care delivery in the united states* (9th ed.). New York: Springer.

Lambrew, J. M. (2007). The state children's health insurance program: Past, present, and future. The Commonwealth Fund, 49, fund report. Retrieved from http://www.commonwealthfund.org/Content/Publications/Fund-Reports/2007/Feb/The-State-Childrens-Health-Insurance-Program--Past--Present--and-Future.aspx

Leavitt, J. K., Chaffee, M. K., & Vance, C. (2002). Learning the ropes of policy and politics. In D. J. Mason, J. K. Leavitt, & M. W. Chaffee (Eds.), *Policy & politics in nursing and health care* (pp. 31–43). St. Louis, MO: Saunders.

Longest, B. B. (1996). *Seeking strategic advantage through health policy analysis.* Chicago: Health Administration Press.

Longest, B. B. (2006). *Health policymaking in the United States* (4th ed.). Chicago: Health Administration Press.

Medicare. (n.d.). General enrollment and eligibility. Retrieved June 1, 2010, from http://www.medicare.gov/MedicareEligibility/home.asp?dest=NAV%7CHome%7CGeneralEnrollment&version=alternate&browser=IE%7C6%7CWinXP&language=English#TabTop

Medicare Payment Advisory Committee. (2010). Data book: Healthcare spending and the Medicare program. Washington, DC: Author.

Nosse, L. J., Friberg, D. G., & Kovacek, P. R. (1999). *Managerial and supervisory principles for physical therapists.* Baltimore, MD: Williams & Wilkins.

Pifer-Bixler, J. (2009). Study: 86.7 million Americans uninsured over the last two years. Retrieved April 1, 2010, from http://www.cnn.com/2009/HEALTH/03/04/uninsured.epidemic.obama

Relman, A. S. (1988). Assessment and accountability: the third revolution in medical care. *New England Journal of Medicine, 319*(18), 1220–1222.

Roper, W. L., Winkenwerder, W., Hackbarth, G. M., & Krakauer, H. (1988). Effectiveness in health care. An initiative to evaluate and improve medical practice. *New England Journal of Medicine, 319*(18), 1197–1202.

Schecter, D. (2010). COBRA laws and EMTALA. Retrieved at http://emedicine.medscape.com/article/790053-overview

Stahl, M. J. (2004). Health Insurance. In *Encyclopedia of Health Care Management* (pp. 259–261). Thousand Oaks, California: Sage Publications Inc.

Sultz, H. A., & Young, K. M. (2009). *Health care USA* (6th ed.). Sudbury, MA: Jones and Bartlett.

Tieman, J. (2003). Medicare won't raise outlier threshold until Oct. ModernHealthcare Website [On-line]. Available: http://www.modernhealthcare.com

The Associated Press. (2009, September 10). Census Bureau: number of Americans without health insurance rises to 46.3 million. *NY Daily News.* Retrieved from http://www.nydailynews.com/money/personal_finance/2009/09/10/2009-09-10_number_of_americans_without_health_insurance_rises_to_463m.html

CHAPTER 27

Pediatric Rehabilitation

Cyndi Cortes

LEARNING OBJECTIVES

At the end of this chapter, the reader will be able to

- Recognize children with special healthcare needs.
- Discuss important legislation affecting services received by children with special healthcare needs.
- Define family-centered care.
- Describe common conditions seen in pediatric rehabilitation settings and their associated conditions.
- Assess nursing interventions for children seen in pediatric rehabilitation settings.

KEY CONCEPTS AND TERMS

Americans with Disabilities Act	Congenital limb deficiency (CLD)	Family-centered care
Arnold-Chiari II malformation (ACM)	Development	Growth
Becker muscular dystrophy (BMD)	Duchenne muscular dystrophy (DMD)	Individualized education plan
Brachial plexus	Dystrophin	Maturation
Cerebral palsy (CP)	Early and Periodic Screening, Diagnosis, and Treatment Act	Myelomeningocele (MMC)
Children with special healthcare needs (CSHCN)	Education for All Handicapped Children's Act	Neuromuscular disorders
Clean intermittent bladder catheterization	Education of the Handicapped Act	Omnibus Budget Reconciliation Act (OBRA)
Cleft lip	Environment	Pediatric rehabilitation
Cleft palate		Social Security Act
		Spina bifida
		Syrinx
		Youth with special healthcare needs

According to the National Survey of Children with Special Health Care Needs, over 10 million children ages 0 through 17, which is almost 14% of the children in the United States, have a special healthcare need (Child and Adolescent Health Measure Initiative, 2005). Not all CSHCN require rehabilitation services, yet all those requiring rehabilitation services meet the definition of CSHCN.

DEFINITION OF POPULATION

There are multiple ways to describe **children with special healthcare needs (CSHCN)**. Definitions may be based on a list of conditions or diagnostic categories, screening questions, functional limitations, or use of ancillary health services (McPherson et al., 1998; Sloper & Turner, 1993; Wallander et al., 1989a; Wallander & Venters, 1995). Because of the variability of approaches in defining CSHCN, the federal Maternal Child Health Bureau's Division of Services for CSHCN formed a work group to develop a new definition of CSHCN. Their definition states that: "children with special health care needs are those who have or are at increased risk for a chronic physical, developmental, behavioral, or emotional condition and who also require health and related services of a type or amount beyond that required by children generally (McPherson et al., 1998, p. 139).

Legislation Affecting CSHCN

Among the first and significant pieces of U.S. federal legislation providing services for CHSHC was the **Social Security Act**, which was signed into law in 1935. States received federal dollars as outlined in the Social Security Act for the purpose of promoting, improving, and developing maternal–child health services, including services for crippled children (Edwards, 1999; Farel, 1997). Title V of the Social Security Act established the Crippled Children Services; the name of the program changed in 1985 to the Program for Children with Special Health Care Needs (Edwards, 1999).

The manner in which states receive funding for services for CSHCN changed with the passage of the **Omnibus Budget Reconciliation Act (OBRA)** in 1981 by creating Maternal and Child Health Services block grants and consolidating programs (Edwards, 1999). OBRA 1989 amended Title V of the Social Security Act by requiring states to spend 30% of the block grant funds on CSHCN and to develop and improve community-based, family-centered, coordinated care for these children and their families (Edwards, 1999; Farel, 1997). Another feature of OBRA 1989 included the provision of any medically necessary service required to treat any condition identified through the **Early and Periodic Screening, Diagnosis, and Treatment Act** would be covered by Medicaid (Farel, 1997).

The **Education of the Handicapped Act** (PL 91-230) defined handicapped children and allocated funds for them (Edwards, 1999). In 1975, PL 94-142, the **Education for All Handicapped Children's Act**, included amendments to PL 91-230 and provided free and appropriate education in the least restrictive environment for children with disabilities over age 5 years regardless of the severity of their cognitive, physical, or psychosocial problems (Easton, Rens, & Alexander, 1999; Edwards, 1999; Farel, 1997; Taggart & Aguilar, 1999; Urbano, 1992). Additionally, PL 94-142 required children with disabilities to have an **individualized education plan** and established due process for questions of eligibility or extent of services offered (Edwards, 1999; Farel, 1997). Schools were also mandated to provide related services such as medical services for diagnosis and evaluation, health services, therapies, transportation, and special education (Farel, 1997; Urbano, 1992). In 1986 the Education for All Handicapped Children Act was amended (PL 99-457) to include children from birth to age 21 years and included the provision of comprehensive, multidisciplinary early intervention services for children with developmental disabilities from birth through age 2 (Blann, 2005; Edwards, 1999; Farel, 1997; Urbano, 1992). PL 99-457 placed emphasis on family-centered care by requiring professionals to involve families in identifying concerns, goals, and intervention strategies for their children (Urbano, 1992).

The **Americans with Disabilities Act** was passed in 1990 and prohibits discrimination on the basis of disability (Easton et al., 1999; Farel, 1997). The Americans with Disabilities Act is divided into four sections and addresses access of employment, services, accommodations, and telecommunications (Edwards, 1999).

Child Growth and Development and Pediatric Rehabilitation

To help children with either congenital or acquired disabilities meet realistic functional and educational goals, it is important to understand the developmental stages through which children typically progress. **Growth, development**, and **maturation** are dynamic processes and are not complete once the young person reaches the age of 21 (Hertzberg, 1999a). Growth occurs at different rates throughout childhood and is generally defined as an increase in physical size (Molnar & Sobus, 1999). Maturation, on the other hand, refers to the internal regulatory process influencing the acquisition of function by organ systems in children and the manifestation of certain skills and abilities (Hertzberg, 1999a). Development is the qualitative refinement of these skills and abilities (Hertzberg, 1999a; Molnar & Sobus, 1999).

There are multiple theories that focus on specific domains of human development. Some of the most common include Erikson's eight stages of psychosocial developmental, Freud's psychoanalytic theory, Kohlberg's theory of moral development, and Piaget's theory of intellectual development. One of the theories of particular salience in rehabilitation is that of motor development. Gessell and his colleagues described developmental stages through which typically developing children progress based on the maturation of the central nervous system (Hertzberg, 1999a; Molnar & Sobus, 1999). Although these theories are not covered here due to space limitations, it is important for pediatric rehabilitation nurses to understand the natural progression of personality, skills, and functional development in children.

Numerous factors influence patient outcomes in **pediatric rehabilitation**. Children with disabilities either have developmental delays or have lost previously acquired skills as a result of their underlying conditions. As children get older the gap between performance and age expectations widens (Hertzberg, 1999a). Outcomes are often enhanced if children receive rehabilitation services either through early intervention for those with congenital disabilities or those injured before age 3 or as soon after an acquired injury as possible (Hertzberg, 1999a). Other factors affecting children's outcomes or prognosis are the severity, extent, and location of the injury. Children with more extensive damage to the affected area (e.g., brain after a traumatic brain injury or the higher lesions in children with myelomeningocele [MMC] or spinal cord injuries) have less favorable outcomes than children with minor traumatic brain injuries or lower level spinal cord lesions (Hertzberg, 1999a; Molnar & Sobus, 1999).

Children's environments also affect their outcomes. **Environment** is described as "the conditions, circumstances, and influences surrounding and affecting the development of an organism" (Hertzberg, 1999b, p. 97). The family is a very important environmental component. There are sociocultural factors that affect families' structures and role relationships. It is essential for the pediatric rehabilitation nurse to consider each child and family unit when developing appropriate nursing interventions (Hertzberg, 1999c).

Family-Centered Care

One aspect of providing care to the pediatric population is that although the child is the patient, care is provided to the family unit as well. Families need to be considered as a partner in their child's care (Fisher, 2001; Milner, Bungay, Jellinek, & Hall, 1996). In pediatrics, the basis of **family-centered care** is the understanding that the family is the child's primary source of both financial and emotional support (American Academy of Pediatrics, 2003) and the focus in on the families and what they consider important in the treatment and care of the CSHCN (Perrin, Lewkowicz, & Young, 2000).

Adult family members typically have hopes and expectations for their children. They may have dreams of their children's future for physical health and wellness and possibly for financial success. For parents of children with congenital or acquired disabilities, these hopes are challenged (Youngblood, 1999). All family members do not respond in the same way. Responses vary within families as well as among the many families with CSHCN. The pediatric rehabilitation nurse and all other healthcare providers need to be able to respond in a culturally sensitive and appropriate manner to any question the family may have.

Nurses are poised to address important issues and concerns of families. There are several needs families of CSHCN have in common (Table 27.1). First, fami-

TABLE 27.1 Common Needs of Families with a Child with Special Needs
Information about their child's condition
Respite care
Increased social support
A strong family network
Emotional and practical support
Assistance with IEP development
Education about normal growth and development, impact of illness on growth and development, realistic expectations regarding outcomes, positioning, safe transfers, bowel and bladder monitoring, administering medications, skin care and prevention of pressure ulcers, use of adaptive equipment, community resources, and impact of the disease on the child and family
IEP, individualized education plan.

lies often request information about their child's condition (Kerr & McIntosh, 2000; King et al., 2002; Perrin et al., 2000). Condition-specific as well as general information for parents and caregivers of CSHCN should be given and explained in terms family members can understand. Additionally, parents frequently request respite care to give them a short, temporary break from their caregiving responsibilities (Milner et al., 1996; Perrin et al., 2000; Sloper & Turner, 1992). Social support has been found to be a protective factor against psychological distress in caregivers and others (Florian & Findler, 2001; Lynch, 1998; Raina et al., 2004; Seltzer, Greenberg, Floyd, & Hong, 2004) and to be a predictor of parents' well-being (Wallander & Varni, 1998; Wallander & Venters, 1995).

Results from a study by Wallander et al. (1989b) indicated that a larger social support network was also related to better maternal physical health. Florian and Findler (2001) found the family network to contribute positively to the mental health of mothers of children with a chronic condition. Other investigators have also noted that informal support from immediate family members was related to personal well-being (Sloper, 1999; Warfield, Krauss, Hauser-Cram, Upshur, & Shonkoff, 1999). Families may not differ in the amount of assistance they receive from relatives, but for families of CSHCN their need for this help is greater (Weisz & Tomkins, 1996). Pediatric rehabilitation nurses are excellent resources for families and can assist them in finding support services close to where they live.

COMMON CONDITIONS IN PEDIATRIC REHABILITATION

Several conditions seen in children necessitate the need for rehabilitation. Common problems discussed in this chapter include cerebral palsy, spina bifida, neuromuscular disorders, craniofacial anomalies, and congenital limb deformities. Nursing interventions for these problems are also discussed.

Cerebral Palsy

Significance of Problem and Pathophysiology

Cerebral palsy (CP) is a leading cause of childhood disability and is the most common condition resulting in severe physical disabilities (Hutton & Pharoah, 2006). According to the 2005 National Survey of Children Special Health Care Needs approximately 2% of CSHCN have the diagnosis of CP (Child and Adolescent Health Measure Initiative, 2005). CP is a nonprogressive disorder typically resulting from damage to an immature brain and primarily affects movement and coordination (Blosser & Reider-Demer, 2009; Hays, 1999a; Jones, Morgan, & Shelton, 2007a; Matthews & Wilson, 1999; Molnar, 1991). The injury can occur during the prenatal, perinatal, or postnatal periods; however, most are prenatal in origin (Matthews & Wilson, 1999).

Etiology of the clinical manifestations often seen can partly be explained by the fragile brain vasculature and physical stresses of prematurity that predispose them to cerebral blood flow compromise (Matthews & Wilson, 1999). The most common cause of CP in children born prematurely is injury to the periventricular white matter of the brain that often results in intraventricular hemorrhage or periventricular leukomalacia (Jones et al., 2007a).

In addition to prematurity, factors associated with an increased risk of a child having CP include complicated labor and delivery, breech presentation, low Apgar scores (less than 3) at 10 minutes, microcephaly, and exposure to maternal infection (Blosser & Reider-Demer, 2009). However, in almost one-third of children with CP there are no known risk factors (Jones et al., 2007a).

Classification of CP

CP is typically classified according to the clinical presentation of the child's motor deficits (Fennell & Dikel, 2001). Depending on the reference, the most common types are spastic, hypotonic, athetoid or dyskinetic, ataxic, and mixed (Blosser & Reider-Demer, 2009; Hays, 1999c;

Jones et al., 2007a; Matthews & Wilson, 1999). Almost three-fourths of children with CP have the spastic type (Matthews & Wilson, 1999). Damage in the brain's corticospinal pathways are described as upper motor neuron injuries and result in spasticity or increased muscle tone (Jones et al., 2007a). Other manifestations of spastic CP include hyperreflexia, clonus, extensor Babinski response, and persistent primitive reflexes (Jones et al., 2007a; Matthews & Wilson, 1999).

> *Depending on the area of the brain that is affected and the extent of the damage, children with CP may also have nonmotor problems, including cognitive or learning deficits or difficulties; neurosensory and/or perceptual disorders; impaired vision, hearing, and/or speech; swallowing or chewing difficulties; and seizures.*
>
> —Cyndi Cortes, author

Spastic CP is also classified topographically, that is, according to limb involvement (Carroll, 2010; Jones et al., 2007a; Matthews & Wilson, 1999). Half the children classified as having spastic diplegia (both lower extremities affected) were born prematurely, between 28 and 32 weeks' gestation, and many have a history of intraventricular hemorrhages (Jones et al., 2007a; Matthews & Wilson, 1999). All extremities, trunk, and oral musculature are involved in persons with spastic quadriplegic CP, often with greater spasticity in the upper extremities than the lower extremities (Jones et al., 2007a; Matthews & Wilson, 1999). Severe periventricular leukomalacia or a history of intraventricular hemorrhage is often seen in children with spastic quadriplegic CP who were born prematurely (Fennell & Dikel, 2001; Jones et al., 2007a). Severe asphyxia during the perinatal period is common in persons diagnosed with spastic quadriplegic CP (Jones et al., 2007a; Matthews & Wilson, 1999). Spastic hemiplegic CP most often occurs as the result of an intrauterine unilateral cerebrovascular event such as a stroke or intraventricular hemorrhage (Fennell & Dikel, 2001; Jones et al., 2007a; Matthews & Wilson, 1999). Dyskinetic CP is attributed to damage to nerve cells outside of the pyramidal tracts in the basal ganglia or thalamus (Jones et al., 2007a; Matthews & Wilson, 1999). There is abnormal regulation of muscle tone, postural control, and coordination manifested by the involuntary athetoid movements of the extremities or dystonic posturing of the trunk as well as the extremities (Fennell & Dikel, 2001; Hays, 1999a; Jones et al., 2007a; Matthews & Wilson, 1999). This group of cerebral palsies accounts for 15% to 22%

of CP cases (Fennell & Dikel, 2001; Jones et al., 2007a) and is attributed to kernicterus in the early postnatal period or to hypoxic-ischemic encephalopathy (Fennell & Dikel, 2001; Hays, 1999a). Ataxia is a type of dyskinetic CP characterized by unsteadiness and uncoordinated movements (Jones et al., 2007a; Matthews & Wilson, 1999) caused by damage to neurons in the cerebellum (Jones et al., 2007a).

Hypotonic CP is manifested as generalized decreased muscle tone that persists through the age of 3 years (Fennell & Dikel, 2001; Jones et al., 2007a). For a person to be classified with this condition, other primary causes of myopathy and neuropathy have to be excluded (Fennell & Dikel, 2001; Jones et al., 2007a). The etiology of hypotonic CP is unclear; however, it has been suggested that it is the result of delayed development of the cerebellum or the maturation of specific muscle fibers (Fennell & Dikel, 2001). There is a subgroup of children with CP that are classified as mixed CP and have characteristics of both spastic and dyskinetic CP (Fennell & Dikel, 2001; Hays, 1999a; Jones et al., 2007a; Matthews & Wilson, 1999).

Diagnosis

Signs and symptoms of a possible diagnosis of CP include tone abnormalities, delayed motor development, and retention of infant reflexes (Hays, 1999a; Jones et al., 2007a; Molnar, 1991). Hypotonia is a precursor of both spasticity and athetosis or dystonia (Jones et al., 2007a; Molnar, 1991). Serial examinations to monitor neurological and motor development are important to track progress and determine the need for diagnostic imaging to diagnose and predict the clinical course (Jones et al., 2007a; Matthews & Wilson, 1999). Children with severe delays and those with known lesions causing brain damage may be diagnosed as early as 6 months of age (Jones et al., 2007a).

Deficits and Other Disorders Associated With CP

Depending on the area of the brain affected and the extent of damage, children with CP may also have nonmotor problems, including cognitive or learning deficits or difficulties; neurosensory and/or perceptual disorders; impaired vision, hearing, and/or speech; swallowing or chewing difficulties, and seizures (Blosser & Reider-Demer, 2009; Jones et al., 2007a; Molnar, 1991). Almost all children diagnosed with spastic diplegic CP ambulate with or without assistive devices and are independent with activities of daily living (Jones et al., 2007a). However, over half the children with spastic diplegic CP have visual deficits, about one-fourth have a seizure disorder,

and approximately 30% have cognitive impairments (Fennell & Dikel, 2001; Jones et al., 2007a; Matthews & Wilson, 1999). In addition to their motor impairments and lack of independence with activities of daily living, children with spastic quadriplegic CP often have comorbidities. Frequently, children with spastic CP need assistance with feeding/eating and have hearing and visual deficits as well as epilepsy, and in the more severely affected mental retardation is also present (Fennell & Dikel, 2001; Jones et al., 2007a; Matthews & Wilson, 1999; Venkateswaran & Shevell, 2008).

Most children with spastic hemiplegic CP are ambulatory but may have an unequal stride length, flexed hip and knee, and an equinus foot (Matthews & Wilson, 1999). They typically are independent with activities of daily living (Hays, 1999a; Jones et al., 2007a; Matthews & Wilson, 1999). Most persons with spastic hemiplegic CP have normal intelligence, but approximately one-fourth have some degree of cognitive impairment (Matthews & Wilson, 1999). Additionally, children with hemiplegia may have visual, sensory, and perceptual deficits (Hays, 1999a; Jones et al., 2007a; Matthews & Wilson, 1999).

Most the children classified as having dyskinetic CP have normal intelligence but often have sensorineural hearing loss and dysarthric speech (Fennell & Dikel, 2001; Hays, 1999a; Jones et al., 2007a; Matthews & Wilson, 1999). Children with ataxic CP may also have difficulties with oral motor control, poor head control, and tremors (Jones et al., 2007a). Ambulatory children with ataxic CP typically have a wide-based, unsteady gait (Hays, 1999a; Jones et al., 2007a).

Children with hypotonia typically have feeding difficulties secondary to their weak facial and oral muscles (Jones et al., 2007a). They may also have learning disabilities that often involve deficits in motor programming, attentional dysfunction, and slowed motor output (Fennell & Dikel, 2001).

Nursing Interventions

Many children with CP have deficits or disorders involving numerous body systems. Professionals from various disciplines often participate in the management of their care. It is important for children with CP as well as all CSHCN to have a primary healthcare provider to monitor general growth and development and to routinely perform complete systemic physical examinations to exclude other disorders (Jones, Morgan, & Shelton, 2007b).

Pediatric rehabilitation specialists are often involved in the care of children with CP, and specific rehabilitation goals include improving function, encouraging functional independence as much as possible, and developing compensatory strategies (Matthews & Wilson, 1999). Children with CP are at risk for developing pressures sores from wearing splints that become too tight or from immobility. Pediatric rehabilitation nurses can teach parents proper positioning techniques, how to perform skin checks, and the initial treatment of skin breakdown (Jones et al., 2007b). Constipation is often experienced by children with CP, and pediatric rehabilitation nurses work with families to develop a bowel management program.

Children with CP have a lifelong developmental disability, not a disease. Families experience financial strains because of their ongoing need for equipment and supplies, the severity of which depends on insurance coverage (Jones et al., 2007b). Some children with CP may be eligible for Supplemental Social Security or other state benefits (Blosser & Reider-Demer, 2009). Having a child with a severe disability can affect the emotional well-being of other family members (Jones et al., 2007b), and nurses can assist families in obtaining respite care and other appropriate services in their communities (Blosser & Reider-Demer, 2009).

Spina Bifida

Significance of Problem and Pathophysiology

Included under the broad heading of neural tube defects are anencephaly, encephalocele, craniorachischisis, and spina bifida (myelodysplasia or MMC) (Kondo, Kamihira, & Ozawa, 2008). **Spina bifida**, also called spinal dysraphism, is a neuroembryological defect due to failure of the neural tube to fuse around the 28th day of gestation (Jorde, 2010; Zipitis & Pachalides, 2003). Approximately 80% of MMCs are located in either the lumbar or lumbosacral region of the spinal column (Boss & Huether, 2010). **MMC** is characterized by the protrusion of meninges, spinal cord, and nerve roots through the vertebral cord (Adzick, 2010; Jorde, 2010). The abnormal development of the spinal cord results in altered motor and sensory nerve function at and below the level of the defect (Molnar & Murphy, 1999; Shaer, 1997).

Yearly, approximately 1,500 infants are born with spina bifida in the United States, which equates to an incidence of 1 per 2,500 live births (Centers for Disease Control and Prevention [CDC], 2009b). The mortality associated with spina bifida has decreased with folate supplementation, but the 5-year mortality rate is 79 per 1,000 spina bifida births and has been reported to be as high as 35% among children who also have a Chiari II malformation (Sutton, 2008). However, about 78% of individuals with spina bifida survive to the age of 17 years (Mitchell et al., 2004).

Current thought is that neural tube defects arise from a combination of genetic and environmental factors (Jorde, 2010; Kondo et al., 2008; Molnar & Murphy, 1999). Environmental risk factors include a family history of spina bifida, low socioeconomic class, diabetes mellitus, maternal obesity, midspring conception, hyperthermia, and in utero exposure to carbamazepine or valproic acid (Kondo et al., 2008; Mitchell et al., 2004; Molnar & Murphy, 1999). Supplemental folic acid (0.4 mg/day) has been shown to reduce the risk of having a child with a neural tube defect (Kondo et al., 2008; Mitchell et al., 2004; Molnar & Murphy, 1999).

Early surgical closure of the defect is the recommended treatment for the infant with MMC (Boss & Huether, 2010). The prognosis depends on the extent of the defect and the success of the prophylactic and acute treatment and management of any complications (Boss & Huether, 2010). Several pediatric neurosurgeons have performed surgical closure of the defect in utero, in which there was a decreased incidence of hindbrain herniation and a decreased need for ventriculoperitoneal shunt placement when compared with infants undergoing surgical closures postnatally (Mitchell et al., 2004; Sutton, 2008).

Deficits and Other Disorders Associated With Spina Bifida

Most people with spina bifida also have deficits is multiple body systems. About 75% to 90% of children born with spina bifida also have hydrocephalus (Boss & Huether, 2010; Jorde, 2010; Thompson, 2009). Placement of a ventriculoperitoneal shunt in infants with both clinical and radiological evidence of hydrocephalus is done at the same time as the MMC repair, but shunt placement is often deferred in cases of moderate ventricular enlargement (Thompson, 2009). Shunt revisions are common and shunt infections are higher in the MMC group than in other children with hydrocephalus (Shaer, 1997; Thompson, 2009). Another neurological condition seen more frequently in children with MMC and hydrocephalus is seizures. Although only 0.2% of children in the general population are reported to have seizures, the prevalence is 17% in the MMC population (Shaer, 1997).

Many children with MMC also have an **Arnold-Chiari II malformation (ACM)**, which is an abnormality in the brain characterized by a low tentorium insertion, herniation of the posterior fossa content into the upper cervical canal, and a small fourth ventricle (Mitchell et al., 2004; Thompson, 2009; Vinck, Maassen, Mullaart, & Rotteveel, 2006). Symptoms of ACM in infants include central apnea and lower cranial nerve dysfunction, whereas older children complain of headache, neck pain, and sensory disturbance in the limbs (Thompson, 2009).

Many individuals with MMC also have cognitive limitations. Approximately 70% of persons with MMC have an IQ of 80 or more, but only 25% to 38% are capable of employment (Thompson, 2009). These cognitive disabilities and language difficulties also adversely affect their ability to live independently (Mitchell et al., 2004). There is evidence that children with hydrocephalus and shunt infections have more cognitive impairments than children without these conditions (Shaer, 1997; Vinck et al., 2006). Vinck and colleagues (2006) investigated the contribution of ACM on the cognitive profile of children with spina bifida. They found a cognitive impairment pattern consistent with cerebellar damage; individuals with ACM demonstrated deficits in verbal memory, verbal fluency, and visual analysis and synthesis (Vinck et al., 2006).

Other neurosurgical complications in children with MMC include the development of a **syrinx** or a tethered cord. A syrinx is the dilation of the fluid channel in the center of the spinal cord that causes deterioration of function, scoliosis, weakness of the upper extremities, or spasticity (Shaer, 1997). A tethered cord develops when the terminal spinal cord remains imbedded in scar tissue after the initial surgical repair and spinal growth continues and traction is exerted on the spinal cord and nerve roots, leading to ischemic injury and neurological deterioration (Shaer, 1997; Thompson, 2009).

Motor paralysis corresponds to the level of the defect as seen on radiographs and is usually the lower motor neuron type, which is manifested as flaccid weakness and the absence of reflexes (Mitchell et al., 2004; Molnar & Murphy, 1999). Independent ambulation is related to the neurological level of the MMC. Individuals with lesions above L-2 are unlikely to ambulate independently because of the lack of quadriceps and iliopsoas muscle function (Thompson, 2009). Motor milestones are delayed even in those that eventually walk and have relatively mild deficits (Shaer, 1997). Although individuals with MMC sacral defects are typically community ambulators, they continue to demonstrate gross motor and balance problems (Schoenmakers, Gulmans, Gooskens, & Helders, 2004). Braces are usually prescribed once children begin to bear weight on their legs and feet (Shaer, 1997).

Children with MMC often have muscle function imbalance in their trunks and lower extremities that may cause hip subluxation or dislocation; spinal deformities including scoliosis, kyphosis, and lordosis; and foot deformities and contractures (Molnar & Murphy, 1999; Shaer, 1997). Over half the children with spina bifida develop some degree of spinal deformity (Molnar & Murphy, 1999; Shaer, 1997; Thompson, 2009). Possible causes include spinal bony anomaly, neuromuscular imbalance, and spasticity with pelvic and hip deformity (Thompson, 2009). The timing of the surgical intervention is based on the child's age and the progression of the deformity because spinal fusion at an early age results in stunted growth of the torso (Molnar & Murphy, 1999; Shaer, 1997). The specific surgical or bracing recommendations and procedures to treat the other orthopedic conditions associated with MMC depend on the clinical manifestations and individual needs of each child.

Kidney function is typically normal in infants born with MMC, but the nerves that control the bladder and sphincter function are not (Shaer, 1997). Typically, the detrusor (bladder) muscle, bladder neck, and external sphincter work synergistically to store and completely evacuate urine (Verpoorten & Buyse, 2008). In individuals with neurogenic bladder sphincter dysfunction, such as those with MMC, there is disordered innervation of the detrusor musculature and external sphincter (Verpoorten & Buyse, 2008). In lower motor neuron injuries, the detrusor is hyporeflexic and the sensation of bladder filling is impaired, bladder volumes are increased leading to retrograde urine flow, and dilatation of the upper urinary tract from reflux is often seen in lower level MMC lesions (Molnar & Murphy, 1999). Individuals with thoracic lesions are more likely to have hypertonic bladders due to the inadequacy of the sphincter closure mechanism, resulting in incontinence (Molnar & Murphy, 1999). These individuals are at increased risk for developing upper urinary tract dysfunction, urinary tract infections, and renal failure if they have high intravesical pressure because the glomerular filtration rate decreases and ureteral drainage deteriorates, which leads to hydronephrosis and/or vesicoureteral reflux (Verpoorten & Buyse, 2008).

Renal damage can occur within the first 6 months of life, which supports maintaining low bladder pressure from birth (deJong, Chrzan, Klijn, & Dik, 2008). During infancy the primary goals of urological management are protection of the upper urinary tracts and control of urinary tract infections (Thompson, 2009). Individuals with spina bifida are at increased risk of either having an overactive pelvic floor or a paralyzed pelvic floor; therefore, it is recommended that bladder activity, capacity, and compliance be monitored yearly with urodynamic studies (deJong et al., 2008). An overactive pelvic floor or insufficient bladder compliance and low capacity is treated with augmentation surgery, **clean intermittent bladder catheterization**, and anticholinergic agents such as oxybutynin (deJong et al., 2008; Verpoorten & Buyse, 2008). However, there are long- and short-term complications associated with bladder augmentation surgery, which should first be explained and discussed with patients and families (Thompson, 2009). Individuals with a paralyzed pelvic floor are incontinent of urine and may benefit from bladder neck surgery to maintain dryness, and detrusor overactivity is treated with medications to increase bladder capacity (deJong et al., 2008; Verpoorten & Buyse, 2008). The creation of a catheterizable stoma may be indicated for those that need to transfer from a wheelchair to perform clean intermittent bladder catheterization; however, as many as half of those who have the surgery report complications (deJong et al., 2008).

Several factors contribute to children with MMC not having control of their bowel functions. Innervation of the muscular layers of the intestines, rectal sphincter, and sensation in the skin of the perirectal area come from the sacral nerves, which are dysfunctional; peristalsis is slowed because the intestinal wall muscles are not well stimulated, which compounds the problem (Shaer, 1997). Although the gastrocolic and inhibitory reflexes are present, the urge to defecate is not (Tobias, Mason, Lutkenhoff, Stoops, & Ferguson, 2008). Constipation is often present due to the increased transit time, which results in too much water being resorbed from the stool (Shaer, 1997; Tobias et al., 2008).

A bowel program or regimen is developed with the children and their caregivers, and a developmental approach is often used. A combination of healthy nutrition with foods high in fiber and sufficient amounts of liquids, exercise or activity, and medications, including stool softeners or laxatives, are used to encourage regularly scheduled bowel movements. When scheduled toileting, diet, activity, and medications do not have the desired results, high-volume saline solution enemas may be used (Tobias et al., 2008). Older children may also benefit from a surgical procedure to create a conduit between the cecum and the skin and an abdominal stoma through which an antegrade colonic enema can be administered (deJong et al., 2008; Tobias et al., 2008).

Many children with MMC are also overweight or obese. Factors contributing to their excessive weight gain include decreased energy expenditure due to muscle paralysis and physical inactivity. (Molnar & Murphy, 1999). They are already at risk for skin breakdown and the development of pressure sores. Obesity increases the risk of decubiti as well as upper extremity stress with physical activity, which leads to being less physically active (Molnar & Murphy, 1999).

Another issue faced by individuals with MMC is latex allergy. Approximately 70% of persons with MMC have tested positive when screened for a latex allergy and about one-fourth have developed overt symptoms (Shaer, 1997). Many products contain latex, and it is important that families receive education materials for themselves and for them to share with others such as school personnel who have contact with and provide care and services for their children.

Nursing Interventions

Pediatric rehabilitation nurses working with children with spina bifida and their families play a significant role in educating them and assisting them to become independent in the areas of skin assessment and care and also with bladder and bowel management (Table 27.2). Most children with spina bifida can learn to assess their skin daily to determine its integrity. This is an important skill to learn because these children are at increased risk for skin breakdown due to immobility, sensory loss, possible altered nutritional status, and the presence of shearing forces, friction, or pressure (Harvey & Kerr, 1999). The pediatric rehabilitation nurse and other healthcare professionals assist the child and family to learn pressure relief techniques, reduce friction and shearing injuries, and maintain passive range of motion (Harvey & Kerr, 1999) There are multiple options for bladder and bowel management programs. Often, the nurse educates families on the particular plan for their child. Teaching typically includes diet and exercise regimens, how to administer pharmacological agents, and how to perform clean intermittent bladder catheterization (Harvey & Kerr, 1999; Mitchell et al., 2004).

Neuromuscular Disorders

Significance of Problem and Pathophysiology

Skeletal muscle weakness is the distinguishing symptom of **neuromuscular disorders** and is attributed to disease of the anterior horn cell, spinal roots, muscular fiber, peripheral nerves, or neuromuscular junction (Hays,

TABLE 27.2   Additional Nursing Strategies in the Care of the Child with a Neuromuscular Disorder

Teaching

- Positioning
- Safe transfers
- Prevention of constipation
- Appropriate nutrition
- Skin assessment and care
- Exercise regimen
- Bowel and bladder management (may include performing CIBC)
- Administration of medication and/or feedings
- Use of adaptive equipment
- Chest physiotherapy and assistive coughing

Other

- Care coordination
- Social support
- Providing emotional support and education
- Referring appropriately to rehab psychologist/psychiatrist
- Assisting with IEP development
- Advocacy and liaison services between the family, school, and community

CIBC, clean intermittent bladder catheterization; IEP, individualized education plan.

1999c). Muscle wasting leads to death of the muscle cells and replacement by fibrosis and fat (CDC, 2009a). Neuromuscular diseases can be hereditary or acquired and can result in abnormalities in one anatomical region or can affect multiple body systems (McDonald, 1999). Discussion of neuromuscular disorders in this chapter focuses on Duchenne and Becker muscular dystrophies.

Duchenne Muscular Dystrophy

Duchenne muscular dystrophy (DMD) is the most common neuromuscular disorder (Blake & Kroger, 2000; CDC, 2009a; Zebracki & Drotar, 2008). It is an X-linked recessive inherited disorder caused by an abnormality at the Xp21 gene loci (McDonald, 1999) and affects approximately 1 in 3,300 to 3,500 live male births (Anderson, Head, Rae, & Morley, 2002; Blake & Kroger, 2000; CDC, 2009a; Poysky, 2007; Yiu & Kornberg, 2008). A small percent of female carriers show manifestations of DMD, and some females are diagnosed with DMD (Bushby et al., 2010a). Mutations in the dystrophin gene result in an absence of **dystrophin** or a nonfunctional dystrophin

protein (Anderson et al., 2002; Poysky, 2007). Dystrophin is the primary protein product and is found in the plasma membrane of all muscle cells (McDonald, 1999). A lack of dystrophin corresponds with poorly anchored skeletal muscle fibers that with repeated contraction tear themselves apart (Carroll, 2010). The dystrophin gene has a high mutation rate, and almost one-third of newly diagnosed cases of DMD are the result of a spontaneous mutation (Anderson et al., 2002). A skewed X (chromosome) inactivation is believed to be the cause of most DMD in females (Bushby et al., 2010a).

The most common presenting symptoms are motor delays such as walking, falling frequently or having difficulty climbing stairs, or an abnormal "waddling" or toe walking gait (Bushby et al., 2010a; Yiu & Kornberg, 2008; Zebracki & Drotar, 2008). DMD is diagnosed around age 5, but muscle weakness is often apparent earlier (Anderson et al., 2002; Bushby et al., 2010a; CDC, 2009a). Another clinical manifestation of DMD and Becker muscular dystrophy (BMD) is the focal increase in the calf circumference due to fat and connective tissue, not to muscle fiber hypertrophy (Carroll, 2010; McDonald, 1999). Another classic symptom exhibited is "Gower's sign" due to proximal weakness of the pelvic girdle that causes children to use their arms to push off from their legs and then proceed to a standing position in a segmented fashion (Bazner-Chandler & Brady, 2009; Bushby et al., 2010a; Carroll, 2010).

In disorders involving injury to muscle fibers, serum creatine kinase levels are elevated. In the early stages of DMD and BMD, creatine kinase values are significantly elevated and may be 50 to 100 times the normal value (McDonald, 1999; Yiu & Kornberg, 2008). As children with DMD and BMD get older, creatine kinase values decrease. Genetic studies are recommended by clinical experts treating patients with neuromuscular diseases. Muscle biopsies provide specific information about the actual molecular size and total or partial absence of dystrophin (Bushby et al., 2010a). The results from these tests allow appropriate information to be given during genetic counseling with patients and families (Bushby et al., 2010a; McDonald, 1999).

Becker Muscular Dystrophy

BMD is similar to DMD, however, it has a later onset and the progression of symptoms is slower and more variable (CDC, 2009a). BMD has the same gene location as DMD. A diagnosis of BMD is suspected when the levels of dystrophin are either 20% to 80% of expected values or there are normal levels of dystrophin and an abnormal molecular weight of dystrophin (McDonald, 1999). Birth prevalence is estimated at 0.5 per 10,000 male births (CDC, 2009a).

Deficits and Other Disorders Associated With DMD and BMD

Muscle weakness is progressive and can be seen in the neck flexors in preschool children with DMD (McDonald, 1999). Independent ambulation is lost, and the use of a wheelchair for mobility occurs between ages 7 and 13 years in children with DMD, whereas those with BMD typically remain ambulatory after age 16 (Bushby et al., 2010a; McDonald, 1999). Musculoskeletal conditions seen in children with DMD include contractures and scoliosis, which in turn adversely affect mobility as well as bed and wheelchair positioning. Orthoses, adaptive equipment, and/or surgery may be required to minimize the development of contractures and deformities (Zebracki & Drotar, 2008). Contractures develop when there is no longer the ability to perform active range of motion and muscles remain in a flexed position. In children with DMD, there is also an imbalance about the joint and fibrotic changes in the muscle (Bushby et al., 2010b). Therefore, joint contractures are seen in most children with DMD over age 13 years in spite of performing range of motion and stretching exercises and wearing appropriate orthotics (Bushby et al., 2005, 2010b; McDonald, 1999).

Most children with DMD develop clinically significant scoliosis (Bushby et al., 2005, 2010b; McDonald, 1999; Yiu & Kornberg, 2008) between ages 12 and 15 years that corresponds with their adolescent growth spurt (McDonald, 1999). Serial spine radiographs should be obtained to monitor the progression of the scoliotic curve (Bushby et al., 2005, 2010b; McDonald, 1999; Yiu & Kornberg, 2008). Spinal deformities are not as common in BMD (McDonald, 1999). Fractures are also common in children with DMD, and those on glucocorticoid treatment have a higher incidence of fractures (Bushby et al., 2010b; Yiu & Kornberg, 2008). Another consideration is that children with DMD report pain that is most often described as aching (Bushby et al., 2010b; McDonald, 1999; Zebracki & Drotar, 2008).

A progressive loss of respiratory muscle strength is part of the natural history of DMD (Bushby et al., 2005, 2010b; McDonald, 1999; Yiu & Kornberg, 2008). The earliest indicators of restrictive pulmonary compromise in DMD are the maximal static airway pressures (McDonald, 1999), and progressive fall in forced vital capacity predicts the development of respiratory failure (Bushby et al., 2005). Children with DMD typically begin to show a linear decline in forced vital capacity between ages 10 and 20 years (McDonald, 1999). Compromised pulmonary function is less problematic in BMD, and forced vital capacity does not usually decline until the third or fourth decade of life in individuals with BMD (McDonald, 1999). Respiratory infections are common in the DMD population and are typically managed with aggressive antibiotic therapy, chest physiotherapy, manual and mechanically assisted cough, as well as noninvasive positive pressure ventilation (Bushby et al., 2005, 2010b; Yiu & Kornberg, 2008). As their respiratory function decreases, assisted ventilation options should be discussed with the family and a plan of care established. Individuals with DMD usually die before age 30 from respiratory or cardiac muscle failure (Blake & Kroger, 2000).

Because dystrophin protein is present in the myocardium and cardiac Purkinje fibers, cardiomyopathy and/or cardiac arrhythmias are frequent complications of DMD and BMD (Bushby et al., 2005, 2010b; McDonald, 1999; Yiu & Kornberg, 2008). Sinus tachycardia is commonly seen in DMD (Bushby et al., 2010b), and ventricular ectopy is a known complication of the condition (Bushby et al., 2005; McDonald, 1999). Clinical experts recommend annual cardiology visits for complete cardiac assessments beginning around 10 years of age (Bushby et al., 2010b; Yiu & Kornberg, 2008). Individuals receiving glucocorticoids require additional hypertension monitoring and potential adjustment in their glucocorticoid dose (Bushby et al., 2010b). The most common electrocardiographic abnormalities in persons with BMD are abnormal Q-waves, right and left ventricular hypertrophy, right bundle branch block, and nonspecific T-wave abnormalities (McDonald, 1999).

There are several gastrointestinal issues in children with DMD. Some of those affected with DMD are thin and have difficulty gaining weight, whereas others are obese (Bushby et al., 2005, 2010b; McDonald, 1999). Many report constipation and may require the use of stool softeners, laxatives, and encouraging more liquids in their diet (Bushby et al., 2005, 2010b; Yiu & Kornberg, 2008). Gastroesophageal reflux and other signs and symptoms of upper gastrointestinal dysfunction are commonly seen with DMD, and acid blockers are routinely prescribed for those taking glucocorticosteroids (Bushby et al., 2010b; McDonald, 1999). Swallowing difficulties may also be experienced as the condition advances. Dysphagia leads to an increased risk of aspiration and the ability to consume (orally) enough nutrition to maintain an appropriate weight (Bushby et al., 2010b).

Numerous studies have been conducted investigating the relationship between the absence of dystrophin and cognitive impairment. The average IQ range for boys with DMD is between 80 and 85, and approximately one-third of boys have IQs less than 70, in the range of mental retardation (Anderson et al., 2002; Poysky, 2007; Yiu & Kornberg, 2008). It has also been found that children with DMD are at increased risk for dyslexia, dyscalculia, and dysgraphia (Poysky, 2007). This population appears to have more deficits in the verbal components of IQ tests, and they demonstrate poorer reading abilities and processing skills when compared with children with other neuromuscular disorders (Blake & Kroger, 2000). Research studies have also shown that boys with muscular dystrophy have social and communication difficulties and are at increased risk for neurodevelopmental disorders including autism spectrum disorder, attention deficit hyperactivity disorder, and obsessive-compulsive disorder (Bushby et al., 2010a; Poysky, 2007). Children with BMD do not typically have the mental changes as seen in children with DMD (Carroll, 2010).

Another area of concern in children with DMD is psychosocial adjustment. It has been observed that poorer adjustment scores occur between ages 8 and 10, which corresponds to the time in the disease process where physical function decreases, and many require the use of a wheelchair for mobility (Poysky, 2007). Overall, adjustment scores improved with age except in the area of peer relations, which became more problematic as boys got older (Poysky, 2007). Pharmacological treatment, in addition to behavior management plans and educational interventions, of moderate to severe psychiatric symptoms is an option to discuss with the children's parents (Bushby et al., 2010a).

Management

A multidisciplinary team approach is recommended in the treatment of individuals with DMD/BMD and in the management of all possible complications associated with these conditions. Physical and occupational therapists often work with children with muscular dystrophies to help maintain muscle function and delay the development of contractures (Bushby et al., 2010a; Yiu & Kornberg, 2008).

The use of steroids has changed the natural history of DMD by prolonging independent ambulation, preventing severe scoliosis, and preserving cardiac and pulmonary function (Bushby et al., 2005, 2010a; McDonald, 1999; Poysky, 2007). There are no established guidelines as to when glucocorticosteroid therapy should be initiated. Cli-

nicians advocate that children receive all recommended immunizations, establish immunity to varicella, and reach a plateau in the area of gaining motor skills before beginning steroid therapy (Bushby et al., 2010a). Other factors influence the decision to add glucocorticoids to the treatment regimen for children with DMD, and all risk factors and adverse side effects should be discussed with parents before the drug is prescribed (Bushby et al., 2010a).

> *The use of steroids has changed the natural history of DMD by prolonging independent ambulation, preventing severe scoliosis, and preserving cardiac and pulmonary function (Bushby et al., 2005, 2010a; McDonald, 1999; Poysky, 2007).*

Nursing Interventions

There are many educational needs of families of children with DMD/BMD. Pediatric rehabilitation nurses have the knowledge and expertise to assist these families to understand the natural progression of the condition and then refer them for needed services in their own communities. Nurses can assist families by teaching appropriate positioning techniques, demonstrating how to transfer their child safely, assisting with monitoring elimination and developing appropriate bowel and bladder plans, teaching chest percussion and assisted cough, and making referral for other support services (Hays, 1999c). An individual education plan should be developed in collaboration with parents and school personnel to address learning problems (Bushby et al., 2010a) Care coordination is often needed as families may be overwhelmed with the day-to-day issues of caring for children with multiple physical and socialemotional needs (see Table 27.2).

> *Skeletal muscle weakness is the distinguishing symptom of neuromuscular disorders and is attributed to disease of the anterior horn cell, spinal roots, muscular fiber, peripheral nerves, or neuromuscular junction.*
>
> —*Cyndia Cortes, author*

Craniofacial Anomalies: Cleft Lip and Cleft Palate

Significance of Problem and Pathophysiology

The most common craniofacial anomalies are **cleft lip** and **cleft palate**. Cleft lip occurs as the result of the embryonic structures surrounding the oral cavity not joining, and cleft palate occurs if the palatal shelves do not fuse (Gaylord & Yetman, 2009). The incidence for cleft lip with or without cleft palate is about 1 per 1,000 births, and the incidence of cleft palate alone is approximately 1 per 2,500 births (Hays, 1999b). Possible etiologies of cleft lip and cleft palate include genetic as well as environmental and lifestyle factors such as parenteral drug use, smoking, and folic acid deficiency (Huether, 2010; Jaruatanasirikul, Chichareon, Pattanapreechawong, & Sangsupavanich, 2008). These factors reduce the amount of neural crest mesenchyme that develops into the face of the embryo, and if the amount is reduced sufficiently, clefting results (Huether, 2010).

Oral clefting may be associated with other congenital anomalies and is seen in several syndromes such as trisomy 13 (Hays, 1999b; Jaruatanasirikul et al., 2008). Cleft lip is caused by the incomplete fusion of the nasomedial or intermaxillary process and is usually located beneath the center of one nostril (Huether, 2010). Cleft palate, on the other hand, results from the failure of the primary palatal shelves to fuse during the third month of gestation (Huether, 2010). Severity of the cleft can range from a small notch in the lip to bilateral clefting of both the lip and the palate resulting in nasal distortion (Hays, 1999b).

Diagnosis

Cleft lip and cleft palate may be diagnosed prenatally with ultrasonography during the last trimester or during the newborn physical assessment (Hays, 1999b). If not diagnosed before an infant's birth, a cleft lip is observed clinically once the face is visible during the birth process (Hays, 1999b). Infants identified with craniofacial anomalies should be referred to a genetic specialist to determine if the defect is related to a specific syndrome (Hays, 1999b).

Deficits and Other Disorders Associated With Cleft Lip or Cleft Palate

There are often dental issues such as supernumerary, deformed, or absent teeth that result from the cleft (Hays, 1999b). Additionally, children may have articulation problems and hearing loss as well as frequent middle ear, nasopharyngeal, and sinus infections (Gaylord & Yetman, 2009; Hays, 1999b; Huether, 2010). Children born with cleft palate are more likely to have hearing difficulties that could be attributed to frequent otitis media (Hays, 1999b). It has also been reported that growth parameters tend to be lower in children with cleft palate with or without cleft lip when compared with children with cleft lip alone (Jaruatanasirikul et al., 2008). Children born with cleft lip and/or cleft palate usually do not have developmental delays unless there were difficulties

with the management of middle ear disease or feeding problems were not resolved early (Hays, 1999b).

Management

Children with cleft lip and cleft palate benefit from a team approach to the management of their multidisciplinary needs. If the palate is intact, infants with a simple cleft lip should be able to nurse; if the lips cannot be pursed, the tongue must work harder (Huether, 2010). For infants with cleft palate to obtain proper nutrition, special nipples and feeding techniques are recommended (Gaylord & Yetman, 2009; Huether, 2010). Surgical repair of cleft lip is usually done within the first 10 weeks of life, and repair of the cleft palate typically occurs before the child's first birthday (Hays, 1999b; Huether, 2010). Evaluation by a speech-language pathologist every 3 months during the first year of life to monitor the child's speech development is recommended (Hays, 1999b).

Nursing Interventions

Pediatric nurses whether in the primary care setting or in a specialty practice are valuable assets to the team caring for the child with cleft lip and /or cleft palate. They assist the parents in establishing a safe and effective nurturing and feeding plan, teach proper feeding positions and techniques, offer anticipatory guidance concerning child growth and development, provide emotional support to families, and refer families for other appropriate services as needed (Hays, 1999b). Consider the situation in Case Study 27.1.

Congenital Limb Deficiencies

Significance and Pathophysiology

Congenital limb deficiency (CLD) occurs when part or all of the limb bud does not form (Gaebler-Spira & Uellendahl, 1999) and is associated with teratogenic exposures, such as thalidomide during pregnancy and chorionic villus sampling prenatally (Gaebler-Spira & Uellendahl, 1999; Hertzberg, 1999c; McGuirk, Westgate, & Holmes, 2001). Infants affected by thalidomide typically have a symmetrical pattern of deficiency or polydactyly, whereas those affected by chorionic villus sampling present with asymmetrical digit loss, constriction rings, and syndactyly (McGuirk et al., 2001). Other causes of CLD or limb reduction defects include hereditary disorders, maternal diabetes, and vascular disruption (McGuirk et al., 2001). The cause of the CLD is not always known or determined. Incidence has reportedly remained stable over the last 30 to 40 years at 26 per 100,000 live births (National Limb Loss Information Center, 2008).

Joan Santiago is a 33-year old new mother whose first child is being adopted from Guatemala. The baby, Lucy, was born with severe cleft lip and cleft palate, which will be surgically repaired after she is brought home to the United States. As a single parent of an infant with special health needs, Joan is concerned about her ability to care for her new daughter. If you were a pediatric rehabilitation nurse, how would you advise Joan regarding her following questions?

Questions

1. What is the best time to do the surgery?
2. What are the long-term implications of Lucy's condition?
3. Are there special things I will need in order to feed her? What do I need to know and where can I get this information? Are there any resources that can help me understand this condition better?
4. Will my daughter ever look normal?
5. What type of rehabilitation will she need after surgery?
6. Are there any support groups in my area for new adoptive mothers who have children with special needs such as this?

The International Society for Prosthetics and Orthotics classification system categorizes all deformities as either transverse or longitudinal (Gaebler-Spira & Uellendahl, 1999). In congenital transverse deficiencies there is complete absence of part of the limb and the appearance is that of a stump seen after an amputation (Jain & Lakhtakia, 2002). These deficiencies are defined according to the last remaining bone segment (Kozin, 2003). A longitudinal bone deficiency has remaining distal portions and is caused by shortening or incomplete bone development (Gaebler-Spira & Uellendahl, 1999; Hertzberg, 1999c).

Many congenital upper limb deficiencies occur as isolated sporadic events and do not have hereditary implications (Gaebler-Spira & Uellendahl, 1999; Hertzberg, 1999c). However, radial deficiency is also seen in five syndromes (Gaebler-Spira & Uellendahl, 1999):

1. Thrombocytopenia with absence of the radius
2. Fanconi syndrome—anemia and leucopenia
3. Holt-Oram syndrome—congenital heart disease
4. Baller-Gerold syndrome—craniosynostosis
5. VACTERL—multiorgan system involvement (Vertebral, Anal atresia, Cardiac, TracheoEsophageal atresia, Renal, Limb)

Fibular longitudinal deficiency is the most common congenital lower limb deficiency (Gaebler-Spira & Uellendahl, 1999).

Management

The goals of treatment for children with limb deficiencies are to make the limb as functional as possible and to promote development and adaptive skills (Hertzberg, 1999b). There are multiple types of prostheses. Often, parents prefer prostheses that look like normal limbs and choose initial prostheses based on appearance instead of on functional qualities; however, once they have adjusted to the limb deficiency, functionality is considered in prostheses selection (Gaebler-Spira & Uellendahl, 1999). Consideration should also be given to the size and weight of the child in relation to that of the prosthesis (Hertzberg, 1999b). Once the child is a preschooler and can operate prosthetic components, the focus should be on selecting the prosthesis that meets the needs of the individual child (Gaebler-Spira & Uellendahl, 1999). Lower extremity prostheses should be fitted when children are ready to pull up to a standing position and should accommodate for changing gait patterns of children (Gaebler-Spira & Uellendahl, 1999).

Nursing Interventions

Parents should be encouraged to treat their children with CLD in the same way they treat a child without a CLD (Gaebler-Spira & Uellendahl, 1999). It has been speculated that children with CLD are at increased risk for psychological and social adjustment problems because of the chronic strain associated with visible physical differences (Bond, Kent, Binney, & Saleh, 1999). Additionally, self-perceived physical appearance is related to depressive and anxious symptoms, which places children with CLD at increased risk for these symptoms (Gaebler-Spira & Uellendahl, 1999). Children with CLD who master developmental tasks and receive positive feedback are more likely to develop positive self-esteem (Hertzberg, 1999b). Bond and colleagues (1999) found that children attending a prosthetic clinic had adjustment scores better than the general population. There were several limitations to this study, and additional research is needed in the area of psychosocial adjustment, not just for children with CLD but for CSHCN in general.

Brachial Plexus Injury

The **brachial plexus** innervates all muscles of the upper extremity except the trapezius (Ruchelsman, Pettrone, Price, & Grossman, 2009). Congenital brachial palsy is believed to occur from trauma to the brachial plexus at birth resulting in stretching, rupture, or avulsion of some, or all, of the cervical and first thoracic nerve roots (Evans-Jones et al., 2003; McAbee & Ciervo, 2006). Paralysis of the upper trunk muscles is seen in C5–6, and infants present with weakness of shoulder elevation and external rotation, absent biceps, and shoulder internal rotation and elbow extension (Ruchelsman et al., 2009). There is also weakness of the triceps, wrist extension, and sometimes thumb weakness in lesions involving C5-6-7 (Ruchelsman et al., 2009). The incidence of congenital brachial palsy is estimated to be between 0.1% and 0.4% of live births (Evans-Jones et al., 2003; Ruchelsman et al., 2009). Several risk factors have been identified and include large birth weight, breech presentation, shoulder dystocia, prolonged second stage of labor, vacuum or forceps delivery, multiparity, and maternal diabetes (Evans-Jones et al., 2003; McAbee & Ciervo, 2006; Ruchelsman et al., 2009).

Recovery prognosis for infants with congenital brachial palsy is associated with the severity of the motor deficit; the less severe the motor deficit, the less likely there will be permanent significant weakness (McAbee & Ciervo, 2006). Many infants have spontaneous ongoing recovery with observation alone (Ruchelsman et al., 2009). The focus of initial therapeutic management is appropriate splinting and careful passive range of motion exercises to prevent contractures and reduce the need for future orthopedic surgery (McAbee & Ciervo, 2006). Several neurosurgical interventions, such as grafting of the affected nerves or nerve transfers, may be appropriate for infants over 3 months old with brachial palsies (McAbee & Ciervo, 2006). However, failure to recover antigravity function of the biceps by 6 months of age is a poor prognostic sign (Ruchelsman et al., 2009).

Common Acquired Conditions in Children

Trauma-related injuries also affect children and youth. This chapter does not include child-specific information on amputations, burns, spinal cord injuries, or traumatic brain injuries because entire chapters in this textbook are devoted to these topics. The same rationale was used in the decision not to include specific pediatric rehabilitation information on childhood cancer and strokes.

ROLE OF THE PEDIATRIC REHABILITATION NURSE

Regardless of their children's diagnoses, parents often report difficulties navigating the healthcare system, being an advocate for their children, understanding the trajectory of the disorder(s), and accessing equipment and services their children need (McNelis, Buelow, Myers, & Johnson, 2007). Caregivers of CSHCN have had to learn a very complicated healthcare system; some have been more successful than others. CSHCN are less likely to receive comprehensive health care and related services than children without special healthcare needs (Strickland et al., 2004), and many families of CSHCN report they have problems obtaining referrals for specialty care.

Nurse as Educator

Nurses working in pediatric rehabilitation have a working knowledge about the various conditions as well as the treatment and pharmacological modalities available for the patients with whom they work. Additionally, both parents and children report not having needed information about their condition and plan of treatment (McNelis et al., 2007; Urbano, 1992). Nurses have access to child-specific data as well as general disease/condition information and can provide detailed educational materials to the CSHCN, their parents, and teachers and other school personnel.

Nurse as Case Manager/Care Coordinator

Care coordination is a comprehensive and collaborative process that assesses plans and implements, coordinates, monitors, and evaluates the needs and available services of CSHCN, who often require multiple referrals to specialty care services (Antonelli & Antonelli, 2004; Kastner, 2004; Strickland et al., 2004). Many parents report that having a professional, such as a nurse, provide knowledgeable and supportive guidance is very satisfying to the family and also to the nurse, and they acknowledged the expert advice they received to help them navigate the healthcare system was beneficial (Burke, Kauffmann, Harrison, & Wiskin, 1999).

Psychosocial Interventions Provided by Nurses

In addition to the typical stressors of parenthood, parents of children with disabilities experience additional stressors related to their children's diagnoses (Burke et al., 1999; Kerr & McIntosh, 2000). Parents of CSHCN also have to cope with uncertainties about their children's

---

BOX 27.1   Web Exploration

Browse the following websites for information and services for CSHCN:

Child and Adolescent Health Measure Initiative (CAMHI)
http://nschdata.org/viewdocument.aspx?item=256

CDC, spina bifida
http://www.cdc.gov/ncbddd/birthdefects/SpinaBifida.htm

National Limb Loss Information Center (2008). Fact Sheet
http://www.amputee-coalition.org/fact_sheets/amp_stats_cause.html

---

health and prognosis as well as the extra workload involved with having a CSHCN (Barnett, Clements, Kaplan-Estrin, & Fialka, 2003). It has been consistently found that families of CSHCN receiving emotional and practical support cope better with both the acute and chronic phases of the child's condition (Barnett et al., 2003; Lynch, 1998; Pearlin, Mullan, Semple, & Skaff, 1990; Weisz & Tomkins, 1996). Talking with other parents who have children with similar disabilities can provide them with emotional support and help them begin to resolve feelings of anxiety, anger, and depression (Kerr & McIntosh, 2000). Nurses working in pediatric rehabilitation can serve as liaisons between families (Box 27.1).

CSHCN exhibit higher rates of behavioral and emotional disorders than children without special healthcare needs (Klassen et al., 2004; Silver, Stein, & Bauman, 1999; Woolfson, 2004).

Woolfson (2004) reported that parents of CSHCN (with cerebral palsy) were five times more likely to report child behavior problems than parents of children without special healthcare needs. Studies investigating factors influencing adjustment or psychological well-being in family caregivers suggest that caregivers of CSHCN who also have behavior problems report poorer adjustment than caregivers of CSHCN who do not have behavior problems (Barakat & Linney, 1992).

ROLE OF THE COMMUNITY AND AGENCIES IN THE LIFE OF A CSHCN

Early Intervention

Early intervention services are provided to children from birth to 3 years of age who have developmental delays or are at risk for delays (Blann, 2005). These services are federally funded entitlement programs administered in each state as part of the Individuals with Disabilities Education Act (Blann, 2005; Edwards, 1999). Children are referred to an early intervention program through "Child Find,"

which is designed to locate, identify, and refer all young children needing early intervention services (Blann, 2005). The goal of early intervention services is to maximize the child's development through therapies, education, nursing, social work, and care coordination services that are child and parent focused (Blann, 2005).

School

Inclusion in school and community activities varies according to the disability. For example, providing school accommodations is relatively easy for those with CLD as opposed to children with more severe conditions. It is important to begin to plan for appropriate educational placement before the CSHCN enters school. Often, the early intervention care coordinator can help with this process. Some CSHCN require psychological assessment because intellectual functioning is often the deciding factor in the most appropriate classroom placement setting (Molnar, 1991). The school should make adaptations to the classroom environment to accommodate the CSHCN as required by law (Molnar, 1991).

Transition to Adulthood

Transitioning to adulthood, including finding adult health care, is often very difficult for **youth with special healthcare needs** and their families. Only one in seven youth with special healthcare needs typically receives all the Maternal Child Health Bureau's recommended service components, and adult healthcare services are generally more fragmented (O'Conner-Von, Looman, Lindeke, Garwick, & Leonard, 2009). Often, CSHCN were enrolled in early intervention programs and received special services through their school systems, but as these children transition into adulthood the availability of services for special needs decreases, and many have difficulty obtaining primary and routine health care. There are multiple obstacles to the process, such as the lack of formalized linkages between agencies and pediatric and adult service providers and a poor understanding of interagency partners (Rearick, 2007). Pediatric rehabilitation nurses can assist these youth and their parents to plan for transition and then guide them through the implementation process (Blomquist, 2007). One approach is for nurses to serve as the transition service coordinator. Nurses in this role assist with care coordination, provide clinical expertise to families, and collaborate with the other professionals involved in the youth's care (Rearick, 2007).

It has been reported that youth with special healthcare needs use the emergency room at almost double the rates of youth without special health care needs

(Blomquist, 2006). Therefore, rehabilitation nurses that work as members of a transition team can also assist the youths and their families to find appropriate primary healthcare services in their communities and educate them on preventive healthcare activities (Blomquist, 2006, 2007). Rehabilitation nurses can work with patients and families to maintain a portable up-to-date medical summary (Blomquist, 2007).

SUMMARY

The content in this focused on CSHCN in a variety of settings. Some of the most common disease processes among children and youth pose enormous challenges for pediatric rehabilitation nurses. Education of the child and family members is essential to obtaining and maintaining positive outcomes in these difficult situations. Family-centered case should be a part of all pediatric rehabilitation nursing interventions.

CRITICAL THINKING

1. What are the individual challenges faced by children and families struggling with Duchenne and Becker muscular dystrophies? In what ways can pediatric rehabilitation nurses help to alleviate some of the inherent difficulties associated with these diseases?
2. When caring for a CSHCN who has been diagnosed with spina bifida, what other considerations, in addition to the early surgical closure of the defect in infants with MMC, can be taken to maximize cognitive, ambulatory, and motor functions?
3. Briefly describe and give examples of the various roles of the pediatric rehabilitation nurse in each of the scenarios presented in this chapter (e.g., cases of spina bifida, MMC, DMD, BMD, and CLD).

PERSONAL REFLECTION

- Imagine you are a first-time parent of a toddler with DMD. What daily struggles would you face? How do you believe these struggles might impact you psychologically, emotionally, and physically? What would you fear most? Need the most help with? Want a rehabilitation nurse to tell you about?
- Which of the healthcare legislation presented in this chapter has the greatest impact on your work in the nursing profession and why?
- What advice would you give to a parent struggling with the daily care that is needed for child with cerebral palsy, specifically spastic CP?

- What resources are available for parents and families who care for a CSHCN?

REFERENCES

Adzick, N. (2010). Fetal myelomeningocele: Natural history, pathophysiology, and in-utero intervention. *Seminars in Fetal & Neonatal Medicine, 15*, 9–14.

American Academy of Pediatrics. (2003). Family-centered care and the pediatrician's role. *Pediatrics, 112*(3 Pt 1), 691–697.

Anderson, J., Head, S., Rae, C., & Morley, J. (2002). Brain function in Duchenne muscular dystrophy. *Brain, 125*, 4–13.

Antonelli, R. C., & Antonelli, D. M. (2004). Providing a medical home: The cost of care coordination services in a community-based, general pediatric practice. *Pediatrics, 113*(5 Suppl), 1522–1528.

Barakat, L. P., & Linney, J. A. (1992). Children with physical handicaps and their mothers: The interrelation of social support, maternal adjustment, and child adjustment. *Journal of Pediatric Psychology, 17*(6), 725–739.

Barnett, D., Clements, M., Kaplan-Estrin, M., & Fialka, J. (2003). Building new dreams supporting parents' adaptation to their child with special needs. *Infants and Young Children, 16*(3), 184–200.

Bazner-Chandler, J., & Brady, M. (2009). Musculoskeletal disorders. In C. Burns, A. Dunn, M. Brady, N. Starr, & C. Blosser (Eds.), *Pediatric primary care* (4th ed., pp. 1001–1034). St. Louis, MO: Saunders Elsevier.

Blake, D., & Kroger, S. (2000). The neurobiology of Duchenne muscular dystrophy: learning from muscle? *Trends in Neurosciences, 23*(3), 92–99.

Blann, L. (2005). Early intervention for children and families with special needs. *MCN. American Journal of Maternal Child Nursing, 30*(4), 263–267.

Blomquist, K. (2006). Health, education, work, and independence of young adults with disabilities. *Orthopaedic Nursing, 25*(3), 168–176.

Blomquist, K. (2007). Health and independence of young adults with disabilities two years later. *Orthopaedic Nursing, 26*(5), 296–309.

Blosser, C., & Reider-Demer, M. (2009). Neurologic disorders. In C. Burns, A. Dunn, M. Brady, N. Starr, & C. Blosser (Eds.), *Pediatric primary care* (4th ed., pp. 634–672). St. Louis, MO: Saunders Elsevier.

Bond, J., Kent, G., Binney, V., & Saleh, M. (1999). Psychological adjustment of children awaiting limb reconstruction treatment. *Child: Care, Health and Development, 25*(4), 313–321.

Boss, B., & Huether, S. (2010). Alterations of neurologic function in children. In K. McCance, S. Huether, V. Brashers, & N. Rote (Eds.), *Pathophysiology the biologic basis for disease in adults and children* (6th ed., pp. 665–693). Marland Heights, MO: Mosby Elsevier.

Burke, S., Kauffmann, E., Harrison, M., & Wiskin, N. (1999). Assessment of stressors in families with a child who has a chronic condition. *MCN. American Journal of Maternal Child Nursing, 24*(2), 98–106.

Bushby, K., Bourke, J., Bullock, R., Eagle, M., Gibson, M., & Quinby, J. (2005). The multidisciplinary management of Duchenne muscular dystrophy. *Current Paediatrics, 15,* 292–300.

Bushby, K., Rinkel, F., Birnkrant, D., et al. (2010a). Diagnosis and management of Duchenne muscular dystrophy, part 1: Diagnosis, and pharmacological and psychosocial management. *Lancet Neurology, 9,* 77–93.

Bushby, K., Rinkel, F., Birnkrant, D., et al. (2010b). Diagnosis and management of Duchenne muscular dystrophy, part 2: Implementation of multidisciplinary care. *Lancet Neurology, 9,* 177–189.

Carroll, K. (2010). Alterations of musculoskeletal function in children. In K. McCance, S. Huether, V. Brashers, & N. Rote (Eds.), *Pathophysiology the biologic basis for disease in adults and children* (6th ed., pp. 1618–1643). Maryland Heights, MO: Mosby Elsevier.

Centers for Disease Control and Prevention (CDC). (2009a). Prevalence of Duchenne/Becker muscular dystrophy among males aged 5–24 years—Four states, 2007. *Morbidity and Mortality Weekly Report, 58*(40), 1119–1122.

Centers for Disease Control and Prevention (CDC). (2009b). What do we know about spina bifida? Retrieved from http://www.cdc.gov/ncbddd/birthdefects/SpinaBifida.htm

Child and Adolescent Health Measure Initiative. (2005). Who are children with special health care needs? National Survey of Children with Special Health Care Needs. Retrieved from http://nschdata.org/viewdocument.aspx?item=256

deJong, T., Chrzan, R., Klijn, A., & Dik, P. (2008). Treatment of the neurogenic bladder in spina bifida. *Pediatric Nephrology, 23,* 889–896.

Easton, J., Rens, B., & Alexander, M. (1999). Psychosocial aspects of childhood disabilities. In G. Molnar & M. Alexander (Eds.), *Pediatric rehabilitation* (3rd ed.). Philadelphia: Hanley & Belfus.

Edwards, P. (1999). Legislation and public policy. In P. Edwards, D. Hertzberg, S. Hays, & N. Youngblood (Eds.), *Pediatric rehabilitation nursing.* Philadelphia: W.B. Saunders.

Evans-Jones, E., Kay, S., & Weindling, A. (2003). Congenital brachial palsy: incidence, causes, and outcome in the United Kingdom and Republic of Ireland. *Archives of Disease in Childhood. Fetal and Neonatal Edition, 88,* F185–F189.

Farel, A. (1997). Children with special health care needs. In J. Kotch (Ed.), *Maternal and child health programs, problems, and policy in public health.* Gaithersburg, MD: Aspen.

Fennell, E., & Dikel, T. (2001). Cognitive and neuropsychological functioning in children with cerebral palsy. *Journal of Child Neurology, 16,* 58–63.

Fisher, H. R. (2001). The needs of parents with chronically sick children: a literature review. *Journal of Advanced Nursing, 36*(4), 600–607.

Florian, V., & Findler, L. (2001). Mental health and marital adaptation among mothers of children with cerebral palsy. *American Journal of Orthopsychiatry, 71*(3), 358–367.

Gaebler-Spira, D., & Uellendahl, J. (1999). Pediatric limb deficiencies. In G. Molnar & M. Alexander (Eds.), *Pediatric rehabilitation* (3rd ed., pp. 331–350). Philadelphia: Hanley & Belfus.

Gaylord, N., & Yetman, R. (2009). Perinatal conditions. In C. Burns, A. Dunn, M. Brady, N. Starr, & C. Blosser (Eds.), *Pediatric primary care* (4th ed., pp. 1035–1079). St. Louis, MO: Saunders Elsevier.

Harvey, J., & Kerr, J. (1999). Health promotion in the disabled child; a nursing perspective. In G. Molnar & M. Alexander (Eds.), *Pediatric rehabilitation* (3rd ed., pp. 179–192). Philadelphia: Hanley & Belfus.

Hays, S. (1999a). Management of central nervous system impairment. In P. Edwards, D. Hertzberg, S. Hays, & N. Youngblood (Eds.), *Pediatric rehabilitation nursing* (pp. 317–336). Philadelphia: W.B. Saunders.

Hays, S. (1999b). Musculoskeletal conditions: Craniofacial anomalies. In P. Edwards, D. Hertzberg, S. Hays, & N. Youngblood (Eds.), *Pediatric rehabilitation nursing* (pp. 337–347). Philadelphia: W.B. Saunders.

Hays, S. (1999c). Neuromuscular disorders. In P. Edwards, D. Hertzberg, S. Hays, & N. Youngblood (Eds.), *Pediatric rehabilitation nursing* (pp. 363–369). Philadelphia: W.B. Saunders.

Hertzberg, D. (1999a). Child growth, development, and maturation. In P. Edwards, D. Hertzberg, S. Hays, & N. Youngblood (Eds.), *Pediatric rehabilitation nursing* (pp. 144–198). Philadelphia: W.B. Saunders.

Hertzberg, D. (1999b). Limb deficiencies in children. In P. Edwards, D. Hertzberg, S. Hays, & N. Youngblood (Eds.), *Pediatric rehabilitation nursing* (pp. 348–362). Philadelphia: W.B. Saunders.

Hertzberg, D. (1999c). Principles of pediatric rehabilitation nursing. In P. Edwards, D. Hertzberg, S. Hays, & N. Youngblood (Eds.), *Pediatric rehabilitation nursing* (pp. 84–111). Philadelphia: W.B. Saunders.

Huether, S. (2010). Alterations of digestive function in children. In K. McCance, S. Huether, V. Brashers, & N. Rote (Eds.), *Pathophysiology the biologic basis of disease in adults and children* (6th ed., pp. 1516–1539). Maryland Height, MOs: Mosby Elsevier.

Hutton, J., & Pharoah, P. (2006). Life expectancy in severe cerebral palsy. *Archives of Diseases in Childhood, 91,* 254–258.

Jain, S., & Lakhtakia, P. (2002). Profile of congenital transverse deficiencies among cases of congenital orthopaedic anomalies. *Journal of Orthopaedic Surgery, 10*(1), 45–52.

Jaruatanasirikul, S., Chichareon, V., Pattanapreechawong, N., & Sangsupavanich, P. (2008). Cleft lip and/or palate: 10 years experience at a pediatric cleft center in southern Thailand. *Cleft Palate-Craniofacial Journal, 45*(6), 597–602.

Jones, M., Morgan, E., & Shelton, J. (2007a). Cerebral palsy: Introduction and diagnosis (Part I). *Journal of Pediatric Health Care, 21*(3), 146–152.

Jones, M., Morgan, E., & Shelton, J. (2007b). Primary care of the child with cerebral palsy: A review of systems (Part II). *Journal of Pediatric Health Care, 21*(4), 226–238.

Jorde, L. (2010). Genes and genetic diseases. In K. McCance, S. Huether, V. Brashers, & N. Rote (Eds.), *Pathophysiology: The biologic basis for disease in adults and children* (6th ed., pp. 126–182). Maryland Heights, MO: Mosby Elsevier.

Kastner, T. A. (2004). Managed care and children with special health care needs. *Pediatrics, 114*(6), 1693–1698.

Kerr, S. M., & McIntosh, J. B. (2000). Coping when a child has a disability: exploring the impact of parent-to-parent support *Child: Care, Health, and Development, 26*(4), 309–322.

King, G., Tucker, M. A., Baldwin, P., Lowry, K., LaPorta, J., & Martens, L. (2002). A life needs model of pediatric service delivery: Services to support community participation and quality of life for children and youth with disabilities. *Physical and Occupational Therapy in Pediatrics, 22*(2), 53–77.

Klassen, A. F., Lee, S. K., Raina, P., Chan, H. W., Matthew, D., & Brabyn, D. (2004). Health status and health-related quality of life in a population-based sample of neonatal intensive care unit graduates. *Pediatrics, 113*(3 Pt 1), 594–600.

Kondo, A., Kamihira, O., & Ozawa, H. (2008). Neural tube defects: Prevalence, etiology and prevention. *International Journal of Urology, 16*, 49–57.

Kozin, S. (2003). Upper extremity congenital anomalies. *Journal of Bone and Joint Surgery, 85A*(8), 1564–1576.

Lynch, S. A. (1998). Who supports whom? How age and gender affect the perceived quality of support from family and friends. *Gerontologist, 38*(2), 231–238.

Matthews, D., & Wilson, P. (1999). Cerebral palsy. In G. Molnar & M. Alexander (Eds.), *Pediatric rehabilitation* (3rd ed.).(pp. 193–218). Philadelphia: Hanley & Belfus.

McAbee, G., & Ciervo, C. (2006). Medical and legal issues related to brachial plexus injuries in neonates. *Journal of the American Osteopathic Association, 106*(4), 209–212.

McDonald, C. (1999). Neuromuscular diseases. In G. Molnar & M. Alexander (Eds.), *Pediatric rehabilitation* (3rd ed.). (pp. 289–330). Philadelphia: Hanley & Belfus.

McGuirk, C., Westgate, M., & Holmes, L. (2001). Limb deficiencies in newborn infants. *Pediatrics, 108*(4), E64.

McNelis, A., Buelow, J., Myers, J., & Johnson, E. (2007). Concerns and needs of children with epilepsy and their parents. *Clinical Nurse Specialist, 21*(4), 195–202.

McPherson, M., Arango, P., & Fox, H. (1998). A new definition of children with special health care needs. *Pediatrics, 102*(1 Pt 1), 137–140.

Milner, J., Bungay, C., Jellinek, D., & Hall, D. M. (1996). Needs of disabled children and their families. *Archives of Disease in Childhood, 75*(5), 399–404.

Mitchell, L., Adzick, N., Melchionne, J., Pasquariello, P., Sutton, L., & Whitehead, A. (2004). Spina bifida. *Lancet, 364*, 1885–1895.

Molnar, G. (1991). Rehabilitation in cerebral palsy. *The Western Journal of Medicine, 154* Rehabiliation Medicine—Adding Life to Years (special issue), 569–572.

Molnar, G., & Murphy, K. (1999). Spina bifida. In G. Molnar & M. Alexander (Eds.), *Pediatric rehabilitation* (3rd ed., pp. 219–244). Philadelphia: Hanley & Belfus.

Molnar, G., & Sobus, K. (1999). Growth and development. In G. Molnar & M. Alexander (Eds.), *Pediatric rehabilitation* (3rd ed.). (pp. 13–28). Philadelphia: Hanley & Belfus.

National Limb Loss Information Center. (2008). Fact sheet: Amputation statistics by cause. Retrieved from http://www .amputee-coalition.org/fact_sheets/amp_stats_cause.html

O'Conner-Von, S., Looman, W., Lindeke, L., Garwick, A., & Leonard, B. (2009). Preparing pediatric nurse leaders for practice. *Nursing Administration Quarterly, 33*(1), 73–77.

Pearlin, L. I., Mullan, J. T., Semple, S. J., & Skaff, M. M. (1990). Caregiving and the stress process: An overview of concepts and their measures. *Gerontologist, 30*(5), 583–594.

Perrin, E. C., Lewkowicz, C., & Young, M. H. (2000). Shared vision: concordance among fathers, mothers, and pediatricians about unmet needs of children with chronic health conditions. *Pediatrics, 105*(1 Pt 3), 277–285.

Poysky, J. (2007). Behavior patterns in Duchenne muscular dystrophy: Report on the Parent Project Muscular Dystrophy behavior workshop 8–9 of December 2006, Philadelphia, USA. *Neuromuscular Disorders, 17*, 986–994.

Raina, P., O'Donnell, M., & Schwellnus, H. (2004). Caregiving process and caregiver burden: conceptual models to guide research and practice. *BMC Pediatrics, 4*, 1.

Rearick, E. (2007). Enhancing success in transition service coordinators use of transformational leadership. *Professional Case Management, 12*(5), 283–287.

Ruchelsman, D., Pettrone, S., Price, A., & Grossman, J. (2009). Brachial plexus birth palsy an overview of early treatment considerations. *Bulletin of the NYU Hospital for Joint Diseases, 67*(1), 83–89.

Schoenmakers, M., Gulmans, V., Gooskens, R., & Helders, P. (2004). Spina bifida at the sacral level: More than minor gait disturbances. *Clinical Rehabilitation, 18*, 178–185.

Seltzer, M. M., Greenberg, J. S., Floyd, F. J., & Hong, J. (2004). Accommodative coping and well-being of midlife parents of children with mental health problems or developmental disabilities. *American Journal of Orthopsychiatry, 74*(2), 187–195.

Shaer, C. (1997). The infant and young child with spina bifida: major medical concerns. *Infants and Young Children, 9*(3), 13–25.

Silver, E. J., Stein, R. E., & Bauman, L. J. (1999). Sociodemographic and condition-related characteristics associated with conduct problems in school-aged children with chronic health conditions. *Archives of Pediatric and Adolescent Medicine, 153*(8), 815–820.

Sloper, P. (1999). Models of service support for parents of disabled children. What do we know? What do we need to know? *Child: Care, Health, and Development, 25*(2), 85–99.

Sloper, P., & Turner, S. (1992). Service needs of families of children with severe physical disability. *Child: Care, Health, and Development, 18*(5), 259–282.

Sloper, P., & Turner, S. (1993). Risk and resistance factors in the adaptation of parents of children with severe physical disability. *Journal of Child Psychology and Psychiatry, 34*(2), 167–188.

Strickland, B., McPherson, M., Weissman, G., van Dyck, P., Huang, Z. J., & Newacheck, P. (2004). Access to the medical home: results of the National Survey of Children with Special Health Care Needs. *Pediatrics, 113*(5 Suppl), 1485–1492.

Sutton, L. (2008). Fetal surgery for neural tube defects. *Best Practice & Research Clinical Obstetrics and Gynaecolology, 22*(1), 175–188.

Taggart, P., & Aguilar, C. (1999). Therapeutic exercise. In G. Molnar & M. Alexander (Eds.), *Pediatric rehabilitation* (3rd ed., pp. 125–152). Philadelphia: Hanley & Belfus.

Thompson, D. (2009). Postnatal management and outcome for neural tube defects including spina bifida and encephalocoeles. *Prenatal Diagnosis, 29*, 412–419.

Tobias, N., Mason, D., Lutkenhoff, M., Stoops, M., & Ferguson, D. (2008). Management principles of organic causes of childhood constipation. *Journal of Pediatric Health Care, 22*(1), 12–23.

Urbano, M. (1992). *Preschool children with special health care needs.* San Diego, CA: Singular Publishing Group.

Venkateswaran, S., & Shevell, M. (2008). Comorbidities and clinical determinants of outcome in children with spastic quadriplegic cerebral palsy. *Developmental Medicine & Child Neurology, 50*, 216–222.

Verpoorten, C., & Buyse, G. (2008). The neurogenic bladder: Medical treatment. *Pediatric Nephrology, 23*, 717–725.

Vinck, A., Maassen, B., Mullaart, R., & Rotteveel, J. (2006). Arnold-Chiari-II malformation and cognitive functioning in spina bifida. *Journal of Neurology, Neurosurgery, and Psychiatry, 77*, 1083–1086.

Wallander, J. L., & Varni, J. W. (1998). Effects of pediatric chronic physical disorders on child and family adjustment. *Journal of Child Psychology and Psychiatry, 39*(1), 29–46.

Wallander, J. L., Varni, J. W., Babani, L., Banis, H. T., DeHaan, C. B., & Wilcox, K. T. (1989a). Disability parameters, chronic strain, and adaptation of physically handicapped children and their mothers. *Journal of Pediatric Psychology, 14*(1), 23–42.

Wallander, J. L., Varni, J. W., Babani, L., DeHaan, C. B., Wilcox, K. T., & Banis, H. T. (1989b). The social environment and the adaptation of mothers of physically handicapped children. *Journal of Pediatric Psychology, 14*(3), 371–387.

Wallander, J. L., & Venters, T. L. (1995). Perceived role restriction and adjustment of mothers of children with chronic physical disability. *Journal of Pediatric Psychology, 20*(5), 619–632.

Warfield, M. E., Krauss, M. W., Hauser-Cram, P., Upshur, C. C., & Shonkoff, J. P. (1999). Adaptation during early childhood among mothers of children with disabilities. *Journal of Developmental and Behavioral Pediatrics, 20*(1), 9–16.

Weisz, V., & Tomkins, A. J. (1996). The right to a family environment for children with disabilities. *American Journal of Psychology, 51*(12), 1239–1245.

Woolfson, L. (2004). Family well-being and disabled children: a psychosocial model of disability-related child behaviour problems. *British Journal of Health and Psychology, 9*(Pt 1), 1–13.

Yiu, E., & Kornberg, A. (2008). Duchenne muscular dystrophy. *Neurology India, 56*(3), 236–247.

Youngblood, N. (1999). Family-centered care. In P. Edwards, D. Hertzberg, S. Hays, & N. Youngblood (Eds.), *Pediatric rehabilitation nursing* (pp. 129–143). Philadelphia: W.B. Saunders.

Zebracki, K., & Drotar, D. (2008). Pain and activity limitations in children with Duchenne or Becker muscular dystrophy. *Developmental Medicine & Child Neurology, 50*, 546–552.

Zipitis, C., & Pachalides, C. (2003). Caring for a child with spina bifida: understanding the child and carer. *Journal of Child Health Care, 7*(2), 101–112.

CHAPTER 28

Gerontological Rehabilitation Nursing

Cheryl A. Lehman
Kristen L. Mauk
Kimberly Hickey

LEARNING OBJECTIVES

At the end of this chapter, the reader will be able to

- Review biological, psychological, and sociological theories of aging.
- Describe the aging process of each physiological system.
- Discuss the impact of normal aging on an older adult's rehabilitation potential.
- Identify unique symptoms often seen in older adults with common illnesses or disease processes.
- Recognize that aging changes partially depend on an individual's health behaviors and preventive health measures.
- Compare aging with an early-onset disability and aging with a disability acquired at an advanced age.
- Apply nursing interventions to promote healthy aging in those with an early-onset disability and those who are aging with a disability acquired at an advanced age.
- Explore web-based and other resources in geriatrics that can be readily used in practice.

KEY CONCEPTS AND TERMS

Baby boomer	Geriatric syndrome	Nonstochastic
Death panel	Gordon's functional health	Palliative care
Elder abuse	patterns	Presbycusis
Elder mistreatment	Hypogeusia	Presbyopia
Era of onset	Hyposmia	Senescence
Generativity versus stagnation	Integrity versus despair	Stochastic

Rehabilitation nursing care of older adults is a subspecialty of rehabilitation nursing that is likely to boom in the next few decades. The Centers for Disease Control and Prevention and the Merck Company Foundation (2007, p. 2) summarized the aging of America this way:

> The current growth in the number and proportion of older adults living in the United States is unprecedented in our nation's history. Two factors—longer lives and aging baby boomers—will double the population of Americans aged 65 or older during the next 25 years. Life expectancy in the U.S. has increased from 47 years for Americans born in 1900 to 77 years for those born in 2001; and baby boomers—those born between 1946

and 1964—will begin to reach age 65 in 2011. By 2030, the number of older Americans is expected to reach 71 million, or roughly 20% of the U.S. population.

With the projected changes in the population, rehabilitation nurses need to be prepared to care for an aging generation. Complaints of chronic illness become more frequent with advanced age, so the need for rehabilitation is often greater among older adults. The U.S. Census Bureau (2008) found that among adults aged 65 years and older, 18.1 million people (51.8%) had a disability and nearly 13 million people (36.9%) reported a severe disability. The purpose of this chapter is to provide the reader with a background on theories of aging, normal aging changes, aging with a disability, common geriatric syndromes, and applicable issues related to older adults in rehabilitation.

THEORIES OF AGING

Aging is a part of living, and yet the prevention of aging has preoccupied humankind for all of known time. Ponce de León tried to find an elixir to prevent aging by seeking the Fountain of Youth, and today there are a myriad of information sources about the "prevention" of aging. Experts in caring for older people have coined the terms "aging with grace" and "successful aging" to reflect the ideal goals in life: to age successfully and with grace. It is possible for all individuals to have a healthy life until **senescence** (the process by which a cell looses its ability to divide, grow, and function, which ultimately ends in cell death) makes life impossible.

A look at the older population shows that as people age, they become more differentiated from one another. The combinations of genetic, socioeconomic, and environment influences are infinite. When a human is born, a few simple tests can give necessary information as to the well-being of that new person. There are, however, multitudes of tests (cognitive, social, economic, psychological, genetic, physiological) available to determine well-being in an older person. These tests reflect the many possible combinations of those biopsychosocial forces that make each older adult unique. Many of these tests are based on a variety of theories of aging within each context. A few of those theories are discussed.

Biological Theories of Aging

Cellular and molecular biologists propose theories to try to explain the aging process and perform research in an attempt to verify their theories. These researchers seek answers to the following questions: What causes aging? How can aging be influenced? Is it possible to prolong life?

Many biological theories of aging have been developed, and they fall into two general categories: Aging is due to random (**stochastic**) forces and aging is preprogrammed or nonrandom (**nonstochastic**). Gerontological specialists tend to favor one type of theory of aging over another based on what is currently known through research.

The biological stochastic error theories of aging refer to random processes that cause errors that alter cell function and cause aging. These biological theories differ on how that cell dysfunction (or senescence) occurs. For example, the nutrition-based stochastic free radical theory of aging proposes that the oxidation of fats, proteins, and carbohydrates creates free electrons that alter cell function. Another stochastic theory of aging, cross-link theory of aging, is based on the premise that over time and with exposure to environmental chemicals and radiation, cross-links form between glucose and protein, resulting in malfunction of the protein. Hematologists and oncologists may subscribe to this theory of aging to explain such conditions as blood dyscrasias and certain cancers attributable to exposure to noxious chemicals. Known cross-linking disorders include cataracts and tough leathery skin.

The somatic mutation theory and the transcription theory can likewise be used to explain unexpected conditions such as autoimmune disorders and cardiac disease. The somatic mutation theory is based on the belief that spontaneous mutations of DNA, RNA, or both result in failure of cell structure or function. The transcription theory proposes a failure of transcription or translation between cells that again results in failure of cell structure or function. The last of the highly subscribed error theories is that of wear and tear. It states that overuse of the body's cells, joints, muscles, and so on with wear-and-tear damage to cells and organs eventually causes senescence of cells, organs, and ultimately death. Osteoarthritis is one condition that exemplifies this theory.

The nonstochastic theories of aging do not have the element of randomness: They are more of a deterministic view of aging. The first of these theories is the programmed senescence theory of aging. This theory states that a biological clock is built into each cell, allowing a specific number of cell divisions before an inevitable and programmed death occurs. Many diseases and conditions attributable to hereditary or genetic predisposition can be explained with this theory. "The link between genes and lifespan is unquestioned. The simple observation that some species live longer than others—humans longer than dogs, tortoises longer than mice—is one convincing piece of evidence" (National Institute of Aging, 2010). The endocrine theory of aging more specifically states that aging occurs because of functional decrements in hormones—cells become less responsive to endocrine stimulation. Menopause is an example of the application of this theory of aging.

Gradual loss of immune competence making the individual susceptible to autoimmune and infectious agents over time is how the immunological theory is explained. Finally, the telomere-telomerase theory of aging espouses that the loss of telomeres (repeated sequences at the end of DNA) and decrease in telomerase function occurs with aging. With each cell division these sequences shorten until the point comes when no more shortening can occur. The cell then enters senescence. Shortened telomeres are found in atherosclerosis, heart disease, hepatitis, and cirrhosis. Interestingly, 90% of cancer cells have been found to possess telomerase. In both normal and cancer cells telomerase prevents the telomere from shortening.

Psychosocial Theories of Development

There are many psychosocial theories of development (Box 28.1). The two most frequently used developmental theories are full-life development theories, which span the course of life from infanthood through the late adult years and place aging as one of the developmental stages in life, albeit the final one, and the mature life theories, which focus only on the psychosocial processes in late adulthood. The psychological full-life development theories of aging assume that development

- Is *predictable and sequential*
- Includes *critical periods* in life
- Includes *normative tasks* to complete
- Involves the *mastery of tasks*

It is agreed within this type of psychological theory of aging that individuals may regress and that the critical periods or stages required for successful aging are clearly delineated.

The most notable of the full-life development theories (the theory of psychosocial development) was developed by Erik Erikson in 1956. It was the first of such theories

---

BOX 28.1   Psychosocial Theories of Aging

- **Sociological theories:** Changing roles, relationships, status, and generational cohort impact the older adult's ability to adapt.
  - **Activity disengagement:** Remaining occupied and involved is necessary to a satisfying later life. Gradual withdrawal from society and relationships serves to maintain social equilibrium and promote internal reflection.
  - **Subculture:** The elderly prefer to segregate from society in an aging subculture sharing loss of status and societal negativity regarding the aged. Health and mobility are key determinants of social status.
  - **Continuity:** Personality influences roles and life satisfaction and remains consistent throughout life. Past coping patterns recur as older adults adjust to physical, financial, and social decline and contemplate death. Identifying with one's age group, finding a residence compatible with one's limitations, and learning new roles postretirement are major tasks.
  - **Age stratification:** Society is stratified by age groups that are the basis for acquiring resources, roles, status, and deference from others. Age cohorts are influenced by their historical context and share similar experiences, beliefs, attitudes, and expectations of life course transitions.
  - **Person–Environment:** Function is affected by ego strength, mobility, health, cognition, sensory, fit perception, and the environment. Competency changes one's ability to adapt to environmental demands.
  - **Gerotranscendence:** The elderly transform from a materialistic/rational perspective toward oneness with the universe. Successful transformation includes an outward focus, accepting impending death, substantive relationships, intergenerational connectedness, and unity with the universe.

- **Psychological theories:** Explain aging in terms of mental processes, emotions, attitudes, motivation, and personality development that is characterized by life stage transitions.
  - **Human need**s: Five basic needs motivate human behavior in a lifelong process toward need fulfillment.
  - Individualism: Personality consists of an ego and personal and collective unconsciousness that view life from a personal or external perspective. Older adults search for life meaning and adapt to functional and social losses.
  - Stages of personality development: Personality develops in eight sequential stages with corresponding life tasks. The eighth phase, integrity versus despair, is characterized by evaluating life accomplishments; struggles include letting go, accepting care, detachment, and physical and mental decline.
  - Life-course/life-span development: Life stages are predictable and structured by roles, relationships, values, and goals. Persons adapt to changing roles and relationships. Age group norms and characteristics are an important part of the life course.
  - Selective optimization with compensation: Individuals cope with aging losses through activity/role selection, optimization, and compensation. Critical life points are morbidity, mortality, and quality of life. Selective optimization with compensation facilitates successful aging.

to be formulated. This theory is not based on research but on Erikson's experience as a psychotherapist. He based the eight theorized socioemotional stages on what he called "psychological crises" that each require resolution before the next stage can be negotiated. There is a stepwise progression through the stages as an individual learns certain things in each stage on which to builtage. Each stage in Erikson's theory is named according to the crisis that must be resolved. The outcome for each stage is also identified. The seventh of the eight stages is the adult stage: **generativity versus stagnation**. Generativity requires that the ego positively identify the needs for giving back to society by raising children; being productive at work; being involved in the community; and guiding, parenting, and monitoring the next generation. Failure to do this can result in stagnation, which is characterized by being unproductive and feeling anger, hurt, and self-absorption. The final and eighth stage of development in Erikson's theory is that of **integrity versus despair**, with the positive outcome of "wisdom." Ego integrity is demonstrated by the older adult's ability to explore life as a retired person who is not identified with an occupation, to contemplate accomplishment, and to feel that life is successful. Despair results if there is feelings of guilt about the past and/or a sense of not accomplishing life goals. Despair can then lead to hopelessness, which is a manifestation of unsuccessful aging.

Examples of mature-life theories are those of Robert Peck (1968) and Bernice Neugarten (1968). Robert Peck theorized that an older adult is required to proceed through three stages of development to reach full psychosocial development:

- Stage 1: Ego differentiation versus work role preoccupation
- Stage 2: Body transcendence versus body preoccupation
- Stage 3: Ego transcendence versus ego preoccupation

This theory states that as a person matures, he or she moves away from "work role preoccupation" (a concept that describes defining oneself through work or an occupation) to the point where one finds new meaning and value to life. This process is called "ego differentiation." In the second stage a person either accepts the limitations that accompanies the aging process (body transcendence) or dwells on diminishing abilities (body preoccupation). Stage 3 is ego transcendence versus ego preoccupation in which elf-examination occurs. If a person believes his or

her life has worthwhile and "life contributions" will live on after death, the person experiences "ego transcendence." Otherwise, the person may feel that he or she has lived a useless life and experience "ego preoccupation."

Bernice Neugarten specifically describes tasks that need to be accomplished for a person to accomplish successful aging:

- Accepting reality and the imminence of death
- Coping with physical illness
- Accepting the necessity of being dependent on outside support while still making independent choices that can give satisfaction

Neugarten's theory of aging has a strong social aspect in that it maintains that a person must remain as active as possible to successfully age. This falls under the category of activity theory. It is postulated that as one ages, the type of activity done in younger years is the type of activity that one will perform in later years. For example, if a person engaged in more social activity than loner activity in younger years, it is anticipated that this is the kind of activity to be seen in their later years.

A final social theory discussed here is the social disengagement theory, the opposite of the activity theory described previously. The social disengagement theory is not without controversy; however, it can be used to explain some patterns seen in aging. This theory includes the following features:

- Both older people and society mutually withdraw from each other.
- A person gradually disconnects from other people in anticipation of death.
- Intrinsic changes in personality occur that allow a person to psychologically withdraw from society's expectations.

One way to assess an older person's theory-based psychological development is to ask questions as described in Marjory **Gordon's functional health patterns**. The health patterns of health perception–health management, self-image–self-concept, and coping beliefs include the following assessment questions (Child Development Institute, 2010):

- How do you rate your health?
- What do you do to maintain your health?
- Describe yourself.
- What assists you with coping?

- What gives you strength?
- What gives you a sense of accomplishment?

NORMAL AGING CHANGES

As the body ages individuals experience a wide variety of changes in bodily systems and their functions. Some of these result from expected "normal" aging, whereas other changes are considered abnormal and may require older adults to use the healthcare system more frequently. Changes generally associated with the aging process are discussed in this section. Significant changes with aging are discussed here in light of the potential impact on rehabilitation.

Cardiovascular

Several significant aging changes in the cardiovascular system can negatively impact an older adult's rehabilitation potential. The heart becomes a less effective pumping muscle and is unable to respond to increased demands placed on it due to lesser cardiac reserve. The blood vessels become less elastic and more tortuous. Arteriosclerosis and atherosclerosis may be present, depending on diet, activity level, and culture. Often, sclerosis of the atrial and mitral valves increases the incidence of heart murmurs, although many persons are asymptomatic (Gallo, Bogner, Fulmer, & Paveza, 2006). With normal aging also comes a decreased maximal heart rate that can lead to fatigue, shortness of breath, and a slower recovery from tachycardia (Heineman, Hamrick-King, & Scaglione Sewell, 2010). It may be more difficult for older adults to engage in intensive therapy due to an overall decline in cardiac function and cardiac output with the onset of exercise (Pue & Wei, 2001) than for younger persons. Peripheral pulses may be diminished. The systolic blood pressure rises with age as the left ventricle works harder to get blood through a stiffer aorta. Because of the higher risk of stroke associated with hypertension, the American Heart Association (2010) recommends that even older adults maintain a blood pressure of less than 120/80. However, some older adults may require a higher blood pressure to achieve adequate cerebral tissue perfusion, so older adults should work with their physician to achieve the ideal blood pressure for them. In addition, safe guidelines for blood pressure during times of exercise should be established for each person.

Myocardial infarction results in greater morbidity among older adults. Heart attacks often present differently in older adults, so rehabilitation nurses should beware of nonclassic symptoms, especially indigestion that is unrelieved by antacids or confusion that comes on suddenly without explanation (Amella, 2004).

Respiratory

Major changes in the respiratory system are due to circulation, structural changes, and alveolar function. Pulmonary circulation is poorer due to a less effective heart pump. Older adults may present with an increased anterior/posterior chest diameter. The more stiff and rigid chest leads to poorer expansion and shallower breathing. The alveoli are flatter and shallower so there is less space for air exchange. Oxygen exchange is less efficient, resulting in less useful oxygen with each breath. There is an overall decrease in tidal volume, expiratory reserve volume, and forced expiratory volume. Although total lung capacity shows no change with normal aging, vital capacity and inspiratory capacity decrease (Heineman et al., 2010). These normal aging changes can adversely affect the older adult's ability to capacity for exercise, even in the absence of any chronic obstruction pulmonary diseases that are also prevalent among this age group.

Gastrointestinal

Many changes in the gastrointestinal system can affect the recovery of patients. With advanced age persons lose teeth and may have dentures. Changes in bones and muscles in the jaw make it harder to chew, and the lack of saliva may make swallowing more difficult (Heineman et al., 2010). Enzymes that break up food are also decreased. For persons who may experience dysphagia due to disorders such as stroke, brain injury, and neurological diseases, these normal aging changes present additional challenges.

There is an increase in complaints of reflux and heartburn as the lower esophageal sphincter becomes more floppy. Peristalsis slows in the esophagus and in the gut, and constipation is common.

Several normal aging changes affect the way the older body responds to medications. Changes in absorption result in medications processed less efficiently and staying in the body longer, which can lead to side effects. Additionally, blood flow perfusion to the liver decreases 30% to 40%, and although there are no significant functional changes in liver, there is decreased drug clearance (Heineman et al., 2010). A general rule for medication dosing in older adults is "start lower and go slower." Rehabilitation nurses should be particularly alert to any side effects appearing with new medications or dosage changes.

Genitourinary

With advanced age, significant changes occur in the renal system. Blood flow to kidneys decreases. Kidneys shrink and lose up to half of the functioning nephrons by the time one is 70. The glomeruli decrease 30% to 40% with age, often resulting in decreased glomerular filtration rate and decreased drug clearance. The Cockcroft-Gault equation to calculate creatinine clearance is a lab value preferred over serum creatinine to evaluate renal function, because it accounts for age, gender, and body weight of the patient (Amella, 2004; Mauk & Hanson, 2010).

Voiding may be more frequent due to decreased bladder capacity, and nocturia is more common. The pelvic muscles have poorer tone, which can contribute to incontinence. However, urinary incontinence is not considered a normal part of aging and should be treated. Pelvic floor muscle exercises (Kegel exercises) in combination with timed or scheduled voiding have shown good success for women, even those with cognitive impairment, with urinary incontinence (Diebold, Fanning-Harding, & Hanson, 2010).

Integumentary

Older adults also experience many changes in the skin, hair, and nails. Skin becomes thinner, drier, less elastic, and more fragile with age. In rehabilitation, older adults who are immobile are more prone to skin breakdown and pressure sores (Gallo et al., 2006). Pigment changes known as age spots appear, and wrinkles are more frequent. Fat distribution changes lead to more fatty tissue on the trunk and less on arms and legs. The hair thins, and male baldness patterns are predominant. The nails become more brittle and prone to breakage. Core body temperature decreases, resulting in cooler extremities. Nurses should evaluate the presence of fever based on the person's baseline temperature versus solely on standard norms (Mauk & Hanson, 2010).

Musculoskeletal

Physical mobility is one of the most important aspects of rehabilitation. Normal aging can interfere with recovery. During the normal aging process muscle mass and strength decrease, but this can be minimized with proper exercise and nutrition. Joints become more fixed and stiff, resulting in decreased range of motion with age. Persons lose bone density with age (decreased bone mass), making fractures more common. Minor changes in balance and coordination can increase the risk for falls and injury. Older adults with hip fracture have a higher morbidity and mortality rate than younger age groups, and at least 50% of elderly persons do not recover their prefracture level of ambulation (Beers & Berkow, 2005). All these changes have obvious implications for those with impaired physical mobility and recovery after fracture or joint replacement surgery.

Neurological

Changes in the neurological system involve the brain and nervous system. The aging brain decreases in size and weight, losing millions of functioning neurons but resulting in no change in intelligence. Plaques and tangles increase with age but do not necessarily manifest as dementia. Slower cognitive processing is normal, and some decline is common but not universal. Most memory functions are adequate for a normal life, with some short-term memory loss being most common. However, a change in mental status is often first indicator of delirium (Amella, 2004) or disease.

With normal aging, involuntary reflexes remain the same. Deep tendon reflexes are unchanged, but voluntary reflexes are slower in response to multiple stimuli. There are slowed motor skills and potential problems with balance and coordination. Sleep changes are significant, with a decrease in stages 3–4 and rapid eye movement sleep. This results in older adults getting less quality sleep (National Sleep Foundation, 2009). There is an increase in sleep disorders with age, and insomnia is most common sleep problem. Finally, thermoregulation is less efficient. The elderly are more susceptible to harm from extremes in temperature.

Sensory

Sensory changes are some of the most obvious with age. The aging eye acquires **presbyopia**, or the inability to focus on near objects. A decreased lens accommodation is also seen, and the lens becomes more opaque with age. Older adults may require more light to see, so nurses need to be sure hallways, bathrooms, and patient rooms are well lit. Smell also decreases with age (**hyposmia**), and there is some decrease in taste (**hypogeusia**) due to atrophied taste buds, but this is thought to perhaps be related to a decrease in smell. Older adults have an increased chance of ear infection, and **presbycusis** (age-related hearing loss) is present in 39% of those over age 75 years (Heineman et al., 2010).

Reproductive

Many significant changes in the reproductive system occur for both men and women. For females estrogen is decreased by 80% with menopause. The average age for menopause among American women is about 51 years (Hall, 2004). In older women the supporting ligaments to the uterus weaken and can contribute to urinary incontinence and uterine prolapse. Vaginal dryness and decreased lubrication as well as thinning of the vaginal wall can lead to pain during sexual intercourse, increase the risk of injury, and pose an increased risk of vaginal infection.

For males fibrosis in the erectile tissue that occurs in the late 50s and decreased testosterone production results in significant changes. With normal aging comes an increased time needed for erection, less full erections and a longer refractory time, as well as less intense orgasms and ejaculation. Fertility is less affected by age, and many men well into their 80s can still father children. Nurses should inquire about sexual activity patterns of rehabilitation patients and do necessary teaching about both contraception (if applicable) and prevention of sexually transmitted infections.

Erectile dysfunction is a common but not a normal part of aging and is often associated with medication use and/or diseases such as diabetes. Rehabilitation nurses should review the list of medications for those that affect libido or sexual function. Changes in the prostate gland are also experienced by most men over the age of 70 and by 90% of men by age 85 (Heineman et al., 2010). About 20% of men experience symptoms associated with benign prostatic hyperplasia, including a decrease in urine stream and increased bladder infections from retention. Nurses should ask about these symptoms upon admission to the rehabilitation unit.

Older adults continue to engage in sexual activity. The frequency of intercourse decreases, but patterns stay the same. Older persons, particularly women, should still be counseled about protection from sexually transmitted disease and HIV, because HIV is on the rise in the older adult population (Hazzard, Blass, Halter, Ouslander, & Tinetti, 2008).

Endocrine and Immune

Hormones are chemical messengers that do not significantly change with age, except for the sex hormones (discussed previously). The thyroid experiences minor changes. For example, thyroid-stimulating hormone may be the high level of normal and the T_3 and T_4 low normal with aging (Heineman et al., 2010). Cortisol levels stay relatively the same with age. Adrenal function is less effective, so there is a decrease in epinephrine in response to stressful stimuli. There are also subtle changes in the regulation of insulin within the body, resulting in impaired glucose tolerance with age.

The endocrine and immune systems are affected by each other in normal aging. Although most hormones do not significantly change with age, the thymus gland experiences some atrophy. The thymus controls T-cell maturation and differentiation, so with advanced age T-cell production decreases and T-cells weaken. This results in a decrease in cell-mediated immunity and a less effective immune system. Older rehabilitation patients may be less able to battle infection and more prone to acquire infection.

AGING AND DISABILITY

The topic of aging and disability actually concerns two different populations of people. The first population includes people who acquire a disabling condition when they are young and then who age *with* the disability. One example of this is a child who acquires cerebral palsy at birth or a baby born with spina bifida. The second population includes older people who acquire a disability when they are older, for example, a woman who has a cerebral hemorrhage at age 85 with damage to the brain. We examine these two populations separately. See Case Study 28.1

Aging *with* a Disability

Historically, young persons with a congenital or acquired disabling condition did not live to become older adults. Life expectancy for persons with Down syndrome has increased from 9 years of age in 1929, to 12 years of age in 1949, to 35 years of age in 1982, to 55 or even older at the present time (Barnhart & Connolly, 2007). There has been a 2,000% increase in life expectancy for persons with spinal cord injury in the past 50 years, compared with 30% for the general, nondisabled population (Fordner, Carruthers & Londner, 2009). Advances in social programs, nutrition, healthcare expertise, and medications, particularly antibiotics, help explain the longer life expectancies. As a result, however, there is currently a generation of persons with a disability who are entering unknown territory, because they will live longer than past generations. The effect of an early-onset disability on aging (or, conversely, the effect of aging on an early-onset disability) is only now being discovered. What is known is that aging with a disability does not follow the norms of aging as experienced by nondisabled people.

> The "20/40 rule" states that functional problems begin to emerge when a person has 20 years duration of disability or is 40 years old, whichever comes first. If the 20/40 rule proves to be true, that would mean the 20-year-old person who was born with a disability would begin functional decline at the age of 20.

CASE STUDY 28.1

Compare the following two individuals who are aging with a disability:

John	Steve
Age 38	Age 38
C-6 complete spinal cord injury	C-6 complete spinal cord injury
Injured at age 8	Injured last month
Medications: many for many years	Medications: none before injury
Activity: wheelchair for 30 years	Activity: wheelchair for 1 month
No athletic activities for 30 years	Many athletic activities until the injury

Questions

1. At the current time, which man could be expected to have each of the following and why?
   a. Excellent renal function
   b. Osteoporosis
   c. Scoliosis
   d. Appropriate muscle mass for age and gender
   e. Overuse syndrome of the shoulders
   f. Higher risk for myocardial infarction
2. Who do you believe will be in better health at age 50 and why?
3. Who will live longer?
4. What nursing interventions at this stage could help each man experience healthier aging? Are the interventions different for John and for Steve?

Currently, 12 million first-generation, early-onset disabled people are in middle and late life. The "norm" for them is atypical aging. They tend to have higher rates of medical and functional problems that begin 20 to 25 years earlier than in those without disability. The "20/40 rule" states that functional problems begin to emerge when a person has 20 years duration of disability or is 40 years old, whichever comes first. These problems include not only a decline in physical function but an increase in medical complications, emotional issues, and changes in caregiver support (Forman et al., 2009). If the 20/40 rule proves to be true, that would mean the 20-year-old person who was born with a disability would begin functional decline at the age of 20.

All persons aging with early-onset disability are likely to have chronic, long-term use of medications, a propensity for renal damage, and a high risk for abuse by others. They are also more likely to leave the work cycle before their peers. The changes in aging experienced with early-onset disability have been theorized as being due to idiopathic accelerated aging, wear and tear, lack of weight bearing, and a sedentary lifestyle. The **era of onset** of a disability may also affect success with aging. A person born with spina bifida in 1949 received different health care, nutrition, and medications throughout his or her life than an identical person born with the same condition in 1997. Thus, although each has disability due to spina bifida, the way in which they age depends on their era of onset.

Aging with Cerebral Palsy

It is now being documented that persons who acquire cerebral palsy at birth have added difficulties associated with aging. These include functional decline, increased bowel and bladder dysfunction, oral motor and dental disorders, osteopenia, and fractures. Other difficulties are an increased risk of falls, contractures, arthritis, scoliosis, and progressive skeletal deformity associated with respiratory disease, sleep problems, pain, and fatigue. Ambulation is likely to decline with aging, and difficulties with balance (standing and sitting) are emerging. Persons with cerebral palsy who are aging are also more likely to die from cancer, circulatory diseases, and respiratory diseases than their nondisabled peers (Jones, 2009; Svien, Berg, & Stephenson, 2008).

Aging with Down Syndrome

Nearly all persons with Down syndrome over the age of 40 display neuropathology consistent with Alzheimer's disease. Also found to be common in this aging population are conductive hearing loss, sleep apnea, and depression. Thyroid dysfunction is not unusual, and obesity is prevalent. There is a higher rate of musculoskeletal disorders associated with aging with Down syndrome, such as arthritis and osteoporosis, as well as cardiovascular disorders such as mitral valve prolapse, deconditioning, and a decline in cardiovascular capacity (Barnhart & Connolly, 2007).

Aging with Spinal Cord Injury

Age-related changes in spinal cord injury have been found to occur as early as 15 years after injury and around 45 years of age (Krause & Coker, 2006). As persons with spinal cord injury age, they experience high rates of shoulder dysfunction, overuse syndrome, and carpal tunnel syndrome. They are more likely to develop pressure ulcers, osteoporosis, and fractures and more likely to have decreases in pulmonary function, insulin resistance, cancer, gallstones, pancreatitis, coronary artery disease, and pain. All these may result in a need for more assistance with self-care, new equipment, and changes in the working and living environments. For example, a person aging with a C-4 spinal cord injury may find that his or her pulmonary function has declined so much due to the aging process that continuous positive airway pressure or bilevel positive airway pressure (BiPAP) is now required at night.

Persons born with spina bifida experience many of the same changes with aging as persons with early-onset spinal cord injury. This population, however, may be more prone to develop latex allergies, due to a lifelong exposure to latex, as well as obesity.

Aging with Traumatic Brain Injury

Not many studies have examined the effects of aging with an early-onset traumatic brain injury. One study found that this population complained of increasing nervousness, arthritis, vision and hearing changes, seizures, and sleep disturbances as they aged (Colantonio, Ratcliff, Chase, & Vernich, 2004). Overall indications are that aging with traumatic brain injury can result in increased social isolation, persistent behavioral problems, continued problems with memory and learning, and decreased occupational function. Other concerns not yet validated by research include the suspicion that aging with traumatic brain injury may decrease driving safety due to reduced sleep, increased fatigue, diminishing reaction times, difficulty with night vision, poorer visual acuity and visual fields, and slow mental processing speed (Brenner, Homaifar, & Schultheis, 2008).

Aging with Multiple Sclerosis

The life expectancy for persons with multiple sclerosis in the United States is 74 years for men and 79 years for women. Persons with multiple sclerosis diagnosed at age 20 are potentially going to live with multiple sclerosis for about 55 years and diagnosed at age 50, for about 20 years. Older individuals with multiple sclerosis have accelerated rates of disability progression compared with younger individuals. Older adults with multiple sclerosis are more likely to have urinary tract infections, septicemia, pneumonia, and cellulitis. They also report having

less freedom and needing more assistance as they age (Finlayson, Van Denend, & Hudson, 2004).

Acquiring a Disability at an Older Age

Persons who acquire a disability at an older age have that disability superimposed on the normal changes of aging, preexisting chronic illnesses, and ongoing changes in socioeconomic status and support systems. Returning to the 20/40 rule, the person who acquires a disability at an advanced age will have functional issues that begin to emerge immediately. It is much more difficult for the 72-year-old diabetic with chronic obstructive pulmonary disease to adapt to a spinal cord injury than it is for a healthy 18-year-old.

Causes of disability in later life include arthritis, dementia, cardiovascular disease, falls, trauma, hypertension, diabetes, cancer, polypharmacy, and social losses. Acquired disability in later life is of major concern because it is directly related to quality of life, ability to remain independent in the community, health services utilization, and burden on family and caregivers.

Some disabilities are more likely to occur in the older adult. For example, rates of traumatic brain injury increase with age over 65, with most related to falls or motor vehicle accidents. Stroke is more prevalent in the older population as well. Rehabilitation can be more difficult with an older adult because of the normal changes of aging such as declines in muscle strength, hearing, vision, and exercise tolerance. Rehabilitation is also impacted by any chronic diseases the patient might have, such as pain syndromes, diabetic neuropathy, and dementia. Social influences, such as aging caregivers, diminishing funding sources, and altered living arrangements, can also impact success with rehabilitation for the older adult.

Interventions to Promote Successful Aging with a Disability

Rehabilitation nurses can intervene to assist both populations to successfully age. Interventions can actually be aimed at four groups:

- Younger age groups without disability
- Younger age groups with disability
- Older adults without disability
- Older adults with a new disability

Tables 28.1, 28.2, 28.3, and 28.4 describe interventions the nurse can use to facilitate healthy aging in these four groups.

TABLE 28.1 Strategies for Promotion of Healthy Aging in the Younger Adult Without Disability			
Young Adult Without Disability	**Primary Prevention**	**Secondary Prevention**	**Tertiary Prevention**

Goal: to prevent injury, disease, and/or disability	Education:
	  Smoking cessation/prevention
	  Injury prevention
	  Safety awareness
	  Alcohol moderation
	  Illicit drug prevention
	  Healthy lifestyle
	    Diet, exercise, weight control
		Screening:
		  Pap smears
		  Breast exams
		  Testicular exams
		  Skin cancer
		  Blood pressure
		  Blood sugar
		  Cholesterol
		  Eyes
		  Ears
		  Teeth	

Source: From © Cheryl Lehman (2010). Used with permission.

TABLE 28.2 Strategies for Promotion of Healthy Aging in the Younger Adult with Disability			
Young Adult With Disability	**Primary Prevention**	**Secondary Prevention**	**Tertiary Prevention**

Goal: to prevent injury, disease, and new disability and manage current disability while preventing and treating secondary complications.	Education:
	  Smoking cessation/prevention
	  Injury prevention
	  Prevention of abuse
	  Safety awareness
	  Alcohol moderation
	  Illicit drug prevention
	  Healthy lifestyle
	    Diet, exercise, weight control
	Preventive activities:
	  Pneumovax
	  Flu vaccine
	  Equipment prescription
	  Adaptive environment
	  Knowledgeable HCP
	  Weight management
	  Skin care
	  Exercise program
	  Education about healthy aging
	  Caregiver training
		Screening:
		  Pap smears
		  Breast exams
		  Testicular exams
		  Blood pressure
		  Blood sugar
		  Cholesterol
		  Eyes
		  Ears
		  Teeth
		  Osteoporosis
		  Weight
		  Skin
			Early recognition and treatment of
			  Overuse syndrome
			    Pressure ulcers
			    Obesity
			    Infection
			    Fractures

HCP, health care provider
Source: From © Cheryl Lehman (2010). Used with permission.

TABLE 28.3   Strategies for Promotion of Healthy Aging in the Older Adult without Disability

Older Adult Without Disability	Primary Prevention	Secondary Prevention	Tertiary Prevention

Goal: to prevent injury, disease and disability while managing chronic diseases.	Education:
	  Smoking cessation/ prevention
	  Injury prevention
	  Prevention of abuse
	  Safety awareness
	  Alcohol moderation
	  Illicit drug prevention
	  Healthy lifestyle
	
	Age-specific interventions:
	  Fall prevention
	  Medication monitoring
	  Socialization
	
	Preventive activities:
	  Pneumovax
	  Flu vaccine
	  Weight management
	  Caregiver training
		Screening:
		  Pap
		  Mammogram
		  Testicular exams
		  Prostate check
		  Blood pressure
		  Blood sugar
		  Cholesterol
		  Eyes
		  Ears
		  Teeth
		  Osteoporosis
		  Weight
		  Depression
		
		Age-specific interventions:
		  Colonoscopy
		  Depression screening
			Early recognition and treatment of Obesity
			
			Age-specific interventions:
			  Chronic disease management

Source: From © Cheryl Lehman (2010). Used with permission.

TABLE 28.4   Strategies for Promotion of Healthy Aging in the Older Adult with Disability

Older with New Disability	Primary Prevention	Secondary Prevention	Tertiary Prevention

Goal: to prevent injury and disease and facilitate adapting to new disability while managing chronic diseases	Education:
	  Smoking cessation/ prevention
	  Injury prevention
	  Safety awareness
	  Alcohol moderation
	  Illicit drug prevention
	  Healthy lifestyle
	
	Age-specific interventions:
	  Fall prevention
	  Medication monitoring
	  Socialization
	
	Preventive activities:
	  Pneumovax
	  Flu vaccine
	  Weight management
	  Caregiver training
	  Caregiver support
	  Equipment prescription
	  Adaptive environment
	  Knowledgeable HCP
	  Education about healthy aging
	  Medication monitoring
		Screening:
		  Pap smears
		  Mammogram
		  Testicular exams
		  Prostate check
		  Blood pressure
		  Blood sugar
		  Cholesterol
		  Eyes
		  Ears
		  Teeth
		  Skin
		  Osteoporosis
		  Weight
		  Depression
		  Caregiver training
		
		Age-specific interventions:
		  Colonoscopy
		  Depression
		  Caregiver support
			Early recognition and treatment of
			  Overuse syndrome
			  Pressure ulcers
			  Obesity
			  Infection
			  Fractures
			  Safety issues
			  Abuse and neglect
			
			Age-specific interventions:
			  Chronic disease management

HCP, health care provider.

Source: From © Cheryl Lehman (2010). Used with permission.

PSYCHOLOGICAL CONSIDERATIONS

Psychological conditions often complicate health, illness, recovery, and rehabilitation in the older adult. These conditions include mood disorders, anxiety disorders, personality disorders, and memory loss.

Depression

Between 1% and 15% of older adults in the community, about 12% of hospitalized older patients, nearly 14% of older adults receiving home health care, and over 40% of nursing home residents have depression (National Institute of Mental Health, 2007; Oppermann, 2010; Snowden, Steinman, & Frederick, 2008). Depression is a major risk factor for suicide and can also affect health and quality of life.

Depressive symptoms can range from dysthymia to mild or major depression to bipolar (or manic-depressive) disorder. Causes of depression in the older adult include health problems, loneliness, isolation, feeling a reduced sense of purpose, social and financial changes within the family, fear, and medications. Health conditions can precipitate depression, as can abuse of alcohol and drugs.

Recognizing depression is sometimes not easy in older adults, because the symptoms may be masked by other illnesses. As many as 75% of older adults who commit suicide have been seen by a healthcare professional in the month before their death (National Institute of Mental Health, 2007). Signs and symptoms of depression in older adults can include weight loss, fatigue, sadness, withdrawal from formerly pleasurable activities, changes in sleep patterns, suicidal thoughts, and abuse of alcohol or drugs. Depression also may be denied by the older adult but present physically as headaches, arthritic pain, or anxiety (HelpGuide.org, 2010).

> As many as 75% of older adults who commit suicide have been seen by a healthcare professional in the month before their death (National Institute of Mental Health, 2007).

Treatment of depression in the older adult begins with recognition of the likelihood of depression. Nurses should be alert for the symptoms of depression and routinely screen for depression in high-risk patients. The Geriatric Depression Scale is often used for such screening and can be found at http://www.merck.com/mkgr/mmg/tables/33t4.jsp. This screen does not diagnose depression but documents many of the symptoms and feelings associated with depression. If the patient screens positive through use of this scale or if the nurse believes the patient may suffer from depression, prompt communication of concerns to the primary care physician is of the utmost importance.

Anxiety Disorders

Anxiety disorders in older adults are "twice as prevalent as dementia among older adults, and four to eight times more prevalent than depressive disorders" (Cassidy & Rector, 2008, p.150). They can cause significant illness and negatively affect the quality of life. Like depression, anxiety disorders can be difficult to diagnose in the geriatric patient. Anxiety disorders in older adults include phobias, obsessive-compulsive disorder, posttraumatic stress disorder, panic disorders, and generalized anxiety disorder. As the person ages the presence of an anxiety disorder increases the likelihood of hospitalization.

> Anxiety disorders in older adults are "twice as prevalent as dementia among older adults, and four to eight times more prevalent than depressive disorders" (Cassidy & Rector, 2008, p.150).

Symptoms of anxiety disorders often mimic the symptoms of depression and physical illnesses, making the disorder that much more difficult to diagnose. These symptoms include changes in sleep patterns, agitation, problems with concentration and memory, chest pain, abdominal pain, headaches, and shortness of breath. Anxiety disorders are often associated with medical illnesses, such as stroke, heart attack, cancer, hypoglycemia, and delirium. Pharmacological treatment begins with an antidepressant such as a selective serotonin reuptake inhibitor, selective norepinephrine reuptake inhibitor, tricyclic, or monoamine oxidase inhibitor. Benzodiazepines are used as last resort treatment only and only in the short term. Psychotherapy is also of benefit.

Personality Disorders

Personality disorders are long-term, maladaptive ways of responding to people and stressful situations. They include paranoia, schizophrenia, psychosis, obsessive-compulsive disorder, borderline personality disorder, and histrionic, narcissistic, antisocial, and avoidant personality disorders. It is thought that as many as 10% of older adults living in the community, and even more in nursing homes, have one of these disorders (American Geriatric Society, 2005).

Personality disorders are sometimes grouped into clusters. Cluster A includes paranoia and schizophrenia. Persons with these disorders often appear to be odd and eccentric. Cluster B includes antisocial, borderline, narcissistic, and histrionic disorders. These people often have dramatic, erratic, and emotional behavior. Cluster C includes the avoidant, dependent, and obsessive-compulsive disorders. These people exhibit anxiety and fear.

Some personality disorders seem to have a genetic cause, some a social cause, but few of the causes are clear. Disruptive behavior secondary to a personality disorder can interrupt rehabilitation and might even dictate discharge to a nursing facility rather than to home. Treatment for personality disorders includes both long-term medications and psychotherapy.

Memory Loss

Mild memory loss can occur with aging. An example of mild memory loss is forgetting a new acquaintance's name or forgetting where you put your keys. The symptoms of memory loss become a concern in several instances:

- When it becomes more difficult to learn new things
- When frequently traveled routes are forgotten
- When "getting lost" occurs more and more frequently
- When the same sentences are repeated over and over in a single conversation
- When how to perform tasks that have been done many times before is forgotten
- When there is trouble with making choices or handling money

Memory loss is problematic when it begins to interfere with daily life. A medical workup is indicated for memory loss to rule out serious conditions such as depression, dementia, stroke, brain injury, and medication effects.

GERIATRIC SYNDROMES

The term "**geriatric syndrome**" is a way to describe how multiple underlying factors contribute to unique health conditions in older adults. These conditions do not fit into discrete disease categories. Geriatric syndromes can limit older adults' abilities to carry out basic daily activities, threaten their independence, and lower their quality of life. Geriatric syndromes are multifactorial and associated with substantial morbidity and poor outcomes (Inouye et al, 2007). They usually involve more than one body system, and one syndrome often contributes to another. For example, the syndrome of malnutrition includes such factors as mood, financial situation, living arrangements, mobility, presence of chronic conditions, and dentition. Malnutrition can lead to dehydration that may, in turn, cause delirium. Likewise, multiple interventions are used to address the overall syndrome of

TABLE 28.5   Geriatric Syndromes

• Polypharmacy	• Failure to thrive
• Dementia	• Sensory impairments
• Instability and falls	• Malnutrition
• Pressure ulcers	• Mood disorders
• Urinary incontinence	• Social isolation
• Iatrogenesis	• Delirium

malnutrition. Highly prevalent syndromes are listed in Table 28.5, and more information on select syndromes can be found in Table 28.6. As the **Baby Boomers** enter their older adulthood in the coming years, it will be more essential for gerontological rehabilitation nurses to recognize and intervene with these syndromes.

OTHER AGING ISSUES

Polypharmacy

Polypharmacy refers to the prescription, administration, or use of more medications than are clinically indicated. No specific number of medications are "too many," but when there are so many medications ordered they are not taken safely or as per order with the right dose by the right route at the right time by the right person, polypharmacy is the diagnosis. Imagine taking the following medications:

Drug "A": 2 pills at meals (8 AM, 12 noon, and 5 PM)
Drug "B": 1 pill at 9 AM
Drug "C": 2 pills every 6 hours (6 AM, 12 noon, 6 PM, and midnight)
Drug "D": 1 pill every 8 hours (8 AM, 4 PM, and midnight).

With just four drugs there are eight different administration times—two administration times that will probably interfere with sleep! There is one drug at each of the following times: 6 AM, 8 AM, 9 AM, 4 PM, 5 PM, and 6 PM and two drugs at noon and midnight.

So, multiple administration times are likely to affect adherence to the treatment plan. Now consider the interactions between multiple drugs. The more drugs that are added to a regimen, the more likelihood there will be a drug interaction with adverse symptoms and perhaps illness. It is also not unusual for a prescriber to order a new drug to treat a side effect of an old drug, for instance, ordering a stool softener to combat the constipation side effects of an opioid. It is not unusual for prescribers to forget exactly why a patient is taking a particular medication, especially if multiple prescribers are involved in the patient's case.

TABLE 28.6   Common Geriatric Syndromes and Complications of Care

Syndrome	General Information	Potential Causes	Diagnosis	Interventions
Delirium	• Acute onset of confusion • Life threatening • Usually reversible • Must be addressed ASAP • May have hyperactivity or hypoactivity related to the delirium • Confusion may come and go • Difficulty focusing • Distractible	• Infection (pneumonia, urinary tract infection) • Myocardial infarction • Pain • Constipation • Medications • Oxygenation • Stroke • Other medical illness	Confusion Assessment Method (CAM) http://consultgerirn.org/uploads/File/trythis/try_this_13.pdf History and physical Labs, x-rays	1. Report change in mental status to physician 2. Help find the cause 3. Treat the cause 4. Maintain safety 5. May need to manage behavior with medications such as Haldol in the short term 6. Help prevent future episodes through ensuring adequate nutrition, hydration, activity, interaction, pain management, glasses, hearing aides, avoiding restraints, minimizing tubes and lines, promoting sleep
Dementia	• Gradual onset • Memory loss • Problems with word-finding, math • Getting lost in familiar places • Not recognizing familiar faces • Decreased attention to grooming	• Vascular dementia • Alzheimer's dementia • Lewy body dementia • Parkinson's disease-related dementia • Pick disease	History and physical Labs, x-rays Mini-mental state exam Psychological testing	1. Referral to specialist 2. Medications may slow but not reverse decline 3. Maintain independence as long as possible 4. Be alert for safety risks, such as wandering, falls 5. Help with memory can include calendars, clocks, stocky notes, signs 6. Long term issues—driving, power of attorney for health-care, power of attorney for business, living will 7. Caregiver support
Falls	Falls with or without injury	• Poor vision • Unable to hear or understand directions • Decreased cognition • Refusal to follow instructions • Cluttered environment • Medications including laxatives, diuretics, antihypertensives, sedatives • Urinary incontinence or urgency • Muscle weakness • Dizziness • Multiple tubes and lines • Hypotension	Fall risk scales such as Morse scale	1. Be aware of risk factors 2. Ensure glasses and hearing aides are in reach and used 3. Ensure belongings and call light in reach 4. Ensure adequate lighting 5. Maintain uncluttered environment 6. Minimize tubes and lines 7. No restraints 8. Answer call lights promptly 9. Consider timed toileting

Syndrome	General Information	Potential Causes	Diagnosis	Interventions

Urinary incontinence	Leakage of urine	• Benign prostatic hypertension (BPH)
		• Stress incontinence
		• Urge incontinence
		• Overflow incontinence
		• Infection
		• Neurogenic bladder (diabetic neuropathy, spinal cord injury)
		• Urinary tract stones
		• Decreased mobility or cognition
		• Medications
			• History of urinary patterns, urgency, frequency, dribbling, difficulty initiating stream, burning, pain
			• Physical exam (male, prostate; female, uterine prolapse)
			• Postvoid residual
			• Urodynamics
			• Urinalysis and culture
				1. Determine cause
				2. Treat according to cause
				  • BPH: medications
				  • Urge, stress: Kegel exercises, fluid intake management, timed voiding
				  • Infection: antibiotics
				  • Stones: medication, lithotripsy
				  • Mobility: strengthening program, toileting program
				  • Cognition: timed toileting
				  • Medication change

Pressure ulcers	Discoloration of skin, redness Skin breakdown	• Pressure • Moisture • Friction • Shear	• Risk assessment (Braden) • Staging • Wound assessment • Investigation of risk factors and causes	1. Decrease risk factors: pressure, friction, shear, moisture 2. Ensure adequate intake of nutritious food and fluids 3. Assist with turning, positioning, out of bed activities 4. Ensure bowel and bladder program implemented
Sleep disorders	Normal changes in sleep due to aging can be complicated by medical illnesses, medications, and other treatments	Normal changes 1. Increased time to fall asleep 2. Changes in ability to stay asleep 3. Early awakening 4. More time in stage 1 and 2 of sleep, decrease in stage 3 and REM sleep as well as total sleep time Chronic insomnia in older adults can lead to • Falls • Cognitive decline • Increased risk of death	History and physical, including evidence of • Sleep apnea • Insomnia • RLS • Narcolepsy Medication review Assess sleep patterns Sleep specialist referral if needed	1. Consistent bedtime 2. Limit naps 3. Use bed for sleep only 4. Avoid caffeine, large meals, tobacco and stimulating activities late in day 5. Relaxation techniques at bedtime 6. Manage environment—noise, lights, interruptions, room temp 7. Toilet at bedtime 8. Low music 9. Massage 10. Provide warmth 11. Provide pain meds as needed 12. Sleep meds as last resort only

(continued)

TABLE 28.6   Common Geriatric Syndromes and Complications of Care *(continued)*

Syndrome	General Information	Potential Causes	Diagnosis	Interventions
Failure to thrive	Gradual physical decline accompanied by apathy and a loss of willingness to eat or drink	Often associated with functional decline, weight loss, depression, impaired cognition May also be associated with medical conditions such as cancer, diabetes, lung disease, stroke, heart failure, and so on or medications such as steroids, beta-blockers, opioids, tricyclic antidepressants, or with polypharmacy Often occurs at the end of life	• History and physical • Medication review • Depression screening • Cognitive screening • Functional assessment • Swallowing evaluation	1. Treatable causes are treated, weighing risks and benefits 2. Interdisciplinary team approach with physical and occupational therapists, speech-language therapist, nurses, physicians, social worker, dietitian

RLS, restless legs syndrome

The following guidelines should be used for medication ordering for the older adult:

- Every medication should be associated with a medical diagnosis.
- Benefits of each medication should outweigh the risks, including the risks of adverse events from drug interactions.
- Caution should be used when medications are ordered to combat the side effects of another drug in use.
- As much as possible, medications should be given in the lowest effective dose for the shortest time possible.
- Long-acting or time-release medications should be given when possible to reduce the frequency of administration.
- All medications for a particular patient should be given on the same schedule, when possible.
- Patients should be asked to bring in all medications being taken when they attend a doctor's appointment or when being admitted to any facility so that medications can be reviewed and screened.

Restraints

It is unfortunate, but not unusual, that restraints are used in many settings as a behavior management plan for older adults to prevent falls and manage agitation. Restraints, however, are rarely indicated and can actually cause, rather than prevent, injury. Geriatric specialty nurses have become adept at successfully using alternatives to restraints, particularly because of the need to emphasize safety and fall prevention in this population. The reader is referred to ConsultGeri.org at www.consultgerirn.org/topics/physical_restraints/want_to_know_more for an excellent and full discussion of restraint use and alternatives to restraints for the older adult.

Advance Directives

There are several important issues to be addressed at the end of life, such as advance directives and living wills. It is not yet the norm that all older adults have completed these important documents, so the nurse is likely to encounter ethical issues if practicing in a setting to which older adults are admitted.

Identification of a decision maker is one aspect of care of the older adult, if there is no advance directive. Decision makers are needed in the rehabilitation setting if the patient is deemed unable to make his or her own informed decisions. These might include decisions about treatment or perhaps discharge location. Decision makers are identified under the laws of the state and most typically begin with the legal spouse. If there is no spouse or if the spouse is incapacitated, then the adult children are the next in line as decision makers. If there are no children, the next in line might be siblings or grandchildren, and so on. If there is no advance directive and no family, the courts are asked to legally appoint a guardian to ensure that decisions are in the best interest of the patient. Caring Connections has copies of each state's advance directives available for download at www.caringinfo.org/stateaddownload. Chapter 25 presents more information on legal aspects of guardianship.

Hospice

Another common issue in care of the older adult is hospice. The website of the National Hospice and Palliative Care Organization can be found at http://www.nhpco.org/templates/1/homepage.cfm.

Patients often wait to enter hospice care until the last days or weeks of life. This is unfortunate, because hospice is not just for the "nearly dead" but can greatly contribute to the quality of life for those at the end of life and their families. Hospice services include psychological support and pain and symptom management. The goal of hospice is not to cure but to assist the patient to have the highest possible quality of life in the time remaining. Likewise, **palliative care** services can assist those who are not eligible for hospice but need a specialized coordinated care team. Palliative care focuses on comfort versus curative medicine but uses a highly skilled team of experts to address the ongoing needs of persons with incurable illnesses.

Death Panel

"**Death panel**" is a term that has recently surfaced with healthcare reform. It refers to a false rumor that the new healthcare reform act would finance panels of people whose job it would be to decide whether others were worthy of life and of receiving costly medical treatment (Rutenberg & Calmes, 2009). The true proposal in the healthcare bill was that Medicare would finance a patient's voluntary consultation with professionals at the end of life to discuss plans for aggressive and potentially life-saving interventions. Misinterpretation, however, necessitated removal of this benefit from the healthcare reform act.

Driving

Driving and older adults is another issue confronting our society, especially as the numbers of older adults increase. Driving is an activity with many strong emotions attached to it. Obtaining that first driver's license when young signals independence, whereas giving up the keys in older age can be a dreaded return to dependence. Losing the "right" to drive may force a senior into social isolation, without an independent method of getting groceries, visiting church or family, or getting to the doctor. Many older adults do not like to depend on others for mobility. Aging, however, brings many factors into play that can make driving unsafe for the older adult, such as changes in vision and hearing, slowed reaction times, and decreased muscle strength. There is no easy answer to this issue; some states mandate retesting at closer intervals in the older adult, and some states do not address the issue at all (Gallo et al., 2006). The burden is often placed upon the healthcare worker to inform the state of potentially unsafe drivers. The following website has a checklist for families to use to evaluate the safety of the older drivers in their family: www.aging-parents-and-elder-care.com/Pages/Checklists/Elderly_Drivers.html.

Healthcare Funding

Funding for medical services seems to be revised every day, as healthcare reform works its way into the system. Private insurance, Medicare, and Medicaid are common sources for healthcare funding for older adults in the United States. Private insurance is often a retirement benefit, or premiums may be privately paid by the individual. Medicare is a health insurance program for people 65 and older, some disabled individuals, and individuals with end-stage renal disease. One restriction for Medicare is that the patient or spouse must have worked for at least 10 years in Medicare-covered employment before it is available to them. Medicare is quite complex and more can be learned at www.medicare.gov/Publications/Pubs/pdf/10050.pdf. Medicaid is jointly funded by the federal and state governments to assist in the provision of adequate medical care to eligible needy persons, including

low income seniors. Each state develops the rules for its citizens, and state-specific information about Medicaid can be obtained from that state's website. The Centers for Medicare & Medicaid oversees both programs at the federal level. Their website has more information about Medicaid rules and coverage (see www.cms.gov/home/medicaid.asp).

ELDER ABUSE AND NEGLECT

Statistics on the abuse, neglect, or mistreatment of older adults are often unreliable, largely due to underreporting of occurrences. However, it is estimated that between 1 and 2 million adults over age 65 have been victims of some type of physical abuse or neglect (National Research Council Panel to Review Risk and Prevalence of Elder Abuse and Neglect, 2003). Up to 5 million persons per year may experience financial exploitation (Fulmer & Greenberg, 2008). Mistreatment of the elderly is a growing problem. Rehabilitation patients are often at higher risk for potential abuse because of their dependence on others for care.

There are several types of **elder abuse**, categorized slightly differently by various authors. Pritchard (1995) named four categories of abuse: physical, psychological, sociological, and legal. Sengstock and Barrett (1992) distinguished six types of abuse or neglect through a useful system (that showed degrees of mistreatment): psycho-

TABLE 28.7   Risk Factors for Elder Mistreatment
Caregiver stress or burden
Depression
Dependence of elder on caretaker
Family history of violence
History of mental illness in caregiver/family member
Increased age
Lack of finances
Physical disability
Poor social support
Shared living arrangement
Social isolation of the older adult
Substance abuse in family members/caretakers
Unsafe living situation

TABLE 28.8   Indications of Possible Elder Abuse
Poor hygiene
Unexplained bruises of various stages of healing
Bruises on inner aspects of body
Broken bones
Skin tears
Poor oral hygiene
Burns
Malnutrition
Dehydration
Depressed mood
Withdrawn, fearful
Cowering
Difficulty sitting down or grimacing when walking/sitting
History of treatment in a variety of facilities and by different providers
Person left alone in the home frequently
Person brought for treatment by someone other than the caregiver
Elder expresses feelings of hopelessness, powerlessness
Elder expresses ambivalent feelings toward family

logical or emotional neglect, psychological or emotional abuse, violation of personal rights, financial abuse, physical neglect, and direct physical abuse. Fulmer and Greenberg (2008) recognized six types of mistreatment labeled physical abuse, emotional/psychological abuse, sexual abuse, financial abuse/exploitation, caregiver neglect, and self-neglect. The major types of elder abuse reported in the United Kingdom are psychological, financial, and physical. Sexual abuse is subsumed under physical abuse in many reports. Other types of abuse include negligence and discrimination.

Women are more likely to be victims of abuse than men. Regardless of the means used to evaluate mistreatment, it can be observed that abuse covers a wide range, such as violations of an older adults' autonomy, financial abuse such as stealing of money or property, neglect of one's basic needs for nutrition or socialization, causing

TABLE 28.9   Strategies for Preventing Elder Mistreatment
Assessment
Observe family interactions, dynamics, and body language to assess risk.
Interview the patient and family or caregiver to find out normal patterns for stress management.
Identify caregivers at highest risk to be abusers, and target interventions to prevent stress from caregiver burden.
Be aware of risk factors and contributing factors.
Interventions
Establish a trusting relationship with the older adult client and caregiver.
Identify possible stressful scenarios and facilitate strategies for families to cope with the situations.
Refer families to resources available in the community.
Strengthen social supports.
Encourage regular respite for the caregiver.
Encourage single patients to stay involved and connected socially.
Perform thorough physical assessments and carefully document findings, including appearance, nutritional state, skin condition, mental/emotional state, attitude and awareness, and need for aids to enhance sensory perception.
Encourage the patient to let a trusted person know where valuable papers are stored.
If abuse is suspected, interview the caregiver and other possible information to confirm or refute suspicions.
Know the laws in your state governing reports of abuse.

BOX 28.2   Web Link to the National Committee for the Prevention of Elder Abuse
Visit http://www.preventelderabuse.org/elderabuse/ and review definitions of elder abuse and the role of professionals in prevention.

BOX 28.3   Web Link to Evidence-Based Geriatric Nursing Practice
Browse the evidence-based geriatric clinical nursing website of The Hartford Institute for Geriatric Nursing, at New York University's College of Nursing at http://consultgerirn.org

BOX 28.4   Web Exploration
American Association of Retired Persons http://www.aarp.org
The official geriatric nursing website of the American Nurses Association (ANA) http://geronurseonline.org
American Society on Aging http://www.asaging.org/index.cfm
The evidence-based geriatric clinical nursing website of The Hartford Institute for Geriatric Nursing, at New York University's College of Nursing http://consultgerirn.org
National Academy on an Aging Society http://www.agingsociety.org/agingsociety
The National Association of Area Agencies on Aging's primary mission is to build the capacity of its members to help older persons and persons with disabilities live with dignity and choices in their homes and communities for as long as possible. http://www.n4a.org
National Council on Aging http://www.ncoa.org
The National Gerontological Nursing Association (NGNA) is dedicated to the clinical care of older adults across diverse care settings. https://www.ngna.org

emotional distress without physical abuse, or extreme violence with the intent of bodily harm.

Several risk factors for elder abuse have been recognized (Table 28.7). In the United Kingdom researchers found the primary risk factors for elder abuse were stress, social isolation, dependency, preexisting relationships, and intergenerational abuse (McGarry & Simpson, 2009). Recognition of the presence of these risk factors is the first step in prevention.

There are several indications of possible **elder abuse** or **mistreatment** (Table 28.8). Detection and prevention are the keys to preventing further abuse. Early reporting is encouraged. McGarry and Simpson encouraged the following process:

- Identifying the indicators of abuse
- Initiating a verbal report to a line manager or other appropriate person, such as a mentor if a nursing student
- Completing a comprehensive written report and documentation

Fulmer (2008) developed a helpful tool for assessment of elder mistreatment. It is available online through the Try This Series from the Hartford Foundation at http://consultgerirn.org/uploads/File/trythis/try_this_15.pdf.

In the United Kingdom once the report is submitted, nurses are kept informed of the progress of the investigation. This is different from the United States where a nurse may report and never know the outcome of the adult protective service inquiry.

Rehabilitation nurses may be more likely than nurses in other specialties to observe elder mistreatment. Patients needing rehabilitation are often those with risk factors such as those discussed earlier. Rehabilitation nurses are also in an ideal position to help prevent or reduce the potential for abuse. Patients should be encouraged to stay active and involved in social activities as much as possible. Older adults should always have access to a telephone and a private place to use it. They should maintain contact with family members and friends who provide positive social support. The nurse can refer patients or clients for help with financial matters if needed and facilitate the involvement of social services and clergy as necessary. In addition, as nurses and social workers perform home evaluations before discharge, the person's surroundings and safety can be evaluated. Table 28.9 provides additional strategies for prevention of elder mistreatment. The reader is encouraged to browse the website in Boxes 28.2 and 28.3 for more information on the topic.

SUMMARY

This chapter has presented an overview of aging, including normal changes with aging, aging and disability, geriatric syndromes, and common issues associated with aging. Rehabilitation nurses will increasingly be challenged to care for aging adults, and knowledge of normal aging and abnormal signs and symptoms is very important. The reader is encouraged to explore the websites listed throughout this chapter for further information on aging.

CRITICAL THINKING

1. It can be challenging for older adults to participate in rehabilitation. Illnesses in older adults may have an atypical presentation, and complications that occur during rehabilitation may not be properly noticed, assessed, and managed. Explore the resources available on delirium at www.consultgerirn.org and ask yourself if the nursing practice in your rehabilitation unit reflects best-practices for management of delirium in older adults.

2. Visit an older adult in your neighborhood. Ask him or her how mobility and access to the environment has changed in the past few years. Assess his or her level of community involvement, transportation resources, and social network. Offer to perform a safety assessment of the home.

3. Explore the resources on older adults at www.rehabnurse.org. Click on Professional resources and then on Caring for Older Adults. Read *Older Adults in Rehabilitation* and consider how your facility might better serve older patients in the rehabilitation setting.

PERSONAL REFLECTION

- Do you believe our society is ready and able to adequately care for older adults with disability? Why or why not?
- Is your community ready and able to care for disabled individuals who are aging?
- Is your family ready and able to care for older relatives who may acquire a new disability?
- How can you apply the concepts in this chapter to your anticipated nursing practice, even if you do not choose to specialize in rehabilitation?
- How might you assist your local community in ensuring that adequate community supports are in place for older adults with disability?
- What volunteer opportunities are available for you to assist with disability prevention at the local, state and national levels?

REFERENCES

Amella, E. J. (2004). Presentation of illness in older adults. *American Journal of Nursing, 104*(10), 40–51.

American Geriatric Society. (2005). Aging in the know: Personality disorders. Retrieved August 26, 2010, from http://www.healthinaging.org/agingintheknow/chapters_ch_trial.asp?ch=35

American Heart Association. (2010). About high blood pressure. Retrieved from http://www.heart.org/HEARTORG/Conditions/HighBloodPressure/AboutHighBloodPressure/Understanding-Blood-Pressure-Readings_UCM_301764_Article.jsp

Barnhart, R.C., & Connolly, B. (2007). Aging and Down syndrome: Implications for physical therapy. *Physical Therapy, 87*(10), 1399–1406.

Beers, M., & Berkow, R. (2005). *The Merck manual of geriatrics* (5th ed.). Whitehouse Station, NJ: Merck.

Brenner, L. A., Homaifar, B. Y., & Schultheis, M. T. (2008). Driving, aging and traumatic brain injury: Integrating findings from the literature. *Rehabilitation Psychology, 53*(1), 18–27.

Cassidy, K.-L., & Rector, N.A. (2008). The silent geriatric giant: Anxiety disorders in late life. *Geriatrics and Aging, 11*(3), 150–156.

Centers for Disease Control and Prevention and the Merck Company Foundation. (2007). *The state of aging and health in America 2007.* Whitehouse Station, NJ: Merck.

Child Development Institute. (2010). Stages of social-emotional development in children and teenagers. Retrieved from http://www.childdevelopmentinfo.com/development/erickson.shtml

Colantonio, A., Ratliff, G., Chase, S., & Vernich, L. (2004). Aging with traumatic brain injury: Long-term health conditions. *International Journal of Rehabilitation Research, 27*(3), 209–214.

Diebold, C., Fanning-Harding, F., & Hanson, P. (2010). Management of common problems. In K. Mauk (Ed.), *Gerontological nursing: Competencies for care* (pp. 454–528). Sudbury, MA: Jones and Bartlett.

Finlayson, M., Van Denend, T., & Hudson, E. (2004). Aging with multiple sclerosis. *Journal of Neuroscience Nursing, 36*(5). Retrieved from http://www.medscape.com/viewarticle/491004_print

Fordner, L. S., Carruthers, D., & Londner, R. B. (2009). What is aging and how is it different with a disability? *Professional Case Management, 14*(5), 270–272.

Fulmer, T. (2008). Elder mistreatment assessment. Retrieved from http://consultgerirn.org/uploads/File/trythis/try_this_15.pdf

Fulmer, T., & Greenberg, S. (2008). Elder mistreatment and abuse. Retrieved from http://consultgerirn.org/topics/elder_mistreatment_and_abuse/want_to_know_more#item_2

Gallo, J. J., Bogner, H. R., Fulmer, T., & Paveza, G. J. (2006). *Handbook of geriatric assessment.* Sudbury, MA: Jones and Bartlett.

Hall, J. (2004). Neuroendocrine physiology of the early and late menopause. *Endocrinology and Metabolism Clinics of North America, 33*(4), 637–659.

Hazzard, W. R., Blass, J. P. Halter, J. D. Ouslander, J. G., & Tinetti, M. E. (2008). *Principles of geriatric medicine and gerontology.* New York: McGraw Hill.

Heineman, J. M., Hamrick-King, J., & Scaglione Sewell, B. (2010). Review of the aging of physiological systems. In K. Mauk (Ed.), *Gerontological nursing: Competencies for care* (pp. 128–231). Sudbury, MA: Jones and Bartlett.

HelpGuide.org. (2010). Depression in older adults and the elderly: Recognizing the signs and getting help. Retrieved August 25, 2010 from http://www.helpguide.org/mental/depression_elderly.htm

Inouye, S. K., Studensky, S., & Tinetti, M. E. (2007). Geriatric syndromes: clinical, research, and policy implications of a core geriatric concept. *Journal of the American Geriatric Society, 55*, 780–791.

Jones, G. C. (2009). Aging with cerebral palsy and other disabilities: Personal reflections and recommendations. *Developmental Medicine and Child Neurology, 51*(Suppl 4), 12–15.

Krause, J. S. & Coker, S. L. (2006). Aging after spinal cord: A 30 year longitudinal study. *Journal of Spinal Cord Medicine, 29*, 371–379.

Mauk, K. L., & Hanson, P. (2010). Management of common illnesses, diseases, and health conditions. In K. Mauk (Ed.), *Gerontological nursing: Competencies for care* (pp. 382–453). Sudbury, MA: Jones and Bartlett.

McGarry, J. & Simpson, C. (2009). Raising awareness of elder abuse in the community practice setting. *British Journal of Community Nursing, 14*, 305–308.

National Institute of Aging. (2010). In search of the secrets of aging. Retrieved August 26, 2010, from http://www.healthandage.com/html/min/nih/content/booklets/in_search_of_the_secrets/p2.htm

National Institute of Mental Health. (2007). Older adults: Depression and suicide facts. Retrieved August 25, 2010 from http://www.nimh.nih.gov/health/publications/older-adults-depression-and-suicide-facts-fact-sheet/index.shtml

National Research Council Panel to Review Risk and Prevalence of Elder Abuse and Neglect. (2003). Elder mistreatment: Abuse, neglect and exploitation in an aging America. Washington, DC: Author.

National Sleep Foundation. (2009). Aging and sleep. Retrieved July 1, 2010, from http://www.sleepfoundation.org/article/sleep-topics/aging-and-sleep

Neugarten, B. N. (1968). The awareness of middle age. In B. N. Neugarten (Ed.), *Middle age and aging: A reader in social psychology* (pp. 93–98). Chicago: University of Chicago Press.

Oppermann, P. (2010). How to recognize and treat depression in the older adult. Retrieved August 25, 2010, from http://www.columbiapsych.com/depression_older.html

Peck, R. (1968). Psychological development in the second half of life. In B. N. Neugarten (Ed.), *Middle age and aging: A reader in social psychology* (pp. 88–92). Chicago: University of Chicago Press.

Pritchard, J. (1995). *The abuse of older people: A training manual for detection and prevention.* London: Jessica Kingsley Publishers.

Pue, K., & Wei, J. (2001). Clinical implications of physiological changes in the aging heart. *Drugs & Aging, 18*(4), 263–276.

Rutenberg, J., & Calmes, J. (2009). False "death panels" rumor has some familiar roots. *New York Times*, Aug. 13, 2009. Retrieved from http://www.nytimes.com/2009/08/14/health/policy/14panel.html?_r=3

Sengstock, M. C., & Barrett, S. A. (1992). Abuse and neglect of the elderly in family settings. In J. Campbell & J. Humphreys (Eds.), *Nursing care of survivors of family violence* (pp. 173–208). St. Louis, MO: Mosby.

Snowden, M., Steinman, L., & Frederick, J. (2008). Treating depression in older adults: Challenges to implementing the recommendations of an expert panel. Retrieved August 25, 2010 from http://www.cdc.gov/pcd/issues/2008/jan/07_0154.htm

Svien, L. R., Berg, P., & Stephenson, C. (2008). Issues in aging with cerebral palsy. *Topics in Geriatric Rehabilitation, 24*(1), 26–40.

U. S. Census Bureau. (2008). Americans with disabilities: 2005. Retrieved from http://www.census.gov/prod/2008pubs/p70–117.pdf

CHAPTER 29

Animal-Assisted Therapy

Rachel M. Easton
Alan Beck

LEARNING OBJECTIVES

At the end of this chapter, the reader will be able to

- Distinguish between animal-assisted therapy, animal-assisted activities, and pet visitation programs.
- Discuss benefits of animal programs and services in rehabilitation settings.
- Identify health and liability requirements associated with animal-assisted therapy and animal visitation programs in healthcare settings.
- Describe research findings of health benefits associated with the human–animal bond.
- Define zoonotic disease and precautions required to minimize disease transmission between animals and humans.

KEY CONCEPTS AND TERMS

Animal-assisted activities (AAA)	Hippotherapy	Pet visitation programs
Animal-assisted therapy (AAT)	Human–animal bond	Staff animal
Assistance animal	One Health	Zoonotic disease

The **human–animal bond** provides social, psychological, and physical health benefits to people who may otherwise be isolated due to emotional, behavioral, or physical problems (Beck & Katcher, 1996; Schaffer, 2008). Because this is an emerging field, there are limitless opportunities for leadership roles in **animal-assisted therapy (AAT)** organizations and projects, and healthcare professionals are uniquely situated to provide community and client education and leadership.

The **One Health** concept is a worldwide strategy for expanding interdisciplinary collaborations and communications in all aspects of health care for humans and animals (Academic Team of the American Veterinary Medical Association [AVMA] One Health Initiative Task Force and Partners, n.d.). Animals are quickly becoming accepted as part of a multidisciplinary healthcare team. Given the inherent risks of working with animals, it is imperative that veterinarians, behaviorists, trainers, and human healthcare professionals work together to minimize risk and to maximize the benefit of AAT (Nolan, 2007).

TYPES OF AAT

Definition

Definitions for AAT and **animal-assisted activities (AAA)** have been established by the Delta Society, a long-standing leader in the development of animal-related therapies since 1977, as well as the Association for Professionals in Infection Control and Epidemiology. (Schaffer 2008) defines AAT as "a goal-directed intervention in which an animal meeting specific criteria is an integral part of the treatment process. AAT is delivered by a health or human service provider working within the scope of his/her profession. AAT is designed to promote improvement in human physical, social, emotional, and/ or cognitive functioning. AATs provide individual or group therapy in a variety of settings and the process is documented and evaluated (p. 76)."

Perhaps most effective with emotional or developmental disabilities, AAT can be used to evaluate the developmental stage of a patient, improve a patient's state of mind, and enhance socialization activities. All these therapies are done with a specific therapeutic goal, such as brain-injured patients whose cognitive recognition can be evaluated by asking them to interact with the dog in specific ways, or poststroke patients whose speech therapy may be enhanced by giving commands to a canine companion.

The goal of any AAA is to enhance quality of life through various educational, recreational, or therapeutic opportunities (Souter & Miller, 2007). In a long-term care setting these activities often provide social interaction that can alleviate distress, depression, and loneliness (Banks, Willoughby, & Banks, 2008; Lutwack-Bloom, Wijewickrama, & Smith, 2005; Souter && Miller, 2007). Studies by Richeson in 2003 and McCabe et al. in 2002, for example, found significant decreases in agitation in Alzheimer's units with residential or visiting dogs.

"Pet therapy" is a general term often used to describe these programs, but this term is not necessarily accurate because not all visiting animals are pets—some may be service animals—and these animals may only be involved in organized activities with residents, not therapies. **Pet visitation programs** are designed to provide companionship, sensory stimulation, and an opportunity for reminiscence. Handlers bring animals to nonambulatory residents and help residents hold and interact with the animals (Appel et al., 2003). Pet visitation programs may address the needs of residents and/or staff that cannot be around the animals due to allergies or phobias. Facilities permitting pet visitation should post notices near the front entrance and at reception alerting visiting pet owners to sign in and out, fill out an animal registration form and owner statement, and informing them that all visiting animals must be licensed, have an identification tag displayed, be clean and parasite free, and be kept on leash or in a carrier (Appel et al., 2003). Facilities should also have a policy in place that should be reviewed and updated at least annually. If there are live-in animals, an additional notice should be posted alerting visitors if the facility has any roaming animals and requiring visiting pets to be on a leash (or in a carrier) and under control at all times while in the facility.

The issue of pets visiting overnight most often comes up with hospice patients facing end-of-life situations or patients in transition between levels of care that need time to find a new home for their pet. The opportunity to say goodbye can be deeply comforting for these patients, and in situations when regular visits from the animal can be arranged, it may help to reduce anxiety. Before granting permission for overnight visitation, the facility should ensure that visiting animals are screened and subject to

the same guidelines as any other visiting animal. Also, a contract should be signed regarding the specifics of care and responsibility for the animal. If there is a roommate that will be affected, permission must be obtained from him or her as well. Visits should all be scheduled through the animal care coordinator when possible (Appel et al., 2003).

Costs associated with this type of visitation are minimal, because animal care and maintenance does not generally happen on the premises. However, signs should be made and posted throughout the facility, and the facility may also want to purchase items such as pet

---

CASE STUDY 29.1

Two of your teenage daughter's friends are talking about their volunteer work at the local animal shelter. You hear them describe how, twice a month, they drive to the shelter, pick up a couple kittens, and take them to the nursing home for the residents to play with for a few hours. They mention that some of the kittens seem stressed and don't look like they enjoy being held or restrained.

Questions

1. As a rehabilitation nurse with knowledge of AAT/AAA, identify what is wrong in this situation.
2. What would you say to these teens, recognizing they are trying to provide a community service?
3. How could you improve on the current situation and still encourage these teens to be involved in this service to older adults? What additional information would you need? What contacts would be required? To whom would you speak to remedy this situation?

In this situation the volunteer needs to be educated regarding the risks of taking young animals with an unknown health status to visit elderly people who may be immunocompromised. The shelter and the volunteer should understand the importance of the animal's signals of stress and discomfort, as well as the risks associated with erratic handling of unpredictable animals. Hopefully, the shelter recommends that all animals visit a veterinarian as soon as possible so they can be health screened and behavior tested before participating in any AAT/AAA programs. In addition, the nursing home should have a protocol and guidelines for AAT/AAA that meets state standards.

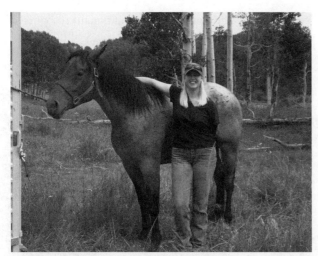

FIGURE 29.1   Animals play an important role in the lives of many persons

gates or towels that can be used during visits (Appel et al., 2003).

The handler is primarily responsible for the visiting animal, but the facility is ultimately responsible for the safety of the residents. Staff members should keep an eye out for trip hazards such as a dog laying in the hallway or stretching in front of doorways, and if a facility is not able to oversee these visits they should not proceed with a visiting animal program (Appel et al., 2003).

A facility decides to provide AAA, AAT, or pet visitation depending on its purpose and the resources available. If the goal is to improve residents' quality of life, then AAAs are indicated. AATs can be used by therapists to help residents achieve specific individual goals. To be considered for AATs, an animal must meet very specific criteria that assist in goal-directed interventions (Schaffer, 2008). AAA or AAT teams can have profoundly positive effects on residents, but the support needed to make these visits a success is often not in place at facilities. Some facilities permit casual animal visits, which are categorized as "nonregistered" because most of them are not associated with an official therapy organization. These animals should still be screened for appropriate temperament, behavior, and sound health, and handlers should still be required to fill out forms and liability statements.

AAAs are more informal activities that simply involve pets and people that provide quality-of-life enhancing opportunities. Both AATs and AAAs can be organized and delivered by specially trained professionals, paraprofessionals, or trained volunteers such as veterinarians, behaviorists, and animal trainers who are equipped to

provide support services to the participating animals and their (Schafer, 2008).

In addition to AAT, AAAs, and pet visitation programs, animals may be used in a variety of other ways (Figure 29.1). These include residential and service animals.

Residential Animals

This group might include staff animals, live-in animals owned by residents, or live-in animals owned by the facility. Live-in animals can be "resident owned" or "facility owned," but in general this type of live-in animal program requires much more care and cost, and responsibilities must be clearly delineated. As long as the animal is part of the facility living environment, the facility is ultimately responsible for ensuring that the animal's care meets general health and hygiene guidelines.

In most cases the resident is the primary caretaker, but some help may be needed from family, friends, or facility staff and should be defined at the time of admission. There should be a written agreement that outlines responsibility for daily care, veterinary care, licensing, grooming, cleanup, and end-of-life considerations. A chart should be maintained for each residential animal within the facility that includes an intake form, care plan, and forms to chart daily activities for the animal. These files should be reviewed at least quarterly by the facility, resident, and the resident's family members as is deemed appropriate (Appel et al., 2003).

More facilities are moving toward the continuing care retirement community model, which ranges from independent living to assisted nursing care. Administrators must determine how the tasks and responsibilities of a residential animal are to be met within each level of care as a resident moves throughout the system. There are many physical and psychological benefits associated with companion animals, and the presence of a familiar animal from home can often ease the transition to life in the facility.

Facilities that would like an animal present during the day but cannot manage a live-in animal, a **staff animal** is a wonderful alternative. Staff animals accompany their owner (a staff member) on part or all of a shift and go home with the staff member at the end of the day. Staff animals must be screened just like any visiting animal for health and temperament requirements. These animals may be included in AAT procedures or simply AAAs, but the staff member should be the main supervisor of the animal at all times while in the facility. A chart and care plan similar to that designed for live-in animals owned by the facility should be created for each staff animal to track the animal's health and behavior. Written objectives should state the purpose of the animal's involvement in facility activities. (These plans and objectives should be reviewed quarterly (Appel et al., 2003).

> *"When older people withdraw from active participation in daily human affairs, the non-human environment in general, and animals in particular, can become increasingly important. Although the potential for significant benefits to a great variety of people exists through association with companion animals, the potential seems great in the elderly, for whom the bond with animal companions is perhaps stronger and more profound than at any other age."*
>
> —Leo Bustad, veterinarian and founder of the People-Pet-Partnership Program in Washington and pioneer for geriatric pet therapy (Bustad & Hines, 198, paragraph 13)

Some specific guidelines for residential animals should include animals having scheduled work times with specifically assigned staff, scheduled rest periods in a quiet place, and frequent bathroom opportunities. The handler should also be familiar with the animal's stress signals, and the animal should spend no more than several hours in the facility in any given day (Appel et al., 2003).

The facility's insurance carrier should be consulted regarding liability, and the insurance company may require proof of the animal's training, behavior, and veterinary care to keep insurance rates as low as possible. Liability will likely vary depending on the extent the animal is in contact with other residents. Staff animals may be excluded from some umbrella liability insurance provided to visiting teams that are nationally registered. As part of the documentation process, the staff member should complete an information form and owner statement, and whenever possible the facility should require staff animals to be registered with a nationally recognized AAA/AAT organization.

Assistance Animals

Assistance animal is the proper term applied to guide, hearing, and other service animals. Assistance animals can perform tasks for people with disabilities such as hearing impairment, physical limitations, emotional disabilities, diabetes, or seizures (Friedmann & Son, 2009). Because these animals are so important to their owners, Title III of the Americans with Disabilities Act of 1990 ruled that these animals have legal access to public places, unlike AAT/AAA animals, which are subject to public rules for all animals (Duncan, 2000; Schaffer, 2008). Service animals are not considered pets, and their purpose is to provide specific benefits to the handler, whereas AAT/AAA animals focus on providing benefits to people besides their handlers (Gammonley et al., 1997).

Assistance animals provide a vital life-improving service to their users, but the animal's welfare must also be considered. Therefore, assistance animals require special attention from veterinarians. Health status, stress level, mobility, and functional capacity should be regularly evaluated by a veterinarian to protect the animal from being overly stressed or overworked. When these animals are hospitalized or removed from the user's care, the change will significantly impact the user's function and physiological status (Friedmann & Son, 2009). Arrangements should be made to ensure the user's safety, as well as physical and psychological needs, and the veterinarian and medical staff should work together to alleviate client distress.

Therapeutic Riding

Therapeutic horseback riding encompasses a variety of equine activities in which people with various disabilities are able to participate. This type of therapy can be an

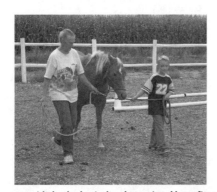 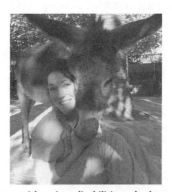

FIGURE 29.2 Horses can provide both physical and emotional benefits to persons with various disabilities, whether a child or adult.

invaluable tool in a patient's physical, psychological, and social development when integrated into a treatment process. A more specific area of therapeutic riding is known as "**hippotherapy**," which uses the movement of a horse as a treatment strategy aimed at improving neuromuscular function (Benjamin, 2000). Therapy sessions led by certified physical, occupational, and speech-language therapists combine riding with exercises intended to improve balance, coordination, posture, and muscle tone (Crawford & Pomerinke, 2003, Schaffer, 2008).

Horseback riding can provide rhythmic and repetitive movements that create a supportive yet dynamic base for the patient. While on the horse, the patient has sensory input through vestibular, proprioceptive, tactile, and visual channels that help them adjust to changes in gait and speed. The horse's walking gait moves the patient in a manner similar to the normal gait of a walking human. The patient has to make small adjustments to maintain stability, which increases trunk strength, posture control, and can enhance sensory and motor systems (Benjamin, 2000) (Figure 29.2).

Each patient is evaluated by medical professionals trained in hippotherapy, and the therapist works with a professional equine handler to manipulate the horse's movement, position, and activities to promote certain functional outcomes. The treatment can be adjusted according to the patient's responses as part of an integrated treatment program (Benjamin, 2000). According to the American Hippotherapy Association, hippotherapy is indicated for children and adults with mild to severe neuromuscular dysfunction (Benjamin, 2000). Hippotherapy may be especially useful as part of a rehabilitation program for sensory integration disorders or speech-language disorders, posttraumatic brain injury, and stroke. Other general impairments, including abnormal muscle tone, balance, coordination, communication, postural symmetry or control, and decreased mobility, may also benefit significantly from this unique equine therapy (Benjamin, 2000). In addition to physical benefits, the emotional bond formed with horses (Figure 29.2) may have a therapeutic effect on well-being and quality of life (AVMA, 2002; Crawford & Pomerinke, 2003).

HUMAN–ANIMAL BOND

Definition

Not only do animals enrich our lives in very obvious ways, but they provide us with distinct physiological, psychological, and social benefits that help keep us healthy and happy. The human–animal bond is prehistoric in its existence but only recently has it developed scientifically as a defined entity (Crawford & Pomerinke, 2003). The AVMA (2002) defines the human–animal bond as "a mutually beneficial and dynamic relationship between people and other animals that is influenced by behaviors that are essential to the health and well-being of both." Currently, over 62% of American households have at least one pet (AVMA, 2002), and over 75% of dog owners say their pet's health is as important to them as their own health (Pfizer Animal Health/Gallup Organization Dog Owner Survey) (Figure 29.3). An American Animal Hospital Association (AAHA) Pet Owner survey (2001) showed that 52% of people are more likely to remember the names of neighbors' pets than the names of the neighbors themselves. And studies have even shown a

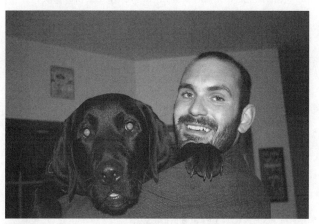

FIGURE 29.3 Dogs are one of the most commonly used animals for AAT.

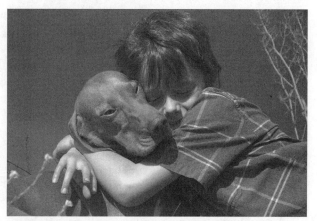

FIGURE 29.4 Pets may play a special role with children

© Jolanta Stozek/Dreamstime.com

link between how people treat animals and how they treat each other. The companionship that comes with our four-legged friends is typically unconditional and unwavering, and the strong bonds that are forged with them are life-changing.

> *"The affection provided by an animal is simple, unconditional, and uncomplicated. Pets are playmates for persons of any age group, provide the security of companionship and are frequently a confidant. These comforting and healing qualities enable animals to be facilitators in therapy."*
>
> —Cornell Companion, Cornell University,
> http://www.vet.cornell.edu/services/companions/bond.htm

Health Benefits for Children

Animals play an important role in stress reduction through a variety of avenues—encouraging physical activity or exercise, providing emotional support, and life balance. Children, for example, are full of energy and playfulness that seems to naturally complement our furry friends. Studies have shown that children with attention deficit hyperactivity disorder may have better focus and a healthier energy outlet when paired with a canine companion. Also, children with special emotional needs can often find comfort and support through their pets (Figure 29.4).

Health Benefits for Older Adults

Pet owners tend to have lower blood pressure, triglycerides, and cholesterol levels. Studies by Friedmann et al. (1980) and Friedmann and Thomas (1995) showed associations with pet ownership and increased survival rates after a heart attack. Animal ownership is often associated with stress reduction, weight control, and having fewer minor health problems. One example of this was seen with Alzheimer's patients allowed to observe fish in a facility fish tank. The study demonstrated improved relaxation, alertness, and eating habits among the participants (Edwards & Beck, 2002). These particular findings were significant because weight loss typically occurs in as many as 50% of people diagnosed with dementia, increasing mortality and speeding disease progression. Weight loss also leads to reduced muscle mass and loss of functional independence, which increases risk of falls, infections, and skin irritations (Edwards & Beck, 2002).

Many older adults also must deal with poststroke rehabilitation. AAT can help stroke victims by encouraging them to use verbal commands to improve communication ability, throwing balls and brushing fur to improve dexterity, and walking dogs through obstacle courses to improve mobility and balance.

Just as with children, animals can help the elderly by providing a sense of security and self-esteem and facilitating play, exploration, and independence. The human–animal bond can have a vastly positive impact on the lonely and emotionally or physically impaired by promoting responsibility, nurturing, loyalty, empathy, and unconditional love. For the elderly, animals provide companionship and support during bereavement, increase levels of activity, improve person-to-person interactions, and ease loss in natural disasters, and they are able to transcend sensory deficits, mental changes, and mobility restrictions that can impede human–human relationships (Allen, 1995) (Box 29.1).

Table 29.1 lists some of the health benefits to seniors with animal companionship. When moving to residential care, there may be significant benefits to elderly persons being allowed to keep their pets. Pets may be the only daily companions for elderly and special needs popu-

---

BOX 29.1 Sample Guidelines for a Residence or Staff Animal in a Healthcare Facility

- Regardless of the ownership of any animal, the healthcare facility assumes overall responsibility for any pets within or on the premises of the facility.
- The healthcare facility ensures that no animal jeopardizes the health, safety, comfort, treatment, or well-being of the patients, residents, or staff.
- A facility employee will be designated, in writing, as being responsible for monitoring or providing the care to the animal and for ensuring the cleanliness and maintenance of the facilities used to house the animal. This rule does not preclude residents, patients, or other individuals from providing care to the pet animals.
- Except for certified assistance animals, animals are not permitted in kitchen areas, in medication storage and administration areas, or in clean or sterile supply storage areas.
- The procedures for maintaining and monitoring the health and behavior of animals kept on the facility's premises must be in accordance with a veterinarian's recommendations. A copy of these recommendations must be maintained in the facility.
- Specific guidelines for animal care may include
  - Frequent bathroom breaks
  - Designated rest periods in a quiet place during the work period
  - Access to water at all times
  - Specified work periods
  - Same designated handler at each visit

TABLE 29.1   Health Benefits for Seniors with Animal Companionship

- Reduced loneliness and isolation of residents in long-term care facilities
- Lower blood pressure
- Fewer doctor visits
- More active daily living with slower deterioration
- Cope better with stressful life events without entering the healthcare system
- Lower triglyceride and cholesterol levels
- Fewer minor health problems
- Better psychological well-being
- Higher 1-year survival rate after coronary heart disease
- Increased social and verbal interactions
- Better physical health due to exercise with pets
- 3% decreased heart attack mortality rate

Source: Appel et al., 2003

lations and therefore occupy the role of physical and emotional caregivers for this group of people. Leaving animals behind during life transitions can create stress and anxiety for pet owners and family members, and acute emotional distress in the form of separation anxiety, guilt, feelings of wrongful loss, and powerlessness can be a source of resistance and conflict for the patient (Allen, 1995).

Physiological Benefits

Recovery From Illness

Research by Friedmann et al. (1980) found the postcoronary survival improved significantly if the patient was a pet owner. Ninety-four percent of pet owners were alive 1 year after hospitalization compared with 43% without pets. It was considered that health benefits could be attributed to dog walking, so to eliminate the confounding factor of physical exercise, dog owners were eliminated from the sample group. The results, however, were the same, suggesting that the intrinsic factor of pet ownership appeared to contribute to patient recovery. In a subsequent study, Friedmann (1982) found that patients were concerned about their pet's welfare while they were hospitalized and often maintained contact with the pet's caretaker. "Owners require frequent reassurance about their pet's welfare during hospitalization, but pets continue to provide a sense of being needed and an impetus for quick recovery for the hospitalized owner" (Friedmann, 1982, p. 347).

Lower Blood Pressure

Talking to people often raises blood pressure, but several studies have shown that talking to people while petting an animal or with an animal present in the room helps to lower blood pressure. A symbiotic relationship between pets and people can result in significant anxiety reduction for patients with mood and psychotic disorders. The study done by Edwards and Beck (2002) providing Alzheimer's patients with a facility fish tank is a perfect example of the real physiological effects of AAT. Many doctors' offices have likewise adopted this simple method of easing patient anxiety by installing aquariums in their waiting rooms.

Increased Self-Care

The basic needs of humans and animals are similar. A secure and safe environment, proper nutrition, shelter, proper hygiene and health conditions, and some degree of interaction with other living beings are innate necessities of most living things. By providing the conditions necessary for the health and happiness of a pet, seniors can learn or be motivated to provide these conditions for themselves. Robert Andrysco (1981) found significant improvement in patient self-care after interaction with a therapy dog.

Psychological Benefits

Pets take a lot of the boredom out of exercise, and they provide companionship, security, and a way to keep busy. A natural boost to both group and individual morale, animals can encourage social interaction, entertainment, and a link to reality when the patient might otherwise be isolated. They are often the center of attention and often provoke laughter. A family pet can often introduce responsibility and teach nurturing behavior to children. All of these benefits ultimately result in an improved sense of well-being and enhanced quality of life for many pet owners (Figure 29.4).

GUIDELINES FOR AAT

Health Screening

Depending on the use of the therapy animal and the people it will be visiting, total wellness screening is an essential aspect of AAT. Physical examinations and behavioral evaluations should all be considered when screening these animals before use in AAT/AAA. Veterinarians can often work closely with participating institutions to follow infectious disease and safe pet guidelines. Because many diseases are transmissible from animals to humans, known as zoonoses, veterinarians play a key role in disease prevention among older adults participating in AAT/AAA (Schaffer, 2008).

Behavior Testing

Behavior testing isn't perfect, but evaluations can be worthwhile when preparing for AAT/AAA. Therapy animals may encounter many situations during AAT/AAA,

TABLE 29.2	Relevant Zoonotic Diseases				
Disease	**Animal Species**	**Organism**	**Category**	**Transmission**	**Symptoms**
Arthropod infections	All mammals	*Sarcoptes* mange mite, *Cheyletiella*	Parasite	Direct contact with infected animals	Temporary dermatitis
Ascaridiasis (roundworm infection)	Dogs, cats	*Toxicara canis, Toxicara cati, Toxascaris leonina*	Parasite	Ingestion of infective eggs in environment	Depends on organ damaged during larval migration—visual, neurological, or tissue damage
Bartonellosis ("cat scratch fever")	Cats	*Bartonella henselae*	Bacteria	Flea contamination through cat scratch, bite	Skin lesions, infection at point of injury, lymphadenopathy, neuroretinitis, aseptic meningitis, bacteremia, peliosis hepatitis, bacillary angiomatosis
Campylo-bacteriosis	Cats, dogs, farm animals, horses	*Campylobacter*	Bacteria	Eating or drinking contaminated food or water or unpasteurized milk and by direct or indirect contact with fecal material from an infected person, animal, or pet	Mild to severe enteritis, watery or bloody diarrhea, fever, abdominal cramps, nausea and vomiting; a rare complication of *Campylobacter* infection is Guillain-Barré syndrome
Crypto-sporidiosis	Calves, lambs, kids, piglets, less commonly cats, dogs, horses	*Cryptosporidium*	Protozoa	Primarily from environmental exposure to raw sewage or contaminated water sources; fecal–oral route	Abdominal pain, self-limiting to severe, watery diarrhea, nausea, vomiting, fever
Dermato-phytosis (such as ringworm)	Cats, cows, dogs, goats, horses, pigs, rabbits, rodents	*Microsporum canis, Trichophyton mentagrophytes*	Fungal	Direct or indirect contact with asymptomatic animals or with skin lesions of infected animals, contaminated bedding	Classic lesions appear as circular alopecia, often with scaling, crusting, or ulceration
Escherichia coli	Cows, dogs, cats	*Escherichia coli*	Bacteria	Ingestion of contaminated food, fecal–oral route	Severe, bloody diarrhea
Giardiasis	Dogs	*Giardia intestinalis*	Protozoa	Ingestion of contaminated water or food, fecal–oral route	Watery, foul-smelling diarrhea, fever, severe abdominal cramps and distention
Hookworm	Cats, dogs	*Ancylostoma*	Parasite	Ingestion of infective eggs or contact with contaminated soil	Pruritic skin lesions; intestinal bleeding; swelling and pain
Influenza	All mammals	*Influenza virus*	Viral	Via aerosol transmission	Fever, muscle aches, headache
Malessezia	Cats, dogs	*Malassezia pachydermatis*	Yeast	Spread by close physical skin or mucosal contact	Otitis externa; identified as a cause of nosocomial infections of infants in intensive care units in hospitals

(Continued)

TABLE 29.2   Relevant Zoonotic Diseases (*continued*)

Disease	Animal Species	Organism	Category	Transmission	Symptoms
Mycobacteriosis	Fish	*Mycobacterium marinum*	Bacteria	Aquarium water: localized infections following access through broken skin	Skin lesions, disseminated disease in immunocompromised patients
Pasteurellosis	Rabbits, rodents, cats, dogs	*Pasteurella multocida*	Bacteria	Bites, scratches (bacteria found in animal mouths)	Cutaneous infections, bacteremia
Plague	Rodents, cats, dogs	*Yersinia pestis*	Bacteria	Transmitted by fleas found on rodents or cats (infected fleas can sometimes be carried by dogs as well), also can be aerogenous contamination by infected cats	In aerogenous infection, pneumonic form of the illness; in percutaneous infection, regional lymphadenomegaly
Psittacosis	Birds	*Chlamydophila psittaci*	Bacteria	Inhalation of dried secretions from infected birds	Fever, headaches, muscle aches, dry cough, pneumonia
Rabies	All animals, mostly wildlife, but human transmission mainly from bats or dogs	Rabies	Virus	Spread through bites and saliva	Irritability, headache, itching or pain at the infection site, fever; progressing signs include muscle spasms of the throat and respiratory tract that can affect breathing and swallowing; other end-stage signs include hallucinations, seizures, paralysis, and death
Rhodococcus equi	Horses	*Rhodococcus equi*	Bacteria	*R. equi* found readily in soil; environmental exposure to humans; exposure to bacteria through horses or farm animals	Pneumonia, pulmonary abscesses
Salmonellosis	Reptiles, birds, cats, dogs, ducklings, chicks, ferrets, fish, horses, rabbits	*Salmonella*	Bacteria	Ingestion of foods contaminated with animal feces; fecal–oral route	Acute gastroenteritis with sudden onset abdominal pain, diarrhea, fever
Tapeworm	Cats, dogs, rabbits, rodents	*Dipylidium*	Parasite	Ingestion of infected flea	Proglottids are passed in feces or found around the anus, causing itching
Toxoplasmosis	Cats	*Toxoplasma gondii*	Protozoa	Primarily ingestion of raw or undercooked infected meat, especially pork, mutton, or goat meat containing the parasite; parasite is also shed in feces of infected cats	Flu-like symptoms, lymphadenopathy

TABLE 29.3   Registered Organizations Related to AAT

Pet Partners (The Delta Society)
http://www.deltasociety.org

Canine Companions for Independence
http://www.cci.org

Therapy Dogs Incorporated
http://www.therapydogs.com

Therapy Dogs International
http://www.tdi-dog.org

Therapet
http://www.therapet.com

Happy Tails Pet Assisted Therapy
http://www.happytailspets.org

North American Riding for the Handicapped Association
http://www.narha.org

American Hippotherapy Association Inc.
http://www.americanhippotherapyassociation.org

and appropriate behavior testing before these situations can go a long way toward making AAT a positive experience for both the animal and the patient. The animal should be tested first through simulations that mimic actual situations they might be placed in given their expected activity.

Programs such as the American Kennel Club and the Canine Good Citizen program can certify animals as "good citizens" only, but only three national organizations are currently able to register therapy animals. Although many programs provide general behavioral evaluation, therapy animals often must show an extra level of social skills and control to meet the challenge of visitations (Schaffer, 2008). Pet Partners (Delta Society) (www.deltasociety.org/Page.aspx?pid=259), Therapy Dogs Incorporated (www.therapydogs.com), and Therapy Dogs International (www.tdi-dog.org) all provide

TABLE 29.4   Additional Resources for Therapeutic Use of Animals in Rehabilitation

Center for the Human–Animal Bond
Purdue University School of Veterinary Medicine
Phone: 765-494-0854
Alan Beck, Director
http://www.vet.purdue.edu/chab

American Medical Equestrian Association (AMEA)
http://asci.uvm.edu/equine/law/amea/amea.htm
North American Riding for the Handicapped Assoc., Inc. (NARHA)
P.O. Box 33150
Denver, CO 80233
Phone: 1-800-369-7433
www.narha.org
The Delta Society
875 124th Avenue NE, Suite 101
Bellevue, WA 98005
Phone: 1-206-226-7357
www.deltasociety.org

Horses and Humans Foundation
P.O. Box 480
Chagrin Falls, OH 44022
Phone: (440) 543-8306
www.horsesandhumans.org

American Hippotherapy Association, Inc. (AHA, Inc.)
9919 Towne Road
Carmel, IN 46032
Phone: 1-877-851-4592 (toll free)
www.americanhippotherapyassociation.org

Canadian Therapeutic Riding Association
P.O. Box 1055
Guelph, Ontario N1H-6J6
Canada
Phone: 519-767-0700

Riding for the Disabled
Avenue R
National Agricultural Centre
Kenilworth
Warwickshire, UK CV8 2LY

The Federation of Riding for the Disabled International
c/o Secretary General Mary Longden
P.O. Box 416
Ascot Vale
Victoria 3032
Australia
Phone: Aus - 61-3-9376-5355
Fax: Aus- 61-3-9376-5944
frdi@rda.org.au

American Veterinary Medical Association (AVMA)
1931 North Meacham Road, Suite 100
Schaumburg, IL 60173-4360
Phone: 800-248-2862
Fax: 847.925.1329
www.avma.org

specific behavior testing with simulations and require a detailed veterinary examination before certification.

Zoonotic Diseases

As previously mentioned, **zoonotic disease** refers to any disease that is transmissible from animals to humans. The transmission of disease is a potential concern in all instances of animal contact; however, precautions can be taken to minimize the risk to more vulnerable populations while maximizing patient-benefiting opportunities (Friedmann & Son, 2009). AAT/AAA is often not allowed in long-term care facilities because of concern about infection, injuries, allergies, and disease transmission, which are especially important to immunocompromised patients such as geriatric patients, HIV/AIDS patients, or patients receiving immunosuppressive therapies (Friedmann & Son, 2009).

In most cases people and animals contract zoonotic infections from the environment simultaneously and independently, not from each other (Hemsworth & Pizer, 2006). Regardless, client education is one of best ways to prevent zoonotic disease transmission (Table 29.2). Several normal precautionary measures include washing hands after animal contact and before handling food and avoiding animal feces and urine in general. These measures alone will help prevent most zoonotic diseases, but immunocompromised patients may need to take extra precautions. Avoid cat scratches and bites to prevent infections with *Bartonella*, a bacteria that can cause serious infection. Also, somebody besides the resident or patient should clean litter boxes and cages, which should be emptied daily and stored away from food preparation areas. When immunocompromised patients must come in contact with animal feces or urine, they should wear gloves when handling. Also of significance is the bacteria *Salmonella*, which is carried by virtually 100% of reptiles. Wearing gloves when handling reptiles or cleaning their habitats should help prevent transmission of this disease.

When at all possible, preventive medicine should be practiced for pets to reduce the possibility of disease transmission to owners. Annual veterinary visits and routine fecal diagnostic testing helps to prevent certain parasite and bacterial disease. However, flea and tick control, current vaccinations, and general pet hygiene should be addressed, especially in situations with immunocompromised owners. More information regarding up-to-date disease control and prevention can be found at the websites listed in Box 29.2.

BOX 29.2   Web Exploration

Browse these resources that provide beneficial information to high-risk individuals:

Centers for Disease Control and Prevention
http://www.cdc.gov/hiv/resources/brochures/print/pets.htm

Healthy Pets for Healthy People
http://www.lgvma.org/hphp/hphp_text.html

PAWS–San Francisco
http://www.pawssf.org

CRITICAL THINKING

1. Examine Table 29.2 and consider the following questions:
   a. What zoonotic diseases are more prevalent in your geographical area and why?
   b. How can a rehabilitation nurse help prevent the spread of animal to human diseases?
   c. Which diseases on the list have received more attention in the media? Why do you believe this is?
2. Can you think of a situation in which a veterinarian might be called on to consult with the interdisciplinary rehabilitation team?
3. What facilities or organizations in your area offer AAT? What guidelines do they use for their program(s)? What types of animals are used?
4. Do you believe certain types of animals are more appropriate for certain situations involving AAT? If so, describe these.

PERSONAL REFLECTION

- Have you ever participated in pet therapy, AAT, or any AAAs? If so, what was this experience like? What were the benefits and drawbacks of this experience for patients?
- Is AAT used at the facility where you work? If so, what types of animals are used? Is the program well received by residents, clients, families, and staff?
- What is the role of the rehabilitation nurse in AAT? What responsibilities does the rehabilitation nurse assume when AAT is part of the rehabilitation program?
- What type of screening protocol should be in place if AAT or "pet therapy" is used in a long-term care facility?

REFERENCES

Academic Team of the AVMA One Health Initiative Task Force and Partners. (n.d.). Appendix E: the academic community brining one health to action: academic summary. Retrieved December 1, 2010, from http://www.avma.org/onehealth/appendix_e.pdf.

Allen, K. M. (1995). Coping with life changes and transitions: The role of pets. *Interactions 13*(3), 5–8.

American Animal Hospital Association Pet Owner Survey (2001). Retrieved July 5, 2010, from http://www.aahanet.org/media/s_pos2001.aspx

American Veterinary Medical Association (AVMA). (2002). *Human-Animal Bond*. Retrieved August 1, 2010, from http://www.avma.org.

Anderson, W. P., Reid, C. M., & Jennings, G. L. (1992). Pet ownership and risk factors for cardiovascular disease. *Medical Journal of Australia, 157,* 298–301.

Andrysco, R. M. (1981). Pet facilitated therapy in a retirement nursing care community. Presentation at the International Conference on the Human/Companion Animal Bond, October 5–7, 1981, Philadelphia.

Appel, L. D., Dapper, N., Elcock, M., et al. (2003). *Animals in residential facilities: Guidelines and resources for success* (1st ed.). Bellevue, WA: Delta Society.

Banks, M. R., & Banks W. A. (2002). The effects of animal-assisted therapy on loneliness in an elderly population in long-term care facilities. *Journals of Gerontology Series A: Biological Sciences and Medical Sciences, 57,* 428–432.

Banks, M. R., Willoughby, L. M., & Banks, W. A. (2008). Animal-assisted therapy and loneliness in nursing homes: Use of robotic versus living dogs. *Journal of the American Medical Directors Association, 9,* 173–177.

Beck, A. M., & Katcher, A. (1996). *Between pets and people: The importance of animal companionship.* West Lafayette, IN: Purdue University Press.

Benjamin, J. (2000). An introduction to hippotherapy. Retrieved from http://www.americanhippotherapyassociation.org/aha_hpot_a_intro.htm

Bustad, L. K. & Hines, L. M. (1983). Placement of Animals with the Elderly: Benefits and Strategies. In A. H. Katcher & A. M. Beck (Eds.) *New Perspectives on Our Lives with Companion Animals.* (pp.351–359). Philadelphia: University Press.

Crawford, J. J., & Pomerinke, K. A. (2003). *Therapy pets: The animal-human healing partnership.* Amherst, NY: Prometheus Books.

Duncan, S. L. (2000). APIC state-of-the-art report: The implications of service animals in health care settings. *American Journal of Infection Control, 28,* 170–180.

Edwards, N. E., & Beck, A. M. (2002). Animal-assisted therapy and nutrition in Alzheimer's disease. *Western Journal of Nursing Research 24,* 697–712.

Fick, K. M. (1993). The influence of an animal on social interactions of nursing home residents in a group setting. *American Journal of Occupational Therapy, 47*(6), 529–534.

Friedmann, E., Katcher, A. H., Lynch, J. J., et al. (1980). Animal companions and one-year survival of patients after discharge from a coronary care unit. *Public Health Reports, 95,* 307–312.

Friedmann, E., Katcher, A. H., & Meislich, D. (1982). When pet owners are hospitalized: Significance of companion animals during hospitalization. A. H. Katcher & A. M. Beck (Eds.), *New perspectives on our lives with companion animals* (pp. 346–350). Philadelphia: University of Pennsylvania Press.

Friedmann, E., & Son, H. (2009). The human-companion animal bond: How humans benefit. *Veterinary Clinics of North America: Small Animal Practice, 39*(2), 293–326.

Friedmann, E., & Thomas, S. A. (1995). Pet ownership. Social support, and one-year survival after acute myocardial infarction in the Cardiac Arrhythmia Suppression Trial (CAST). *American Journal of Cardiology, 76,* 1213–1217.

Gammonley, J., Howie, A., Kirwin, S., Zapf, S., Frye, J., & Freeman, G. (1997). *Animal-assisted therapy: Therapeutic interventions.* Renton, WA: Delta Society.

Hemsworth, S., & Pizer, B. (2006). Pet ownership in immunocompromised children—A review of the literature and survey of existing guidelines. *European Journal of Oncology Nursing, 10,* 117–127.

Lutwack-Bloom, P., Wijewickrama, R., & Smith, B. (2005). Effects of pets versus people visits with nursing home residents. *Journal of Gerontological Social Work, 44,* 137–159.

McCabe, B.W., Baun, M. M., Speich, D., & Agrawal, S. (2002). Resident dog in the Alzheimer's special care unit. *Western Journal of Nursing Research, 24,* 684–696.

Nolen, R.S. (2007). AMA adopts one-health policy. *Journal of American Veterinary Medical Association, 231,* 353, 357.

Richeson, N. E. (2003). Effects of anima-assisted therapy on agitated behaviors and social interactions of older adults with dementia. *American Journal of Alzheimer's Disease and Other Dementias, 18,* 353–358.

Schaffer, C. B. (2008). Enhancing human-animal relationships through veterinary medical instruction in animal-assisted therapy and animal-assisted activities. *Journal of Veterinary Medical Education, 35*(4), 503–510.

Serpel, J. (1991). Beneficial effects of pet ownership on some aspect of human health and behavior. *Journal of the Royal Society of Medicine 84,* 717–720.

Souter, M. A., & Miller, M. D. (2007). Do animal-assisted activities effectively treat depression? A meta-analysis. *Anthrozoos, 20,* 167–180.

Siegel, J. M. (1990). Stressful life events and use of physician services among the elderly: The moderating role of pet ownership. *Journal of Personality and Social Psychology, 58*(6), 1081–1086.

CHAPTER 30

Life Care Planning: A Unique Practice Area for Nurses

Susan Wirt
Ava G. Porter

LEARNING OBJECTIVES

At the end of this chapter, the reader will be able to

- Define life care planning.
- Describe the role of the rehabilitation nurse in life care planning.
- Explain the recommended preparation and clinical background for nursing practice in life care planning.
- Recognize situations where a life care plan is routinely warranted.
- Identify steps for developing a life care plan.
- Discuss five of the essential components of a life care plan.
- Explore options for certification in the unique practice area of life care planning.

KEY CONCEPTS AND TERMS

American Association of Nurse Life Care Planners	Clients	Polytrauma
	Damages	Quality of life
Case management	Life care plan (LCP)	Spinal cord injury

Regardless of where one practices rehabilitation nursing, exposure to individuals who have sustained life-altering injuries or illnesses is at the core. Such conditions as acquired brain injury, **spinal cord injury**, amputation, burns, and multiple sclerosis are frequently seen by the rehabilitation nurse, and these very same conditions comprise many of the situations where **a life care plan (LCP)** is requested. The experiences of working with these individuals, or **clients**, requires the rehabilitation nurse to use the nursing process (assess, diagnose, plan, implement, and evaluate). The practice of life care planning; however, goes one step further: It requires rehabilitation nurses, based on their unique knowledge of the patient and family, resources, and illness trajectories, to anticipate the prognoses and life-long care needs for their clients. The life care planner anticipates and plans for potential complications for which the client is at risk. Prevention of or, at the very least, reduction of the severity of anticipated complications is a primary goal of any LCP.

LIFE CARE PLANNING DEFINED

Life care planning has several recognized definitions, and the following definition has gained widest acceptance in the field of rehabilitation: "A dynamic document based upon published standards of practice, comprehensive assessment, data analysis and research, which provides an organized concise plan for current and future needs with associated costs, for individuals who have experienced catastrophic injury or have chronic health care needs" (Weed & Beren, 2007, p. 1223). The **American Association of Nurse Life Care Planners** provided this statement (n.d.):

> The Nurse Life Care Planner utilizes the nursing process in the collection and analysis of comprehensive client specific data in the preparation of a dynamic document. This document provides an organized, concise plan of estimated reasonable and necessary (and reasonably certain to be necessary), current and

future healthcare needs with the associated costs and frequencies of goods and services. The nurse life care plan is developed for individuals who have experienced an injury or have chronic healthcare issues.

Mauk and Mauk summarized the LCP as a "comprehensive document designed to help meet the long-term financial and health needs of a person who has experienced a catastrophic injury" (2010, p. 786).

An LCP outlines not only the specific services and resources the client can reasonably be expected to require over the course of his or her lifetime but also incorporates realistic cost projections for these services and resources. It is not at all unusual to plan for one's retirement with the assistance of a financial planner. Similarly, when facing a life-altering condition that has lifetime or long-term implications, it is critical to consider and include the financial impact of the future life care necessities. Without such consideration for realistic cost projections, it becomes impossible to prepare for the financial impact of lifelong care and services.

HISTORY OF LIFE CARE PLANNING

Deutch and Raffa (1981) in their publication, *Damages in Tort Actions*, first referenced the practice of life care planning and identified it as a guide for establishing **damages** in civil litigation. This multivolume text, still in publication with biannual updates, is commonly used by attorneys in the practice areas of personal injury, wrongful death, and property damage to assist with defining compensatory and punitive damages. Deutch and Sawyer (1985) followed with *A Guide to Rehabilitation*. This text not only addressed specific medical conditions encountered during the rehabilitation process but also outlined concepts and formats for developing LCPs. Additionally, it provided multiple resources for the practicing life care planner as well as samples of LCPs. Although the practice of life care planning continues to play a significant role in the legal arena, the practice has evolved into a valuable resource for all areas of rehabilitation, discharge planning and teaching, **case management**, and healthcare funding guidance (Deutsch, Allison, & Cimino-Ferguson, 2005).

The first documented training in the process and practice of life care planning was done by Dr. Paul M. Deutch in 1986. Over 100 rehabilitation professionals, including nurses, attended to learn more about the practice. In the early 1990s Susan Riddick-Grisham was the first nurse to train other nurses about the practice of life care planning. She was also the only nurse involved in establishing the curriculum for the first national training program offered by the Rehabilitation Training Institute. In the mid-1990s another nurse, Patti McCollom, established the first professional organization for nurses practicing in life care planning, the Academy of Nurse Life Care Planners. At the encouragement of other rehabilitation professionals, she later evolved the organization into a multidisciplinary organization and changed the name to the International Academy of Life Care Planners. This group subsequently became a specialty section of the International Association of Rehabilitation Professionals. Later, Kelly Lance, a nurse, established a nurse-only professional organization for the practice of life care planning, the American Association of Nurse Life Care Planners (Weed & Berens, 2009).

ROLES OF THE REHABILITATION NURSE IN THE UNIQUE PRACTICE OF LIFE CARE PLANNING

Rehabilitation nurses have numerous role responsibilities in professional practice, including the three main roles for professional nursing practice identified by the American Association of Colleges of Nursing (AACN, 2008): (1) provider of care; (2) designer, manager, and coordinator of care; and (3) member of the profession. These three major roles will be discussed her in relation to life care planning.

In the provider role rehabilitation nurses who practice life care planning provide *indirect* "care in and across all environments" (AACN, 2008, p. 9). Rehabilitation nurses act as patient advocates and educators who work in partnerships with the client and family (caregivers) "in order to foster and support the patient's active participation in determining healthcare decisions" (AACN, 2008, p. 8). The rehabilitation nurse holistically focuses on the client's and family's values and goals as they evaluate and manage aspects of the environment to support the client's well-being. In the provider role the rehabilitation nurse "uses research findings and other evidence in designing and implementing (a plan of) care that is multidimensional, high quality, and cost effective" (AACN, 2008, p. 9).

The practice of life care planning most clearly exemplifies the designer, manager, and coordinator of care role. Skills of communication and collaboration with the client, family, caregivers, and healthcare delivery team are mandatory. To ensure **quality of life** and health, future life care projections require the planner to be aware of and sensitive to the client's individual goals. Complex sets of health and wellness issues, expertise from multiple multidisciplinary team members, client and family values, and community resources must all be considered as the LCP is developed. Nurses with rehabilitation nursing certification demonstrate the competencies required to develop and manage an LCP; thus, transition into the practice area of life care planning can be readily made by most rehabilitation nurses.

Once the LCP has been prepared, the rehabilitation nurse/life care planner assumes a primary role as an educator. The LCP is the "road map" for the future to be used by the client, family, caregivers, and multidisciplinary team members. Educating all parties about the plan ensures coordinated delivery of appropriate care in a timely manner. The presence of an LCP increases overall accountability of all parties included in the plan as well as certain future barriers to the delivery of care (Leksin, Lew, Queen, Reeves, & Bleiberg, 2007). Educating the client and family (caregivers) allows them to assume greater responsibility and independence in future care and achievement of outcomes.

Nursing practice in life care planning is congruent with Dorothea E. Orem's self-care deficit nursing theory, which proposes that nursing systems and individual nursing interventions are designed to meet an individual's health-derived or health-associated limitations in self-care or dependent care (Taylor, 2006). Nursing interventions can include offering information, resources, and tools necessary for restoration of health or ability to carry out required self-care. The nurse's role in helping the client to achieve or maintain a level of optimal health and wellness is to act as an advocate, redirector, support person, teacher, and facilitator of an environment conducive to therapeutic development (Taylor, 2006).

A principle or tenet of life care planning is that the plan must be preventative in nature, thereby minimizing the frequency, duration, and severity of any potential complication (Deutsch et al., 2005). However, there are numerous situations where a progressive deterioration of function can be anticipated despite provision of preventative care. One example of this is the individual with a spinal cord injury and resultant paraplegia. Use of the upper extremities for locomotion and transfers will, over time, put increased stress on upper extremities, including the joints of the shoulders, elbows, and wrists. Coupled with the aging process, it is likely an individual will develop pain in the upper extremities commonly associated with overuse syndrome or nerve entrapment (Winkler, 2008). Treatment options for either condition include medication and/or surgical intervention, both of which will have potential impact on independence. The rehabilitation nurse must be aware of this in development of the LCP because it will impact recommendations for wheelchairs (manual versus power chair) and other assistive modifications in the client's home environment to provide for support in personal care and activities of daily living.

Healthy lifestyle and wellness promotion are integral components of an LCP. The negative impact of obesity or smoking on the individual who has not sustained a catastrophic injury or other chronic illness is well documented. Combined with the functional losses of an individual with either a catastrophic injury or chronic illness, unhealthy lifestyle behaviors increase the risk, duration, and severity of complications. Therefore, the LCP should include activities and services to promote a healthy lifestyle.

The impact of social and emotional support on health has measurable impact on morbidity and mortality as well as self-reported outcomes of some diseases (Reblin & Uchino, 2008). Social support can promote healthy behaviors and is regularly used as a tool to reduce or cease unhealthy behaviors, as in the case of Alcoholics Anonymous. There is also some evidence that being a support provider leads to improved health and reduction of stress (Brown, Nesse, Vinokur, & Smith, 2003). The life care planner considers the issues of social and emotional support when identifying services and interventions for the client.

As might be expected, clients who most typically require the services of a life care planner have numerous healthcare providers involved in their care. It is not unusual to have several medical specialists, a psychologist and/or social worker, a dietitian, as well as speech, physical, and occupational therapists. Development of the LCP benefits when each member of the multidisciplinary team is given the opportunity to provide his or her input and expertise. There may also be situations where the client has not benefited from specialty evaluations appropriate to the injuries or illness. In that case it is appropriate for the life care planner to arrange for such evaluations and then incorporate the additional information into the client's LCP. In these circumstances the LCP pulls all information together in one place and should be shared with the providers as well as the client and family, allowing for a more cohesive approach to future care.

Given the relative newness of the practice of life care planning, it is distinctly possible that members of the multidisciplinary team of providers may be unfamiliar with the practice. This provides yet another opportunity for the rehabilitation nurse to fulfill the role of educator. Attorneys, judge, and jurors often seek out information and education provided by the life care planner regarding the nature of the injury (or injuries), functional abilities, anticipated impact of aging, necessary care, and the projected costs and economic impact of the outlined care and services.

PREPARATION AND CLINICAL BACKGROUND FOR NURSING PRACTICE IN LIFE CARE PLANNING

The professional rehabilitation nurse is uniquely qualified to enter the practice of life care planning for several reasons. First, the nature and scope of healthcare challenges that must be considered for the catastrophically injured or chronically ill client are regularly experienced in the rehabilitation setting. Second, the rehabilitation process involves a team of multidisciplinary providers; therefore, collaboration with all members of the team is customary and routine. As Weed (1999) stated, "life care plan development involves data collection, resource development, and planning strategies in an interdisciplinary rehabilitation environment" (p. 448). Third, rehabilitation nurses by nature are inclined to practice from a holistic framework that considers all aspects of human responses to debilitating injury or illness.

As noted previously, the LCP is a tool used with great regularity in the legal arena. The rehabilitation nurse who transitions into this area of practice will likely find that attorneys, both for the plaintiff and defense, call on them to help assess damages. If this is the case, the life care planner will benefit from additional training in the area of public speaking. Again, working in this capacity allows the life care planner to be an "educator" to the parties involved, including the attorneys, judges, and jurors. It should be noted that although the nurse life care planner may develop the LCP from the perspective of health needs, the services of a professional economist are generally used to assign values to each of the categories of the LCP to come up with a usable numerical figure of predicted costs over the person's lifetime. Such an economist uses standard formulas to determine and calculate present and future costs associated with the person's condition in events where attorneys intend to use the LCP to substantiate asking for certain amounts of money in a settlement dispute, such as in the case of catastrophic injury in which one party is accused of causing long-term harm to another.

Nurses are held in high regard by the public and are consistently ranked as the most honest and ethical profession (Saad, 2008). With so much emphasis on education, this high regard and public trust reinforces the suitability of the rehabilitation nurse in the role of life care planner. Rehabilitation, medical, and nursing research is continually adding to the body of knowledge that the life care planner needs to ensure the client's plan is comprehensive and evidence based. The life care planner must stay involved in professional organizations where such information is disseminated, review appropriate and reliable publications and websites, and continually network with other colleagues in the field. Nurses should seek out current articles from peer-reviewed journals that can be accessed via online databases such as CINAHL, PubMed, MEDLINE, or Cochrane. Cochrane reviews offer the combined results of the world's best healthcare research studies and are recognized as the gold standard in evidence-based health care.

It is equally important to recognize one's own areas of strength and weakness, such as working with adult versus pediatric clients. In working with children, "the life care planner must focus on the child's future growth and development and project the child's needs into adulthood and across a potentially long lifetime" (Riddick-Grisham, 2004, p. ix). Should the opportunity arise to work with a client outside the nurse's area of knowledge and expertise, the life care planner may elect to retain the services of another nurse with specialty experience in working with that particular client population. Clearly, this requires that the life care planner have access to additional resources that may be identified through professional groups and organizations as well as local community providers. Another option is to refuse to accept referrals for clients who fall outside the life care planner's area of knowledge and expertise; however, the downside is lost opportunities for future growth and professional development. There are some specialized training programs for rehabilitation nurses who are interested in transition to the practice of life care planning that is discussed in more detail later in this chapter under Certification.

When establishing the costs for various procedures, interventions, and testing, a basic knowledge of coding and billing is most helpful. An LCP does not seek to identify what amount any particular payment source is willing to pay or reimburse a medical provider. Instead, it seeks to identify what the actual charge or billed amount for the service or item will be. The rationale for this is that the payer is very likely to change in the course of the client's life. Even if the payer does not change, there are frequent changes to what may or may not be covered under some plans as well as the portion or percentage the client may be required to pay out of pocket. Most medical providers (physicians, therapists, hospitals, etc) use specialized coding to communicate the specifics of what types of patients they are treating and what services are provided for those patients. These codes, including ICD-10 (*International Classification of Diseases*), CPT (current procedural terminology), HCPCS (healthcare common procedural coding system), and DRGs (diagnosis-related groups), allow for consistency in classifying and comparing medical conditions, interventions, associated charges, and, in some instances, the allowed reimbursement by an insurance company or other payment source. Knowledge of these codes allows the life care planner to ensure the most accurate information is being requested when a future procedure or service is planned (Maniha, 2008).

Situations Benefiting From LCPs

Patients who most typically benefit from the services of a life care planner are in situations where detailed knowledge of the individual's future care and associated costs are beneficial. This may include persons with catastrophic injury from an accident or those with chronic illness. Table 30.1 lists common medical conditions that often benefit from the services provided by a life care planner. Table 30.2 lists common nursing diagnoses used by nurse life care planners.

The demand for life care planning has increased as significant numbers of wounded military personnel have returned home from combat with severe traumatic injuries, often resulting in **polytrauma** (Pomeranz, Shaw, Yu, & Moorhouse, 2008). Polytrauma often results from explosive devices and refers to two or more serious, and

TABLE 30.2 Common NANDA Nursing Diagnoses Addressed by a Nurse Life Care Planner	
Mobility, impaired physical	Home maintenance, impaired
Mobility, impaired bed and/or wheelchair	Falls, risk for
Walking and/or transfer ability, impaired	Injury, risk for
Autonomic dysreflexia, risk for	Infection, risk for
	Protection, ineffective
Anxiety and/or fear	Trauma, risk for
Coping, ineffective	Skin integrity, risk for impaired
Self-concept, readiness for enhanced	Sexuality pattern, ineffective
Hopelessness and/or powerlessness	Communication, impaired verbal Communication, readiness for enhanced
Urinary elimination, impaired	Caregiver role strain, risk for
Bowel incontinence	
Constipation	Role performance, ineffective
Swallowing, impaired	
Nutrition, impaired	Social interaction impaired
Self-care deficit, bathing, dressing, feeding, and/or toileting	Social isolation
	Knowledge, deficient
Sensory perception, disturbed	Knowledge, readiness for enhanced
Comfort, impaired	Therapeutic regimen management, ineffective
Pain, chronic	Therapeutic regimen management, readiness for enhanced
Aspiration, risk for	
Ventilation, impaired spontaneous	

Source: NANDA, North American Nursing Diagnosis Association.

TABLE 30.1   Medical Diagnoses Commonly Associated with Life Care Plans
• Spinal cord injury
• Chronic pain
• Acquired brain injury
• Multiple sclerosis
• Burns
• Vision and/or hearing loss
• Amputations
• Minors with developmental delays or other handicapping conditions
• Multiple fractures
• Individuals with handicapping conditions who have been deemed incompetent and unable to make decisions

possibly life-threatening, injuries leaving significant impairment and disability (Pomeranz, et al., 2008). "The successful rehabilitation and community integration of veterans who have sustained polytrauma have become an important mandate for the Veteran's Administration (VA) Medical Centers" (Pomeranz, et al., 2008, p. 321). Use of a life care planning approach has changed the perspective of the Veterans Administration system from viewing each episode of care as singular and independent to "viewing each as a part of the ongoing dynamic process of improving the quality of life for the patients with polytrauma" (Leksin, et al., 2007, p. xxvi). The work of the nurse life care planner is essential to this approach.

Certification

Rehabilitation nurses "are members of the profession and in this role are advocates for the client and the profession. The use of the term 'professional' implies the formation of a professional identity and accountability for one's professional image" (AACN, 2008, p. 9). Acquiring specialized professional certification is one way to develop and demonstrate an appropriate set of knowledge, skills, and values in the specialty practice area of life care planning.

Although two current certifications exist specific to the practice area of life care planning, Certified Nurse Life Care Planner and Certified Life Care Planner, these are not mandated by any regulatory bodies. As previously noted in this chapter, most experienced rehabilitation nurses have the knowledge and expertise required for entry into the practice of life care planning. Information on additional training and specialized certification can be found in Box 30.1

DEVELOPING AN LCP

Regardless of the specialty area in which a nurse practices, the steps of the nursing process are consistently the same—assessment, diagnosis, planning, implementation, and evaluation. An LCP addresses more than just the medical interventions. It is a comprehensive list of services necessary to promote long-term health and function to allow the client to pursue health, vocational, and leisure activities of importance to the individual. Table 30.3 lists the essential areas addressed in an LCP.

The process or key steps involved in the development of an LCP is similar; however, the assessment phase typically involves review of extensive medical records from multiple care providers and interviews with the client/patient, family members, caregivers, and medical providers. The assessment phase includes research of resources and review of the literature to identify evidence-based standards of nursing and medical practice for all the recommendations included in the plan.

Planning care is essentially the preparation of the LCP report, which is far more comprehensive and all-inclusive than a more typical short-term plan of care. Implementation involves educating the client, care providers, and other members of the multidisciplinary team; however, the actual implementation of the LCP is typically not performed by the rehabilitation nurse who has prepared the report. Instead, it is often a case manager and/or the client along with his or her community-based care providers who implement the LCP.

Finally, the nursing process calls for evaluation of the LCP. The rehabilitation nurse who is practicing life care planning recognizes that many unforeseen medical issues arise in the life of any individual. Although these issues may have a direct impact on the recommendations and allocations in the LCP, there is not always a means for evaluation of the LCP. This step of the process can be dictated by the referral source and the reason the LCP was requested. If it is being used as tool in litigation, once the legal issues are resolved the life care planner may not have the opportunity to interact with the client again and thus would not be able to evaluate the overall effectiveness of the LCP.

SUMMARY

Life care planning is an emerging field for which rehabilitation nurses are uniquely suited. Developing a LCP may be beneficial for those with catastrophic injuries or long term illnesses to help predict future costs of lifetime care. The LCP is often used in a court of law to help determine award amounts in settlements for wrongful injury. Rehabilitation nurses interested in becoming life care planners have a variety of options for training and certification, and this specialty lends itself well to those who prefer independent and challenging practice.

BOX 30.1
Browse these websites related to certification as a life care planner:
http://www.law.capital.edu/LCP
http://lcp.dce.ufl.edu
http://ichcc.org
http://www.kelynco.com
http://www.cnlcpcertboard.org

CRITICAL THINKING

1. Browse the websites in Box 30.1 regarding certification as a life care planner. What are general requirements of certification in this specialty area? Which of the certifications is more geared toward nurses? Which requires the most education or training?
2. Consider the concept of certification in life care planning. If is it not required, what would be the benefits

TABLE 30.3 Essential Areas of an LCP

Medical care: This includes routine diagnostic testing such as renal ultrasounds to evaluate renal function, lab tests, and common medical procedures as required based on the nature of the disability.

Surgical care: Some, but not all, clients face additional future surgeries.

Nursing care: This category includes such services as skilled nursing and/or unlicensed assistive personnel as deemed applicable. It may also include the services of a nurse case manager when indicated.

Facility/residential care: This category includes such things as placement in an assisted living, residential, or skilled care facility where applicable.

Therapy services: This category includes such things as physical, occupational, and speech therapies as well as psychology and counseling both immediate as well as services potentially needed over an individual's lifetime as his or her needs change.

Medications: This category is used to outline reasonable regimens of medications as prescribed and episodic medications that are likely to be used after surgical interventions. One must also have familiarity with the metabolism of the client's medications as well as the impact of the aging process on hepatic and renal function. These issues may substantiate the need for laboratory testing to alter medications or dosages in the long term.

Transportation: Should the client require assistive devices for locomotion, these devices may require special vehicles or at the very least vehicular modifications. Additionally, consideration should be given to the travel experienced by the client for any and all medical or surgical care. Special rates for mileage reimbursement for medical transportation are outlined by the Internal Revenue Service and can be found at http://www.irs.gov/newsroom/article/0,,id=216048,00.html/.

Leisure and health maintenance: An LCP should cover specific recommendations that would make access to wellness resources as well as identify any special maintenance programs that are indicated for the individual based on his or her disability. Examples of this might include identification of a fitness center with a lift to provide ease in transfer from a wheelchair into the pool or willingness to add a lift if one is not currently available.

Durable medical equipment and supplies: This category can include such items as prosthetics, orthotics, specialized catheters, suctions equipment, dressing supplies, walkers, canes, lotions and creams, and aides to independent function. One should also consider the maintenance of any piece of equipment to facilitate safety and longevity. This category can be further subdivided as indicated. For example, if the client requires ventilator support, this can be outlined and addressed in a completely separate category.

Wheelchairs: This category not only includes a wheelchair but specialized seating to prevent pressure ulcers as well as maintenance to improve the longevity of the items. When preparing a, LCP for a pediatric case consideration must also be given to the child's physical growth and development because this further dictates when replacement chairs should be provided. Finally, this category can consider specialized chairs for leisure activities or they may be included in the leisure and health maintenance category.

Education: When addressing a child, young adult, or other individual who is enrolled or planning to enroll in some form of education, this category should be addressed. Special modifications that may be required in the physical environment, support persons, etc. can be included in this category. Additionally, specialized training that may be beneficial could be included in this area. For example, the individual who sustained extensive burns would benefit from attending burn conferences such as those provided by the Phoenix Society (http://www.phoenix-society.org).

Vocational rehabilitation: This category would be included if the individual's disability had impact on an existing or a planned career. Many rehabilitation nurses are not qualified to address this area and will consult with a vocational rehabilitation expert who provides a separate assessment and report.

of certification? Can anyone become a life care planner? What would make rehabilitation nurses better well suited for this area of practice?

3. Google "life care planner" and see what pops up. What do you find that life care planners charge for their services? Compare this with what you know about other specialties and the amount of preparation required to work in that capacity.

PERSONAL REFLECTION

- Think of a patient for whom you have cared who had catastrophic injuries. How might he or she have benefited from the services of a life care planner?
- Do you know any nurses who are life care planners? Consider contacting them and finding out more about what they do.

- Would you, as a rehabilitation nurse or student nurse learning about rehabilitation nursing, be interested in life care planning as a job? What steps would you need to take to be prepared for this role? What personal strengths and weakness would make you well suited, or not, for such a job?

REFERENCES

American Academy of Nurse Life Care Planners. (n.d.). Life care planning. Retrieved August 1, 2010, from http://www.aan-lcp.org

American Association of Colleges of Nursing (AACN). (2008). *The essentials of baccalaureate nursing education for professional nursing practice*. Washington, DC: Author.

Brown, S. L., Nesse, R. M., Vinokur, A. D., & Smith, D. M. (2003). Providing social support may be more beneficial than receiving it: Results from a prospective study of mortality. *Psychological Science 14*, 320–327.

Deutsch, P., Allison, L., & Cimino-Ferguson, S. (2005). Life care planning assessments and their impact on quality of life in spinal cord injury. *Topics in Spinal Cord Injury Rehabilitation, 10*, 135–145.

Deutsch, P., & Raffa, F. (1981). *Damages in tort actions*. New York: Matthew Bender and Company.

Deutsch, P., & Sawyer, H. (1985). *A guide to rehabilitation*. New York: Matthew Bender and Company.

Leksin, G., Lew, H., Queen, H., Reeves, D., & Bleiberg, J. (2007). Adaptation of life care planning to patients with polytrauma in a VA inpatient setting: Implications for seamless care coordination. *Journal of Rehabilitation Research & Development, 44*, xxiii–xxvi.

Maniha, A. (2008). Research to another level: Medical coding and the life care planning process: Part 1. *Journal of Life Care Planning, 7*, 61–72.

Mauk, K. L. & Mauk, J. M. (2010). Trends that impact gerontological nursing. In K. L. Mauk (Ed.) *Gerontological Nursing: Competencies for Care*. (pp. 782–796). Sudbury, MA: Jones and Bartlett Learning.

Pomeranz, J. L., Shaw, L. R., Yu, N. S., & Moorhouse, M. D. (2008). Polytrauma and life care planning: Managing the complex interaction of multiple injuries. *Work, 31*, 310–326.

Reblin, M., & Uchino, B. (2008). Social and emotional support and its implication for health. *Current Opinion in Psychiatry, 21*, 201–205.

Riddick-Grisham, R. (2004). *Pediatric life care planning and case management*. Atlanta, GA: CRC Press.

Saad, L. (2008). Nurses shine, bankers slump in ethics ratings. Retrieved September 8, 2010, from http://www.gallup.com/poll/112264/nurses-shine-while-bankers-slump-ethics-ratings.aspx

Taylor, S. G. (2006). Dorothea E. Orem, self care deficit theory of nursing. In A. M. Tomey & M. R. Alligood (Eds.), *Nursing theorists and their work* (6th ed., pp. 267–296). Philadelphia: Mosby Elsevier.

Weed, R. O., & Berens, D. E. (2007). Life care planning after TBI: Clinical and forensic issues. In N. Zasler, D. Katz, & R. Zafonte (Eds.), *Brain injury medicine* (pp. 1223–1241). New York: Demos.

Weed, R. O., & Berens, D. E. (2009). *Life care planning & case management handbook* (3rd ed.). Atlanta, GA: CRC Press, Taylor & Francis LLC.

Winkler, T. (2008). Spinal cord injury and aging. Retrieved July 1, 2010, from http://emedicine.medscape.com/article/322713-print

RE: Robert Miller, Sr.
DOB: 01/28/1920
SSN: 222-33-4444
DOI: 04/20/2006
PRIMARY DIAGNOSES: Weakness, debilitation, dysphasia,
dysarthria, fracture C5 vertebra (healed), fracture right
humerus (healed), depressive disorder, intermittent incontinence

LIFE CARE PLAN
Medical Care
August 28, 2007

Wirt & Associates
P.O. Box 8
Catawba, VA 24070
(540) 529-3631
(540) 384-5162 (fax)

DESCRIPTION	Year initiated/ replacement schedule	Purpose/Rationale	Cost per item	Cost per year
Quarterly follow up with Pamela McClure-Smith, MD	2007, throughout lifetime	Monitor medications, renal and liver function, assess need for home care, urology consults, etc	$85.00 per visit	$ 255.00 per year*
Complete blood count (CBC) and Comprehensive metabolic panel (CMP)	2007, throughout lifetime	Monitor renal and liver function for side-effects of medications and/or problems with elimination	CBC $37.00 CMP $46.00 TOTAL $83.00	$ 83.00**
Bi-annual follow up with Finnie Green, MD, urologist	2007, throughout lifetime	Due to chronic and persistent problems with urinary incontinence and infections follow up is warranted to further monitor renal function and appropriately treat infections	$95.00 per visit	$ 190.00
Urinalysis with culture and sensitivity, twice per year	2007, throughout lifetime	Evaluate urinary infections and identify appropriate treatment	$361.00 per sample	$ 722.00 per year
Totals this page				$1,250.00 per year

* This figure reflect the cost of 3 visits per year. Mr. Miller should have an annual medical evaluation for routine health care assessment annually. The impact of the motor vehicle collision require that he be seen at least 3 times per year over and above the routine baseline
** This figure reflects the cost of lab testing once per year. Mr. Miller would be expected to have annual baseline lab work completed as part of a routine health care assessment. As a result of the multiple medications he will use for the reminder of his lifetime, he should have his lab testing repeated at least one more time per year.

RE: Robert Miller, Sr.
DOB: 01/28/1920
SSN: 222-33-4444
DOI: 04/20/2006
PRIMARY DIAGNOSES: Weakness, debilitation, dysphasia,
dysarthria, fracture C5 vertebra (healed), fracture right
humerus (healed), depressive disorder, intermittent incontinence

LIFE CARE PLAN
Medications and Nutritional Needs
August 28, 2007

Wirt & Associates
P.O. Box 8
Catawba, VA 24070
(540) 529-3631
(540) 384-5162 (fax)

DESCRIPTION	Year initiated/ replacement schedule	Purpose/Rationale	Cost per item	Cost per year
Jevity 1 nutritional supplement	2006, throughout lifetime	Meet nutritional needs Mr. Miller cannot do orally	$370.00 per month	$ 4,440.00
Jevity feeding bags, tubing and other pump supplies	2006, throughout lifetime	Allows slow administration	$584.00 per month	$ 7,008.00
Metoprolol, 50 mg, twice per day	2006, throughout lifetime	Beta-blocker, reduces risk of MI	$23.59 per month	$ 283.08
Pepcid AC		Reduces gastric acid production, enhances digestion and reduces risk of ulcers	$22.69 per month	$ 272.28
Aspirin, 81 mg, once per day		Cardiac protective, mild anti-coagulant to reduce risk of DVT	$2.51 per month	$ 30.12
Totals this page				$12,033.48

RE: Robert Miller, Sr.
DOB: 01/28/1920
SSN: 222-33-4444
DOI: 04/20/2006
PRIMARY DIAGNOSES: Weakness, debilitation, dysphasia,
dysarthria, fracture C5 vertebra (healed), fracture right
humerus (healed), depressive disorder, intermittent incontinence

LIFE CARE PLAN
Nursing Care/Therapy Services
August 28, 2007

Wirt & Associates
P.O. Box 8
Catawba, VA 24070
(540) 529-3631
(540) 384-5162 (fax)

DESCRIPTION	Year initiated/ replacement schedule	Purpose/Rationale	Cost per item	Cost per year
Skilled nursing care, 2 visits per day	2007, throughout lifetime	Provide medication administration, tube feeding, skin assessment, continence assessment, change PEG tube dressing,	$55.00 per visit = $110.00 per day	$40,040.00 per year
CNA, daily visit	2007, throughout lifetime	Assist with transfers, bathing, dressing and toileting needs. Provide safety monitoring when Mrs. Miller is out of the house	$16.00 per hr M-F ($64.00 per day = $320.00 per week) $17.00 per hr S & S ($68.00 per day = $136.00 per week) Total = $456.00 per week	$23,712.00 per year
Physical therapy – 3 visits	2007 – one time occurrence	Vehicle transfer instruction	$135.00 per visit	$ 405.00* (one time, non-recurring)
Totals this page				$63,752.00 per year for nursing care $ 405.00* (one time)

* Mr. and Mrs. Miller need additional instruction and practice with the PT to improve independence in car transfers

RE: Robert Miller, Sr.
DOB: 01/28/1920
SSN: 222-33-4444
DOI: 04/20/2006
PRIMARY DIAGNOSES: Weakness, debilitation, dysphasia, dysarthria, fracture C5 vertebra (healed), fracture right humerus (healed), depressive disorder, intermittent incontinence

LIFE CARE PLAN
Durable Medical Equipment
August 28, 2007

Wirt & Associates
P.O. Box 8
Catawba, VA 24070
(540) 529-3631
(540) 384-5162 (fax)

DESCRIPTION	Year initiated/ replacement schedule	Purpose/Rationale	Cost per item	Cost per year
Shower bench	2007	Current shower bench shows sign of rust and should be replaced with one that does not rust for safety purposes	$138.95	$138.95 (one time purchase)
Swivel seat	2007	Assist with car transfers	$141.95	$141.95 (one time purchase)
Seating cushion	2007	Fluid and air cushion can be used in wheelchair, recliner or car to help reduce risk of skin breakdown associated with pressure	$232.00	$232.00 (one time purchase)
Totals this page				$512.90 *
* These items should last throughout Mr. Miller's lifetime				

RE: Robert Miller, Sr.
DOB: 01/28/1920
SSN: 222-33-4444
DOI: 04/20/2006
PRIMARY DIAGNOSES: Weakness, debilitation, dysphasia, dysarthria, fracture C5 vertebra (healed), fracture right humerus (healed), depressive disorder, intermittent incontinence

LIFE CARE PLAN
Incontinence Supplies
August 28, 2007

Wirt & Associates
P.O. Box 8
Catawba, VA 24070
(540) 529-3631
(540) 384-5162 (fax)

DESCRIPTION	Year initiated/ replacement schedule	Purpose/Rationale	Cost per item	Cost per year
External catheter and night time collection bag	2006, throughout lifetime	Assist with keeping Mr. Miller dry throughout the night reducing risk of skin breakdown and maintaining good hygiene	External catheter = $55.50 per month Tubing & bag = $ 3.49* per month Total = $58.99	$ 707.88
Absorbent undergarment	2006, throughout lifetime	Prevent soiling of clothing and seating surface when incontinence occurs	$57.99** per month	$ 695.88
Totals this page				$1,403.76
* Collection bag can be cleaned, dried and reused for approximately one month, and then it should be replaced.				
** Provides for up to 3 changes per day				

RE: Robert Miller, Sr.
DOB: 01/28/1920
SSN: 222-33-4444
DOI: 04/20/2006
PRIMARY DIAGNOSES: Weakness, debilitation, dysphasia, dysarthria, fracture C5 vertebra (healed), fracture right humerus (healed), depressive disorder, intermittent incontinence

LIFE CARE PLAN
Cost Summary
August 28, 2007

Wirt & Associates
P.O. Box 8
Catawba, VA 24070
(540) 529-3631
(540) 384-5162 (fax)

Category	Annual or One-Time only Costs
Medical Care	$ 1,250.00 annually
Nursing Care & Therapy Services	$63,752.00 annually $ 405.00 one-time only
Medications & Nutritional Needs	$12,033.48 annually
Incontinence Supplies	$ 1,403.76 annually
Durable Medical Equipment	$ 512.90 one-time only
Grand totals	$78,439.24 annually $ 917.90 one time only

APPENDIX B

RE: C. Ellis DOB: 09/23/1922 DOI: 03/11/2006	**LIFE CARE PLAN** **Medical Care** September 19, 2008			Wirt & Associates P.O. Box 8 Catawba, VA 24070 (540) 529-3631 (540) 384-5162 (fax)
PRIMARY DIAGNOSES: Fall, fracture of Left hip, subsequent with surgical repair, Post-operative hypoglycemia, hypotension, & hypoxia				
DESCRIPTION	Year recommended/initiated	Purpose/Rationale	Cost per item	Cost per year/episode
Bi-annual follow up with primary care physician*	2008, thru lifetime	Ms. Ellis would have been expected to see her PCP twice per year for monitoring and evaluation of her pre-existing health conditions, however, the additional impact of the March 2006 events justify additional follow up. Home care needs would be further assessed during these visits.*	$100.00/visit	$200.00/year
Totals this category				$200.00/year thru life
* This reflects 2 additional visits per year over the expected 2 that would have been expected for routine care, bringing the annual total of visits to 4 per year.				

RE: C. Ellis DOB: 09/23/1922 DOI: 03/11/2006	**LIFE CARE PLAN** **Home Health Nursing and Therapies** September 19, 2008			Wirt & Associates P.O. Box 8 Catawba, VA 24070 (540) 529-3631 (540) 384-5162 (fax)
PRIMARY DIAGNOSES: Fall, fracture of Left hip, subsequent with surgical repair, Post-operative hypoglycemia, hypotension, & hypoxia				
DESCRIPTION	Year recommended/initiated	Purpose/Rationale	Cost per item	Cost per year/episode
Skilled nursing evaluation and monthly follow up, throughout lifetime	2008	Establish and coordinate home care treatment, bowel and bladder program, direct services of CNAs, provide education to Ms. Ellis and family as indicated	$100.00/visit	$ 1,200.00/year thru life
CNA/Attendant care, 16 hours per day	2008	Provide AM and PM care, implement bowel and bladder program, assist with transfers, follow thru with daily therapy/home exercise program	$10.00/hour × 16 hours = $160.00/day × 5 days per week (M-F) = $800.00/week + $10.00/hr × 8 hours per day = $80.00 × 2 days/week (Sat & Sun) = $160.00/week TOTAL = $960.00/week	$49,920.00/year thru life
Home based physical therapy, 3 × per week × 8 weeks	2008	Focus on strength, endurance and weight bearing to improve independence with ambulation and transfers	$100.00/visit = $300.00/week × 8 weeks = $2,400.00*	$ 2,400.00*
Totals this category				$51,120.00/year thru life $ 2,400.00*
* One-time only				

RE: C. Ellis
DOB: 09/23/1922
DOI: 03/11/2006

LIFE CARE PLAN
Medical Equipment and Supplies
September 19, 2008

Wirt & Associates
P.O. Box 8
Catawba, VA 24070
(540) 529-3631
(540) 384-5162 (fax)

PRIMARY DIAGNOSES: Fall, fracture of Left hip, subsequent with surgical repair,
Post-operative hypoglycemia, hypotension, & hypoxia

DESCRIPTION	Year recommended/initiated	Purpose/Rationale	Cost per item	Cost per year/episode
Lightweight wheelchair	2008	Provide ease in mobility and community access	$900.00*	$ 900.00*
Pressure relief/reduction chair cushion	2008	Reduce risk of skin breakdown	$325.00/year	$ 325.00/year thru life
Rolling shower chair	2008	Allow access to shower and commode	$228.50*	$ 228.50*
Bedside commode	2008	Allow ease of access for toileting needs at night	$120.00*	$ 120.00*
Rolling walker	2008	Mobility around home	$110.00*	$ 110.00*
Hoyer lift	2008	Ease in transferring from bed to sitting reducing the risk of injury to caregivers	$1,700.00*	$1,700.00*
Totals this category				$3,058.50* $ 325.00/year thru life
* One time purchases only				

RE: C. Ellis
DOB: 09/23/1922
DOI: 03/11/2006

LIFE CARE PLAN
Home Modifications
September 19, 2008

Wirt & Associates
P.O. Box 8
Catawba, VA 24070
(540) 529-3631
(540) 384-5162 (fax)

PRIMARY DIAGNOSES: Fall, fracture of Left hip, subsequent with surgical repair,
Post-operative hypoglycemia, hypotension, & hypoxia

DESCRIPTION	Year recommended/initiated	Purpose/Rationale	Cost per item	Cost per year/episode
Addition of a wheelchair-accessible area with drive way to entrance	2008	Several modifications will need to be made to make Ms. S.'s home safe for Ms. Ellis, however, it is not feasible to make an existing bedroom or bathroom accessible. Instead, an addition will need to be added to the home in the back with a drive that will allow safe access to the residence	Pending receipt of plans and cost projections from contractor	Pending–to be supplemented with contractors plans and cost projections
Totals this category				

RE: C. Ellis
DOB: 09/23/1922
DOI: 03/11/2006

LIFE CARE PLAN
Cost Summary
September 19, 2008

Wirt & Associates
P.O. Box 8
Catawba, VA 24070
(540) 529-3631
(540) 384-5162 (fax)

PRIMARY DIAGNOSES: Fall, fracture of Left hip, subsequent with surgical repair,
Post-operative hypoglycemia, hypotension, & hypoxia

Category	Annual or One-time only costs
Medical Care	$ 200.00/year thru lifetime
Home Health	$51,120.00/year thru lifetime $ 2,400.00*
Medical Equipment and Supplies	$ 325.00/year thru lifetime $ 3,058.50*
Home Modifications	Pending–to be supplemented upon receipt of contractors projections
Totals	$51,645.00/year thru lifetime $ 5,458.50*
* One time purchases or costs only.	

APPENDIX C

RE: Ryan W. S.	**LIFE CARE PLAN**	Wirt & Associates
DOB: 05//30/1979	**Medical Care**	P.O. Box 8
SSN: 222-33-4444	April 29, 2008	Catawba, VA 24070
DOI: 10/23/2005		(540) 529-3631
PRIMARY DIAGNOSES: Spinal cord injury, paraplegic T4		(540) 384-5162 (fax)
ASIA C (some motor and sensory return)		

DESCRIPTION	Year recommended/initiated	Purpose/Rationale	Cost per item	Cost per year/episode
Annual evaluation by physiatrist	2008, throughout lifetime	Update rehabilitation needs, guidance for medications and other evaluations such as therapy services, wheelchair seating evaluation	$177.00/year	$ 177.00/yr
Annual evaluation by neuro-urologist	2008, throughout lifetime	Assess renal and bladder status, obtain updated testing, recommend changes to bladder routine	$177.00/year	$ 177.00/yr
Bi-annual follow up with local urologist	2008, throughout lifetime	Monitor renal and bladder status, implement urologic treatment defined by neuro-urologist.	$95.00/visit	$ 190.00/yr
Bi-annual follow up with local primary care physician	2008, throughout lifetime	Implement treatment plan defined by physiatrist, obtain blood work as indicated as well as provide prescriptions	$83.00/visit	$ 166.00/yr
Psychological evaluation	Undetermined	Provide support services during adjustments to future life-style changes associated with his SCI	$400.00*	$ 400.00* (one time only)
Complete Blood Count (CBC), Complete Metabolic Panel (CMP), Urinalysis with Culture & Sensitivity (UA + C & S)	2008, bi-annually throughout lifetime	Monitor renal, liver and cardiac status, evaluate potential urinary infections	CBC = $37.00 CMP = $46.00 UA + C & S = $333.00 Blood draw = $15.00	$ 862.00/yr

RE: Ryan W. S.	**LIFE CARE PLAN**	Wirt & Associates
DOB: 05//30/1979	**Medical Care**	P.O. Box 8
SSN: 222-33-4444	Page 2	Catawba, VA 24070
DOI: 10/23/2005		(540) 529-3631
PRIMARY DIAGNOSES: Spinal cord injury, paraplegic T4–T7		(540) 384-5162 (fax)
ASIA C (some motor and sensory return)		

Renal ultrasound & urodynamic studies	2008, annually throughout lifetime	Detailed assessment of renal and bladder function	Renal Ultrasound = $638.00 Urodynamic studies = $4,194.00	$4,832.00/yr
Dexa-scan	2008, every 2 years throughout lifetime	Mr. S. is at risk for osteoporosis due to his non-weight bearing status. He will need a baseline dexascan to assess bone density and help define treatment plan	$408.00/test	$ 204.00/yr
Totals this category				$ 400.00* $6,608.00/yr

* Additional services (and charges) may be incurred depending on results and recommendations of evaluation

RE: Ryan W. S. DOB: 05//30/1979 SSN: 224-41-1103 DOI: 10/23/2005 PRIMARY DIAGNOSES: Spinal cord injury, paraplegic T4 ASIA C (some motor and sensory return)	**LIFE CARE PLAN** **Medications** April 29, 2008			Wirt & Associates P.O. Box 8 Catawba, VA 24070 (540) 529-3631 (540) 384-5162 (fax)
DESCRIPTION	Year recommended/initiated	Purpose/Rationale	Cost per item	Cost per year/episode
Vesicare, 10 mg, once daily	2008, throughout lifetime	Relaxes overactive bladder	$5.33/pill	$ 1,945.45.00/yr
Cymbalta, 60 mg, once daily	2008, throughout lifetime	Neuropathic pain	$4.17/pill	$ 1,522.05/yr
Nexium, 40 mg, once daily	2008, throughout lifetime	Reduce gastric acid production, reduce upset associated with multiple medications	$4.93/pill	$ 1,799.45/yr
Buspirone, 10 mg, 4×/day	2008, throughout lifetime	Anti-anxiety medication	$0.25/pil = $1.00/day	$ 365.00/yr
Clonazepam, 0.25 mg/ 4×/day	2008, throughout lifetime	Anti-anxiety medication	$0.86/day	$ 313.90/yr
Baclofen, 20 mg, 6 tablets per day	2008, throughout lifetime	Anti-spasticity medication, controls muscle spasms associated with SCI	$4.38/day	$ 1,598.70/yr
Baclofen, 10 mg, 2×/day	2008, throughout lifetime	Controls muscle spasms	$0.94/day	$ 343.10/yr
Tizanidine, 4 mg, 8 tablets/day	2008, throughout lifetime	Anti-spasticity – muscle relaxant	$9.52/day	$ 3,474.80/yr
Didronel, 400 mg	2008 (expected to be discontinued at next follow with physiatrist)*	Decreases development of heterotopic bone formation	$21.42/day	$ 7,818.30/yr
Ultram ER, 300 mg, once daily	2008, throughout lifetime	Pain management	$9.10/day	$ 3,321.50/yr
Tramadol, 50 mg, 2×/day	2008, throughout lifetime	Pain management	$0.52/day	$ 189.80/yr
Lyrica, 50 mg, once daily	2008, throughout lifetime	Pain management	$2.65/pill	$ 967.25/yr
Benazepril, 10 mg, once daily	2008, throughout lifetime	Improves kidney function, lower blood pressure	$0.75/pill	$ 273.75/yr
Nitrofurantion, 100 mg, once daily	2008, throughout lifetime	Antibiotic to help reduce risk of urinary tract infections	$1.98/pill	$ 722.70/yr

RE: Ryan W. S. DOB: 05//30/1979 SSN: 224-41-1103 DOI: 10/23/2005 PRIMARY DIAGNOSES: Spinal cord injury, paraplegic T4 ASIA C (some motor and sensory return)	**LIFE CARE PLAN** **Medications** Page 2 April 29, 2008			Wirt & Associates P.O. Box 8 Catawba, VA 24070 (540) 529-3631 (540) 384-5162 (fax)
DESCRIPTION	Year recommended/initiated	Purpose/Rationale	Cost per item	Cost per year/episode
Unisom, 50 mg, 2 pills at night	2008, throughout lifetime	Sleep aid	$0.16/day	$ 58.40/yr
Cranberry pill, 2×/day	2008, throughout lifetime	Helps decrease risk of urinary tract infection	$0.14/day	$ 51.10/yr
Magic Bullet suppository, every other day	2008, throughout lifetime	Component of bowel program	$0.02/suppository	$ 3.65/yr
Vitamin D, 1×/day*	2008*	Reduce risk of osteoporosis	$0.20/pill	$ 73.00/yr
Fosamax, 70 mg + D*, 1×/week	2008, throughout lifetime*	Mr. S. has not begun Fosamax yet, but it is expected that at the time of his next physiatry evaluation, he will undergo a dexascan to assess his bone density then begin Fosamax + D.	$12.95/pill	$ 673.40/yr
Totals this category				$17,624.00/yr**

* Dr. Alfano, the physiatrist following Mr. S. has indicated that he will discontinue the Didronel at the next appointment, then initiate
  Fosamax to help reduce the risk of osteoporosis associated with non-weight bearing. As Vitamin D is included with the Fosamax,
  Mr. S. will be able to discontinue that supplement.
** This total does not include the ongoing costs of Didronel and Vitamin D but does include the annual cost of Fosamax.

RE: Ryan W. S. DOB: 05//30/1979 SSN: 222-33-4444 DOI: 10/23/2005 PRIMARY DIAGNOSES: Spinal cord injury, paraplegic T4 ASIA C (some motor and sensory return)	**LIFE CARE PLAN** **Wheelchairs & Supplies** April 29, 2008			Wirt & Associates P.O. Box 8 Catawba, VA 24070 (540) 529-3631 (540) 384-5162 (fax)
DESCRIPTION	**Year recommended/initiated**	**Purpose/Rationale**	**Cost per item**	**Cost per year/episode**
Wheelchair seating evaluation and assessment	2010, then periodically as needed	Provide input and information regarding most appropriate wheelchairs and custom seating to prevent skin breakdown	$988.00*	$ 988.00* (one time only)
Ultra-light wheelchair, anti-tippers, pop-off wheels,adjustable back, hill holders, etc	2005, replace in 5 years (next new purchase in 2010), then every 10 years afterwards	Provide mobility in the community. This will also be used as a back up when power chair is not available or is having maintenance work.	$2,600.00 × 5 purchases	$ 13,000.00 (over lifetime)
Wheelchair maintenance	2006, annually except year of new purchases when warranty is in effect	Provide new cushions, covers, tires, straps, etc as needed	$260.00/year, except year of new purchases	$260.00/yr × 40.9 yrs = $ 10,634.00 (over lifetime)
Power chair	2010, replace every 5 years	At 10 years post-injury, providing a power chair will reduce the risk of upper extremity overuse problems such as carpal tunnel syndrome and rotator cuff tear	$12,000.00 × 9 purchases	$108,000.00 (over lifetime)
Power chair maintenance	2011, annually except year of new purchase when warranty is in effect	Provides for safety of operation of the power chair including replacement parts such as batteries, tires, etc	$1,200.00/year, except year of new purchases	$1,200.00/yr × 33.9 yrs = $ 40,680.00 (over lifetime)
Rolling shower chair	2008, replace every 3 years	Ease of access to toileting and showering	$1,700.00 × 15 purchases	$ 25,500.00 (over lifetime)

RE: Ryan W. S. DOB: 05//30/1979 SSN: 222-33-4444 DOI: 10/23/2005 PRIMARY DIAGNOSES: Spinal cord injury, paraplegic T4–T7 ASIA C (some motor and sensory return)	**LIFE CARE PLAN** **Wheelchairs & Supplies** Page 2			Wirt & Associates P.O. Box 8 Catawba, VA 24070 (540) 529-3631 (540) 384-5162 (fax)
DESCRIPTION	**Year recommended/initiated**	**Purpose/Rationale**	**Cost per item**	**Cost per year/episode**
Maintenance of shower chair	2009, annually except year of new purchase	Provides for safety of shower chair	$170.00/year, except year of new purchases	$170.00/yr × 30.9 = $ 5,253.00 (over lifetime)
Totals this category				$204,055.00 (over lifetime)

* For purposes of this LCP, this charge has only been added one time. Additional evaluations may be indicated should Mr. S. have a significant change in his weight or begin to develop problems with skin breakdown in pressure areas. Should more frequent evaluations be necessary additional costs would be incurred.

RE: Ryan W. S. DOB: 05//30/1979 SSN: 222-33-4444 DOI: 10/23/2005 PRIMARY DIAGNOSES: Spinal cord injury, paraplegic T4 ASIA C (some motor and sensory return)	**LIFE CARE PLAN** **Medical Equipment & Supplies** April 29, 2008			Wirt & Associates P.O. Box 8 Catawba, VA 24070 (540) 529-3631 (540) 384-5162 (fax)
DESCRIPTION	**Year recommended/initiated**	**Purpose/Rationale**	**Cost per item**	**Cost per year/episode**
CVS Soft cloths	2008, throughout lifetime	Used to aid in personal care before and after bowel and bladder program	$8.97/week	$ 466.44/yr
CVS Latex free gloves	2008, throughout lifetime	For bowel program and suppository insertion	$7.99/week	$ 415.48/yr
CVS lubricating jelly	2008, throughout lifetime	Bowel program	$3.79/month	$ 45.48/yr
Urinary drainage bag	2008, throughout lifetime	Urine collection	$0.39/day	$ 142.35/yr
Avant gauze sponges	2008, throughout lifetime	Cleanings, wound care, etc	$6.99/month	$ 83.88/yr
Advance plus Hollister catheterization kit	2008, throughout lifetime	Bladder program– intermittent catheterization program	$5.02/day	$1,832.30/yr
Red rubber urinary catheter, 14 French	2008, throughout lifetime	Intermittent urinary catheterization program	$0.93/day	$ 339.45/yr
Mattress overlay	2008, replace annually throughout lifetime	Reduces risk of skin breakdown	$300.00/purchase	$ 300.00/yr
Totals this category				$3,625.38/yr

RE: Ryan W. S.
DOB: 05//30/1979
SSN: 222-33-4444
DOI: 10/23/2005
PRIMARY DIAGNOSES: Spinal cord injury, paraplegic T4
ASIA C (some motor and sensory return)

LIFE CARE PLAN
Health Maintenance
April 29, 2008

Wirt & Associates
P.O. Box 8
Catawba, VA 24070
(540) 529-3631
(540) 384-5162 (fax)

DESCRIPTION	Year recommended/initiated	Purpose/Rationale	Cost per item	Cost per year/episode
Physical therapy evaluation	2008, annually through out lifetime	Guide and direct independent exercise program, update wheelchair seating as needed	$188.00	$188.00/yr
Fitness membership	2008, throughout lifetime	Provide access to exercise equipment and pool for strength and fitness. Also provides a health- focused environment and access to other resources as indicated	$54.00/month	$648.00/yr
Totals this category				$836.00/yr

RE: Ryan W. S.
DOB: 05//30/1979
SSN: 222-33-4444
DOI: 10/23/2005
PRIMARY DIAGNOSES: Spinal cord injury, paraplegic T4
ASIA C (some motor and sensory return)

LIFE CARE PLAN
Transportation
April 29, 2008

Wirt & Associates
P.O. Box 8
Catawba, VA 24070
(540) 529-3631
(540) 384-5162 (fax)

DESCRIPTION	Year recommended/initiated	Purpose/Rationale	Cost per item	Cost per year/episode
Wheelchair modifications to van	2007, then each time new vehicle is purchased*	Hand-controls, wheelchair tie down, electric lift to ease access in wheelchair	Undetermined*	Undetermined
Mileage to and from medical appointments	2008, throughout lifetime	Trips to and from UVA to see physiatrist and neuro-urologist are 246 miles round trip. Trips to and from local medical providers (PCP and urologist) are 18 miles round trip	246 × 2 = 492 miles × $0.505/mile** = $248.46 18 × 4 = 72 miles x $0.505/mile** = $36.36	$248.46/yr + $ 36.36/yr $284.82/yr
Handicapped parking decal	2008, throughout lifetime	Provides closer parking when out in community	$5.00/yr	$ 5.00/yr
Totals this category				$289.82/yr

* The costs to modify a vehicle and make it wheelchair accessible as well as adapt hand controls will vary depending on the make and model of the vehicle. Future charges for this will be incurred if/when a new vehicle is purchased but the frequency of this cannot be predicted.
** Based on IRS mileage allowance for 2008.

RE: Ryan W. S.
DOB: 05//30/1979
SSN: 222-33-4444
DOI: 10/23/2005
PRIMARY DIAGNOSES: Spinal cord injury, paraplegic T4
ASIA C (some motor and sensory return)

LIFE CARE PLAN
Medical Equipment & Supplies
April 29, 2008

Wirt & Associates
P.O. Box 8
Catawba, VA 24070
(540) 529-3631
(540) 384-5162 (fax)

DESCRIPTION	Year recommended/initiated	Purpose/Rationale	Cost per item	Cost per year/episode
CVS Soft cloths	2008, throughout lifetime	Used to aid in personal care before and after bowel and bladder program	$8.97/week	$ 466.44/yr
CVS Latex free gloves	2008, throughout lifetime	For bowel program and suppository insertion	$7.99/week	$ 415.48/yr
CVS lubricating jelly	2008, throughout lifetime	Bowel program	$3.79/month	$ 45.48/yr
Urinary drainage bag	2008, throughout lifetime	Urine collection	$0.39/day	$ 142.35/yr
Avant gauze sponges	2008, throughout lifetime	Cleanings, wound care, etc	$6.99/month	$ 83.88/yr
Advance plus Hollister catheterization kit	2008, throughout lifetime	Bladder program— intermittent catheterization program	$5.02/day	$1,832.30/yr
Red rubber urinary catheter, 14 French	2008, throughout lifetime	Intermittent urinary catheterization program	$0.93/day	$ 339.45/yr
Mattress overlay	2008, replace annually throughout lifetime	Reduces risk of skin breakdown	$300.00/purchase	$ 300.00/yr
Totals this category				$3,625.38/yr

GLOSSARY

75% rule: Devised to separate inpatient rehabilitation from acute care, Medicare devised a list of eight diagnoses to determine which patients were most likely to qualify for acute inpatient rehabilitation. A rehabilitation hospital or unit, to bill for TEFRA payments, had to demonstrate that 75% of the patients admitted were diagnosed with one of those eight diagnoses.

Absorption: The process of being absorbed.

Acceptance and Action Questionnaire: A tool used to detect avoidance coping characterized by both active and passive attempts to avoid thoughts, feeling, memories, and bodily sensations the individual considers negative.

Ace wrapping: The process of using an ace bandage to wrap an extremity to provide support and decrease swelling.

Acquired brain injury: See **traumatic brain injury (TBI)**.

Activation of prior knowledge: Occurs as the brain searches for "hooks" (frame of reference based on prior knowledge) on which to hang new information.

Active range of motion: Extent of movement within a given joint that the person can perform solely on his or her own.

Activities of daily living (ADLs): Also known as self-care, these are activities such as feeding, grooming, bathing, upper and lower extremity dressing, and toileting.

Activity-based restorative therapies: Evidence-based tools used for neurological recovery in spinal cord injury, thought to promote recovery through regeneration of nerve cells.

Activity limitations: Problems in a person's performance of everyday functions such as communication, self-care, mobility, learning, and behavior (U.S. Department of Health and Human Services).

Acute rehabilitation: A comprehensive program of coordinated, integrated, interdisciplinary services provided under the direction of physicians qualified in rehabilitation.

Adaptation: Recovery through which an individual suffering from a disabling or functionally limiting condition, whether temporary or irreversible, participates to regain maximal function, independence, and restoration.

Adaptive equipment: Designed to help compensate for a client's limitations in strength, range of motion, mobility, dexterity, speech, and other skills most of us take for granted.

Adolescent Coping Scale: Measures coping in adolescent populations to identify productive and nonproductive strategies.

Adult learning theory: Developed by Knowles, emphasizes prior knowledge and partnerships in learning.

Advance directive: Legal document that conveys an individual's decisions regarding end-of-life care and treatment.

Advanced practice registered nurse (APRN): An umbrella term used to describe those nurse roles of certified registered nurse anesthetist, certified nurse midwife, clinical nurse specialist, and nurse practitioner; conducts comprehensive assessment and integrates education, research, and consultation into clinical practice.

Advocacy: Championing the needs and interests of another.

Affect: Appearance of emotion in a person's tone of voice, facial expression, and other nonverbal behavior.

Afferent: Conduction of nerve impulses toward the central nervous system.

Agitation: Extreme emotional disturbance.

Agnosia: Series of perceptual deficits that describe a marked indifference to or lack of awareness of the paralyzed side of the body and disregard to the environment on the affected side.

Albumin: Serum lab value commonly used to measure overall nutritional health in the body.

Allodynia: Pain from something that is not usually painful.

Alteration in comfort: Due to phantom pain or postoperative residual limb pain.

Ambiguous loss: Feelings of not being certain of a person's absence or presence, such as whether a loved one is dead or alive, dying, or recovering or when an injured loved one does not seem the same as before they were injured.

Ambulatory aids: Walkers, crutches, and/or wheel-chairs.

American Association of Nurse Life Care Planners: A nurse-only professional organization for the practice of life care planning.

Americans with Disabilities Act (ADA): Enacted in 1990 to mandate that people with disabilities are afforded legal protection and are provided with essential public services.

American Nurses Association Code of Ethics: The code of conduct that guides nursing practice within the United States and defines the ethical obligations and duties of individuals who have entered into and practice within the profession of nursing.

Amino acid: Protein provides a source of these, which are necessary for the body to build and repair its tissues.

Amputation: Partial or complete surgical removal of a limb as the result of an injury, intolerable pain, gangrene, vascular obstruction, uncontrollable infection, or congenital anomalies.

Anabolism: Process of storing or using protein for tissue building.

Andragogy: Emphasizes a learner-centered approach with an equitable balance between the teacher and learner.

Anergia: Impairment of initiation in which the patient begins an action either slowly or not at all and requires external cueing to move through the steps involved in a familiar activity.

Aneurysm: An abnormal bulge in a blood vessel due to a weakened vessel wall.

Angina pectoris: Chest pain or discomfort due to a temporary interruption of blood to the heart muscle.

Animal-assisted activity (AAA): Any activity in which the goal is to enhance quality of life through various educational, recreational, or therapeutic opportunities with the use of animals.

Animal-assisted therapy (AAT): A goal-directed intervention in which an animal meeting specific criteria is an integral part of the treatment process (Schaffer).

Anorexia: Lack or loss of appetite resulting in weight loss.

Anorexia nervosa: Weight less than 85% of that expected for height. The anorexic has an altered body image and sees him- or herself as fat, thereby curtailing food intake.

Anosagnosia: A cognitive impairment that causes a lack of knowledge or insight into one's own illness, injury, or medical condition.

Anterior cord syndrome: Occurs when there is damage to the anterior spinal artery, typically caused by bone fragments or a herniated disc and resulting in paralysis and loss of pain, temperature, and touch sensation.

Anxiety:

Aphasia: Impairment of language functions after brain damage, specifically, the disturbed capacity to decode (interpret) and encode (formulate, express) conventional, meaningful symbols.

Appraisal:

Apraxia: Lack of ability to perform previously learned motor skills either on command or by imitation.

Apraxia of speech: Neurological disorder characterized by loss of the ability to sequence syllables into sounds, despite having the desire and the physical ability to perform the movements.

Areflexic: In the areflexic bladder there is damage to the reflex arc This lower motor neuron disorder produces a flaccid, atonic bladder because of injury to the S2–4 segments. Patients have involuntary voiding, no sensation, and overflow incontinence.

Arnold-Chiari II malformation (ACM): An abnormality in the brain characterized by a low tentorium insertion, herniation of the posterior fossa content into the upper cervical canal, and a small fourth ventricle.

Articular cartilage: The cartilage that covers the articular part of bones.

ASIA impairment scale: Developed by the American Spinal Cord Injury Association (ASIA), a classification system for the evaluation and assessment of SCI that defines the function of motor and sensation below the level of injury.

Aspiration pneumonia: Pneumonia that can occur due to the inability to swallow.

Assistance animal: Performs tasks for people with disabilities such as hearing impairment, physical limitations, emotional disabilities, diabetes, or seizures.

Assistive device: Devices that assist a person in the ability to walk or perform other activities of daily living.

Association of Rehabilitation Nurses (ARN): Established in 1974 by Susan Novak, an organization that seeks to promote quality rehabilitation. Its stated mission is to promote and advance professional rehabilitation nursing practice through education, advocacy, collaboration, and research to enhance the quality of life for those affected by disability and chronic illness.

Association of Rehabilitation Nurses Competency Assessment Test (ARN-CAT): Provides multiple-choice online tests in 16 assessment areas and can be used as a tool by nursing leadership to evaluate the proficiency of rehabilitation nurses.

Asthma: A chronic respiratory disease characterized by recurring attacks of labored breathing, chest constriction, and coughing.

Ataxia: Inability of muscles to perform synchronized movements.

Atrial fibrillation (AF): A cardiac dysrhythmia in which the heart quivers or fibrillates, not beating in normal sinus rhythm.

Attention process training: A cognitive remediation to help stroke survivors with attention deficits.

Attention: Focused awareness.

Autoimmune disorders: Disorders in which autoimmune antibodies destroy receptors or peripheral myelin, such as Gullain-Barré syndrome.

Automated peritoneal dialysis: A type of peritoneal dialysis typically undertaken overnight in which a small machine performs the dialysis exchanges while the person sleeps.

Autonomic dysreflexia: Caused when stimuli sent to the brain via the spinal cord cannot reach the message center. Sensory receptors are blocked, but the stimuli continue and the impulses build, producing a reflex arteriolar spasm through the autonomic nervous system, leading to arteriole vasoconstriction and elevated blood pressure, with massive vasodilatation to the heart and the brain.

Autonomy: Duty to allow the individual the right to make his or her own decision.

Avascular necrosis: Death of bone tissue due to ischemia or loss of blood supply.

Baby boomers: Persons born between 1946 and 1964.

Beck Depression Inventory: A common tool to measure depression.

Becker muscular dystrophy (BMD): With the same gene location as Duchenne muscular dystrophy but with a later onset and slower and more variable progression of symptoms, a diagnosis is suspected when the levels of dystrophin are either 20% to 80% of expected values or

there are normal levels of dystrophin and an abnormal molecular weight of dystrophin.

Benchmarking: The standard of best practices by which healthcare settings and processes can be measured or judged.

Beneficence: The duty to do good.

Berg Balance Scale: Grades function and mobility tasks on a four-point scale. Assistive devices such as walkers and canes are not allowed. There is a maximum score of 56, and anything less than 46 points means the person tested is a fall risk. Examples of items assessed include ability to stand unsupported, transfer from one chair to another, picking up an object off the floor, and standing on one leg.

Bioethics: Branch of ethics concerned with issues surrounding health care and the biological sciences.

Biographical disruption: Concept of illness and disability as disrupting the life course of an individual's life plot or biography.

Bladder: The storage place in the body for urine.

Bladder tapping: A technique used to stimulate voiding.

Blast injury: An injury that creates pressure changes within the body (especially in cavities that are air filled), causes items in the environment to become lethal projectiles, propels the body in space, and exposes the body to other toxins, burns, and trauma from falling debris.

Bobath: Therapy for survivors with injuries to the central nervous system, adults with stroke, and hemiplegia whose concept is based on the brain's ability to reorganize and recover after neurological insult (neuroplasticity).

Body image disturbance: Change in how the client perceives him- or herself.

Bony prominences: Those areas on the body where specific pressure points occur that could result in pressure ulcers.

Brachial plexus: Innervates all muscles of the upper extremity except the trapezius.

Braden Scale for Predicting Pressure Ulcer Risk: Most commonly used scale to assess for pressure ulcer risk and consists of six subscales that are scored from 1 to 3 or 4 points. See also **Norton scale**.

Brain attack: See **cerebrovascular accident** and **stroke**.

Brown-Sequard syndrome: Occurs when there is damage to one side of the spinal cord, usually due to a penetrating injury or tumor. On the damaged side there is loss of motor function, proprioception, and vibratory sense below the level of the injury, whereas on the opposite side there is loss of pain and temperature sensation.

Bulimia: Eating binges and purging are characteristic but weight is often normal. Excessive exercise, laxative use, appetite suppressants, and diuretic medications may be used.

Burns: Damaged or injured tissue due to exposure to heat or fire.

Cachexia: Progressive wasting of fat and muscle even in the presence of a satisfactory intake of food and fluids due to severe metabolic dysfunction.

Cancer: A chronic and complex set of diseases that affects every age group but more commonly affects people older than 65 years.

Caritas consciousness relationship: A caring relationship that is transpersonal in nature, meaning it involves both a giving and receiving interaction between the nurse and the patient.

Case management: Coordination of health care, including advocacy for patients and families, communication between other team members and insurance companies.

Case manager: Coordinates implementation of treatment plan; communicates insurance benefit information to patient/families and the team and optimal use of available benefits; advocates for services; acts as liaison between patient, hospital, and payer; and provides updated information to insurance companies.

Catabolism: Breaking down of protein for use as energy when needed, via the Krebs cycle.

Catastrophizing: Characterized by unrealistic and excessively negative self-statements in response to pain.

Cauda equina: That part of the spinal cord below L1–2, where it becomes a loose collection of nerves that resembles a horse's tail.

Central cord syndrome: A hyperextension injury to the cervical region in older adults in which motor deficits are greater in the upper extremities than in the lower.

Central poststroke pain syndrome (CPSP): A neuropathic pain disorder caused by damage to the central nervous system.

Central sleep apnea: Multiple episodes of sleep apnea characterized by cessation of efforts to breathe.

Cerebral palsy (CP): A leading cause of childhood disability and the most common condition resulting in severe physical disabilities, CP is a nonprogressive disorder typically resulting from damage to an immature brain and primarily affects movement and coordination.

Cerebrovascular accident: A nontraumatic brain injury caused by disruption in blood flow to part of the brain from either occlusion of a blood vessel (ischemic stroke) or rupture of a blood vessel (hemorrhagic stroke). Also known as stroke or brain attack.

Certification: Professional recognition of skills in a specialty practice developed and maintained by professional organizations.

Certified registered rehabilitation nurse (CRRN): The credential for certified rehabilitation nurses.

Charcot-Marie-Tooth (CMT) disease: The most common inherited neuromuscular disorder that results from mutations in genes that either code for proteins that comprise peripheral myelin or in proteins that aid in maintaining axonal health.

Children with special healthcare needs (CSHCN): Children who have or are at increased risk for a chronic physical, developmental, behavioral, or emotional conditions and who also require health and related services of a type or amount beyond that required by children generally.

Cholesterol: Lipid compound found exclusively in animal tissue that can be ingested or produced by the body. The body requires cholesterol to produce certain hormones, cell walls, and bile acids for digestion.

Chondrocytes: A primary component of articular cartilage (the other being the **extracellular matrix**), these are the main cells within the articular cartilage and are responsible for the synthesis and breakdown of the ECM, which is a continuous process in normal joint function.

Chronic bronchitis: Diagnosed when a patient has excessive airway mucous secretion leading to a persistent, productive cough. One of the two major diseases of the lung grouped under chronic obstructive pulmonary disease.

Chronic disease: Conditions that continue indefinitely, such as asthma, diabetes, and renal disease. See also **chronic illness**.

Chronic illness: Conditions that continue indefinitely, such as asthma, diabetes, and renal disease. See also **chronic disease**.

Chronic illness trajectories: More than the medical course of illness, the trajectory of chronic illness is linked with people's individual expectations, so that each person defines his or her illness course differently. Individuals' views of their trajectories, along with shifting social relations, affect personal identity, and efforts to maintain social relationships and build new ones contribute to a changed sense of identity.

Chronic kidney disease (CKD): Chronic renal disease characterized by progressively worsening kidney function.

Chronic obstructive pulmonary disease (COPD): Term used for two closely related diseases of the respiratory system: chronic bronchitis and emphysema. In many cases these diseases occur together, although there may be more symptoms of one than the other. COPD gets gradually worse over time.

Chronic sorrow: A persistent and pervasive phenomenon of sorrow whose chronic and recurrent nature is seen as a natural response to a tragic event.

Chronic wounds: Features include protracted phases of healing, lysis of cells before remodeling occurs (cellular senescence), deficiency of growth factor receptor sites, reduced fibrin and growth factor production, and high level of enzymes in the wound.

Chronicity: Relating to chronic or long-term, particularly with relationship to an ongoing illness that may require rehabilitation or prolonged periods of care.

Clasp knife phenomenon: Finding observed in those with upper motor neuron disease and is characterized by rigidity on contraction of a muscle.

Clean intermittent bladder catheterization:

Cleft lip: Embryonic structures surrounding the oral cavity do not join.

Cleft palate: Palatal shelves do not fuse.

Client: The recipient of care; sometimes used interchangeably with the term "patient"

Clinical nurse leader: A nurse leader with a graduate degree or higher in nursing, management, policy, or administration.

Closed head injuries: Brain injuries that are nonpenetrating, such as those resulting from a blow to the head.

Cognition: Mental processes of knowing and thinking.

Cognitive dissonance: Social theory that addresses the level of discomfort felt when what one does differs from what one believes.

Cognitive load theory: A universal set of learning principles that are proven to result in efficient instructional environments as a consequence of leveraging human cognitive learning processes (Clark et al.).

Collaboration: The process used by the interdisciplinary team to communicate and work together for shared goals.

Collaborative discussion: Demands communication skill and an ability to transcend professional jargon, shed the expectation of physician dominance, and become comfortable with blurred professional boundaries.

Commission on Accreditation of Rehabilitation Facilities (CARF): Implemented in 1966 as an independent, nonprofit accreditor of rehabilitation services. Their stated mission is to promote the quality, value, and optimal outcomes of rehabilitation services (CARF International).

Communication: One of three domains of disability categorized by the U.S. Census Bureau describing such deficits as blindness, deafness, or a speech disorder. See also **mental** and **physical**.

Community settings: Outpatient rehabilitation therapy that occurs in therapy gymnasiums housed in freestanding facilities or in acute care or rehabilitation hospitals.

Compassion fatigue: Emotional residue from caring for those who have suffered from traumatic events.

Competencies: Establishes standards, knowledge, and core essential skills needed to perform a particular profession, job, or role.

Complementary and alternative medicine (CAM): Group of diverse medical and healthcare systems, practices, and products that are not generally considered part of conventional medicine.

Complex regional pain syndrome: Complications include diffuse distal limb pain, loss of function, and autonomic dysfunction.

Complication: A negative sequalea of an illness or injury.

Concussion: Temporary loss of consciousness resulting from a blow to the head.

Confabulation: A function of impaired recall for what is actually happening day to day and an attempt to construct an account of what is going on by using information that is actually recalled but is out of the current context.

Conflicts of death: Past wars in which more soldiers died as compared with wars of the current day in which survivals rates are higher.

Congenital limb deficiency (CLD): Part or all of the limb bud does not form.

Consciousness: Awareness.

Consolidated Omnibus Budget Reconciliation Act (COBRA): Signed into law in 1986, under COBRA any employee who works for an employer with 20 or more employees for 50 days of the year or more is qualified to continue temporary insurance coverage at group rates.

Constipation: More than 3 days with no bowel movement.

Constraint-induced movement therapy: A technique that combines active training with the affected arm by constraining the unaffected arm. This type of relearning functional skills is associated with changes in cortical physiology by overcoming learned nonuse of the affected limb.

Continuous ambulatory peritoneal dialysis: A type of peritoneal dialysis that requires the individual to manually change the dialysate in the peritoneal cavity four or five times each day, every day of the year.

Contusion: Bruising of cerebral tissue.

Conus medullaris: Distal end of the spinal cord.

Coping: Constantly changing cognitive and behavioral efforts to manage specific external and/or internal demands that are appraised as taxing or exceeding the resources of the person (Lazarus & Folkman).

Coronary angioplasty: Percutaneous coronary intervention in which a balloon is inflated within the coronary artery to crush the plaque into the walls of the artery.

Coronary artery bypass graft surgery: A surgery in which the diseased segment is bypassed using an artery or vein harvested from elsewhere in the body.

Coronary artery disease (CAD): The single leading cause of death in the United States, CAD is caused by atherosclerosis, with narrowing of the coronary arteries due to the build up of plaque. Also called **coronary heart disease**.

Coronary heart disease: See **coronary artery disease (CAD)**.

Coup/contrecoup: Injuries that result from acceleration/deceleration of the brain within the skull at the moment of impact. The brain crashes into the skull by motion toward the impact area (**coup**) and then rebounds to the opposite side of the skull (**contrecoup**).

Cultural diversity: Differences that occur between human societies and cultures.

Cultural imperialism: Applying the provider's culture to the client.

Culturally competent care: Provision of care that considers the patient or client's culture as an integral part of treatment.

Culturally congruent care: Care consistent or congruent with a patient's cultural beliefs and practices.

Culture: Integrated patterns of human behavior that include the language, thoughts, actions, customs, beliefs, and institutions of racial, ethnic, social, or religious groups.

Culture care accommodation and/or negotiation: One of three action modes of Leininger's Culture Care Theory to guide nurses when making transcultural care decisions or taking actions. See also **culture care preservation and/or maintenance** and **culture care repatterning and/or restructuring**.

Culture care preservation and/or maintenance: One of three action modes of Leininger's Culture Care Theory to guide nurses when making transcultural care decisions or taking actions. See also **culture care accommodation and/or negotiation** and **culture care repatterning and/or restructuring**.

Culture care repatterning and/or restructuring: One of three action modes of Leininger's Culture Care Theory to guide nurses when making transcultural care decisions or taking actions. See also **culture care preservation and/or maintenance** and **culture care accommodation and/or negotiation**.

Current level of function: A person's ability in the present time to perform certain daily tasks or activities.

Cystic fibrosis (CF): An inherited disease that causes thick, sticky mucus to be formed, affecting the lungs, pancreas, and other organs.

Daily Spiritual Experiences (questionnaire)

Damages: A monetary award made to compensate for injury or loss.

Death panel: Term that has recently surfaced with healthcare reform that refers to a false rumor that the new healthcare reform act would finance panels of people whose job it would be to decide whether others were worthy of life and of receiving costly medical treatment. The true proposal in the healthcare bill was that Medicare would finance a patient's voluntary consultation with professionals at the end of life to discuss plans for aggressive and potentially life-saving interventions.

Debridement: The process by which debris is removed from the wound, thus preparing the wound bed for granulation and eventual closure.

Deep vein thrombosis (DVT): A blood clot in a vein, usually in a lower extremity.

Defecation: Removal of solid waste from the bowel.

Degenerative disorders: Generally associated with the impairment or loss of motor neurons; degenerative conditions worsen over time without a return to baseline symptomatology.

Delirium: An acute confusional state often due to medication, environmental, toxic, or metabolic factors.

Dementia: Diffuse decline in cognitive functioning that especially affects memory, executive functions, visuospatial functioning, and processing speed.

Demyelination: The process by which the myelin sheath that assists with the conduction of nerve impulses is harmed or destroyed.

Department of Defense: DoD, is the oldest and largest government agency that is in charge of the military and a large civilian force that defends the United States.

Depression: A negative emotion associated with feelings of sadness and hopelessness that, when prolonged, may lead to decreased quality of life, functional decline, and disability.

Detrusor: A muscle in the bladder formed by smooth muscle fibers.

Detrusor sphincter dyssynergia: The result of lack of synchrony between the detrusor muscle and the external sphincter.

Development: Qualitative refinement of skills and abilities.

Diagnosis-related group (DRG):

Dietitian: Oversees patient's nutritional status, works with physician to provide necessary dietary requirements, and provides patient/family education on diets.

Dimensions of adaptability:

Diplopia: Double vision.

Disability: The general term used to represent the interactions between individuals with a health condition and barriers in their environment (U.S. Department of Health and Human Services).

Disability culture: A sense of community and identify shared by persons with disablities.

Disaccharides: Simple carbohydrates.

Disorientation: Reduced awareness or confusion with respect to person, time, place, and reason or purpose.

Dispositional optimism: Belief in positive outcomes in the future.

Distractibility: Inattention, in which focus is drawn away by environmental or other stimuli.

Doctorate of nursing practice: Considered to be a terminal practice doctorate degree and proposed for future programs preparing the clinical nurse specialist and nurse practitioner.

Do not resuscitate (DNR): A request by the patient to not receive cardiopulmonary resuscitation in the event his or her heart stops or he or she stops breathing while at the hospital.

Duchenne muscular dystrophy (DMD): The most common neuromuscular disorder, it is an X-linked recessive inherited disorder caused by an abnormality at the Xp21 gene loci.

Dynamic alignment: Adjusting the alignment between a prosthesis and the limb to optimize the gait characteristics so they are as effortless and natural as possible.

Dynamic balance: Ability to maintain balance with movement or perturbations.

Dynamic Gait Index: Test that acts as a predictor for falls by assessing a person's ability to walk with changing task demands, such as walking while turning the head horizontally, stepping over obstacles, and going up and down stairs. A score of less than 19 (out of a possible 24) means that a person is at risk for falls. This test is usually performed for patients already walking on their own, and an assistive device may be used.

Dysarthria: Impairment in speech as a result of reduction in muscle strength, speed, range of motion, and/or coordination.

Dysphagia: Impaired swallowing.

Dysphonia: Voice impairment.

Dystrophin: Primary protein product found in the plasma membrane of all muscle cells.

Dysvascular: Compromised circulation.

Early and Periodic Screening, Diagnosis, and Treatment Act: The provision provided by OBRA 1989 that any medically necessary service required to treat any condition identified through this Act would be covered by Medicaid.

Eaton-Lambert syndrome: Autoimmune antibodies destroy presynaptic calcium channels, leading to a loss of functional channels and a decrease in the release of acetylcholine.

Education for All Handicapped Children's Act: Amended the Education of the Handicapped Act to provide free and appropriate education in the least restrictive environment for children with disabilities over age 5 years regardless of the severity of their cognitive, physical, or psychosocial problems.

Education of the Handicapped Act: Defined handicapped children and allocated funds for them.

Educator: Responsible for assessing educational needs, developing and implementing a plan to meet those needs, and evaluating the desired outcomes and goals accomplished.

Effective care: Services are based on scientific knowledge and provided to all who could benefit and refraining from providing services to those not likely to benefit.

Efferent: To carry away from the central nervous system.

Efficient care: Avoids waste, including waste of equipment, supplies, ideas, and energy.

Elaboration and rehearsal: When the working memory integrates old and new information, transforming it into new and expanded schemas.

Elder abuse: Physical, financial, or emotional mistreatment of older adults.

Elder mistreatment: A more politically correct term for elder abuse; can also encompass physical or emotional neglect of older adults and violation of personal rights.

Emboli: Clots that can travel from the heart or extracranial arteries to the brain.

Embolic stroke: An emboli in the brain travels to and blocks a small blood vessel, causing a stroke.

Emotion-focused behavior: Avoidance efforts are used to divert away from thoughts and feelings caused by stress; these maladaptive behaviors result in poor outcomes.

Emotional intelligence: The ability to perceive emotions, to access and generate emotions so as to assist thought, to understand emotions and emotional knowledge, and to reflectively regulate emotions to promote intellectual growth (Mayer & Salovey).

Emotional lability: Uncontrollable episodes of laughter, crying, or both.

Emphysema: Permanent destruction of the alveoli, the tiny elastic air sacs of the lung, because of irreversible destruction of a protein in the lung called elastin, which is important for maintaining the strength of the alveolar walls. One of the two major diseases of the lung grouped under chronic obstructive pulmonary disease.

Encoding: Places information into permanent storage.

End-stage renal disease (ESRD): Stage 5 chronic kidney disease in which KRT is required to prevent death.

Environment: The conditions, circumstances, and influences surrounding and affecting the development of an organism (Hertzberg).

Environmental factors: Policies, systems, social contexts, and physical barriers or facilitators that affect a person's participation in activities, including work, school, leisure, and community events (U.S. Department of Health and Human Services).

Epidural hematoma: Bleeding between the dura and the skull.

Era of onset: The era in which a person experiences a disability determines how well he or she ages with that disability due to advances in medicines, therapy, and so on.

Erectile dysfunction: The decreased ability of a man to achieve and maintain an erection.

Ethnic culture: Comprised of a particular groups' beliefs, values, and social norms.

Ethnic minority groups: Groups of persons who are outside of the majority; usually includes persons from African American, Hispanic, Pacific-Islander, and Asian Americans.

Ethnohistory: Using historical documents to study ethnographic groups and customs.

Evidence-based practice: The conscientious, explicit, and judicious use of current best evidence to make decisions and integrate clinical expertise and resources for the care of individual patients (DiCenso, Guyatt, & Ciliska).

Existential spirituality: Not directly related to a specific place of worship or an agreed on set of ideals but rather refers to a worldview or perspective in which persons seek purpose in their life and come to understand their life as having meaning and value.

Expertise reversal effect: When a given teaching strategy that works well for a novice is likely to depress learning for a person with more expertise. Instructional strategies, such as directed learning, are used to manage cognitive load for novices, helping the working memory to organize information. Experienced learners do not need this support. It burdens the working memory and depresses learning.

Extracellular matrix (ECM): A primary component of articular cartilage (the other being chondrocytes), it consists of water, collagen, and aggrecan and provides tensile strength yet allows for force disbursement and deformation.

Extraneous load: Mental work that is irrelevant to the learning task at hand. See also **cognitive load theory**.

Extrinsic load: Relevant load imposed by the teaching strategies used to improve learning outcomes. See also **cognitive load theory**.

Exudate: Fluid that collects due to inflammation or injury.

Family-centered care: Because the family is the child's primary source of both financial and emotional support, the family is involved in what they consider important in the treatment and care of their child.

Family Crisis Oriented Personal Evaluation Scale: Measures the degree of faith and religious belief in relation to medical care.

Fee for service (FFS): Provider bills an insurance company for services provided and negotiates payment after the services are provided.

Five stages of death and dying: Phases individuals experience in coping with disability and disease; they are shock, denial, anger, depression, and finally acceptance and adjustment.

Focal injuries: Injuries that occur in a specific area of the brain, such as contusion of brain tissue, intracranial hemorrhage, or hematoma.

Functional assessment measures: Various tests used by the nurse to asses functioning.

Functional capacity: An important factor in deciding who is appropriate for cardiac rehabilitation, with factors such as age, pulmonary status, and other systemic illnesses influencing the decision.

Functional independence measure (FIM): Commonly used throughout the rehabilitation world as a measurement of disability, the FIM is an 18-item instrument graded on a nominal 1 to 7 scale in terms of how much assistance a person needs regarding tasks ranging from ambulation and tub/shower transfers to communication and bladder management.

Functional mobility: Ability to move from one position in space to another and includes bed mobility, transfers, ambulation, wheelchair mobility, stairs, and driving.

Gait belt: Plastic or cloth straps that wrap around the patient's waist, closest to his or her center of gravity, to promote safety if the patient were to lose his or her balance.

Galveston orientation and amnesia test: Valid and reliable 10-question test for determination of the extent of posttraumatic amnesia.

Generativity versus stagnation: The seventh of the eight stages of Erickson's full-life development theory, this stage states that generativity requires that the ego positively identify the needs for giving back to society by raising children; being productive at work; being involved in the community; and guiding, parenting, and monitoring the next generation. Failure to do this can result in stagnation, which is characterized by being unproductive and feeling anger, hurt, and self-absorption.

Geragogy: The art and science of helping older adults learn by compensating for age-related changes in function.

Geriatric rehabilitation nurse: Nurses with knowledge and experience in the principles of rehabilitation and care of the elderly.

Geriatric syndrome: A way to describe how multiple underlying factors that do not fit into discrete disease categories contribute to unique health conditions in older adults.

Glasgow coma scale (GCS): Comprises three tests, eye, verbal, and motor responses, to estimate consciousness.

Goals of independence: Those overriding objectives and goals that move a persons towards self-sufficiency and self-care.

Gordon's functional health patterns: A way to assess an older person's theory-based psychological development by asking questions based on health patterns of health perception–health management, self-image–self-concept, and coping beliefs.

Grief: Sorrowful emotions that occur after a loss.

Grieving: The process of mourning and bereavement that occurs after a loss.

Group dynamics: The interactions, roles, and relationships between members in a group.

Growth: Occurs at different rates throughout childhood and is generally defined as an increase in physical size.

Guardian: Person who has the legal authority and duty to care for another's person or property.

Guardian ad litem: One who usually only appears in court for an incapacitated individual to handle legal matters.

Guardianship: A tool developed to care for those who may not be able to make decisions in a cogent manner in which a guardian is appointed by a court to make those decisions.

Guillain-Barré syndrome (GBS): A process in which the body begins to produce antibodies that attack peptides contained within peripheral myelin, resulting in progressive loss of function; also called acute idiopathic polyneuritis.

Handicap: External or societal limitation on the individual who has the disability.

Headache: Pain occurring in the head.

Health belief model: States that learners are more receptive to changes in behavior if there is belief that the risk is real and personal, that it will negatively affect them, that benefits of action outweigh barriers to action, and if they are confident they can take that action to improve the situation.

Health disparities: Differences between groups of people that affect how frequently a disease occurs in a group, how many people become sick, and how often the disease causes death.

Health literacy: Degree to which individuals have the capacity to obtain, process, and understand basic health information and services needed to make appropriate health decisions (Healthy People 2010).

Health maintenance organizations (HMOs): Created in the late 1980s by healthcare insurance companies as a way to contain costs by implementing such controls as a gatekeeper process, a network of preferred providers, and a capitated payment system.

Health-related quality of life:

Heart failure (HF): Inability of the heart to supply the blood and oxygen needed to the body.

Hemiparesis: Weakness on one side of the body

Hemiplegia: Paralysis on one side of the body

Hemispatial inattention: Inability or reduced ability to attend to one side of space and of the body (also called "neglect").

Hemodialysis: Receiving dialysis via the vascular system.

Hemorrhagic injuries: Injuries resulting from bleeding into a space.

Hemorrhagic stroke: Process by which weakened cerebral blood vessels rupture and spill blood into nearby intracranial spaces or brain tissue.

Heterotopic ossification: Development of bone outside the skeleton.

Hip arthroplasty: Replacement of the hip joint.

Hip precautions: Routine instructions given to patients after a hip replacement to avoid dislocation of a prosthesis and other complications; generally includes avoiding crossing the legs and extreme bending after surgery, as well as weight bearing specifications.

Hippotherapy: A more specific area of therapeutic riding in which the movement of a horse is used as a treatment strategy aimed at improving neuromuscular function.

Holistic care: Comprehensive care that considers all aspects of the person such as psychosocial, biophysical, cultural, and spiritual.

Home health care rehabilitation nurse: An example of a nursing position that denotes both a role and a setting for practice, the rehabilitation nurse in home health care acts as an advocate for clients and their families as they move from the hospital or facility to the home and the community, promoting autonomy and independence.

Homonymous hemianopsia: Hemianopsia refers to one half of the visual field of each eye, and homonymous indicates the loss is on the same side of each eye.

Hospital-acquired condition: A complication or problem acquired in the hospital settings.

Human–animal bond: A mutually beneficial and dynamic relationship between people and animals that is influenced by behaviors that are essential to the health and well-being of both (American Veterinary Medical Association).

Human sexual response: Kaplan (1990), building on early work by Masters and Johnson, identified a triphasic model of human sexual response. The three phases are desire, excitement, and orgasm.

Hydrogenated: In a saturated fat one bond is between the two carbon atoms and one is with a hydrogen atom.

Hyperkinesia: Excess of movement—more movement or more rapid movement than is appropriate or necessary for the situation.

Hypersomnia: An increased sleep propensity with excessive daytime sleepiness and/or increased sleep needs.

Hypogeusia: Decrease in the ability to taste.

Hyposmia: Decrease in the sense of smell.

Illness mode: Pertaining to the sick role or acute sickness.

Immune mediated: Conditions resulting from abnormal activity of the body's immune system.

Impact analysis: The process of assessing the merits or magnitude of a proposed alternative when comparing outcome versus cost.

Impaired physical mobility: Impaired physical ability for independent movement within the environment.

Impairment: Relates to the part that is affected. For example, eyes, ears, legs, or speech may be impaired.

Improvised explosive devices (IEDs): A homemade bomb or device to kill or injure others.

Impulsivity: Initiation of an action apparently without thought and in which the action is unwise, inappropriate, or dangerous.

Incongruence: Not in agreement; disharmonious; inequality

Incontinence: The involuntary leakage of urine.

Incontinence-associated dermatitis: A skin condition moat often seen in the rehabilitation population due to incontinence.

Individual with a disability: A person who has a physical or mental impairment that substantially limits one or more major life activities (Americans with Disabilities Act).

Individuals with Disabilities Act: Provides eligible children with disabilities a free appropriate public education in the least restrictive environment.

Individualism: A perspective that holds high the expectation of self-care and values independence.

Individualized education plan: Developed in collaboration with parents and school personnel to address learning problems.

Inflammatory phase: The first phase in would healing, characterized by edema, erythema, hyperemia, and pain. This phase lasts from 4 to 6 days. See also **proliferative phase** and **maturation phase**.

Informed consent: Voluntary permission given by an individual for a procedure, treatment, or research participation; for informed consent to be valid, the person must be competent to give permission, be informed and have questions answered, and not be coerced to participate.

Informed decision: A choice made when the person making the decision has been fully informed of risks, benefits, and possible outcomes of a particular choice.

Inner strength: The capacity to build self through a developmental process that positively moves an individual through challenging life events.

Innervation: The distribution of nerves across the body.

Inpatient rehabilitation facility: A place where rehabilitation services are provided in a an inpatient setting and where 24 hour per day nursing care is available.

Insight: Understanding the inner nature of things.

Instrumental activities of daily living: Activities that may be more cognitively challenging or require more mobility, such as writing checks, shopping, housekeeping, and many other purposeful life tasks.

Integrity versus despair: The eighth and final stage of Erickson's full-life development theory, this stage is based on the positive outcome of "wisdom." Ego integrity is demonstrated by the older adult's ability to explore life as a retired person who is not identified with an occupation, to contemplate accomplishment, and to feel that life is successful. Despair results if there is feelings of guilt about the past and/or a sense of not accomplishing life goals. Despair can then lead to hopelessness, which is a manifestation of unsuccessful aging.

Intercessory prayer: Interceding with a higher power through prayer to ask that a certain request be granted.

Interdisciplinary model: This model uses a more collaborative approach in that team members work together in goal setting, treatment, decision making, and ongoing problem solving to ensure continuity of care and a more holistic approach. May also be referred to as an interprofessional model.

Interdisciplinary team (IDT): Knowledgeable specialists who work together, share common goals, and collaborate to help clients reach their personal goals.

International Classification of Functioning, Disability, and Health (ICF): Developed by the World Health Organization, the ICF provides a model that represents individual function as a relationship between health conditions and contextual factors. It focuses on components of health and provides a framework for understanding chronic illness and disability as complex products of dynamic interactions between several health domains and personal and environmental contextual factors.

International Normalized Ratio: An internationally recognized lab value that measures clotting time of the blood; used commonly to regulate blood thinners in patients.

Intimacy: A sense of closeness or knowledge of another; can include physical and emotional closeness as well as sexual expressions.

Intracerebral hemorrhage (ICH): Small vessels deep in the brain burst and bleed into brain tissue, putting pressure on tissue and causing vessel tearing, brain shifting, and herniation.

Intracranial pressure: Pressure within the brain.

Intraparenchymal: Into the tissues.

Intraparenchymal hemorrhage: Intraaxial (within brain tissue) hemorrhages that usually result from trauma or hemorrhagic stroke.

Intraventricular: Into the ventricular spaces where cerebrospinal fluid is produced and stored.

Intraventricular hemorrhage: Intraaxial (within brain tissue) hemorrhages that usually result from trauma or hemorrhagic stroke.

Intrinsic load: Amount of mental work required on the part of the learner by the complexity of the content to be learned. See also **cognitive load theory**.

Ischemic stroke: Stroke in which the blood vessel becomes occluded, interrupting blood flow to the brain and depriving neurons and other cells of essential nutrients, including oxygen.

Justice: The duty to treat all fairly or act in a manner such that risks and benefits are distributed equally.

Kidney: Filters materials such as electrolytes, glucose, water, and small proteins from the body.

Kidney transplantation: Operation in which a donor kidney is placed in the iliac fossa and native kidneys are not normally removed. Immunosuppression is required to prevent rejection.

Knee arthroplasty: Replacement of the knee joint.

Knee immobilizer: A long, orthopedic brace that prevents both medial/lateral movement and flexion/extension.

Knowledge deficit: Absence of information or skills for disability management, usually due to the lack of previous experience with the disability.

Lacunar infarction: Result of blood flow blockage to very small arterial vessels. Also called small vessel thrombosis.

Language: Communication of thoughts and feelings through gestures, symbols, signals, or vocal inflection.

Language barrier: Barriers in understanding that occur when the language is different between the healthcare provide and the patient/family.

Leininger's Culture Care Theory: Includes three action modes to guide nurses when making transcultural care decisions or taking actions: (1) culture care preservation and/or maintenance, (2) culture care accommodation and/or negotiation, and (3) culture care repatterning and/or restructuring.

Leininger's Sunrise Enabler: Relates to Leininger's Sunrise model that guide culturally competent care.

Lethargic: Slow in behavior.

Levels of assist: Amount of effort expended by the person assisting the client.

Lewin's Change Theory: A theory that suggests change occurs in three phases: unfreezing, freezing, and refreezing.

Lewy bodies: Abnormal proteins.

Liaison nurse: Completes preadmission evaluations and arranges for admission of clients to services or programs along the rehabilitation continuum of care.

Licensed practical nurse/licensed vocational nurse: Technical nurses, generally with one year of nursing training, that provide daily care for patients or residents.

Life care plan (LCP): A projection of costs of medical and associated care over a person's lifetime used to identify costs in personal injury cases and insurance or reinsurance cases and may be used as tool to guide clients, family's healthcare plans, insurance expenditures, or settlement costs.

Life changes and losses: Changes and losses that naturally occur with chronic illness and disability.

Life span: The continuum from birth to death.

Life thread model: Supports a view of stroke as a time of transition rather than simply of loss. Using the metaphor of "threads" as stories that represent past lives and future plans, after stroke people must manage the life threads, find a "new me," and learn new rules in an unfamiliar world.

Liner: A type of wrap used after amputation that is shaped like the residual limb and is of a thicker material; it is donned with the prosthesis.

Lived experience: Examining a phenomena from an individual's personal experience and meanings of that experience.

Living will: A written document that sets forth the types of medical treatments or life-sustaining measures the patient wants or does not want in the event the person has a terminal illness and is unable to communicate. Also known as a healthcare declaration or healthcare directive.

Locus of control: Social psychology theory describing personal beliefs regarding the amount of control one has over one's own health and the ultimate outcomes from injury or illness.

Loss of consciousness (LOC): A common sign or symptom of TBI seen at the time of or shortly after injury which can last from minutes to hours or days.

Loss of the assumptive world: When chronic illness or disability cause such traumatic loss that assumptions of the world are shattered, along with the ability to believe or assume.

Low-density-lipoprotein (LDL) cholesterol: Harmful cholesterol.

Lower motor neuron (LMN): Spinal cord injuries that represent damage to the motor neurons connecting the spinal cord to muscle fibers and that typically demonstrate an areflexic (flaccid) motor pattern. Injuries at L-1 and below (lumbar and sacral injuries) are considered to be LMN injuries.

Lung cancer: Second most commonly diagnosed cancer in males and females and the most common cause of cancer death.

Maceration: Tissue damage resulting from continued exposure to moisture.

Macronutrients: Major nutrients used by the body: protein, carbohydrates, and fats.

Mainstreaming: Including individuals with disabilities in the education system, accessibility requirements, and equal opportunity hiring requirements.

Malnutrition: Poor health or lack of nutrients needed for good health.

Managed care: A system that influences or controls utilization of services and costs of services (Kovner & Knickman).

Manual muscle test: Used to isolate each muscle group to check the strength of a muscle and graded on a scale of 0 to 5, ranging in the ability to lift the muscle against the pull of gravity or hold against maximal resistance.

Maturation: Internal regulatory process influencing the acquisition of function by organ systems in children and the manifestation of certain skills and abilities.

Maturation phase: Third and final phase of wound healing, this is when the wound matures, scar forms, and the wound contracts or remodels. This phase can last from about 21 days to 2 years. See also **inflammatory phase** and **proliferative phase**.

Mauk model of poststroke recovery: A six-phase model focusing on the process of stroke recovery in which the phases may be experienced simultaneously, in different proportions, and over long periods of time: the six phases are agonizing, fantasizing, realizing, blending, framing, and owning.

Meaning reconstruction: Postulates that symptoms of bereavement and response to loss have individual meaning to people and are central to the grieving process.

Mechanical lifts: Used for clients who are too dependent or heavy to safely transfer manually.

Medicaid: Healthcare coverage for the poor, administered by state governments.

Medical model: The medical model, which drives health and illness practice in the Western world, views disability and chronic illness solely as the consequence of impairment of an individual's body or mind structures and functions.

Medical power of attorney: Allows the patient to choose an individual to make medical decisions on his or her behalf when the patient is unable to do it him- or herself.

Medicare: Healthcare coverage for senior citizens, administered by the federal government.

Medigap: Private insurance that picks up where Medicare drops off, covering the 20% of the incurred expenses.

Mental: One of three domains of disability categorized by the U.S. Census Bureau describing such deficits as learning disability or Alzheimer's disease. See also **communication** and **physical**.

Metabolism: The set of chemical reactions that happen in the body to maintain life and health.

Metacognition: One's knowledge about how one thinks, reasons, and knows.

Micronutrients: Vitamins, minerals, and trace elements needed for growth and maintenance.

Micturition reflex: When the bladder has 250 to 300 mL of urine, the bladder contracts and the internal sphincter relaxes by activating the spinal reflex arc.

Mild brain injury: Injury occurring from direct contact or acceleration/deceleration and having the characteristics of no loss of consciousness or brief loss of consciousness of 20 minutes or less, mild posttraumatic amnesia, and a Glasgow coma scale score > 13.

Mitrofanoff appendicovesicostomy: A surgical procedure that creates a stoma in the lower abdomen using a length of intestine or the appendix.

Mobility: Ability to move spontaneously and independently within the environment and to do purposeful activities such as caring for one's self.

Moderate brain injury: Injury occurring from direct contact or acceleration/deceleration and having the characteristics of loss of consciousness longer than 20 minutes, posttraumatic amnesia, Glasgow coma scale score of 9–12, and cerebral edema and cerebral hemorrhages may be seen on neuroimaging tests.

Modified Ashworth Scale: A scale of 0 to 4 used to evaluate spasticity.

Moment of impact injury: Result of acceleration/deceleration of the brain within the skull at the moment of impact. Further described as **coup/contrecoup** injuries.

Monounsaturated fatty acids (MUFAs): Fatty acids that have a single double bond in the fatty acid chain; found in natural foods (such as red meat, olives, avocados) along with saturated fats.

Motivational interviewing: A strategy that facilitates self-efficacy and self-responsibility by focusing on the client's readiness to change and reflects the transformational model of change by recognizing that change is not a discrete behavioral activity but rather a process that occurs over time.

Motor neuron: Efferent neurons that control the contraction of muscles related to movement.

Multidisciplinary model: Team members usually work independently to accomplish discipline-specific goals and may not directly communicate with all team members regarding care planning. Communication is more vertical than lateral, and team members do not usually participate in team conferences.

Multiple sclerosis (MS): A disorder that evolves from an immune-mediated inflammatory demyelinating process that leads to progressive and degenerative changes in neurological function.

Muscle spasms: A tightening of the muscle in response to firing neurons.

Myasthenia gravis: A condition in which antibodies destroy postsynaptic acetylcholine receptors, leading to a slow decrease in the number of receptors and eventually reaching the point at which acetylcholine can no longer bind effectively.

Myelomeningocele (MMC): Characterized by the protrusion of meninges, spinal cord, and nerve roots through the vertebral cord.

Myocardial infarction (MI): Interruption of blood supply to part of the heart, causing heart cells to die. Also known as a heart attack.

Narrative repair: Because illness and disability have an overwhelming impact, lives and biographies lose continuity, necessitating their repair and reconstruction.

Narrative representations: Regarding chronic illness and disability, personal narratives relate not just the course of illness but rather how lives are altered by illness.

Nasogastric (NG) tube: A tube inserted through the nose into the stomach for feeding, typically used on a short-term basis.

National Pressure Ulcer Advisory Panel (NPUAP): A regulatory agency with specific interest in wound care and healing.

Necrotic (devitalized) tissue: Tissue that is dead.

Neglect syndrome: Deficit in awareness of one side of a space or one side of the body opposite to the lesion.

Neurogenic bladder dysfunction: A variety of lower urinary tract disorders caused by disease or disruption of neurological function.

Neuromuscular disorders: Distinguished by skeletal muscle weakness, these diseases can be hereditary or acquired and can result in abnormalities in one anatomical region or can affect multiple body systems.

Neuroplasticity: Ability of the brain to rearrange the connections between its neurons and alter its behavior in response to new information, sensory stimulation, development, damage, or dysfunction.

Nonessential proteins: Those proteins manufactured by the body.

Nonmalfeasance: The duty to do no harm.

Nonstochastic: Nonrandom.

Norton scale: A systemic risk assessment for pressure ulcer formation. See also **Braden Scale for Predicting Pressure Ulcer Risk.**

Nurse: A healthcare professional who collaborates with the interdisciplinary healthcare team to provide safe and competent care to acute and chronically ill persons, families, or communities.

Nurse–patient communication: Communication between the nurse and the patient.

Nurse-sensitive indicators: Indicators of patient outcomes sensitive to interventions that may be independently initiated and performed by nurses.

Nutrients: Three classes of these are needed by humans: protein, carbohydrates, and fats.

Obtunded: State of reduced consciousness or mental capacity.

Occupational therapist: Assists the patient in gaining maximal function in areas of activities of daily living.

Omnibus Budget Reconciliation Act (OBRA): Passed in 1981, this Act changed the manner in which states received funding for services for children with special healthcare needs by creating Maternal and Child Health Services block grants and consolidating programs.

One Health: Worldwide strategy for expanding interdisciplinary collaborations and communications in all aspects of health care for humans and animals.

Operation Enduring Freedom (OEF): Conflicts in the Middle East.

Operation Iraqi Freedom (OIF): Conflicts in the Middle East.

Optimism: Positive thinking; cheerfulness.

Outcome measures: Quality measures that consider the results of care, such as morbidity and mortality resulting from a disease.

Outcomes management: Assessment of data and identification of preferred interventions that lead to the desired clinical outcome.

Outcomes measurement: Evaluation of the results of programs, processes, or interventions and their comparison with the intended results.

Outcomes research: Seeks to understand the results of specific healthcare practices and interventions.

Overflow incontinence: Occurs when the bladder is overdistended with underactive or acontractile detrusor muscle activity.

Palliative care: Care focusing on comfort versus curative medicine for persons with incurable illnesses.

Paralympic: The equivalent of Olympic but for persons with (especially physical) disabilities.

Paraplegia: Paralysis involving two limbs.

Parasympathetic: The part of the Autonomic Nervous System that returns the body to homeostasis, or rest and relaxation.

Parkinson's disease: Pathogenic process behind Parkinson's disease is not well understood but is characterized by the accumulation of abnormal proteins known as Lewy bodies within neurons. Disease is characterized by muscle rigidity and tremor.

Passive range of motion: Extent of movement within a given joint when a therapist moves the joint while the client is relaxed.

Patient Self-Determination Act: Enacted in 1990, it requires all medical facilities that accept Medicare or Medicaid funding to provide counseling for patients on advance directives.

Pediatric rehabilitation: Rehabilitation of children.

Pediatric rehabilitation nurse: An RN who must possess both rehabilitation specialty and generalist pediatric skills.

Peer groups: A group comprised of those with similar experiences and interests, and usually of similar age.

Peer visitor: An amputee who has had training by the Amputee Coalition of America in peer support.

People with disabilities: People identified as having an activity limitation or who use assistance or who perceive themselves as having a disability (U.S. Department of Health and Human Services).

Perceived Support From God Scale: Measures support derived from a dynamic, communicative exchange between individuals and God.

Percutaneous endoscopic gastrostomy (PEG) tube: Inserted directly into the stomach, this tube is the preferred type for long-term enteral nutrition.

Percutaneous endoscopic jejunostomy tube: Surgically placed through a stab wound from the outside directly into the jejunum for long-term nutrition support, for emptying of the stomach after surgery, or if an NG tube is not tolerated.

Peritoneal dialysis: Introducing 2 to 3 liters of a sterile dextrose-containing solution (dialysate) into the peritoneal cavity.

Perseveration: The inability, or simply the difficulty, of switching attention from one idea or response to another.

Personal tragedy model: Disadvantage and reduced quality of life to the point where disability is understood as an individual and family tragedy. Through this lens, chronic illness and disability are viewed as medical issues and as personal problems. People are "victims" of their impairments and are "confined by" and "suffering from" their conditions.

Pet visitation programs: Programs designed to provide companionship, sensory stimulation, and an opportunity for reminiscence.

Phantom limb pain: Feeling of pain in a limb, or portion of a limb, that is no longer there.

Phenomenological approaches: Frameworks describing illness and disability as being experienced primarily as disruptions to the lived body rather than as bodily impairments; chronic illness and disability redefine individuals' relationships to their worlds.

Physiatrists: Doctor of physical medicine and rehabilitation.

Physical: One of three domains of disability categorized by the U.S. Census Bureau describing such deficits as spinal cord injury, arthritis, or stroke. See also **communication** and **mental**.

Physical Medicine and Rehabilitation: A new field of medicine that focuses on the restoration of patient capabilities.

Physical therapist: Works with patients to improve gross motor skills.

PLISSIT model: The most widely cited model for practitioners to use when addressing sexual concerns of patients and their partners. The PLISSIT acronym stands for the levels of intervention by members of the rehab team, which include **P**ermission (encouraging patients and their partners to voice sexual concerns), **L**imited **I**nformation (providing information for overcoming sexual problems by giving patients and their partners pamphlets, video resources, and information about helpful Websites), **S**pecific **S**uggestions (treatments for vaginal dryness, erectile dysfunction, and/or vaginal dryness, adopting comfortable positions for intercourse, methods of managing spasticity during intercourse), and **I**ntensive **T**herapy (marital or sex therapy, which requires special training).

Poikilothermic: Body temperature varies with the temperature of their environment.

Point of service: A type of employer-funded insurance that allows the insured to receive health care at providers outside the network, albeit with higher copays and deductibles.

Polysaccharides: Complex carbohydrates.

Polytrauma: Two or more injuries to physical regions or organ systems, one of which may be life threatening, resulting in physical, cognitive, psychological, or psychosocial impairments and functional disability (Veterans Administration).

Polytrauma rehabilitation center: A rehabilitation facility specializing in care of those with multiple traumatic injuries such as TBI, burns, and amputation, often occurring after blast injuries acquired during wartime.

Polytrauma–TBI system of care: Developed by the VHA, this system of care provides specialized rehabilitation care for veterans and service members with polytrauma and TBI.

Polytrauma triad: A triad of symptoms: chronic pain, posttraumatic stress disorder, and postconcussive syndrome.

Polyunsaturated fatty acids (PUFAs): Fatty acids that contain more than one double bond; found in oils such as vegetable, soy, and sunflower.

Postconcussion syndrome: Formerly called "concussion," in this syndrome symptoms can go unrecognized until they begin to interfere with activities of daily living; headache is the cardinal symptom.

Post-polio syndrome (PPS): After the acute illness of polio has passed, a significant number of individuals develop new symptoms such as fatigue, weakness, pain, and atrophy.

Poststroke depression (PSD): Depression after stroke.

Posttraumatic amnesia: A common sign and symptom of TBI seen at the time of or shortly after injury which lasts for varied lengths of time.

Posttraumatic stress disorder (PTSD): A severe anxiety disorder that can develop after exposure to any event that results in psychological trauma, such as those events involved in war.

Pragmatics: Regarding social behavior, the ability to act in ways that are appropriate and socially acceptable.

Prealbumin: A serum blood test/value used to diagnose malnutrition or risk of malnutrition.

Predialysis: Stage 4 chronic kidney disease.

Preferred provider organization: The most liberal form of healthcare insurance, it allows individuals to freely choose their providers. Financial incentives and lower deductibles and copays to receive care within a selected network of providers still remain.

Prehension: Ability to use one or more digits or replacement digits against an opposing thumb or replacement thumb.

Presbycusis: Age-related hearing loss.

Presbyopia: Inability to focus on near objects.

Pressure relief: Moving the body to ensure the weight of the person's body is now on a completely different location to give the area that was just receiving pressure a chance to recover.

Pressure ulcer: Caused by unrelieved pressure on soft tissue between bony prominences and the sitting or lying surface.

Prevention: Strategies used to stop a disease or injury from arising in the first place.

Primary appraisal: The initial personal judgment regarding the relevance to one's life of the chronic illness or disability.

Primary injuries: Injury that occurs from the initial insult.

Prior level of function: The abilities and activity level of a person prior to injury or illness.

Problem-focused behavior: Adaptation is used and results in improved outcomes.

Process measures: Quality measures that track performance of a particular action.

Professional geriatric care manager: One who guides and provides resource for families of older adults and others with chronic needs and issues related to aging.

Professional subculture: A group of people who are part of a larger subculture but whom identify themselves with a smaller group who are members of a profession that share common values and beliefs.

Proliferative phase: The second phase in wound healing, in which the defect is filled and wound edges begin to contract. This phase lasts generally from 4 to 24 days or longer. See also **inflammatory phase** and **maturation phase**.

Proning: A position used to prevent hip flexure contractures in which clients are urged to prone (lie on their stomach).

Proprioception: Knowledge of the position of limb and joint in space.

Proprioceptive neuromuscular facilitation: A technique originally developed in the 1940s for polio patients and based on neurophysiological mechanisms; specific objectives are increasing range of motion, improving voluntary movement, and improving gait training skills.

Prospective payment system (PPS): A method of paying based on foreseen costs rather than billed costs.

Psychiatric advance directive: A legal document used to declare in advance one's desires regarding the psychiatric or mental health treatment they wish to receive. Also referred to as a declaration for mental health treatment.

Psychogenic erections: Erections that result when messages are passed down the spinal cord from the brain to the sacral area.

Psychologist: A health professional who studies the mind and assists patients and clients to deal with life problems; often focuses on behavior modification and counseling.

Ptosis: Drooping eyelids.

Pulmonary embolism (PE): A blood clot that has traveled from another part of the body to the lungs.

Quality measure: Quantification of the degree to which a desired healthcare process or outcome is achieved or the extent that a desirable structure to support healthcare delivery is in place (Institute of Medicine).

Quality of life: The term used to collectively capture a person's sense of life satisfaction, enjoyment, and well-being.

Rancho Los Amigos scale of cognitive recovery: An evaluation tool created by the Rancho Los Amigos National Rehabilitation Center that describes stages of recovery typically seen after a brain injury.

Reasonable accommodation: A modification or change made to allow a qualified disabled person to participate in his/her job functions; part of a Federal law to prohibit discrimination against persons with disability in the workplace.

Receptor: A structure that receives information.

Reconfiguring the future: Transition to well-being is depicted as a function of meaning reconstruction and the reconfiguration of new life plots.

Reflexic: Relating to working reflexes and associated activity.

Reflexogenic erections: Erections that result from direct stimulation of the genital area.

Rehabilitation: A process to restore mental and/or physical abilities lost to injury or disease, in order to function in a normal or near-normal way (National Cancer Institute).

Rehabilitation delivery system: The way rehabilitation care is organized and provided.

Religious spirituality: A relationship with God or a higher power typically seen among individuals who attend organized services within a community.

Researcher: Develops and maintains the knowledge base for nurses who care for individuals/families and groups with physical disability and chronic illness.

Resilience: The ability to overcome or bounce back after injury or insult.

Resource utilization groups: Provides a fixed payment based on anticipated costs for skilled services.

Retrieval: Getting schema from long-term memory and placing it back into working memory for utilization and further learning.

Rheumatoid arthritis: A systemic autoimmune disease that affects the synovial joints.

Rigid dressing: A hard plastic device that serves to protect the freshly sutured limb while maintaining knee extension.

Risk: The probability of something happening; in healthcare, usually risk refers to the potential for hazard, injury, or other negative outcome.

Roy's Adaptation Model: Model set forth by Sister Callista Roy that demonstrates how persons adapt to stress.

Safe care: Service that avoids injuries to patients from the care that is intended to help.

Safe patient handling: Protocols designed to decrease injury to workers, increase safety and comfort for patients, decrease chance for litigation related to injuries, decrease lost work and wages due to injury, and decrease workers' compensation claims.

Schema: Meaningful relationships and patterns found in conceptual and factual knowledge.

Scotomas: Blind spots in the visual field.

Secondary appraisal: Evaluation by the individual of the adequacy of his or her abilities and resources to manage the chronic illness or disability.

Secondary injuries: Result from the swelling and homeostatic responses to the initial brain injury.

Self-care: A deliberate, learned act of provided care for oneself.

Self-care deficit: Decreased ability to perform activities of daily living.

Self-efficacy: The confidence that one can perform the behaviors needed to reach one's goals.

Senescence: Process by which a cell looses its ability to divide, grow, and function, which ultimately ends in cell death.

Severe brain injury: Injury involving loss of consciousness > 6 hours, prolonged posttraumatic amnesia, and Glasgow coma scale score < 8. There can be intracranial or subdural hemorrhage, tearing and shearing of brain tissue, or penetration of brain tissue by an object or projectile, with deficits seen on neuroimaging tests.

Sexuality: How people express themselves as sexual beings.

Shared primary language: A common language shared with others.

Shifting perspectives model: As an illness experience progresses and contexts change, individuals' perspectives shift.

Shoulder arthroplasty: Replacement of the shoulder joint.

Shoulder subluxation: A partial or incomplete dislocation due to changes in the anatomy of the shoulder joint.

Shrinker: A type of wrap used after amputation on the residual limb to control edema and reshape the limb.

Skilled nursing facility (SNF): An institution that provides skilled nursing care and rehabilitation services.

Skin integrity: The intactness and condition of the skin.

Sleep disordered breathing (SDB): A group of disorders characterized by abnormal respirations or pauses in breathing.

Sleep–wake disorders (SWDs): A group of disorders characterized by fragmented or interrupted sleep.

Social construction model: Emphasizes the central roles played by language, social interaction, values and beliefs, power relationships, and culture in the construction of meaning in human contexts.

Social model: Emphasizes the collective, structural, and social origins of disability, such as discrimination, oppression, and barriers to participation, rather than the individual, personal, and medical origins.

Social Security Act: Signed into law in 1935, as outlined in the Act, states received federal dollars for the purpose of promoting, improving, and developing maternal–child health services, including services for crippled children.

Social worker: Focuses on psychosocial support; prepares patients and families for discharge; identifies supportive services and resources needed after discharge; and links patient and family to community physicians, services, home health care, long-term care facilities, and medical equipment providers.

Societal changes: Modifications or alterations that occur at the societal level.

Somatosensation: Bodily sensation and perception.

Somnolent: Sleepy.

Spasticity: Velocity-dependent increase in tonic stretch reflexes (muscle tone) in resistance to muscle stretch that develops after an upper motor neuron injury within the central nervous system.

Speech-language pathologist (SLP): Evaluates and treats cognition, communication, swallowing disorders, and hearing deficits.

Sphincter: Muscles that control excretion of the urine from the bladder through the urethra.

Spina bifida: A neuroembryological defect due to failure of the neural tube to fuse around the 28th day of gestation. Also called spinal dysraphism.

Spinal cord injury: Damage to the spinal cord.

Spinal Cord Lesion Coping Strategies Questionnaire: Measures specific coping mechanisms of acceptance, fighting spirit, and social reliance used by respondents.

Spinal Cord Lesion Emotional Wellbeing Questionnaire: Measures emotional consequences to the spinal cord injury and evaluates the positive emotional outcomes of personal growth and the negative outcomes of helplessness and intrusion.

Spinal shock: Observed in the initial phases of spinal cord injury and defined as the absence of spinal reflex activity below the level of the injury.

Spiritual blessing: The belief in certain cultures that a child with a developmental disability or certain impairments has god-like qualities and is therefore a blessing.

Spiritual care: Mindful presence expressed in a truly caring manner.

Spiritual distress: When one is searching for the meaning or purpose behind the events of life.

Spirituality: A sense of making meaning through connectedness to a power greater than oneself, to others and the environment, and within oneself.

Staff animal: These animals accompany their owner (a staff member) on part or all of a shift and go home with the staff member at the end of the day; they are used in facilities that would like an animal present during the day but cannot manage a live-in animal.

Stage models: A series of stages people need to pass through to cope and adjust adequately to the changes and losses associated with chronic illness and disability.

Stakeholder: A person with a vested interest in an organization, company, or project.

State children's health insurance program (SCHIP):

Static balance: Balance while being still.

Stochastic: Random.

Stress incontinence: Leakage of urine with coughing, sneezing, laughing, or other activity.

Stroke: A nontraumatic brain injury caused by disruption in blood flow to part of the brain from either occlusion of a blood vessel (ischemic stroke) or rupture of a blood vessel (hemorrhagic stroke). Also known as cerebrovascular accident or brain attack.

Stroke syndromes: A collection of symptoms that, when found together, are characteristic of stroke.

Structure measures: Quality measures that track whether a particular mechanism or system is in place.

Stuporous: State of reduced consciousness.

Subacute rehabilitation: For those patients who do not meet criteria for acute rehabilitation but nevertheless need a 24-hour care rehabilitation environment. Patient placement into subacute rehabilitation is determined by an acute functional disability, a recent 3-day acute care hospitalization, a qualifying diagnosis, medical or surgical condition that limits the stamina required for participation in more intensive rehabilitation, and the ability to participate in at least 1 hour of therapy per day.

Subarachnoid hemorrhage: Bleeding into the subarachnoid space caused by rupture of a vessel in the protective lining of the brain.

Subculture: A group of people who are part of a larger culture, but who separate themselves from the larger culture because of shared or common beliefs and values.

Subdural hematoma: Bleeding between the dura and arachnoid membranes.

Suprapubic triggers: Prompts used to stimulate spontaneous voiding via the intact reflex arc, such as tapping over the pubic area, squeezing the glans penis, stroking the thigh, pulling the pubic hair, or running water over the pubic area.

Synovial joint: A joint that allows for movement.

Synovial membrane: Located on the inner surface of the joint capsule, which encloses the synovial capsule, and covers any ligaments or tendons that pass through the joint.

Syrinx: Dilation of the fluid channel in the center of the spinal cord that causes deterioration of function, scoliosis, weakness of the upper extremities, or spasticity.

Tax Equity and Fiscal Responsibility Act (TEFRA): With the advent of PPS in the inpatient hospitals in 1983 a system for payment for acute inpatient rehabilitation was needed. Under TEFRA inpatient rehabilitation units and hospitals were excluded from the diagnosis-related group system and paid at a per diem rate with a maximum ceiling.

Team competence: Derives from the ability of multiple disciplines to behave as a single system.

Terminally ill: A condition in which the person's illness has no cure and will end his or her life.

Tetraplegia: Formerly referred to as quadriplegia, paralysis involving four limbs.

Therapeutic use of self: Delivering spiritual care by engaging oneself in the interaction, being aware that spiritual care must be patient led, not nurse directed.

Thompson Model of Care Congruence: Illustrates how the care process should proceed and, using the Leininger enablers, allows for a mechanism to work through differences.

Thrombotic stroke: Fatty deposits, or plaques, clog and gradually block blood flow to the brain, causing a stroke.

Thrombus: Blood clot that forms in an area previously damaged by atherosclerosis.

Total joint replacement: Removal of a damaged joint that is then replaced with an artificial joint.

Transcultural care decisions and actions: Care decisions and actions that take into account a patient's culture.

Transfemoral: Above the knee.

Transfer: The ability to move one's body from one position in space to another, such as going from the wheelchair to the bed, toilet, or tub bench.

Transhumeral: Classification when 50% to 90% of the humerus remains after amputation.

Transient ischemic attack: Sudden loss of neurological function with complete recovery usually within 24 hours.

Transition in chronic illness: Moving from one place to another in the acute-chronic illness continuum towards long-term care.

Transition theory: Emphasizes the movement from one state or stage to another or changing into something different when adapting to chronic illness and disability.

Transradial: Below the elbow.

Transtibial: Below the knee.

Transurethral sphincterotomy: A procedure used to make an incision in the urinary sphincter in which the goal is to decrease the pressure in the bladder and allow it to empty more completely.

Traumatic brain injury (TBI): A complex injury that occurs when there is disruption of brain tissue resulting from an impact to the head in which the head hits, is hit by, or is penetrated by an object. Also called **acquired brain injury**.

Tremor: Repetitive often regular oscillatory movements.

Triglyceride: Chemical name for fats in the body or in food. It consists of three fatty acids and a glycerol molecule.

Uninhibited bladder: Persons with this kind of bladder have a lesion or interruption somewhere along the cortical regulatory tract.

Union of Physically Impaired Against Segregation: Group that arose as part of the disability movement that focused attention on the environmental barriers and social oppression of individuals with disability. Their goal is to replace segregated facilities with opportunities for people with impairments to participate fully in society, to live independently, to undertake productive work, and to have full control over their lives.

Upper motor neuron (UMN): Spinal cord injuries that represent damage to the motor pathways between the cerebral cortex and the conus medullaris and that typically demonstrate a reflexic (spastic) motor pattern. Injuries sustained at T-11 to L-1 and above (cervical and thoracic injuries) are considered to be UMN injuries.

Urethra: Extending from the bladder to the outside of the body, the way in which urine exits the bladder.

Urge incontinence: Sudden and strong sensation to void without the ability to delay urination.

Vaginal dryness: A condition commonly associated with advanced age in females; lack of normal lubrication of the vagina that can cause discomfort during sexual intercourse.

Veracity: The duty to be truthful and provide the person served with adequate information necessary to make an informed decision.

Veterans Health Administration (VHA): An organization created to promote and organize the care of military veterans.

Viagra (sildenafil): A medication used to help achieve and maintain penile erection.

Videofluoroscopic swallow study: Use of radiological techniques to visualize the swallowing process; most often used to diagnose dysphagia in those with swallowing difficulties; sometimes called a barium swallow.

Wars of disabilities: Our wars of today in Iraq and Afghanistan in which wounded soldiers have higher survival rates and the need for rehabilitation services is increased.

Weight bearing as tolerated: The patient is permitted to bear as much or little weight as he/she can comfortably tolerate.

Well-being: State of being happy, healthy, or prosperous.

Wheelchair sports teams: Groups of athletes who play sports in wheelchairs.

Working memory: The part of the brain that provides temporary storage and manipulation of information during complex cognitive tasks.

Wound healing: The process by which an injury to the skin or underlying tissues repairs itself.

Youth with special healthcare needs: Older children who have or are at increased risk for a chronic physical, developmental, behavioral, or emotional conditions and who also require health and related services of a type or amount beyond that required by older children generally.

Zoonotic disease: Any disease that is transmissible from animals to humans.

INDEX

Boxes, figures, and tables are indicated with b, f, and t following the page number.

A

AAA (animal-assisted activities), 460–462
AACN (American Association of Colleges of Nursing), 472
AAT. *See* Animal-assisted therapy
Abilities, emphasizing, 2, 2*t*, 7
Absorption of nutrients, 85
Abuse and neglect. *See also* Discrimination
  by caregivers, 282
  drug. *See* Substance abuse
  elder, 453–455, 454–455*t*, 455*b*
  in institutions, 32, 171
  sexual, 163–164, 171
Academic settings, 74–77
Academy of Nurse Life Care Planners, 472
Acceptance and Action Questionnaire, 203
Acceptance and adaptation, 39, 202–203
Accessibility of resources/opportunities
  environmental barriers to, 17
  healthcare access, 414, 415
  in ICF model, 34
  legal and ethical issues and, 396–398, 397*t*
  older adults and issues of, 19
  settings for care and, 24
Accidents. *See* Trauma
Acetylcholine, 345–346, 349
Ace wrapping, 302
ACM (Arnold-Chiari II malformation), 423–424
Acquired brain injury. *See* Traumatic brain injury
Activation of prior knowledge (in learning), 179–180, 180*f*
Active assistive range of motion, 290
Active range of motion, 137, 290–291
Activism, defined, 381. *See also* Advocacy
Activities of Daily Living (ADLs). *See also* Mobility; Self-care;
   specific disabilities or diseases
  adaptive equipment and, 144
  definition of disability and, 14–15, 15*t*
  mobility/function and, 136, 145
Activity-based restorative therapies, 282
Activity intolerance diagnosis, 145
Activity limitations. *See also* Activities of Daily Living
  defined, 14
  in dimensions of adaptability, 42
  in ICF model, 34–35, 35*f*
  skin integrity and, 102, 103*t*, 104, 108*t*
Acute pain, 116–117
Acute rehabilitation
  for neurological disorders, 354
  payment systems and, 409–410
  for SCI, 271, 271*f*
  settings of, 23
ADA. *See* Americans with Disabilities Act

Adaptation. *See also* Coping; *specific disabilities/diseases*
  amputation and, 301, 312–314. *See also* Prosthetics
  education of clients and, 177–178
  equipment for. *See* Equipment
  as goal of rehabilitation, 2, 2*t*
  models of, 35, 43–44, 44*f*, 44*t*, 202
  recovery and, 2, 6–7, 43
  theories of, 18, 36–43, 42*f*, 202
Adaptive equipment. *See* Equipment
ADLs. *See* Activities of Daily Living
Administrative nursing roles, 72–74
Adolescent Coping Scale, 203
Adolescents. *See* Pediatric rehabilitation
Adult learning theory, 184, 184*b*
Advance directives, 390, 391–394, 392*b*, 449, 453. *See also*
   Terminal illness
Advanced practice registered nurses (APRNs), 55, 57*t*, 69, 77–80
Advocacy. *See also* Legal issues
  activism and, 381
  ARN, 6, 6*b*
  community education and prevention, 196
  coping strategies and, 208
  defined, 64
  ethical issues and, 403
  health promotion for disabled and, 16–17
  by managers/administrators, 73
  by nurse educators, 75
  nurse's roles in, 64–69, 71, 78–79
  by researchers, 77
AF (atrial fibrillation), 236–237
Affect
  affective domain, 196
  defined, 150*b*, 157
  disorders in TBI, 258
Afferent neurons, 349
African American populations
  amputation in, 301
  cardiac disease in, 336
  CKD in, 361
  coping strategies, 37, 203, 205
  health disparities and, 378
  SCI in, 270
  stroke in, 216, 217
Age-related issues. *See also* Gerontological rehabilitation;
   Pediatric rehabilitation
  in CF, 341
  child development, 419–420
  in COPD, 340
  in degenerative neurological disorders, 355
  nursing roles and, 67
  nutrition and, 97

Age-related issues (*cont.*)
in osteoarthritis, 285
in SCI, 282
sexuality and, 163–164, 164*t*
skin integrity and, 102, 103*t*
theories of aging, 438–441, 439*b*
Agitation and brain injury, 150*b*, 156, 156*t*
Agnosia, 226–227, 227*t*
Agriculture Department Food Guide Pyramid, 98
AHA. *See* American Heart Association
Airway management. *See* Pulmonary disease/complications
Albumin, 88–89, 89*b*
Alcohol consumption
avascular necrosis and, 285
cancer and, 364
in chronic disease risk, 17, 179
ICH and, 217
Native Americans and, 411
older adult health and, 19
SDB and, 238
sexual dysfunction and, 162, 167
stroke and, 217, 218*t*
Alertness. *See* Consciousness
Allergies. *See* Asthma; Latex allergy and spina bifida
Allodynia, 279
ALS. *See* Amyotrophic lateral sclerosis
Alteration in comfort, 313–314
Alternative medicine. *See* Complementary and alternative
medicine
Alzheimer's disease, 124, 131, 131*t*. *See also* Delirium/dementia
Amantadine (Symmetrel), 354, 354*t*
Ambiguous loss, 321
Ambulation. *See* Mobility
Ambulatory aids, 301
American Academy of Nurse Practitioners, 78, 79, 82
American Academy of Physical Medicine and Rehabilitation,
4, 4*t*
American Association of Colleges of Nursing (AACN), 472
American Association of Critical Care Nurses, 73
American Association of Nurse Life Care Planners, 471–472
American Board of Physical Medicine and Rehabilitation, 4, 5*t*
American Geriatrics Society, 70, 70*b*, 82
American Heart Association (AHA), 218, 221, 332, 334, 334*b*,
441
American Indians. *See* Native Americans
American Medical Directors Association of long-term care
facilities, 171
American Nurses Association (ANA)
ARN and, 5, 9
Code of Ethics, 210, 387–388, 388*t*
Magnet Recognition Program, 64, 73
nursing roles and, 70, 70*b*, 71, 82
safe lift protocols, 143
American Nurses Credentialing Center (ANCC), 68, 69, 82, 338
American Organization of Nurse Executives (AONE), 73
American Physical Therapy Association, 143
American Red Cross Institute for Crippled and Disabled Men,
3, 4*t*

American Society for Parenteral and Enteral Nutrition
(ASPEN), 98
American Spinal Cord Injury Association (ASIA) Impairment
Scale, 271, 285–286
American Stroke Association (ASA), 218, 221, 245*t*, 246
Americans with Disabilities Act (ADA 1990)
activism and, 381
disability definition, 14–15
history and description of, 4, 5*t*, 17, 419
right to life issues and, 397*t*, 398
Amino acids, 84–85
Amish populations and culture care, 376, 376*b*
Amnesia, 258, 259, 262, 322. *See also* Memory
Amputation, 296–316
causes, 297, 297*t*
in children, 297, 298
complications and comorbidities, 303
defined, 296
diagnoses, outcomes, and interventions, 311–314, 313*b*
education of clients on, 301, 309–313, 310–311*t*, 313–314*b*
IDT roles in, 300–303, 300*t*, 302*f*
incidence and statistics, 297–298, 297*b*
in older adults, 297, 298
pain management, 304, 313–314
polytrauma and, 299, 319, 319*t*, 324
prevention, 298
prosthetics and, 300*t*, 301, 303, 303*t*, 305–309, 305–309*f*
psychological aspects of, 299–300
reassessment, 304–305
risk factors, 298
Amyotrophic lateral sclerosis (ALS), 344, 345*t*, 349, 351, 352
ANA. *See* American Nurses Association
Anabolism, 85
Analgesics, 133, 133*t*, 279, 304
Anatomy and physiology. *See also* Pathophysiology
bowel, 130
neuroanatomy and function, 148–149
of SCI, 270–271, 270*f*
skin, 101–104, 102–103*f*, 103*t*
speech, 152
traumatic brain injury, 256, 256*f*, 257*t*
urinary tract, 121–122, 122*f*
ANCC. *See* American Nurses Credentialing Center
Andragogy, 184, 184*b*
Anergia, 150*b*, 156
Anesthetics, 240, 241*t*
Aneurysm, 217
Anger
prevention and detection of, 208–209
in stages of adaptation, 202
Angina pectoris, 332–333
Angiotensin-converting enzyme inhibitors, 334, 335*t*, 361
Angiotensin II receptor blockers, 334, 335*t*, 361
Animal-assisted activities (AAA), 460–462
Animal-assisted therapy (AAT), 460–470
guidelines for, 464*b*, 465–469, 466–468*t*, 469*b*
human-animal bond, 463–465, 463*f*, 464*b*, 465*t*
poststroke, 248

types of, 460–463, 461–462f
Anomic aphasia, 229, 230t
Anorexia nervosa, 87, 373. *See also* Eating disorders
Anosagnosia, 155
Anterior cord syndrome, 273–274
Antibiotic treatment for skin wounds, 110, 114, 115–116t
Antibodies in autoimmune disorders, 345–346
Anticholinergic medications
    bladder management and, 127, 425
    constipation and, 133, 133t
    for pulmonary disease, 339
    sexual dysfunction and, 167, 168t
    for tremor, 357
Anticoagulants, 217, 236, 292, 334, 335t
Anticonvulsives. *See also* Antiepileptics
    amputation and, 304
    constipation and, 133, 133t
    for CPSP, 240, 241t
    for SCI pain, 279
    sexual dysfunction and, 167, 168t
    for spasticity, 353, 353t
    in TBI, 263
Antidepressants
    amputation and, 304
    constipation and, 133, 133t
    CPSP and, 240, 241t
    PSD and, 233–234, 234t
    for SCI pain, 279
    sexual dysfunction and, 167, 168t
    sleep disorders and, 239, 239t
Antiepileptics, 138, 139, 239–240, 240t, 262. *See also* Anticonvulsives
Antihypertensives, 167, 168t
Anti-inflammatory medications, 278, 279
Antiparkinsonians, 133, 133t
Antiplatelets, 334, 335t
Antiseizure medications. *See* Antiepileptics
Antiviral medications, 354, 354t
Anxiety. *See also* Psychological well-being
    as mood state, 157
    in older adults, 448
    prevention and detection of, 208–209
    SCI and, 280
    sexuality issues and, 161
    in stages of adaptation, 202
    in TBI, 258, 259
AONE (American Organization of Nurse Executives), 73
Aphasias, 148–149, 150b, 152, 153t, 170–171, 171b, 229, 230t, 242–243. *See also* Speech and language impairments
Appraisal and adaptation, 35–38, 38b, 42
Approach coping strategy, 37–38
Apraxia
    of speech, 149, 150b, 152, 231
    stroke and, 226, 226t, 229, 231
APRNs. *See* Advanced practice registered nurses
Architectural Barriers Act (1968), 4, 5t
Areflexic bladder, 125, 125f, 127, 129, 276
Areflexic bowel, 131t, 132, 274–275

Army Wounded Warrior Program, 328. *See also* Veterans and war
ARN. *See* Association of Rehabilitation Nurses
ARN-Competency Assessment Test (CAT), 10–11, 10t, 65, 67, 68, 146
Arnold-Chiari II malformation (ACM), 423–424
Arrhythmias, 236–237
Arteriolar pressure and skin integrity, 102, 103t
Arteriovenous malformation, 217
Arthritis, 165–166t, 168, 288–289, 378, 379t
Arthritis Self-Management Program, 183
Arthroplasty, 286–287
Articular cartilage, 284
ASA. *See* American Stroke Association
ASIA Impairment Scale, 267, 285–286
Asian populations
    cardiac disease in, 332
    coping strategies, 37
ASPEN (American Society for Parenteral and Enteral Nutrition), 98
Aspiration
    pneumonia, 237
    with tube feeding, 94
Assessment. *See also* Diagnoses; Outcome evaluation (management, measurement, research)
    amputation, 301, 304–305
    bladder management, 125, 126t
    bowel management, 132, 274
    cancer, 364–365, 365t
    CKD, 361–362
    cognitive, 228–229, 228t, 229f, 259–262, 259–262t, 260b, 264t
    COPD, 340–341
    coping strategies, 203–204
    CP, 421–422
    depression, 233, 447–448
    dysphagia, 92–93, 237
    of elder abuse, 454, 455t
    joint replacement, 292
    language and communication, 231–232
    learning needs/abilities, 185–186, 190, 190t, 192–193
    mobility, 137–138, 137–138t, 141f
    neurological disorders, 352–353
    nutritional, 88–89, 89b, 92
    payment systems and, 403
    of SCI, 271, 274, 285–286
    skin integrity, 104–107, 106–107t
    spasticity, 222, 222b
    spiritual, 206–207
    TBI, 259–262, 259–264t, 260b, 262b, 323, 323t
    terminal illness, 368
Assistance animals, 462. *See also* Animal-assisted therapy
Assistive devices. *See* Equipment
Assist levels, 137, 137t
Association of Rehabilitation Nurses (ARN)
    certification/competencies, 5–6, 5t, 10–11, 10t, 64, 65. *See also* Certified rehabilitation registered nurse (CRRN) credential
    definitions of rehabilitation nursing, 9–10, 9t

Association of Rehabilitation Nurses (ARN) (*cont.*)
   history of, 5–6, 5*t*
   quality care promotion, 17
   resources available through, 5–6, 5–6*b*, 20*b*, 146, 169, 169*t*
   role descriptions. *See* Nursing roles
   safe lift protocols, 143
   settings for practice, 22, 22*t*
Assumptive world theory, 36, 41, 44, 44*f*
Asthma, 339*t*, 341
Ataxia. *See also* Gait
   neurological disorders and, 347, 350, 352, 355*t*
   stroke and, 221
Atherogenesis/atherosclerosis. *See* Cardiovascular problems;
      Stroke
Atrial fibrillation (AF), 236–237
Atrophic vaginitis/urethritis, 123, 124*t*
Atrophy in neurological disorders, 349, 350, 352
Attention, 149, 150*b*, 179, 180*f*, 227, 228. *See also* Consciousness;
      Memory
Attention process training, 243
Attitudes. *See* Beliefs
Auditory impairment. *See also* Speech and language
      impairments
   aging and, 442
   agnosia and, 226–227, 227*t*
   culture and, 381–382
   polytrauma and, 319, 319*t*, 325
Autobiographical memory, 154
Autoimmune disorders, 344–347, 350–351, 353. *See also specific
      disorders*
Autolytic debridement, 109–110
Automated peritoneal dialysis, 361
Autonomic dysreflexia, 129–130, 130*b*, 130*t*, 274, 278
Autonomous bladder/bowel. *See* Areflexic bladder; Areflexic
      bowel
Autonomy principle, 24, 371, 374, 391. *See also* Independence
Avascular necrosis, 289–290
Avoidance coping strategy, 37–38, 203
AW2 (U.S. Army Wounded Warrior Program), 328
Awareness. *See* Consciousness

B
Baby Boomers, 437, 449
Baclofen (Lioresal), 128, 222–223, 277–278, 279, 353, 353*t*
Balance
   assessment of, 138, 139, 146
   in Parkinson's disease, 349
   in stroke, 218, 221
   in TBI, 259
Bandages. *See* Topical treatment
Barriers to optimal quality of life. *See also* Legal issues
   barriers to learning, 177, 192
   social/environmental factors, 17
   social model of, 31, 31*f*
Barrier wipes, 111, 112*t*
Basic nutrients. *See* Nutrients, essential
Beck Depression Inventory, 208
Becker muscular dystrophy (BMD), 426–427

Behavior. *See also* Cognition and behavior
   behavioral coping strategies, 38. *See also* Coping
   modification. *See* Education of clients and families
   testing for therapy animals, 465
Beliefs. *See also* Ethical considerations; Frameworks for chronic
      illness, disability, adaptation, and coping; Spirituality
   learning abilities/needs and, 182–183, 183*f*, 186
   pain control and, 208
Benchmarking, 24, 24*t*
Benedikt syndrome, 218, 220*t*
Beneficence principle, 24, 387
Benzodiazepines
   falls and, 138, 139
   for phantom limb pain, 304
   for sleep disorders, 239, 239*t*
   for spasticity, 223, 353, 353*t*
Berg Balance Scale, 138, 139, 146
Best practice. *See* Competencies, certification, and education;
      Evidence-based practice
Beta-blockers, 334, 335*t*
Bethanechol (Urecholine), 128
Bioethics, 389–390
Biographical disruption, 33, 40, 43
Biological dressings, 114, 116
Biological theories of aging, 438–439
Biomedical frameworks for chronic illness/disability, 29–31,
      30*b*, 31*f*
Biopsychosocial frameworks for chronic illness/disability, 29–
      30, 33–35, 35*f*, 36*b*, 39. *See also* Psychosocial issues; Social
      frameworks for chronic illness/disability
Birth defects. *See* Congenital anomalies
Blacks. *See* African American populations
Bladder management, 121–130. *See also* Kidneys
   aging and, 442, 448–449, 451*t*
   anatomy of urinary tract, 121–122, 122*f*
   bladder tapping, 276
   complications in, 128–130, 128*f*, 130*b*, 130*t*
   falls and, 138
   in neurological disorders, 354, 355*t*
   nursing interventions, 125–127, 126*b*, 126*t*
   pathophysiology of urinary tract, 122–125, 123–124*t*, 125*f*
   in SCI, 124, 125, 127–130, 275–276, 276*b*
   sexual issues and, 171
   in spina bifida, 424–425
   in stroke, 124, 126, 232
   TBI and, 258, 263, 263*t*
Blast injuries, 317–318, 319, 319*t*. *See also* Polytrauma
Bleeding
   cancer tumors and, 364
   in hemorrhagic stroke, 217
   in traumatic brain injuries, 258
Blindness. *See* Visual impairment
Blood pressure. *See* Hypertension; Hypotension
Blood vessel occlusion/rupture. *See* Cardiovascular problems;
      Stroke
Blue Cross/Blue Shield, 405
BMD (Becker muscular dystrophy), 426–427
Bobath approach, 241–242

Body image issues, 87, 95, 299, 312

Body mass. *See* Obesity and weight management

Body mechanics, 140–142

Body structures/functions (ICF model), 34–35, 35*f*

Body temperature regulation, 111, 258, 279

Bony prominences, in skin assessment, 105. *See also* Pressure ulcers

Botox (Botulinum toxin), 127, 222, 242, 353–354

Bowel management, 130–135. *See also* Constipation
    aging and, 441
    anatomy of bowel, 130
    in muscular dystrophy, 427
    neurogenic characteristics and treatments, 130–134, 131–133*t*, 133*b*
    in neurological disorders, 354, 355*t*
    in polytrauma, 319, 319*t*
    in SCI, 130–131, 131*t*, 132, 133, 274–275, 275*b*
    sexual issues and, 171
    in spina bifida, 131*t*, 132, 425
    in stroke, 131, 131*t*, 133, 232
    TBI and, 258, 263, 263*t*

Brachial plexus injury, 431

Braden Scale for Predicting Pressure Ulcer Risk, 104

Brain
    anatomy and function, 148–149, 256, 256*f*, 257*t*
    injury/dysfunction. *See* Cognition and behavior; Stroke; Traumatic brain injury

Brain attack. *See* Stroke

Brainstem, 256, 257*t*

Brain Trauma Foundation, 91

Breathing problems. *See also* Oxygen therapy; Pulmonary disease/complications
    asthma and, 339*t*, 341
    COPD and, 339*t*, 340–341
    in muscular dystrophy, 431
    in SCI, 277, 277*f*
    sexual issues and, 169, 170*f*
    sleep disordered breathing, 238–239, 239*t*

Broca's aphasia, 229, 230*t*, 242

Broken bones. *See* Fractures

Bronchitis, chronic, 340

Brown-Sequard syndrome, 273

Bulimia, 87. *See also* Eating disorders

Burns, 91, 323–324, 323*b*, 324*t*

Bury, M., 33, 36

C

Cachexia, 364, 369

CAD. *See* Coronary artery (heart) disease

Calcium alginate dressings, 111, 114*t*

Calcium channel blockers, 334, 335*t*

Calcium requirements, 90, 95

Calculi, 129

CAM. *See* Complementary and alternative medicine

Cancer, 363–367
    assessment and screening, 364–365, 365*t*
    CKD and, 359
    diagnoses, 365, 366*t*
    education of clients/families, 367
    epidemiology, 363
    ethical issues, 367
    interventions, 366–367, 366*t*
    lung, 339*t*, 341–342
    outcomes, 367
    pathophysiology, 364
    prevention, 364
    risk factors and warning signs, 364
    sexual issues and, 165, 165*t*

Capacity determination, 395–396

Carbamazepine (Tegretol), 240, 240–241*t*, 263

Carbohydrates, 85

Cardiovascular problems, 332–338. *See also* Diabetes; Hypertension; Myocardial infarction; Stroke
    aging-related, 441
    amputation and, 304
    CAM and, 378, 379*t*
    cardiac rehabilitation, 336–338, 337*b*
    cardiomyopathy, 332, 334
    coronary artery disease, 332–333, 333*f*, 334, 335*t*
    education and, 192, 193–195*b*, 340, 342
    ethical issues, 342
    heart failure, 332, 333–334, 334*b*, 336
    in joint replacement, 288
    muscular dystrophy and, 427
    nursing competencies, 342
    nutritional needs, 89, 90*b*
    outcome evaluation, 342
    in polytrauma, 319, 319*t*
    prevention, 335–336
    risk factors and warning signs, 335, 335*t*
    sexual issues and, 167, 168*b*, 169
    symptoms of, 336
    with TBI, 258, 263, 263*t*
    treatment of, 334–335, 334*b*, 335*t*

Caregivers. *See also* Family
    caregiving experience, 380
    education of, 178, 183
    effects of disability on, 8
    levels of assist and, 137, 137*t*
    patient handling safety for, 141, 142–145
    roles of, 385
    SCI and, 281–282
    stroke and, 232, 235, 244, 247*t*

Carel, H., 38–39, 42

Care provider nursing role, 64

CARF. *See* Commission on Accreditation of Rehabilitation Facilities

Caring, art of, 200–214. *See also* Spirituality
    adaptation models, 202. *See also* Adaptation
    coping strategies and scales, 203–204. *See also* Coping
    culture of caring, 210–211, 380–382
    efficacy evaluation, 209–210
    ethical considerations, 210
    interdisciplinary team and, 206–207
    meaning, purpose, and significance, 200–201, 205–206, 210
    nursing interventions and, 207–208, 207*b*, 207*t*

Caring, art of (*cont.*)
  outcomes and, 204–205
  in polytrauma, 321–322
  preventing/detecting emotional problems, 208–209, 209*b*
  spiritual care, 201–202, 208–209
Caring Theory (Watson), 202, 211
Caritas consciousness relationship, 202
Carryover ability, 155
Case Management Society of America (CMSA), 71
Case managers/management
  amputation and, 300, 300*t*
  as interdisciplinary team members, 54*f*, 55, 56*t*
  life care planning and, 472
  nursing roles of, 69, 70–72
  sexual issues and, 162
CAT. *See* ARN-Competency Assessment Test
Catabolism, 85
Catastrophizing, 208
Catheterization
  bladder dysfunction and, 125, 126–127, 129
  poststroke, 232
  in SCI patients, 275–276
  sexual relationships and, 162
  in spina bifida patients, 425
Caucasians. *See* White populations
Cauda equina injury, 131*t*, 132, 271, 274
CDC. *See* Centers for Disease Control and Prevention
Census Bureau (U.S.), 14–15
Centers for Disease Control and Prevention (CDC), 17, 18, 20*b*,
    179, 262, 262*b*
Centers for Medicare and Medicaid Services (CMS). *See*
    Medicaid/Medicare
Central cord syndrome, 273
Central nervous system stimulants, 358, 358*t*
Central neurogenic bladder, 125
Central poststroke pain syndrome (CPSP), 240–241, 241*t*
Central sleep apnea, 238–239
Cerebellum, 256, 256*f*, 257*t*
Cerebral hemorrhage. *See* Hemorrhagic stroke
Cerebral palsy (CP)
  aging with, 444
  bladder dysfunction and, 124
  in children, 420–423
  sexual issues and, 169
Cerebral stroke syndromes, 218–219, 218–219*t*
Cerebrospinal fluid rhinorrhea/otorrhea, 258
Cerebrovascular accident. *See* Stroke
Certification. *See* Competencies, certification, and education
Certified rehabilitation registered nurse (CRRN) credential
  for case managers, 71
  for direct care providers, 64
  for geriatric nurses, 69
  history of, 5, 5*t*
  for liaison nurses, 67
  requirements for, 11
Cervical spine injuries, 271, 271*f*
CF (cystic fibrosis), 339*t*, 341
Changes with chronic illness/disability. *See also* Adaptation

change theory, 184–185, 184*t*, 185*b*, 202, 211
  life changes and losses, 36
  in sense of identity, 32, 33, 36, 40–43
  transition theory on, 41
Chaplains, 55, 57*t*
Charcot-Marie-Tooth (CMT) disease, 344, 345*t*, 350, 351, 357*b*
Chemical debridement, 109–110
Cheyne Stokes breathing, 238–239
Children with special healthcare needs (CSHCN), defined, 422.
    See also Pediatric rehabilitation
Chinese traditional medicine, 378
Cholesterol, 85–86, 89
Chondrocytes, 288
Chorea, in Huntington's disease, 349
Chronic bronchitis, 340
Chronic illness/disease, defined, 17–18, 28–29. *See also specific*
    illnesses/diseases
Chronic illness trajectories, 32–33
Chronicity, 14–21. *See also* Frameworks for chronic illness,
    disability, adaptation, and coping
  aging population and, 18–19, 19*b*
  chronic illness/disease, 17–18, 18*t*
  defined, 18
  disability definition and, 14–16, 15–16*t*, 28–29
  health promotion and, 16–17
  as rehabilitation principle, 6
  role of healthcare practitioners and, 19–20
Chronic kidney disease (CKD), 359–363, 362*t*
Chronic obstructive pulmonary disease (COPD), 339*t*, 340–341
Chronic sorrow, 39–40
Chronic wounds, defined, 104. *See also* Pressure ulcers
Cialis (tadalafil), 167
Circulation problems. *See* Cardiovascular problems
CKD (chronic kidney disease), 359–363, 362*t*
Clasp knife phenomenon, 348–349, 352
Classifications. *See* Assessment
CLD (congenital limb deficiency), 429–430
Clean intermittent bladder catheterization, 425
Cleansing wounds, 109
Cleft lip/palate, 428–429
Client-family teaching, 25. *See also* Education of clients and
    families
Clients, defined, 471. *See also* Patients
Clinical history. *See* History and physical examination
Clinical nurse leaders, 72
Clinical nurse specialists (CNSs), 78–79. *See also* Advanced
    practice registered nurses
Clinician role, 66
Closed head injuries, 255
Clots, blood. *See* Cardiovascular problems; Stroke
CMS (Centers for Medicare and Medicaid Services). *See*
    Medicaid/Medicare
CMSA (Case Management Society of America), 71
CMT (Charcot-Marie-Tooth) disease, 344, 345*t*, 350, 351
CNSs (clinical nurse specialists), 78–79. *See also* Advanced
    practice registered nurses
COBRA (Consolidated Omnibus Budget Reconciliation Act of
    1986), 407

Code of Ethics (ANA), 210, 391–392, 392t
Cognition and behavior, 148–160. *See also* Education of clients and families; Neurological conditions
assessment of, 228–229, 228t, 229f, 259–262, 259–262t, 260b, 264t
cognition defined, 149, 150b
cognitive coping strategies, 38, 203
consciousness, attention, and executive control, 149–152, 150b
CP and, 422
dementia. *See* Delirium/dementia
impulse control, 155–157, 156t
insight and judgment, 155
management of impairments, 158–159
memory. *See* Memory
muscular dystrophy and, 428
neuroanatomy and function, 148–149
in neurological disorders, 359–360t, 361
sexual issues and, 169, 171–172
speech and language, 148–149, 150b, 151–154, 153t
spina bifida and, 424
in stroke, 151, 227–229, 228t, 229f, 243
in TBI, 258, 259–262, 259–262t, 260b, 262b
Cognitive deficits. *See* Cognition and behavior
Cognitive dissonance theory, 183
Cognitive domain, 196
Cognitive load theory, 181–182, 181f, 182b
Collaboration, 52. *See also* Interdisciplinary teams
Collaborative discussion, 55
Collagenase, 114, 115t
Coma. *See* Glasgow coma scale
Commission for Case Management Certification, 71
Commission of Chronic Diseases/Illness, 18
Commission on Accreditation of Rehabilitation Facilities (CARF), 17, 52, 52b, 60, 177, 388
Communication. *See also* Cognition and behavior; Education of clients and families; Speech and language impairments
with clients/families, 158, 186, 189
cultural issues in, 375, 377, 377f
disability, defined, 15, 16t
falls prevention and, 139
in interdisciplinary teams, 53–54, 53f, 55, 57–59, 265
in safe lifting and promoting ambulation, 143
sexual issues and, 161, 162, 164, 166, 170–171, 171b
spiritual issues and, 204, 207, 208–209, 210
Community reintegration/reentry, 2, 2t, 7, 121, 246–248, 262. *See also* Independent living
Community settings for care, 23–24, 432–433, 432b
Compassionate care. *See* Caring, art of
Compassion fatigue, 321–322
Compensatory techniques. *See* Adaptation
Competencies, certification, and education. *See also* Efficacy of care; Nursing roles
for advanced practice nurses, 78, 79
ARN certification, 5–6, 5t, 10–11, 10t, 64, 65. *See also* Certified rehabilitation registered nurse (CRRN) credential
in cardiac and pulmonary rehabilitation, 338, 342

for case managers, 71–72
certification, defined, 64
competencies, defined, 65
for direct care providers, 1, 63–64
for geriatric healthcare, 19, 69–70
of interdisciplinary team, 57–59, 57b
for liaison nurses, 66, 67
for life care planning, 474–476, 475t, 476b
for managers/administrators, 72–74
nurse educators and, 74–75, 193
for pediatric nurses, 67–68
polytrauma and, 320, 320b
for researchers, 76
skin integrity and, 117
Complementary and alternative medicine (CAM)
history and usage of, 378, 379t
for SCI pain treatment, 280–281
spirituality and, 204
Complete spinal cord injuries, 273, 281
Complex regional pain syndrome (CRPS), 258
Complications
in amputation, 304
in bladder management, 128–130, 128f, 130b, 130t
falls. *See* Falls
incontinence and, 123
in joint replacement, 287–288
maladaptive coping and, 203–204
of myocardial infarction, 333, 333f
of neurological disorders, 354, 355–356t
in older adults, 69
poststroke, 223–224, 232–234, 236–241, 239–241t
pressure ulcers. *See* Pressure ulcers
prevention of, 2, 2t, 8–9
psychological. *See* Psychological well-being
in SCI, 271
in TBI, 258–259
in tube feeding, 94
Composite dressings, 111, 112t
Concussion, 258, 259, 326, 327
Conduction aphasia, 229, 230t
Confabulation, 150–151, 150b
Confidence. *See* Self-efficacy
Confidentiality. *See* Ethical considerations; Privacy
Conflicts
of death, 318
ethical. *See* Ethical considerations
of interpretation, 380
Confusion. *See* Disorientation
Congenital anomalies, 297, 298, 332, 334. *See also* Pediatric rehabilitation; *specific anomalies*
Congenital limb deficiency (CLD), 429–430
Consciousness. *See also* Cognition and behavior; Glasgow coma scale; Rancho Los Amigos scale of cognitive recovery
defined, 149, 150b
impairments of, 149–152, 150b
loss in brain injury, 258
Consolidated Omnibus Budget Reconciliation Act (COBRA 1986), 407

Consortium on Spinal Cord Medicine, 127, 130, 130*b*
Constipation. *See also* Bowel management
    with neurological conditions, 89–90
    in older adults, 96
    prevention of, 132–133, 133*b*, 133*t*
    in stroke patients, 232
    in uninhibited bowel, 131, 131*t*
Constraint-induced movement therapy, 242
Content memory, 154–155
Contextual factors (ICF model), 34–35, 35*f. See also*
    Environmental factors
Continuous ambulatory peritoneal dialysis, 361
Continuous positive airway pressure (CPAP), 238–239
Contractures
    amputation and, 301, 302–303
    in muscular dystrophy, 431
    preventive care and, 9
    in stroke, 221–222
Contrecoup/coup injuries, 256–257
Control
    locus of, 183
    loss of with illness/disability, 33, 36, 42
Contusion, brain, 258
Conus medullaris syndrome, 274
Coordination
    assessment of, 138
    in Parkinson's disease, 353
    in stroke, 218, 221
COPD. *See* Chronic obstructive pulmonary disease
Coping. *See also* Adaptation
    of family members, 8
    principles of rehabilitation and, 6, 7
    spirituality and, 205–206, 208
    strategies and scales, 203–204, 208
    theories of, 36–38, 38*b*, 202
Coronary angioplasty, 334, 336
Coronary artery bypass graft surgery, 334
Coronary artery (heart) disease (CAD), 332–333, 333*f*, 334, 335*t.*
    See also Myocardial infarction
Corticosteroids, 267
Costs. *See* Financial issues
Cough, chronic. *See* Chronic obstructive pulmonary disease
Coumadin (warfarin), 236–237, 288, 334, 335*t*
Coup/contrecoup injuries, 256–257
CP. *See* Cerebral palsy
CPAP (continuous positive airway pressure), 238–239
CPSP. *See* Central poststroke pain syndrome
Craig handicap assessment and reporting technique, 262, 262*b*
Cranial nerves, 92
Craniofacial anomalies, 428–429
Credé maneuver, 125, 127, 128
Critical thinking, defined, 65
CRPS (Complex regional pain syndrome), 258
CRRN. *See* Certified rehabilitation registered nurse (CRRN)
    credential
CSHCN (children with special healthcare needs), defined, 418.
    See also Pediatric rehabilitation

Cultural issues, 373–384. *See also* Race and racial issues; Social
    issues
    in adaptation/coping, 40, 203
    aging and, 18
    in amputation, 299–300
    in appraisal and coping strategies, 37
    in cardiac disease, 335
    competence and, 375–378, 376*b*, 379*f*
    complementary/alternative medicine. *See* Complementary
        and alternative medicine
    cultural change, 381
    cultural diversity, defined, 374
    cultural expressions of care, 376
    cultural imperialism, 382–383
    culturally competent care, defined, 377
    culturally congruent care, defined, 376
    cultural role, 381
    cultural values, beliefs, attitudes, and actions, 380
    culture, defined, 375
    culture of caring, 210–211, 376–378
    disability culture, 378–382, 381–382*b*
    diversity in the U.S., 374–375, 375*b*
    in education/learning, 178, 182–183, 183*f*, 186
    holistic approach and, 8
    IDT culture, 59
    nursing culture, 382–383, 383*f*
    nutrition and, 97
    preservation and accommodation, 376
    in psychosocial frameworks, 33
    in social models, 31, 32
    spirituality and, 207, 209
Current level of function, 138
Cylert (pemoline), 354, 354*t*
Cystic fibrosis (CF), 339*t*, 341

D
Daily Spiritual Experiences questionnaire, 208
Damages, in life care planning, 472
Danaparoid, 236
Dantrolene sodium (Dantrium), 128, 223, 353, 353*t*
Deafness. *See* Auditory impairment
Death. *See also* Terminal illness
    conflicts of, 318
    dying and stages of, 202
    panels, 453
    rates and causes. *See* Epidemiology and mortality statistics
Debridement, 109–111
Declarative memory, 154
Deep vein thrombosis (DVT), 236, 288
Defecation, defined, 130. *See also* Bowel management
Degenerative neurological disorders, 344, 347–350, 351, 353.
    See also specific disorders
Dehydration. *See* Fluids
Delirium/dementia
    ambiguous loss and, 321
    causes of and care for, 157–158
    defined, 150*b*, 151
    flat affect and, 157

geriatric syndromes and, 448–449, 450t
neurological disorders and, 357
sexual issues and, 165, 171
stroke and, 227
transient incontinence and, 123, 124t
uninhibited bowel and, 131
Dementia. *See* Delirium/dementia
Demyelination, 344, 345–346, 350
Denial
in SCI, 281
in stages of adaptation, 202
Depakene/Depakote (valproic acid), 240, 240t
Department of Agriculture Food Guide Pyramid, 98
Department of Defense (DOD), 317
Department of Health and Human Services. *See* U.S.
Department of Health and Human Services
Department of Veterans Affairs. *See* Veterans Administration
(VA) and Veterans Health Administration (VHA)
Depression. *See also* Psychological well-being
amputation and, 299
coping/adaptation and, 202, 203
dementia/delirium vs., 158
as mood state, 157
neurological disorders and, 344
in older adults, 447–448
poststroke (PSD), 233–234, 234–235t, 239
prevention and detection of, 208–209
SCI and, 280, 281
sexual issues and, 168, 168t
in TBI, 258
Dermatitis, 101, 114
Desire, in triphasic sexual response, 165. *See also* Sexuality
and disability
Detrusor muscle and sphincter dyssynergia
bladder management and, 122, 123, 124, 127, 128
in SCI, 275, 276
Development. *See* Age-related issues
Diabetes
amputation and, 297–298, 297t, 301, 304
bladder dysfunction and, 125, 129
bowel dysfunction and, 131t, 132
CAM and, 378, 379t
as CKD cause, 360, 361
sexual issues and, 165–166t
stroke and, 90, 216, 218t, 219, 232, 246
Diagnoses. *See also* Assessment
in amputation, 311–314
of cancer, 365, 366t
of CKD, 362, 362t
of cleft lip/palate, 429
of CP, 422
LCPs and, 475, 475t
of mobility level, 145–146
of MS, 347
of neurological disorders, 354, 355–356t
payment systems and, 409–410
problem identification and, 187, 187b
of SDB/SWDs, 238

of speech/language disorders, 152–154, 153t, 231–232
in TBI, 263, 264b
of terminal illness, 368, 368t
Diagnosis-related groups (DRGs), 409
Dialysis, 364–365
Diazepam (Valium), 128, 353, 353t
Diet. *See* Nutrition
Dietitians as interdisciplinary team members, 53–54f, 55, 57t,
84, 96, 300t
Diffuse injuries (brain), 257
Digestion. *See* Bladder management; Bowel management;
Nutrition
Digital stimulation, 132, 274
Dignity, as goal of rehabilitation, 2, 2t
Digoxin, 167, 168t
Dilantin (phenytoin), 240, 240t
Dimensions of adaptability, 42–43
Diminished bodily capacity, 42
Diplopia, 346
Disability culture, 381–382
Disability, defined, 14–16, 15–16t, 17, 28–29, 380. *See also*
Frameworks for chronic illness, disability, adaptation,
and coping
Disaccharides, 85
Discrimination. *See also* Americans with Disabilities Act;
Cultural issues
advocacy and legislation against, 16–17, 381, 396–398
social frameworks of, 31–32
Disease. *See* Chronic illness/disease, defined; Chronicity
Disorientation, 149–151, 150b, 218, 262. *See also* Delirium/
dementia
Disparities, health, 374, 415
Dispositional optimism, 207
Distractibility, 150b, 151
Ditropan (oxybutynin chloride), 128
Diuretics, 133, 133t, 334, 335t
Diversity. *See* Cultural issues
Dizziness
in SCI, 278
in stroke, 218
in TBI, 258–259
DMD (Duchenne muscular dystrophy), 426
DNR. *See* Do not resuscitate (DNR) orders
Doctorate of nursing practice degrees, 72–73
Documentation. *See also* Life care plan (LCP) and
planning
falls prevention and, 139
of learning activities, 192, 193–195b
safety devices and, 144
third-party payment and, 23
DOD (Department of Defense), 317
Domains of learning, 196
Do not resuscitate (DNR) orders, 392, 393
Dopamine, 349, 353
Dopaminergic agents, 239
Down syndrome, 444
Dressings. *See* Topical treatment
DRGs (diagnosis-related groups), 409

Driving
  older adults and, 453
  poststroke, 246, 248
Drugs. *See* Alcohol consumption; Medications; Smoking and
    tobacco use; Substance abuse
Duchenne muscular dystrophy (DMD), 426
DVT. *See* Deep vein thrombosis
Dying, stages of, 202
Dynamic alignment, 307
Dynamic balance, 138
Dynamic Gait Index, 138, 139, 146
Dysarthria, 150*b*, 152, 153*t*, 229, 231, 231*t*, 243
Dysarthria-clumsy hand stroke syndrome, 218, 220*t*
Dysphagia
  aging and, 441
  in muscular dystrophy, 427
  neurological disorders and, 354, 356*t*
  nutrition and, 90–93, 92*b*, 96, 96*f*, 97*t*
  stroke and, 233, 237
  TBI and, 259
Dysphonia, 346, 354, 356*t*. *See also* Speech and language
    impairments
Dyspnea, 334, 339
Dyssynergia, 123, 127, 128
Dystrophin, 426–428
Dysvascular conditions, 301. *See also* Diabetes

E
Early and Periodic Screening, Diagnosis, and Treatment Act
    (1989), 419
Eastern Cooperative Oncology Group Performance Status
    Scale, 365, 365*t*
Eating disorders, 87, 95, 369. *See also* Nutrition
Eaton-Lambert syndrome, 344, 345–346, 345*t*, 350, 357*b*
ECM (extracellular matrix), 288–289
Economic issues. *See* Financial issues
Edema
  in amputation, 302, 302*f*
  in brain injuries, 257
  in SCI, 272
Education for all Handicapped Children's Act (1975), 419
Education of clients and families, 176–199. *See also* Advocacy
  on aging with disability, 445–447*t*
  on amputation, 301, 309–313, 310–311*t*, 313–314*b*
  on cancer, 367
  on cardiac disease, 336, 338
  on CKD, 363
  on cleft lip/palate, 429
  community education and prevention, 196
  coping and, 203–204
  evaluation of learning, 192–193
  as goal of rehabilitation, 2, 2*t*
  health literacy, 177, 178–179, 178*b*
  holistic approaches and, 8
  on joint replacement, 291, 291*b*
  learning process, 179–181, 180*f*
  learning theories/models, 181–185, 181*f*, 182*b*, 183*f*, 184–185*b*,
    184*t*, 196

  on muscular dystrophy, 428
  need for education, 177–178
  on neurological conditions, 354–356, 357*b*
  nurse's roles in, 64–69, 71, 74, 78–79, 435
  on nutrition, 97
  of older adults, 19, 69
  in pediatric rehabilitation, 431–432
  peer education, 193
  on polytrauma issues, 319–320, 320*b*, 324–326
  prevention and, 179, 179*t*
  on pulmonary disease, 340, 341–342
  on SCI, 275
  on settings for care, 25
  on sexual issues. *See* Sexuality and disability
  on skin integrity issues, 111, 117
  on spina bifida, 429
  on stroke, 232, 236, 238, 240, 243–246, 244*b*, 245*t*, 247*t*
  teaching interventions, 188–191, 189*b*, 190*t*
  teaching process, 185–188, 186–188*b*
  technology use in, 191–192, 191*b*, 193–195*b*
  on terminal illness, 369, 369*t*
  on traumatic brain injury, 265–266
  in women to women model, 18
Education of healthcare practitioners. *See* Competencies,
    certification, and education
Education of the Handicapped Act (1970), 419
Educator nursing role, 74–76, 193
Efferent neurons, 349
Efficacy of care. *See also* Competencies, certification,
    and education; Outcome evaluation (management,
    measurement, research)
  AAT and, 464–465
  effective care, defined, 413
  interdisciplinary team and, 58–60
  spiritual care and, 209–210
Efficient care, defined, 413
Elaboration and rehearsal (in learning), 180, 180*f*
Elder abuse/mistreatment. *See* Abuse and neglect
Elderly patients. *See* Gerontological rehabilitation
Electrical stimulation, 279–280, 282–283, 304
Elimination. *See* Bladder management; Bowel management
Emboli/embolic stroke, 217, 236, 288
Emergency Medical Treatment and Active Labor Act
    (EMTALA 1986), 411
Emotional intelligence, 59
Emotional lability, 234
Emotional needs/responses. *See* Affect; Psychological well-
    being; Sexuality and disability
Emotion-focused behavior/coping strategies, 37, 203
Emphysema, 340
Employment
  disability and. *See* Vocational rehabilitation
  insurance and, 459, 407
EMTALA (Emergency Medical Treatment and Active Labor
    Act of 1986), 411
Encoding ability, 155, 180, 180*f*
Endocrine problems, 123, 124*t*, 258, 443

End-of-life decisions, 357, 389–394, 392b. *See also* Advance
 directives
End-stage renal disease (ESRD), 359–361
Enemas, 133–134. *See also* Suppositories
Enteral nutrition, 91, 93–94, 94t, 98
Environmental factors. *See also* Social issues
 adaptation and, 39, 42
 in communicating with patients, 158
 coping strategies and, 38, 38b
 defined, 14
 in delirium, 151
 environmental context and culture, 376, 377–378
 environment, defined, 420
 in falls, 138
 in models of disability, 16–17, 34–35, 35f
 in pediatric rehabilitation, 420
 in SCI and body temperature, 279
 in sleep disorders, 238, 239
 in spina bifida, 423
Enzymatic debriding agent, 110, 114, 115t
Epidemiology and mortality statistics
 amputation, 297–298
 arthritis, 288, 289
 brachial palsy, 431
 burns, 323
 cancer, 363
 cardiac disease, 332, 332b, 333, 334
 children with special needs, 418
 CKD, 359–360
 CLD, 429
 cleft lip/palate, 428–429
 CP, 421
 neurological disorders, 345, 345t
 older adults, 437
 pulmonary diseases, 338, 340, 341
 SCI, 269–270, 269f, 277, 278
 spina bifida, 423
 stroke, 216
 TBI, 255–256, 322–323
 terminal illness, 367–368
Epidural hematoma, 258
Epilepsy. *See* Antiepileptics; Seizures
Episodic memory, 154
Equipment. *See also* Technology; *specific equipment*
 adaptive, 144, 275, 282–283
 assistive devices, 143, 308
 for lifting, 142, 143
 orthotics, 242
 patient safety devices, 144–145
Era of onset, defined, 444
Erectile dysfunction, 162, 166–168, 166t, 168t, 280–281, 443
Erickson's theory of development, 439–440
Esophageal swallowing phase, 93
ESRD (end-stage renal disease), 359–361
Essential proteins, 84–85
Ethical considerations, 386–401. *See also* Legal issues
 advance directives, 390, 391–394, 392b
 in amputation, 299, 2993b
 in cancer, 367
 in cardiac and pulmonary disease, 342
 in CKD, 363
 defining ethics, 386–387
 dilemmas in, 389–390
 guardianship, 394–396, 395t
 for the incompetent and dying, 390–391
 models for decision making, 386–387
 in neurological disorders, 356–357
 Olmstead decision, 397t, 398–399
 patient restraints and, 144–145
 professional code of conduct, 387–389, 388t, 389b
 right to life issues, 396–399, 397t
 in settings for care, 24
 spiritual care and, 210
 in terminal illness, 370
Ethnicity. *See also* Race and racial issues
 ethnic culture, defined, 380
 ethnic minority groups, defined, 374
 ethnohistory, 376
European Pressure Ulcer Advisory Panel, 104–105, 109
Evacuation of the bowel, 132. *See also* Bowel management
Evaluation. *See* Assessment; Outcome evaluation (management,
 measurement, research)
Evidence-based practice. *See also* Outcome evaluation
 (management, measurement, research)
 advanced practice nurses and, 79
 ARN focus on, 10
 CARF standards of, 17
 case managers and, 71–72
 defined, 65
 in geriatric nursing, 69–70, 70b
 joint replacement and, 295, 295b
 liaison nurses and, 67
 managers/administrators and, 73
 nurse educators and, 75
 in pediatric nursing, 68
 researchers and, 76, 77
 SCI and, 282–283
 settings for care and, 25
 sexuality issues and, 163, 171
 in stroke treatment, 241
 teaching/learning strategies and, 179
Examination. *See* History and physical examination
Excitement, in triphasic sexual response, 165
Executive control impairments, 149–152, 150b, 158, 228, 229,
 243
Exercise. *See also* Lifestyle factors; Mobility
 for amputation, 302
 cancer and, 367
 cardiac disease and, 335–336, 335t, 337–338
 CKD and, 361, 363
 fecal incontinence and, 232
 for joint replacement, 288–291, 295
 in older adults, 19
 for pulmonary rehabilitation, 340
 sexual function and, 167
 stroke and, 219, 241–242

Existential spirituality, defined, 201
Expertise reversal effect, 181–182
External urethral sphincter, 122
Extracellular matrix (ECM), 284–285
Extraneous load, 181, 181*f*
Extremities. *See* Amputation; Joints and joint replacement
Extrinsic load, 181, 181*f*
Exudate in wounds, 111
Eye problems. *See* Visual impairment

F
Facilities for care. *See* Settings for care
Failure to thrive (geriatric syndrome), 448–449, 452*t*
Falls
    amputation and, 304
    geriatric syndromes and, 448–449, 450*t*
    incontinence and, 123, 138
    in older adults, 19, 138–139, 139*t*
    in Parkinson's patients, 90
    risk assessment/prevention of, 138–140, 139–140*t*, 145–146, 223–224, 224*t*
    in stroke patients, 223–224, 224*t*
Family. *See also* Caregivers; Education of clients and families; Sexuality and disability; Social issues
    affects of illness/disability on, 8, 18, 178
    amputation and, 300, 311
    changes in relationships with illness/disability, 36
    dementia and, 158
    end-of-life decisions and. *See* End-of-life decisions
    family-centered care, 420, 420*t*
    history of disease. *See* Genetics
    in inappropriate behavior modification, 172
    in interdisciplinary team, 51, 52, 53–54, 53–54*f*, 55, 59
    memory impairments and, 154
    in pediatric rehabilitation, 420, 420*t*, 423, 428
    polytrauma and, 320–321
    in selection of setting for care, 25
    support of disabled person, 35
    in TBI care, 265
    therapists, 328
    in transition theory, 41
Family Caregiver Alliance, 244, 245*t*
Family Crisis Oriented Personal Evaluation Scale, 203
Fatigue
    cancer and, 366–367
    CKD and, 362
    compassion, 321–322
    in neurological disorders, 350, 352–353, 354–355*t*
    sexual issues and, 165, 168
    in TBI, 259
Fats/fatty acids, 85
Fat-soluble vitamins, 86, 86*t*
Fears. *See* Anxiety
Fecal incontinence. *See* Bowel management
Feeding. *See* Nutrition
Feeding tubes, 93–94, 94*t*, 237
Fee for service (FFS), 406
Females. *See* Gender and gender issues

FFS (fee for service), 406
Fiber, 89, 90, 132, 133, 232
FIM. *See* Functional Independence Measure
Financial issues. *See also* Payment systems
    adaptive equipment and, 144
    in cardiac and pulmonary disease, 342
    in CP, 423
    in life care planning, 473–475
    mobility/function and, 138
    for older adults, 19, 95, 453
    in polytrauma, 321
    poverty and disability, 381
    prevention and, 179
    prosthetics and, 307–308
    renal disease costs, 360
    rising costs problem, 414
    self-efficacy and, 183
    stroke costs, 216
    TBI costs, 323
    in treating the whole person, 8
First Nations. *See* Native Americans
Five stages of death and dying, 202
Fluids
    aspiration pneumonia and, 237
    for bowel management, 132, 133, 232, 275
    for calculi management, 129
    dysphagia and, 233
    nutrition and, 87
    SCI and, 279
    TBI and, 257
Foam dressings, 111, 113*t*
Focal injuries (brain), 257
Food. *See* Nutrition
Food Guide Pyramid (U.S. Department of Agriculture), 98
Foot prostheses, 307, 307*f*
Formulas for tube feeding, 94, 94*t*
Fractures
    aging and, 442
    in muscular dystrophy, 427
    outcome evaluation and, 24
    in polytrauma, 324
    preventing in older adults, 19
    spinal, 271. *See also* Spinal cord injuries
    TBI and, 258
Frameworks for chronic illness, disability, adaptation, and coping, 28–50. *See also specific theories/models*
    adaptation, 38–43, 42*f*
    appraisal and adaptation/coping, 35–38, 38*b*
    biomedical frameworks, 29–31, 30*b*, 31*f*
    biopsychosocial frameworks, 29–30, 33–35, 35*f*, 36*b*, 39
    chronic illness vs. disability, 28–29
    individual model of disability, 16
    interdisciplinary team models, 53–55, 53–54*f*, 53*b*
    models based on interpretive frameworks, 43–44, 44*f*, 44*t*
    psychosocial frameworks, 29–30, 32–33, 34*b*, 36, 41, 43–44
    social frameworks, 16–17, 29–30, 31–32, 31*f*, 32*b*
Friction and skin integrity, 102, 103*t*, 104, 108, 108*t*
Frontal lobe, 256, 256*f*, 257*t*

Functional assessment measures, 262. *See also* Assessment
Functional capacity, 336
Functional incontinence, 123
Functional Independence Measure (FIM), 90, 137, 262, 262*b*
Functional limitations. *See also* Cognition and behavior;
    Mobility; *specific limitations/impairments*
    assessment of, 137–138, 137–138*t*, 262
    with cancer, 364–365, 365*t*
    with CKD, 362–363
    defined, 14–15, 15*t*
    diagnoses and interventions, 145–146
    in dimensions of adaptability, 42
    in ICF model, 34–35, 35*f*
    with polytrauma, 322
    with SCI, 271, 272–273
    with stroke, 221–228, 226*t*
    with TBI, 262
Functional mobility, defined, 136. *See also* Mobility
Function, promoting. *See also* Adaptation; Community
    reintegration/reentry; Mobility; Outcome evaluation
    (management, measurement, research)
    in amputation patients. *See* Prosthetics
    assessment of function, 137–138, 137–138*t*
    in cancer patients, 371
    compensation, 38, 42
    diagnoses and interventions, 145–146
    as goal of rehabilitation, 2, 2*t*, 136
    in stroke patients, 241–248, 245*t*, 247*t*
    in TBI patients, 265–266

G
GABA compounds, 233, 234*t*
Gabapentin. *See* Neurontin
Gait. *See also* Ataxia; Balance
    belts, 142
    evaluation, 137–138, 139, 146
    neurological disorders and, 349, 354, 355–356*t*
    training, 242, 296
Galveston orientation and amnesia test, 262, 262*t*
Gamma-aminobutyric acid (GABA) compounds, 233, 234*t*
Gastrointestinal problems. *See* Bowel management; Nutrition
Gastrostomy tubes, 93–94
Gauze dressings, 111, 112–113*t*
GBS. *See* Guillain-Barré syndrome
GCS. *See* Glasgow coma scale
Gender and gender issues. *See also* Cultural issues; Sexuality
    and disability
    adaptation and, 40
    arthritis and, 285
    in bladder management, 275–276
    in CKD, 363
    inner strength in women, 205
    SCI and, 269, 275–276, 278
    stroke and, 216, 218*t*, 233
    TBI and, 256, 323
Generativity vs. stagnation (developmental stage), 440
Genetics
    of aging, 438–439

cancer and, 364
    in cardiac and pulmonary diseases, 334, 338, 340
    CKD and family history, 361
    cystic fibrosis and, 341
    genetic testing, 399
    of muscular dystrophy, 426
    in neurological disease, 350, 351, 354
    in osteoarthritis, 289
    spina bifida and, 423
Genitourinary problems. *See* Bladder management; Sexuality
    and disability
Geragogy, 184, 184*b*
Geriatric syndromes, 448–449, 449–452*t*
Gerontological rehabilitation, 437–458. *See also* Medicaid/
    Medicare
    AAT in, 463–464, 464*b*, 465*t*
    aging and disability, 443–445, 445–447*t*
    aging changes, normal, 441–443
    aging theories, 438–441, 439*b*
    for amputation, 297, 298
    bladder management, 123, 123*t*, 126, 129, 133
    cancer and, 364
    chronicity and, 18–19, 19*b*
    elder abuse/neglect, 453–455, 454–455*t*, 455*b*
    future of healthcare and, 415
    geriatric syndromes, 448–449, 449–452*t*
    nutrition and, 95–96, 97
    psychological issues in, 208, 445–448
    role of rehabilitation nurse and, 67, 69–70, 70*b*, 82–83
    for SCI, 282
    settings for care, 25
    sexuality issues and, 163, 164–166, 171
    for stroke, 216, 218*t*, 227
    for traumatic brain injury, 256
Gerontological Society of America (GSA), 19, 20*b*
Glasgow coma scale (GCS), 259–260, 259*t*, 260*b*, 326
Global aphasia, 229, 230*t*, 243
Glucocorticoids, 427, 428
Goals of rehabilitation. *See also* Principles of rehabilitation;
    specific disabilities/disorders
    in AAT/AAA, 460
    abilities emphasis and, 7
    in cancer rehabilitation, 366
    in cardiac rehabilitation, 338
    general, 2–3, 2*t*
    goals of independence, 382
    learning and setting of, 188, 188*b*
    mobility, 136, 140, 140*t*, 141*f*
    in pulmonary rehabilitation, 341
    quality of healthcare and, 413
Gordon's functional health patterns, 440–441
Grief and grieving
    amputation and, 298–299, 312–313
    effects of disability on family and, 8
    loss of the assumptive world and, 36
    theories and models of, 39–41, 44, 44*f*
Group dynamics/learning, 52, 191
Group Visit program, 183

Growth
    of children, 419
    factors, 114, 116
    hormone, 114, 115*t*
GSA (Gerontological Society of America), 19, 20*b*
Guardian ad litem, 394
Guardianship, 394–396, 395*t*
Guillain-Barré syndrome (GBS)
    assessment, 352
    education of clients/family on, 348–356, 357*b*
    interventions and management, 353
    pathophysiology, 344, 345, 345*t*, 346
    risk factors and warning signs, 350, 351

H
Halo braces, 271, 271*f*
Handicap, defined, 380
Handling patients. *See* Safety
Hand prosthetics, 308–309, 308–309*f*
Harassment, sexual, 171–173
The Hartford Institute for Geriatric Nursing (New York
    University College of Nursing), 69–70, 70*b*, 83
HCAs (heterocyclic antidepressants), 233, 234*t*
Headache
    autonomic dysreflexia and, 278
    in stroke, 217, 218
    in TBI, 258–259
Head injury. *See also* Spinal cord injuries; Traumatic brain
    injury
    bladder management and, 126
    bowel management and, 131
    closed, 255
    Parkinson's disease and, 355
    sexual issues and, 165, 168–170
Health
    belief model, 182, 183*f*
    disparities, 374, 415
    domains (ICF model), 34–35, 35*f*
    within illness concept, 38–39, 42
    literacy, 177, 178–179, 178*b*
    promotion. *See* Education of clients and families;
        Well-being
Health Insurance Portability and Accountability Act (HIPAA),
    300
Health maintenance organizations (HMOs), 405–406, 406*f*
Health-related quality of life, 206. *See also* Quality of life
Healthy People 2010: Objectives for Improving Health (U.S.
    Department of Health and Human Services), 14, 16, 20*b*,
    59, 178
Hearing impairment. *See* Auditory impairment
Heart
    attack. *See* Myocardial infarction
    disease. *See* Cardiovascular problems
    failure (HF), 332, 333–334, 334*b*, 336
    rhythm abnormalities, 236–237
Height and weight assessment, 88, 89*b*, 95
Hemiparesis, 221
Hemiplegia, 221, 223, 241

Hemispatial inattention, 150*b*, 151–152, 225
Hemodialysis, 360
Hemorrhage. *See* Bleeding
Hemorrhagic brain injuries, 258
Hemorrhagic stroke, 216, 217. *See also* Stroke
Heparin/heparinoids, 236, 288
Heterocyclic antidepressants (HCAs), 233, 234*t*
Heterotopic ossification, 278, 324
HF (heart failure), 332, 333–334. *See also* Cardiovascular
    problems
Hip. *See also* Joints and joint replacement
    arthroplasty, 286
    precautions, 289
HIPAA (Health Insurance Portability and Accountability Act),
    300
Hippotherapy, 462–463, 462*f*
Hispanic populations
    amputation in, 297
    CKD in, 361
    health disparities and, 374
    SCI in, 270
    stroke in, 216
History and physical examination. *See also* Assessment
    amputation, 301
    bowel management, 132
    joint replacement, 288
    neurological disorders, 352
    skin integrity, 104
    stroke, 217, 218*t*, 224, 233
History of disease. *See* Genetics
History of rehabilitation
    attitude toward disability and, 32
    interdisciplinary team and, 1, 51–52, 52*b*
    joint replacement, 283
    life care planning, 472
    payment systems and. *See* Payment systems
    rehabilitation nursing, 3–6, 4–5*t*
HMOs (health maintenance organizations), 405–406, 406*f*
Holistic care. *See also* Animal-assisted therapy; Caring, art of;
    Interdisciplinary teams
    adaptation and, 39, 42
    culture and. *See* Cultural issues
    interdisciplinary model and, 54
    philosophy of rehabilitation and, 1
    in polytrauma, 321, 327
    principles of rehabilitation and, 6, 8
    role of rehabilitation nurses and, 9–10
    Rusk on, 4
    spirituality and, 201–202, 204, 206–207, 211
Homan's sign, 236
Home health care rehabilitation
    nurses, 66
    payment systems and, 410
    setting for care, 23–24
Homonymous hemianopsia, 225
HOPE spiritual assessment tool, 206–207
Horses in therapy, 462–463, 462*f*
Hospice, 453

Hospitals
    hospital-acquired conditions, 100
    information on, 192
Hospital Survey and Construction Act (1946), 5t
H₂ blocking agents, 167, 168t
Human-animal bond. *See* Animal-assisted therapy
Human sexual response, 165. *See also* Sexuality and disability
Humor, benefits of, 209, 209b
Huntington's disease, 344–345, 345t, 349, 351, 357b
Hydration. *See* Fluids
Hydrocolloid dressings, 111, 112t
Hydrogel dressings, 111, 113t
Hydrogenated fatty acids, 85
Hydronephrosis, 128, 128f
Hyperalgesia, 279
Hyperkinesia, 150b, 157
Hyperlipidemia, 219, 246
Hyperosmotics, 133
Hyperreflexia. *See* Autonomic dysreflexia
Hypersomnia, 238, 239
Hypertension. *See also* Cardiovascular problems
    AAT and, 464–465
    in autonomic dysreflexia, 129–130, 278
    incidence of, 332
    in older adults, 441
    stroke and, 90, 216, 217, 218t, 219, 246
    in TBI, 258
Hypnotics, 239, 239t
Hypogeusia, 442
Hyposmia, 442
Hypotension, 257, 278–279
Hypotonic cerebral palsy, 422
Hypoxia/hypoxemia, 216, 257, 333

I

IADLs. *See* Instrumental Activities of Daily Living
ICF. *See* International Classification of Functioning, Disability and Health
ICH (intracerebral hemorrhage), 217, 218
IDEA. *See* Individuals with Disabilities Act
Identity. *See* Body image issues; Changes with chronic illness/disability
IDTs. *See* Interdisciplinary teams
IEDs (improvised explosive devices), 318, 319
IHS (Indian Health Service), 411
Illness mode, 386. *See also* Chronic illness/disease, defined; Chronicity
Immune system. *See also* Autoimmune disorders
    aging and, 438–439, 443
        immune-mediated central demyelination, 344
        immunization and neurological disorders, 346, 350
        skin integrity and immunosuppression, 102, 103t, 109
Impact analysis, 24, 24t
Impaired physical mobility diagnosis, 145, 316. *See also* Mobility
Impairment, defined, 380. *See also specific impairments*
Implantable devices, 282–283
Impotence. *See* Erectile dysfunction

Improvised explosive devices (IEDs), 318, 319
Impulsivity, 150b, 155–157, 156t
Incapacitation determination, 395–396
Incidence. *See* Epidemiology and mortality statistics
Incidental pain, defined, 117
Incomplete syndromes (SCI), 273–274, 281
Incongruence, cultural, 383
Incontinence. *See also* Bladder management; Bowel management
    in older adults, 19, 123, 123t, 442, 448–449, 451t
    skin wounds and, 101, 114
    stroke and, 232
    urinary, defined, 122
Incontinence-associated dermatitis, 101, 114
Independence. *See also* Independent living; Self-care
    adaptation and, 7, 40
    bladder management and, 126, 127
    in children with disabilities, 422–423, 425
    as goal of rehabilitation, 2, 2t, 382
    mobility/function and, 90, 136, 137, 137t
    of older adult patients, 69
    SCI and, 272–273, 274
Independent living. *See also* Community reintegration/reentry
    model, 31
    sexuality and disability in, 168–171, 168b, 169t, 170f, 171b
Indian Health Service (IHS), 411
Indicators of outcome. *See* Outcome evaluation (management, measurement, research)
Individualism, attitudes on, 381
Individualized education plans, 419
Individual model of disability, 16
Individuals with Disabilities Act (IDEA 1975), 397t, 398
Individual with a disability, defined (ADA), 17. *See also* Disability, defined
Indwelling catheters, 127, 275–276
Infants. *See* Pediatric rehabilitation
Infarction. *See* Myocardial infarction; Stroke
Infection
    cancer and, 364
    in joint replacements, 287–288
    neurological disorders and, 346, 350
    polytrauma and, 319, 325, 326
    skin integrity and, 102, 103t, 110–111
    transient incontinence and, 123, 124t
    urinary tract. *See* Urinary tract infection
Inflammatory phase of wound healing, 103
Informed consent, 387. *See also* Ethical considerations
Informed decisions, 25. *See also* Education of clients and families
Inherited conditions. *See* Genetics
Inner strength, 205
Innervation, 345
Inorgasmia, 165
Inpatient Rehabilitation Facilities (IRFs), 5t, 6, 409. *See also* Settings for care
Insight impairments, 150b, 155
Insomnia, 238, 239, 259
Institute of Medicine (IOM), 75, 207, 412–413

Instrumental Activities of Daily Living (IADLs)
  adaptive equipment and, 144
  definition of disability and, 15, 15t
Insurance. *See* Payment systems
Integrity versus despair (developmental stage), 440
Integumentary poststroke complications, 241
Intercessory prayer, 204
Intercourse, sexual. *See* Sexuality and disability
Interdisciplinary practice model, 53–54, 54f
Interdisciplinary teams (IDTs), 51–62. *See also* Holistic care;
    Nursing roles; *specific team members*
  in amputation care, 300–303, 300t, 302f
  benefits and challenges, 55
  in bladder/bowel management, 232
  caring/spirituality and, 206–207
  characteristics of effective, 58, 58b
  in cognition/behavior improvement, 148, 158
  competence of, 58–59
  in educating clients, 177, 185–186, 191
  evaluating effectiveness of, 59–60
  goals of, 2–3, 2t
  history and background, 1, 51–52, 52b
  holistic approaches of, 8
  home care and, 66
  in joint replacement care, 288
  in life care planning, 473–474
  members of/roles in, 2, 10, 55–58, 56–57t, 57b
  nutrition management and, 96–97, 96–97t
  in polytrauma, 327–328, 327b
  safe lift protocols and, 143
  in settings for care, 23
  sexual issues and, 162–163
  skin integrity education, 117
  in TBI care, 265, 265t
  team models, 53–55, 53–54f, 53b
Intermittent catheterization, 126–127, 275–276
Internal urethral sphincter, 122
International Academy of Life Care Planners, 472
International Classification of Functioning, Disability and
    Health (ICF), 34–35, 35f, 40, 42
International Normalized Ratio, 237
Interpretation, defined, 29. *See also* Frameworks for chronic
    illness, disability, adaptation, and coping
Interventions. *See specific disabilities/diseases*
Intervertebral disk problems, 131t, 132
Interviewing. *See* Communication; Motivational interviewing
Intimacy, defined, 161. *See also* Sexuality and disability
Intracerebral hemorrhage (ICH), 217, 218
Intracranial pressure, 217
Intraparenchymal hemorrhage, 217, 258
Intravenous nutrition. *See* Parenteral nutrition
Intraventricular hemorrhage, 217, 258
Intrinsic load, 181, 181f
IOM. *See* Institute of Medicine
IRFs. *See* Inpatient Rehabilitation Facilities
Iron requirements/supplements, 86, 89, 91, 95, 133, 133t
Irrigation of wounds, 110
Ischemic stroke, 216–217. *See also* Stroke

J
Jobs. *See* Nursing roles; Vocational rehabilitation; Work settings
Joint Commission
  on cultural issues, 375
  on falls prevention, 139–140
  on IDTs, 52, 52b, 60
  on nutrition, 88
  on spiritual care, 201–202
Joints and joint replacement, 283–295
  assessment, 288
  complications, 287–288
  implications for total replacement, 284–286
  outcome evaluation for replacement, 24, 291, 291b
  pathophysiology, 284
  prosthetics, 287
  rehabilitation modalities, 288–291, 290f, 295
  stroke effects on, 222–223
  surgical approaches to replacement, 286–287
Judgment impairments, 155
Justice principle, 24, 363, 387

K
Karnofsky Performance Status scale, 364–365, 365t
Kegel exercises, 125–126, 126b
Keppra. *See* Levetiracetam
Kidneys
  anatomy/physiology, 121, 122f, 446
  hydronephrosis, 128, 128f
  kidney stones, 129
  polytrauma injury, 319, 319t
  renal disease, 359–363, 362t
  replacement therapy (KRT), 359–363
  spina bifida and function of, 424–425
  transplantation, 361
Knee. *See also* Joints and joint replacement
  arthroplasty, 286
  immobilizer, 301
  prosthetic, 306, 306f
Knowledge deficit, 145, 316. *See also* Education of clients and
    families
Knowles adult learning theory, 184, 184b
KRT (kidney replacement therapy), 359–363

L
Laboratory nutritional tests, 88–89, 89b
Lacunar infarction, 216–217, 220t
Language. *See also* Communication
  barriers, 380
  brain function and, 148–149
  conception of disability and, 32
  culture and, 376, 380, 381–382
  impairments. *See* Speech and language impairments
Lateral scoot transfer, 142
Latex allergy and spina bifida, 425, 444
Laws. *See* Legal issues
LCP. *See* Life care plan (LCP) and planning
LDL cholesterol. *See* Low-density-lipoprotein (LDL) cholesterol
Leadership. *See* Manager nursing roles

Learning. *See* Competencies, certification, and education; Education of clients and families

Legal issues. *See also* Advocacy; Competencies, certification, and education; Ethical considerations; *specific legislation*
  documentation and, 192
  end-of-life decisions. *See* End-of-life decisions
  in financing of healthcare. *See* Payment systems
  guardianship, 394–396, 395t
  legislative action, 381
  life care planning and, 472
  in pediatric care, 398, 419
  pressure ulcer incidence and, 100
  rehabilitation legislation, 3–4, 4–5t, 6b, 17, 67, 318, 381
  right to life issues and legislation, 396–399, 397t

Leininger
  Culture Care Theory, 376–378, 376b, 377f
  Sunrise Enabler, 377, 377f

Leisure activities poststroke, 248
Lethargic state, 149, 150b
Levels of assist, 137, 137t
Levels of consciousness, 149, 150b
Levetiracetam (Keppra), 240, 240t, 353, 353t
Levitra (vardenafil), 167
Levodopa, 90
Lewin's Change Theory, 184, 184t, 202, 211
Lewy bodies, 349
Liaison nurse, 66–67
Licensed nurses (practical and vocational), 64. *See also* Competencies, certification, and education

Life care plan (LCP) and planning, 471–478
  defined, 71, 471–472
  developing an LCP, 476, 477t
  history of, 472
  nursing roles in, 472–474
  preparation for practice in, 474–476, 475t, 476b

Life changes and losses, 36. *See also* Changes with chronic illness/disability
Life narrative. *See* Narrative
Life span and disability culture, 381
Lifestyle factors. *See also* Adaptation; Prevention; *specific factors (e.g., Nutrition)*
  in cancer, 364
  in cardiovascular disease and stroke, 89, 335–336, 335t, 338, 342
  in chronic disease/illness, 17, 179
  in CKD, 361
  in pulmonary disease, 338, 340, 342
  in sexual issues, 162, 167
  in weight control, 88

Life thread model, 43
Lifting. *See* Transfers
Limbs. *See* Amputation; Joints and joint replacement
Liners (for residual limbs), 302, 302f
Linoleic acid, 85
Lioresal. *See* Baclofen
Lipid-lowering agents, 167, 168t
Lipids, 85, 89
Listening. *See* Caring, art of; Communication
Literacy, health, 177, 178–179, 178b

Lived experiences, 381
Living loss, 39–40
Living wills, 390, 392, 392b
LMNs. *See* Lower motor neurons (LMNs)
LOC. *See* Loss of consciousness
Locked-in syndrome, 218, 220t
Locus of control theory, 183
Long-term memory, 154, 180
Long-term/subacute settings for care, 23, 171
Loss. *See also* Grief and grieving
  ambiguous, 321
  of the assumptive world. *See* Assumptive world theory
  chronic illness/disability as, 29, 35–36, 39–40, 44, 44f
Loss of consciousness (LOC), 258, 259, 322. *See also* Consciousness
Lou Gehrig's disease. *See* Amyotrophic lateral sclerosis
Loving care. *See* Caring, art of
Low-density-lipoprotein (LDL) cholesterol, 85–86, 89
Lower motor neurons (LMNs)
  diseases of, 348, 349
  injury, 271–273, 274
Lung cancer, 339t, 341–342. *See also* Pulmonary disease/complications
Lyrica (pregabalin), 240, 279, 353, 353t

M
Maceration, 105, 111
Macronutrients, 85. *See also specific macronutrients*
Mafenide acetate, 114, 115t
Maggots, debridement using, 110–111
Magnetic resonance imaging (MRI) techniques, 347, 347f
Magnet Recognition Program (ANA), 64, 73
Mainstreaming, 381
Males. *See* Gender and gender issues
Malnutrition, 84, 87–88, 233
Managed care, 52, 53b, 410–411. *See also* Payment systems
Management. *See specific disabilities/diseases*
Manager nursing roles, 69, 72–74. *See also* Case managers/management
Manual muscle test, 137, 138t, 146
Marketing, nursing roles in, 66–67
Masturbation, dealing with in public, 172
Maturation
  of children, 419
  phase of wound healing, 104
Mauk model of poststroke recovery, 43, 44t
Meaning. *See* Reconstruction of meaning; Spirituality
Mechanical debridement, 109–110
Mechanical lifts, 143
Mechanics of the body, 140–142
Medicaid/Medicare. *See also* Payment systems
  history and description of, 5t, 6, 408–410
  institutionalization vs. community care, 399
  Medigap, 407–408
  older adults and, 453
  pressure ulcer costs and, 100
  reform, 415
  supply/demand for healthcare and, 403

Medical Library Association, 191
Medical model, 30–31, 31f, 53, 53f
Medical power of attorney, 392–393
Medications. *See also specific medications*
  for atrial fibrillation, 236–237
  bladder control, 124–125, 127, 128
  bowel management, 133–134, 133t, 275
  CAM and, 378
  for cardiac disease, 334, 335t
  for CKD, 360, 361
  for CPSP, 240, 241t
  delirium and, 151, 158
  for depression. *See* Antidepressants
  dysphagia and, 92
  falls and fractures and, 138, 139, 431
  immunosuppression, pressure ulcers and, 109
  mood and, 157
  for muscular dystrophy, 428
  for neurological disorders, 353–355, 353–354t
  nutrition in elderly and, 95
  older adults and, 441, 449
  pain, 117, 240, 279, 304, 366
  for Parkinson's disease, 90
  for pulmonary disease, 339–340
  in SCI, 271, 275, 278, 279
  seizure, 239–240, 240t
  sexual issues and, 166, 167, 168t, 172
  for spasticity, 222–223, 277–278
  stroke risk and, 217
  for SWDs, 239, 239t
  in TBI, 262–263
  topical wound, 114, 115–116t
  transient incontinence and, 123, 124t
  for venous thromboembolism, 236
Medigap, 407–408
Melatonin receptor agonists, 239, 239t
Memory. *See also* Cognition and behavior
  aging and, 448
  assessment, 229
  impairments, 150–151, 154–155, 158–159, 169, 227–228. *See also* Amnesia; Delirium/dementia
  learning and, 179–181, 180f, 189–190, 196
  remediation of deficits in, 243
Men. *See* Gender and gender issues
Mental illness/disability. *See also* Psychological well-being
  defined, 15, 16t, 18
  Olmstead decision and, 398–399
  psychiatric advance directives and, 393–394
Merck Institute of Aging and Health (MIAH), 18–19, 20b
Metabolism, 86. *See also* Nutrition
Metacognition. *See* Executive control impairments
Methylphenidate (Ritalin), 354, 354
MI. *See* Myocardial infarction
MIAH (Merck Institute of Aging and Health), 18–19, 20b
Micronutrients, 84, 85, 85t. *See also specific micronutrients*
Micturition reflex, 122. *See also* Bladder management
Mild brain injury, 259, 323, 323t
Military patients. *See* Veterans and war

Mineral nutrient requirements, 86, 91
Mini Mental State Examination, 228–229, 228t
Minority cultures, defined, 374. *See also* Cultural issues
Minority group model, 31
Mistreatment. *See* Abuse and neglect
Mitrofanoff appendicovesicostomy, 127
MMC (myelomeningocele). *See* Spina bifida
Mobility, 136–147. *See also* Activity limitations; Exercise; Functional limitations
  amputation and, 301, 312. *See also* Prosthetics
  assessment, 137–138, 137–138t
  CKD and, 362–363
  CP and, 421–422
  defined, 136
  diagnosis and outcomes, 145–146
  falls and. *See* Falls
  goals of therapy, 140, 140t, 141f
  interventions, 140–142, 145–146
  of joints. *See* Joints and joint replacement
  muscular dystrophy and, 426–427
  neurological disorders and, 354, 355–356t
  nurse's role, 145
  safe patient handling, 141, 142–145
  SCI and, 272–273
  sexual issues and, 169, 169t, 170f
  skin integrity and, 102, 103t, 104, 108t, 276
  spina bifida and, 424
  stroke and, 221–227, 222b, 224t, 226f, 226t, 241, 246–248
  TBI and, 258, 263, 263t
  transient incontinence and, 123, 124t
Modafinil (Provigil), 239, 354, 354t
Model, defined, 29. *See also* Frameworks for chronic illness, disability, adaptation, and coping; *specific models*
Moderate brain injury, 259, 323, 323t
Modified Ashworth Scale, 222, 222b
Moisture and skin integrity, 102, 103t, 104, 108t, 111
Moment of impact injuries, 256–257
Monounsaturated fatty acids (MUFAs), 85–86
Mood. *See* Affect
Morbidity. *See* Epidemiology and mortality statistics
Mortality. *See* Death
Motivational interviewing, 185, 185b, 192
Motor control. *See* Mobility
Motor injuries/disorders. *See specific injuries and disorders*
Motor neurons, 345. *See also* Degenerative neurological disorders
Moving patients. *See* Transfers
MRI (magnetic resonance imaging) techniques, 347, 347f
MS. *See* Multiple sclerosis
MUFAs (monounsaturated fatty acids), 85–86
Multidisciplinary model, 53, 53f
Multiple sclerosis (MS)
  aging with, 445
  assessment of, 352
  bladder dysfunction and, 124, 125
  bowel dysfunction and, 131, 131t, 132
  depression and, 203
  diagnoses, 354, 355t

education of clients/families on, 354–355, 357*b*

incidence of, 345, 345*t*

interventions and management, 353

nutrition and, 89, 90*b*

pathophysiology of, 344, 345, 346–347, 347*f*, 350–351

sexual issues and, 165, 169–170, 169*t*

Mupirocin calcium, 114, 116*t*

Muscle

atrophy, 349, 350, 352

relaxants, 133, 133*t*, 279, 353, 353*t*. *See also specific relaxants*

spasms. *See* Spasticity

tests, 137, 138*t*, 146

Muscular dystrophy, 426–427

Musculoskeletal deficits/disorders. *See* Mobility; Neurological conditions; *specific disorders*

Musculoskeletal pain, 279

Musculoskeletal rehabilitation

joint replacement, 288–291, 295

in older adults, 442

stroke, 241–242

Myasthenia gravis

assessment, 352–353

education of clients/family on, 354–356, 357*b*

pathophysiology of, 344, 345, 345*t*, 346, 346*f*

risk factors and warning signs, 350–351

Myelomeningocele (MMC). *See* Spina bifida

Myocardial infarction (MI). *See also* Cardiovascular problems

aging and, 441

CAD and, 332–333, 333*f*

embolic stroke and, 217, 218*t*, 236

sexual issues and, 168, 168*b*

N

Narcotics, 279

Narrative

in models of adaptation, 43–44

repair, 40

representation, 33

spiritual care and, 205

Nasogastric (NG) tube, 93, 94, 237

National Academy of Certified Case Managers, 71

National Alliance for Caregiving (NAC), 244, 245*t*

National Aphasia Association, 244, 245*t*

National Association of Clinical Nurse Specialists, 79, 83

National Association of Professional Geriatric Care Managers, 69, 70, 70*b*

National Cancer Institute, 2

National Cholesterol Adult Treatment Panel, 89

National Family Caregiver Association (NFCA), 244, 245*t*

National Guidelines Clearing House, 146

National Institute for Occupational Safety and Health, 143

National Institute of Neurological Disorders and Stroke, 218

National Institute of Nursing Research (NINR), 69, 77, 83

National Institute on Aging (NIA), 19, 19*b*

National Institutes of Health (NIH), 338

National Kidney Foundation, 361

National League for Nursing (NLN), 75, 83

National Organization of Nurse Practitioner Faculties, 79, 83

National Patient Safety Foundation (Partnership for Clear Health Communication), 178, 178*b*

National Pressure Ulcer Advisory Panel (NPUAP), 91, 104–105, 109, 117

National Stroke Association (NSA), 218, 244, 245*t*

Native Americans

cardiac disease in, 332

CKD in, 361

IHS and, 411

Nausea

in stroke, 217

in TBI, 258

NCA. *See* National Alliance for Caregiving

Necrotic tissue, 109–111, 289–290. *See also* Pressure ulcers

Negative pressure wound therapy, 114

Neglect. *See* Abuse and neglect

Neglect syndrome. *See* Hemispatial inattention

Nerves/neurons

blocks for spasticity, 223, 357

disorders of. *See* Neurological conditions

stimulation. *See* Electrical stimulation

swallowing and, 91–92

Neural tube defects. *See* Spina bifida

Neurodevelopmental treatment, 241–242

Neurogenic bladder dysfunction, 122–123, 124–125, 125*f*, 126*t*, 128

Neurogenic bowel, 130–134, 131–133*t*, 133*b*, 274–275, 275*b*

Neurological conditions, 344–358. *See also* Cognition and behavior; *specific neurological injuries/disorders*

aging and, 442

assessment, 352–353

in children, 425–428, 426*t*

dysphagia and, 92

education of clients/family, 354–356, 357*b*

ethical issues, 356–357

incidence/prevalence, 345, 345*t*

interventions/management, 353–354, 353–356*t*

motor speech disorders and, 152

nutritional needs, 89–91, 90*b*

pathophysiology, 345–350, 346–347*f*

prevention, 351

risk factors and warning signs, 350–351

sexual issues and, 165, 169, 170

TBI and, 258, 259, 263, 263*t*

Neuromuscular disorders, 425–426, 426*t*. *See also specific disorders*

Neurontin (gabapentin), 240, 240*t*, 279, 353, 353*t*

Neuropathic pain, 116–117, 240–241, 279

Neuroplasticity, 219–220

Neuropsychologists, 55, 56*t*

New York University College of Nursing. *See* The Hartford Institute for Geriatric Nursing (New York University College of Nursing)

NFCA. *See* National Family Caregiver Association

NG tube. *See* Nasogastric (NG) tube

NIA (National Institute on Aging), 19, 19*b*

NIH (National Institutes of Health), 338

NINR. *See* National Institute of Nursing Research

Nitrates, 334, 335*t*

Nitro-paste/pills, 278

NLN (National League for Nursing), 75, 83

N-methyl-D-aspartate antagonists, 240, 241*t*

Nociceptive pain, 116–117

Nonadherent dry dressings, 111, 113*t*

Nonadherent moist dressings, 111, 112*t*

Nonessential proteins, 85

Nonmalfeasance principle, 387

Nonstochastic forces in aging, 438

Normality, concepts of, 31

Norton scale, 104

Nosocomial pneumonia, 237–238

NPs. *See* Nurse practitioners

NPUAP. *See* National Pressure Ulcer Advisory Panel

NRIs (selective noradrenaline reuptake inhibitors), 233, 234*t*, 240

NSA. *See* National Stroke Association

Nurse-patient communication. *See* Communication

Nurse practitioners (NPs), 77–79, 96. *See also* Advanced practice registered nurses

Nurse-sensitive indicators, 24, 24*t*

Nursing homes. *See* Settings for care; Skilled nursing facilities (SNFs)

Nursing roles, 63–83. *See also* Competencies, certification, and education; Interdisciplinary teams
    advanced practice nurses, 77–80
    in advocacy, 64–69, 71, 78–79
    in amputation, 300, 300*t*
    in cancer rehabilitation, 365
    care provider, 9–10, 9*t*, 19–20, 64
    case manager, 54*f*, 55, 56*t*, 70–72
    educator role, 74–76, 193
    in elder abuse prevention, 454–455
    geriatric rehabilitation nurse, 19–20, 69–70, 70*b*
    in health literacy, 178–179
    home health/home care, 66
    in interdisciplinary team, 53–54*f*, 55, 56–57*t*, 58, 59
    in life care planning, 472–474
    manager/administration, 72–74
    mobility and, 145
    nurse liaison, 66–67
    nursing culture and interventions, 382–383
    in nutrition management, 97
    in pain management, 117
    pediatric rehabilitation nurse, 67–68, 83, 431–432
    in policy-making process, 412
    in polytrauma, 319, 321, 327
    rehabilitation across life span, 67
    researcher, 76–77
    sexual issues and, 162–163
    teaching and advocacy, 64–66

Nutrients, essential, 84–86, 86*t*, 94

Nutrition, 84–99. *See also* Lifestyle factors
    aging and, 95–96, 445
    altered states of, 87–88, 88*f*
    assessment, 88–89, 89*b*, 105
    basic, 84–86, 86*t*
    CAM and, 378, 379*t*
    cancer and, 364
    cardiac disease and, 335, 335*t*
    cleft lip/palate and, 429
    constipation prevention and, 133
    dysphagia and, 91–93, 92*b*, 233
    educating patients/families, 97
    enteral, 91, 93–94, 94*t*
    interdisciplinary management, 96–97, 96–97*t*, 96*f*
    parenteral, 91, 94–95
    polytrauma and, 325
    rehabilitation situations and, 89–91, 90*b*
    SCI and, 275
    skin integrity and, 102, 103*t*, 104, 105, 108, 108*t*
    stroke and, 89, 90, 233, 237
    TBI and, 263, 263*t*
    water, 87

O

Obesity and weight management
    amputation and, 298
    cancer and, 364
    in cardiac disease and stroke, 89, 217–219, 218*t*, 335–336, 335*t*
    CKD and, 361
    neurological conditions and, 89–90
    nutrition and, 87–88, 88*f*, 89*b*, 95
    sexual function and, 167
    spina bifida and, 425

Objectives, 188, 188*b*. *See also* Goals of rehabilitation

OBRA (Omnibus Budget Reconciliation Act of 1981 and 1989), 419

Obtunded state, 149, 150*b*

Occipital lobe, 256, 256*f*, 257*t*

Occupational therapists (OTs) and therapy
    amputation and, 300, 300*t*
    as interdisciplinary team members, 53–54*f*, 55, 56*t*
    joint replacement and, 293
    mobility/function promotion and, 136
    muscular dystrophy and, 428
    nutrition management and, 96
    sexual issues and, 162
    stroke and, 222, 225

Ocular impairment. *See* Visual impairment

OEF. *See* Operation Enduring Freedom

OIF. *See* Operation Iraqi Freedom

Older adults. *See* Gerontological rehabilitation

Olmstead decision (1999), 397*t*, 398–399

Omega 3 fatty acids, 85

Omega 6 (linoleic acid), 85

Omnibus Budget Reconciliation Act (OBRA 1981, 1989), 419

One Health concept, 460

Operation Enduring Freedom (OEF), 317–318, 327

Operation Iraqi Freedom (OIF), 317–318, 321

Opioids/opiates
    amputation and, 304
    for cancer pain, 366
    constipation and, 133, 133*t*

for CPSP, 240, 241*t*
    sexual dysfunction and, 167, 168*t*
Oppressed minority model, 31
Oppression. *See* Discrimination
Optimism, 206, 207
Oral swallowing phase, 92–93
Orgasm, in triphasic sexual response, 165. *See also* Sexuality
    and disability
Orientation. *See* Disorientation
Orthopedic injuries, 324–325. *See also* Amputation; Joints and
    joint replacement
Orthostasis, 278–279
Orthotics, 242
Osteoarthritis, 288–289. *See also* Arthritis
OTs. *See* Occupational therapists (OTs) and therapy
Outcome evaluation (management, measurement, research).
        See also Efficacy of care; Evidence-based practice
    in amputation, 311–314
    for cancer, 367
    in cardiac and pulmonary rehabilitation, 340, 342
    certification and, 64
    for CKD, 363
    of client education, 178, 192–193
    for interdisciplinary team, 59–60
    for joint replacement, 24, 291, 291*b*
    of mobility, 145–146
    in pediatric rehabilitation, 419–420
    quality measures, 412–414
    for SCI, 272–273
    in settings for care, 24, 24*t*
    spirituality and, 204–205, 207, 209–210
    for stroke, 24, 220–221
    in terminal illness, 369
Outcome measures, 412
Outpatient care. *See* Community settings for care
Overflow incontinence, 123
Overnutrition, 87–88, 88*f*
Oxybutynin chloride (Ditropan), 128
Oxygen, lack of. *See* Cardiovascular problems; Hypoxia/
    hypoxemia
Oxygen therapy
    for breathing disorders, 239
    mobility and, 143–144
    for pulmonary disease, 339–340
    sexual issues and, 169, 170*f*
    for skin wounds, 114

P
Packing strip dressings, 111, 113*t*
Pad dressings, 111, 113*t*
Pain and pain management
    in amputation, 304, 313–314
    CAM and, 378, 379*t*
    in cancer patients, 364, 366
    for joint replacement, 288
    in neurological disorders, 350, 354*t*
    in polytrauma, 325, 326–327
    psychosocial/spiritual factors in, 208
    in SCI patients, 208, 277–278, 279–280, 281

sexual issues and, 165, 165*t*, 168
    skin integrity and, 110, 116–117
    in stroke patients, 222, 223, 240–241, 241*t*
    in TBI patients, 258
Palliative care, 360, 366, 367–369, 453
Paperwork. *See* Documentation
Paralympic, 382
Paralysis. *See* Spinal cord injuries; *specific types of*
Paralyzed Veterans of America, 130, 130*b*
Paraplegia
    bowel dysfunction and, 131*t*, 132
    defined, 272
    incidence of, 270
    nutrition and, 88, 90
    skin integrity and, 9
Parasympathetic nerves, 122
Parenteral nutrition, 91, 94–95, 98
Parents. *See* Family
Parietal lobe, 256, 256*f*, 257*t*
Parkinson's Disease. *See also* Delirium/dementia
    assessment, 352
    bladder dysfunction and, 124
    bowel dysfunction and, 131, 131*t*
    diagnoses, 354, 356*t*
    education of clients/families on, 355, 357*b*
    genetics and, 351
    incidence of, 345, 345*t*
    interventions and management, 353
    nutrition and, 90, 90*b*
    pathophysiology of, 344, 349–350, 351
    sexual issues and, 165, 169–170
Participation (ICF model), 34–35, 35*f*
Partnership for Clear Health Communication (National Patient
    Safety Foundation), 178, 178*b*
Passive range of motion, 137, 290–291
Pastoral care. *See* Spirituality
Pathophysiology
    cancer, 364
    cardiac diseases, 332–334
    CKD, 360–361
    cleft lip/palate, 428–429
    joint replacement, 284
    neurological disorders, 344–350, 346–347*f*
    neuromuscular disorders, 425–426
    pulmonary diseases, 340, 341
    spina bifida, 423
    terminal illness, 368
    traumatic brain injury, 256–258
    urinary tract, 122–125, 123–124*t*, 125*f*. *See also* Incontinence
Patient history. *See* History and physical examination
Patient Protection and Affordable Care Act (2010), 67, 403
Patients. *See also* Education of clients and families; *specific*
        populations
    as interdisciplinary team members, 51–54, 53–54*f*, 55, 59
Patient Self-Determination Act (1990), 390–391
Payment systems, 402–417. *See also* Financial issues; Medicaid/
    Medicare
    for acute rehabilitation, 23
    assessment and accountability, 403

Payment systems (*cont.*)
  Blue Cross/Blue Shield, 405
  COBRA, 407
  for community-based care, 23–24
  cost containment, 403
  documentation and, 192
  employer-funded insurance, 405, 407
  future of, 415
  growth and development, 403
  healthcare financing overview, 403–404, 405*f*
  health policy and, 402–403, 411–415
  HMOs, 405–406, 406*f*
  managed care, 52, 53*b*, 406–407
  Medicaid and Medicare. *See* Medicaid/Medicare
  Medigap, 407–408
  PPS, 5*t*, 6, 410
  pre-20th century, 404
  private financing, 403, 404, 404*f*
  public financing, 404, 404*f*, 408
  reform attempts, 408
  75% rule, 409–410, 410*b*
  for special groups, 410–411
  stakeholders in, 412, 413*t*
  TEFRA and, 409
  uninsured and, 411
  workers' compensation, 405
PCS. *See* Postconcussion syndrome
PE. *See* Pulmonary embolism
Pedagogy, 184, 184*b*. *See also* Competencies, certification, and
    education; Education of clients and families
Pediatric Nursing Certification Board, 68
Pediatric rehabilitation, 418–436
  AAT in, 463, 463*f*
  for amputation, 297, 298, 309
  for brachial plexus injury, 431
  for CF, 341
  child development and, 419–420
  for CLD, 429–430
  for cleft lip/palate, 428–429
  community agencies and, 432–433, 432*b*
  coping strategies and, 203–204
  for CP, 421–423
  definition of population, 418
  family-centered care in, 420, 420*t*
  insurance for children. *See* Medicaid/Medicare; State
    children's health insurance program
  legal issues in, 398, 419
  for neuromuscular disorders, 425–428, 426*t*
  nutrition and, 87, 95, 97
  pediatric rehabilitation nurses, 67–68, 83, 435–436
  sexual development of children, 163–164, 164*t*
  for spina bifida, 423–425
  for TBI, 256, 322–323
  transdisciplinary model and, 55
PEEK readiness to learn assessment, 186, 186*b*
Peer
  groups, 382
  visitors, 300

PEG tube. *See* Percutaneous endoscopic gastrostomy (PEG)
    tube
Pelvic floor exercises, 125–126, 126*b*
Pemoline (Cylert), 354, 354*t*
People with disabilities, defined, 14–15, 17
Perceived Support From God Scale, 205–206
Perceptions. *See* Beliefs; Sensory perception
Percutaneous endoscopic gastrostomy (PEG) tube, 93–94, 237
Percutaneous endoscopic jejunostomy tube, 94
Performance standards. *See* Competencies, certification, and
    education
Peritoneal dialysis, 360–361
Perseveration, 150*b*, 151
Personal factors (ICF model), 34–35, 35*f*
Personality disorders, 448
Personal tragedy model, 31
Perspectives model. *See* Shifting perspectives model
Petrolatum gauze dressings, 111, 112*t*
Pet visitation programs, 460. *See also* Animal-assisted therapy
Phantom limb pain, 304, 313–314
Pharmacological agents. *See* Medications
Pharyngeal swallowing phase, 93
Phenol injections, 223
Phenomenological approaches, 33, 39. *See also* Psychosocial
    issues
Phenytoin (Dilantin), 240, 240*t*
Philosophy of rehabilitation, 1–2, 4, 205–206
Photography, in assessment, 105
Physiatrists/physicians
  acute rehabilitation and, 23
  amputation and, 300, 300*t*
  APRNs and, 78–79
  case managers and, 71
  in community reintegration, 246
  in IDTs, 51, 53–54*f*, 55, 56–57*t*, 58
  nutrition management and, 96
  sexual issues and, 162
Physical activity. *See* Exercise
Physical disability, defined, 15, 16*t*
Physical examination. *See* History and physical examination
Physical Medicine and Rehabilitation, 52
Physical therapists (PTs) and therapy
  amputation and, 300–302, 300*t*
  heterotopic ossification and, 278
  in interdisciplinary team member, 53–54*f*, 55, 56*t*
  joint replacement and, 288–289
  mobility/function promotion and, 136, 137, 140, 140*t*, 141*f*,
    142
  muscular dystrophy and, 432
  nutrition management and, 96
  sexual issues and, 162
  spasticity and, 222
  wound treatment and, 114
Physicians. *See* Physiatrists/physicians
Physiology. *See* Anatomy and physiology
Pineal gland, 256, 257*t*
Pituitary gland, 256, 257*t*
Planning. *See* Life care plan (LCP) and planning

PLISSIT model, 162, 280
Pneumonia and stroke, 237–238
Poikilothermia, 279
Point of service insurance plan, 411
Policy. *See* Legal issues
Polio. *See* Post-polio syndrome
Polypharmacy, 449
Polysaccharides, 85
Polytrauma, 317–331
    amputation and. *See* Amputation
    blast injuries, 317–318, 319, 319*t*
    burns and, 323–324, 323*b*, 324*t*
    centers, 5*t*, 6
    defined, 317
    IDTs and, 327–328, 327*b*
    LCPs and, 475
    military response to, 328
    nursing implications for, 326–327
    pain and, 325, 326–327
    PTSD and, 325
    rehabilitation center (PRC), 321
    sensory impairments and, 325
    as specialty area, 1
    system of care, 318–322, 319*t*
    TBI and, 317–319 322–323, 322*b*
    triad, 326
    wounds and, 325, 326
Polytrauma-TBI system of care, 318
Polyunsaturated fatty acids (PUFAs), 85
Positioning and amputation, 302–303
Postconcussion syndrome (PCS), 259, 323
Post-polio syndrome (PPS), 344–345, 345*t*, 350, 351, 352, 357*b*
Poststroke depression (PSD), 233–234, 234–235*t*, 239
Posttraumatic amnesia (PTA), 258, 259, 322
Posttraumatic stress disorder (PTSD), 258, 325, 326
Power of attorney, 392–393
PPS. *See* Post-polio syndrome; Prospective payment systems
Pragmatic behavior, 150*b*, 157
Prayer, 204, 205, 207, 207*b*. *See also* Spirituality
PRC (polytrauma rehabilitation center), 321
Prealbumin, 88–89, 89*b*
Predialysis, 360
Preferred provider organizations, 407
Pregabalin (Lyrica), 240, 279, 353, 353*t*
Pregnancy, nutrition during, 95
Prehension, 308
Premature ejaculation, 165
Preoral swallowing phase, 92
Presbycusis, 442
Presbyopia, 442
Pressure relief, 276
Pressure ulcers. *See also* Skin integrity
    assessment, 104–107, 106–107*t*
    care and treatment of, 108–116, 111*b*, 112–116*t*
    factors influencing, 101–103, 102–103*f*, 103*t*, 108, 108*t*
    geriatric syndromes and, 452–453, 455*t*
    nutrition and, 91
    pain management, 110, 116–117

phases of healing, 103–104
prevalence and cost of treating, 100–101
prevention of, 8–9, 100–101, 108, 108*t*
in stroke patients, 241
Prevention
    AAT and, 469, 469*b*
    of amputation, 298
    of autonomic dysreflexia, 278
    of cancer, 364
    of cardiovascular disease, 335–336
    for chronic illnesses, 17
    of CKD, 361
    of complications. *See* Complications
    of constipation, 132–133, 133*b*, 133*t*
    of COPD, 340
    educating clients on, 179, 179*t*
    of effects of immobility, 136
    of emotional/psychological problems, 203, 208–209, 209*b*
    health promotion and, 16
    life care planning and, 473
    of malnutrition with stroke, 233
    of neurological disorders, 351
    older adults and, 19
    of orthostasis, 279
    of secondary strokes, 219, 246
Primary appraisal, 37, 38
Primary injuries (brain), 256–257
Principles of rehabilitation, 6–9, 391. *See also* Goals of
        rehabilitation
Prior knowledge, 179–180, 180*f*, 186. *See also* Education of
        clients and families
Prior level of function, 137–138
Privacy
    amputation and, 299–300
    sexual issues and, 171, 172–173
ProAmatine, 279
Problem-focused behavior/coping strategies, 37, 203
Procedural memory, 154–155
Procedural pain, defined, 117
Process measures, 412
Professional geriatric care manager, 69
Professional practice. *See* Competencies, certification, and
        education; Ethical considerations; Evidence-based
        practice; Nursing roles
Professional subculture, 383
Proliferative phase of wound healing, 103–104
Proning and amputation, 302–303
Proprioception, 305
Proprioceptive neuromuscular facilitation, 242
Prospective payment systems (PPS), 5*t*, 6, 410
Prostate gland, 123
Prosthetics
    amputation and, 300*t*, 301, 303, 303*t*, 305–309, 305–309*f*
    for CLD, 430
    for joint replacement, 287
Protein requirements, 84–85, 88–89, 89*b*, 90, 91, 95
Provigil (modafinil), 239, 354, 354*t*
PSD. *See* Poststroke depression

Psychiatric advance directives, 393–394
Psychogenic erections, 281
Psychological well-being. *See also* Anxiety; Coping; Depression;
 Mental illness/disability; Psychosocial issues; Spirituality;
 Stress
 AAT and, 465
 adaptability and, 42
 advance directives and, 393–394
 in amputation, 287–300, 312–313
 cancer and, 364, 367
 cardiac rehabilitation and, 336
 in CKD, 362–363
 education of clients and, 176, 196
 neurological disorders and, 351
 in older adults, 208, 445–448
 in polytrauma, 318, 320–322, 324, 324t, 325, 327–328
 pulmonary rehabilitation and, 340, 342
 in SCI, 280, 281
 skin integrity and, 101
 in TBI, 258
 in terminally ill patients, 368–369
 transient incontinence and, 123, 124t
Psychologists
 amputation and, 300, 300t
 as interdisciplinary team members, 53–54f, 55
 polytrauma and, 327–328
Psychomotor domain, 196
Psychosocial issues. *See also* Biopsychosocial frameworks for
 chronic illness/disability; Caring, art of; Psychological
 well-being; Social frameworks for chronic illness/disability
 in CLD, 430
 in development/aging, 419, 439–441, 439b
 in muscular dystrophy, 428
 in pediatric nursing, 431–432
 in polytrauma, 320–322, 324, 324t
 psychosocial frameworks for chronic illness/disability, 29–
  30, 32–33, 34b, 36, 41, 43–44
 psychosocial learning models/theories, 182–185, 183f, 184–
  185b, 184t
 in stroke, 233–234, 234–235t
 in TBI, 263, 264t
Psychostimulants, 233, 234t
PTA. *See* Posttraumatic amnesia
Ptosis, 346, 346f, 351
PTs. *See* Physical therapists (PTs) and therapy
PTSD. *See* Posttraumatic stress disorder
PUFAs (polyunsaturated fatty acids), 85
Pulmonary disease/complications, 338–343. *See also* Breathing
 problems
 aging and, 441
 asthma, 339t, 341
 chronic obstructive pulmonary disease, 339t, 340–341
 cystic fibrosis, 339t, 341
 education of family/client, 340, 341–342
 ethical issues, 342
 lung cancer, 339t, 341–342
 nursing competencies, 342
 nursing interventions, 341–342
 outcome evaluation, 344, 346

 in polytrauma, 319, 319t
 pulmonary rehabilitation, 339–340
 risk factors, 338, 340
 in SCI, 277
 of stroke, 237–239, 239t
 symptoms/consequences of, 338–339, 339t, 340–341
 of TBI, 258–259, 263, 263t
Pulmonary embolism (PE), 236, 292
Pure motor stroke syndrome, 218, 220t
Pure sensory stroke syndrome, 218, 220t
Purpose in life, 205–206
Pylons, 306–307

Q

Quadriplegia. *See* Tetraplegia
Quality measures, 412
Quality of care, 412–414. *See also* Competencies, certification,
 and education
Quality of life. *See also* Outcome evaluation (management,
 measurement, research); *specific disabilities/diseases*
 AAT and. *See* Animal-assisted therapy
 adaptation and, 39, 42
 life care planning and, 472
 medical model and, 31
 prevention and, 179
 principles of rehabilitation and, 6
 promotion of optimal, 16–17
 restoring, as goal of rehabilitation, 2, 2t
 Rusk on, 4
 spirituality and, 204–205, 206
Quinlan case, 390

R

Race and racial issues. *See also* Cultural issues
 in cardiac disease, 332
 in CKD, 361, 363
 in coping, 37, 203, 205
 diversity in the U.S., 374–375
 health disparities and, 415
 in SCI, 270
 in stroke, 216, 218t
Rancho Los Amigos scale of cognitive recovery, 150b, 156, 156t,
 259–261, 260–261t, 264–265
Range of motion (ROM), 137, 241, 293–295
Reasonable accommodations, 398
Reauthoring the self, 40
Recall. *See* Memory
Receptors, immune, 345
Recognition, 155
Reconfiguring the future, 44, 44f
Reconstruction of meaning, 39, 40, 44, 44f. *See also* Adaptation
Records. *See* Documentation
Recovery. *See* Adaptation; Function, promoting; Outcome
 evaluation (management, measurement, research)
Reeducation. *See* Education of clients and families
Reentry. *See* Community reintegration/reentry
Reflexic bladder, 125, 276
Reflexic bowel, 131t, 132, 274–275
Reflexogenic erections, 281

Reflux (bladder), 125, 125f, 128
Rehabilitation Act (1973), 4, 396–398, 397t
Rehabilitation, defined, 1, 2, 2t
Rehabilitation delivery system, 378
Rehabilitation facilities. See Settings for care
Rehabilitation Learning Readiness Assessment Guide (RLRAG), 190, 190t
Rehabilitation nursing, defined, 1, 9–10, 9t. See also Nursing roles
Rehabilitation Nursing Foundation, 76
Reimbursement. See Payment systems
Reintegration. See Community reintegration/reentry
Relationships. See Caring, art of; Communication; Family; Interdisciplinary teams; Sexuality and disability; Social issues
Religious spirituality, defined, 201. See also Spirituality
Remote memory, 154
Renal problems. See Kidneys
Reproduction. See Sexuality and disability
Researcher nursing role, 76–77. See also Evidence-based practice
Residential animals, 461. See also Animal-assisted therapy
Residual limb, 301
Resilience, 34, 35, 42, 381. See also Adaptation
Resource accessibility. See Accessibility of resources/opportunities
Resource utilization groups, 410
Respiratory problems. See Pulmonary disease/complications
Responsibilities. See Nursing roles
Responsiveness. See Consciousness
Restlessness, 156–157
Restorying a life, 40
Restraints, 144–145, 449
Restructuring. See Adaptation
Retrieval of memories, 180, 180f, 189–190
Rheumatoid arthritis, 289
Rights, patient. See Ethical considerations
Rigid dressings, 301–302
Rigidity, muscle. See Spasticity; Tremors
Risk factors. See also Complications; specific disabilities/diseases; specific risk factors
    for falls, 138–139, 139t, 145, 223–224
    health literacy and, 178–179
    older adults and, 69
    skin integrity and, 101, 102–103, 103t, 104, 108, 108t
Ritalin (methylphenidate), 354, 354t
RLRAG (Rehabilitation Learning Readiness Assessment Guide), 190, 190t
Roles of healthcare practitioners. See Interdisciplinary teams; Nursing roles
ROM. See Range of motion
Romantic relationships. See Sexuality and disability
Roy's Adaptation Model, 202

S
Safety. See also Falls
    education and, 178–179, 196
    falls and, 224, 224t
    of mechanical debridement, 110

nurse's role in, 73, 75, 78
    in patient handling, 141, 142–145, 146
    post joint replacement, 289
    safe care, defined, 413
    sexuality in rehabilitation facilities and, 171
    TBI and, 264t, 265–266
Saline
    in bowel management, 133
    in wound treatment, 109, 110, 111, 114–115t
Saturated fats, 85
Schema (in learning), 180
SCHIP. See State children's health insurance program
Schools and disabled children, 432
SCI. See Spinal cord injuries
Scoliosis, 427
Scotomas, 352
Screening. See Assessment
SDB. See Sleep disordered breathing
Secondary appraisal, 37
Secondary complications. See Complications
Secondary injuries (brain), 256, 257
Secondary strokes, 219, 246
Sedatives, 239, 239t
Sedentary lifestyle. See Exercise; Lifestyle factors
Segregation, movement against, 17
Seizures
    poststroke, 239–240, 240t
    in TBI, 258, 259, 262–263
Selective noradrenaline reuptake inhibitors (NRIs), 233, 234t, 240
Selective serotonin reuptake inhibitors (SSRIs), 233, 234t, 240
Self-care. See also Activities of Daily Living; Independence; specific aspects of self-care
    AAT and, 465
    amputation and, 310, 310–311t
    cultural issues and, 381
    deficit, in amputation, 312
    deficit theory, 473
    as goal of rehabilitation, 2, 2t
    philosophy of rehabilitation and, 1–2
    principles of rehabilitation and, 6
    self-efficacy and, 183
    stroke and, 221
Self-efficacy, 18, 182–183, 184b, 185, 190
Self, sense of. See Body image issues; Changes with chronic illness/disability
Senescence, defined, 438
Senior citizens. See Gerontological rehabilitation
Sensory perception. See also specific sensory deficits
    aging and, 442
    brain injury and, 149, 151, 258
    falls and, 138
    polytrauma and, 319, 319t, 325
    skin integrity and, 102, 103t, 104, 108t, 276
    stroke and, 218, 224–227, 226–227t, 226f
Serotonin and noradrenaline uptake inhibitors (SNRIs), 233, 234t
Settings for care, 22–27. See also Work settings
    acute rehabilitation settings, 23

Settings for care (*cont.*)
  ARN list of, 22, 22*t*
  client-family teaching and, 25
  community settings, 23–24
  ethical considerations, 24
  evaluation of outcomes and, 24, 24*t*
  evidence-based practice and, 25
  for geriatric care, 25, 69
  long-term/subacute settings, 23, 171
  payment practices for IRFs, 5*t*, 6
  polytrauma, 321
  sexual relationships and, 168–171
75% rule, 409–410, 410*b*
Severe brain injury, 259, 323, 323*t*
Sexuality and disability, 161–175
  in children, 163–164, 164*t*
  evidence-based practice and, 163
  in independent living, 168–171, 168*b*, 169*t*, 170*f*, 171*b*
  in older adults, 164–165, 442–443
  public masturbation, dealing with, 172
  in rehabilitation facilities, 171
  SCI and, 165, 168–169, 169*t*, 280–281
  sexually explicit materials, 172–173
  sexually inappropriate behavior, 157, 171–172
  stroke and, 165, 165–166*t*, 169–170, 235–236
  TBI and, 263, 264*t*
  triphasic sexual response, 165–166, 165–166*t*
  vaginal dryness and erectile dysfunction, 166–168, 168*t*, 280–281
Shared primary language, 381–382
Shattered assumptions theory, 36
Shear and skin integrity, 102, 103*t*, 104, 108, 108*t*
Shifting perspectives model, 41–42, 42*f*
Shock, in stages of adaptation, 202
Shoes and prosthetics, 307
Shortness of breath. *See* Breathing problems
Short-term memory, 154
Shoulder
  arthroplasty, 286–287. *See also* Joints and joint replacement
  pain syndrome, 241
  subluxation, 223, 241
Shrinkers, 302
Side effects of medications
  sexual dysfunction and, 167, 168*t*
  for spasticity, 222–223
Signs and symptoms. *See specific disorders/diseases and symptoms*
Sildenafil (Viagra), 166, 167
Silver-impregnated dressing, 114, 116*t*
Silver sulfadiazine, 114, 115*t*
Skilled nursing facilities (SNFs), 23, 24, 410
Skin integrity, 100–120. *See also* Pressure ulcers; Wounds
  aging and, 442
  amputation and, 301, 302
  anatomy and physiology of skin, 101–104, 102–103*f*, 103*t*
  assessment, 104–107, 106–107*t*
  education, 117
  general wound care, 108–111, 111*b*

pain management, 116–117
  prevention, 108, 108*t*
  at risk populations, 101
  SCI and, 276–277
  spina bifida and, 425
  TBI and, 259
  treatment modalities, 111–116, 112–116*t*
Skull fracture, 258. *See also* Traumatic brain injury
Sleep disordered breathing (SDB), 238–239, 239*t*
Sleep-wake disorders (SWDs), 238–239, 239*t*
Sliding board transfer, 142
Slings for shoulder subluxation, 223, 241
SLPs. *See* Speech-language pathologists
Smoking and tobacco use
  amputation healing and, 304
  cancer and, 364
  cardiovascular disease and stroke and, 89, 218*t*, 219, 246, 335, 335*t*
  chronic disease and, 17, 179
  CKD and, 361
  health of older adults and, 19
  pressure ulcer risk and, 102
  pulmonary disease and, 338, 339, 340
  sexual dysfunction and, 162, 167
SNFs. *See* Skilled nursing facilities
SNRIs (serotonin and noradrenaline uptake inhibitors), 233, 234*t*
Social frameworks for chronic illness/disability, 16–17, 29–30, 31–32, 31*f*, 32*b*. *See also* Biopsychosocial frameworks for chronic illness/disability; Psychosocial issues
Social issues. *See also* Cultural issues; Environmental factors; Family; Social frameworks for chronic illness/disability
  adaptation and, 39, 41, 42–43
  aging population issues, 18–19, 441
  in aging theories, 439*b*, 440
  appraisal and, 37
  cancer and, 364
  changes in relationships with illness/disability, 36
  CKD and, 363
  cognitive impairments and, 157
  coping and, 202, 203, 206
  health belief model and, 182, 183*f*
  health literacy and, 178
  holistic approaches and, 8
  life care planning and, 473
  mobility/function and, 138
  social adaptability, 42–43
  social construction model (U.S.), 31–32
  social model (U.K.), 16–17, 31–32, 31*f*
  societal changes, 385
Social Security Act (1935, 1965), 408, 419
Social workers
  amputation and, 300, 300*t*
  as interdisciplinary team members, 53–54*f*, 55, 57*t*
  joint replacement and, 289
Society of Pediatric Nurses, 68, 83
Socioeconomic factors. *See* Financial issues; Social issues
Socks, prosthetic, 306, 306*f*

Soft tissue injury. *See* Pressure ulcers
Somatic pain, 117
Somatosensation, defined, 150*b*, 151
Somnolent state, 149, 150*b*
Sorrow. *See* Grief and grieving
Spasticity
    in CP, 421–422
    in neurological disorders, 352, 353–354, 353*t*
    in SCI, 272, 277–278
    sexual issues and, 169
    skin integrity and, 102, 103*t*
    in stroke, 222–223, 222*b*
Spastic neurogenic bladder, 125
Speech and language impairments. *See also* Aphasias; Apraxia
    cognition and, 148–149, 150*b*, 151–154, 153*t*, 158
    myasthenia gravis and, 346
    in neurological disorders, 354, 356*t*
    sexual relationships and, 170–171, 171*b*
    in stroke, 218, 229–232, 230–231*t*, 242–243
    in TBI, 259, 263, 264*t*
Speech-language pathologists (SLPs)
    cleft lip/palate and, 429
    in communicating with patients, 158
    diagnosis of disorders, 152, 231, 237
    hemispatial inattention and, 151–152
    as interdisciplinary team members, 54*f*, 55, 56*t*
    oral nutrition and, 90, 93, 96
    sexual issues and, 162
    in treating stroke patients, 242–243
Sphincterotomy, 276
Sphincters, urinary tract, 122. *See also* Bladder management
Spina bifida, 131*t*, 132, 423–425, 444
Spinal cord injuries (SCI), 269–286. *See also* Hemiplegia;
      Neurological conditions; Paraplegia; Tetraplegia
    acute phase of, 271, 271*f*
    aging with, 282, 444
    anatomy/physiology of, 270–271, 270*f*
    assessment, 271, 274, 285–286
    autonomic dysreflexia, 278
    bladder dysfunction and, 124, 125, 127, 128–130, 275–276,
      276*b*
    bowel dysfunction and, 130–131, 131*t*, 132, 133, 274–275,
      275*b*
    caregiver roles, 281–282
    coping strategies, 203, 206
    epidemiology/incidence of, 269–270, 269*f*
    functional outcomes, 272–273
    hemiparesis, 221
    heterotopic ossification, 278
    history of rehabilitation and, 3, 6
    incomplete syndromes, 273–274
    level of injury, 271–273
    life care planning and, 475
    nutritional needs, 90, 90*b*
    orthostasis, 278–279
    pain management, 208, 279–280
    in polytrauma, 319, 319*t*
    pressure ulcers and, 101

    psychological issues and, 281
    research and trends, 282–283
    respiration and, 277, 277*f*
    sexual issues and, 165, 168–169, 169*t*, 280–281
    skin integrity and, 276–277
    spasticity and, 277–278
    thermoregulation, 279
Spinal Cord Lesion Coping Strategies Questionnaire, 203
Spinal Cord Lesion Emotional Wellbeing Questionnaire, 203
Spinal shock, 271
Spirituality. *See also* Cultural issues
    coping and, 203
    definitions of, 201–202
    IDTs and, 206–207
    meaning, purpose, and significance, 200–201, 205–206, 210
    nutrition and religious beliefs, 97
    outcomes and, 204–205
    spiritual blessing concept, 380
    spiritual care, 201–202, 207–209, 207*b*, 207*t*
    spiritual distress, 210
    terminal illness and, 368–369
Splinting, 222, 223, 241
Sponge dressings, 111, 113*t*
Sports, adaptive, 248
Squat pivot transfer, 142
SSEEO (Stroke Survivors Empowering Each Other), 244, 245*t*
SSRIs (selective serotonin reuptake inhibitors), 233, 234*t*, 240
Staff animals, 461, 464*b*
Stage models, 39
Staging pressure ulcers, 105, 106–107*t*
Stakeholders, 25, 387, 412, 413*t*
Standards and Scope of Rehabilitation Nursing Practice (ARN),
    64, 69
Standards of practice. *See* Competencies, certification, and
    education; Evidence-based practice
Stand pivot transfer, 142
State children's health insurance program (SCHIP), 6, 404, 411
Static balance, 138
Statistics on incidence. *See* Epidemiology and mortality statistics
Stem cell therapy, 282, 399
Steroids, 271, 353, 427, 428
Stimulants
    antidepressant, 233, 234*t*
    for bowel management, 133
    central nervous system, 358, 358*t*
    for sleep disorders, 239
Stochastic forces in aging, 442
Stomas, 127
Stool impaction, 123, 124*t*, 129. *See also* Bowel management
Stool softeners, 133
Stories. *See* Narrative
Strength training in joint replacement, 290–291
Stress. *See also* Posttraumatic stress disorder
    appraisal of chronic illness/disability and, 37
    incontinence, 123
    learning abilities and, 177
    neurological disorders and, 351, 354, 355
    SCI pain and, 280

Stretching poststroke, 222, 223
Stroke, 215–254
    bladder management and, 124, 126, 232
    bowel management and, 131, 131t, 133, 232
    caregiver issues, 232, 235
    cognition and, 151, 227–229, 228t, 229f, 243
    defined, 216
    education on, 243–246, 244b, 245t, 247t
    grief of patients and family members, 8
    history of rehabilitation and, 3, 6
    impact of, 216
    language/communication deficits, 229–232, 230–231t,
        242–243
    medical complications poststroke, 236–241, 239–241t
    models of recovery/transition, 43–44, 44f, 44t
    musculoskeletal and motor deficits, 221–224, 222b, 224t,
        241–242
    neuroplasticity, 219–220
    nutritional needs, 89, 90, 233
    outcome evaluation/predictors, 24, 220–221
    psychosocial issues, 233–234, 234–235t
    rehabilitation, 241–248, 244b, 245t, 247t
    risk factors, 217–218, 218t, 219
    secondary strokes, 219, 246
    sensory perception deficits, 224–227, 226–227t, 226f
    sexual issues and, 165, 165–166t, 169–170, 235–236
    syndromes, 218–219, 218–220t
    types of, 216–217
    warning signs of, 217, 218
Stroke Family Caregiving for African Americans, 244, 245t
Stroke Survivors Empowering Each Other (SSEEO), 244, 245t
Structure measures, 412
Stuporous state, 149, 150b
Subacute rehabilitation, 23
Subarachnoid hemorrhage, 217, 258
Subcultures, 381, 383
Subdural hematoma, 258
Subluxation, shoulder, 223, 241
Substance abuse, 217, 218t, 246. *See also* Alcohol consumption;
    Smoking and tobacco use
Suction socket, 306
Sunrise Enabler, Leininger's, 377, 377f
Supplements, nutritional, 87, 95, 133, 133t, 378, 379t. *See also*
    Enteral nutrition; Parenteral nutrition
Support networks. *See* Family; Social issues; Spirituality
Suppositories, 131, 131t, 132, 133–134, 274–275
Suprapubic catheters, 127
Suprapubic triggers, 125
Suprasacral neurogenic bladder, 125
Surgery. *See also* Amputation
    for bladder problems, 127
    for cardiac disease, 334
    for cleft lip/palate, 429
    for closure of pressure ulcers, 116, 276–277
    for CPSP, 240–241
    joint replacement, 290–291
    nutrition and, 91
    for SCI, 271

    for spina bifida, 423, 424
        surgical debridement, 109–110
Swallowing problems. *See* Dysphagia
SWDs. *See* Sleep-wake disorders
Swelling. *See* Edema
Symmetrel (amantadine), 354, 354t
Symptoms. *See specific disorders/diseases and symptoms*
Syndromes, stroke, 218–219, 218–220t
Synergy, 221
Synovial joint/membrane, 284
Syrinx, 424

T
Tactile impairment, 226–227, 227t. *See also* Sensory
    perception
Tadalafil (Cialis), 167
Taft-Hartley Act (1947), 405
Tax Equity and Fiscal Responsibility Act (TEFRA 1983), 409
TBI. *See* Traumatic brain injury
Teaching. *See* Competencies, certification, and education;
    Education of clients and families
Team approach. *See* Interdisciplinary teams
Team competence, 58–59
Technology. *See also* Equipment
    healthcare, 414–415
    use in teaching, 191–192, 191b, 193–195b
Teens. *See* Pediatric rehabilitation
TEFRA (Tax Equity and Fiscal Responsibility Act of 1983), 409
Tegretol. *See* Carbamazepine
Temperature. *See* Body temperature regulation
Temporal dimension of adaptation, 43
Temporal lobe, 256, 256f, 257t
TENS. *See* Transcutaneous Electrical Nerve Stimulation
Terminal illness, 367–370, 368–369t, 369b. *See also* End-of-life
    decisions
Testing. *See* Assessment
Tethered cord, 424
Tetraplegia
    bowel dysfunction and, 131t, 132
    defined, 272
    incidence of, 270
    nutrition and, 88, 90
    sexuality issues and, 169
Thalamic pain. *See* Central poststroke pain syndrome
Thalamus, 256, 257t
Theory, defined, 29. *See also* Frameworks for chronic illness,
    disability, adaptation, and coping; *specific theories/models*
Therapeutic recreation (TR), 55, 56t
Therapeutic riding, 462–463, 462f
Therapeutic use of self, 207
Therapy/therapists. *See specific kinds of therapy/therapists*
Thermoregulation. *See* Body temperature regulation
Thinking. *See* Cognition and behavior
Third-party payers. *See* Payment systems
Thompson Model of Care Congruence, 383, 383f
Thrombotic stroke, 216–217, 236. *See also* Stroke
Thrombus, defined, 216
Tilt tables, 279

Time and memory, 154
Tiredness. *See* Fatigue
Tissue injury. *See* Pressure ulcers
Tizanidine (Zanaflex), 223, 279, 353, 353t
Tobacco use. *See* Smoking and tobacco use
Toileting. *See* Bladder management; Bowel management
Topical treatment
  in amputation, 301–302
  in wound care, 110, 111–114, 112–116t
Total join replacement. *See* Joints and joint replacement
TR. *See* Therapeutic recreation
Tracheostomy tubes, 237–238
Trail Making test, 229, 229f
Transcortical motor aphasia, 229, 230t
Transcortical sensory aphasia, 229, 230t, 243
Transcultural care decisions and actions, 376. *See also*
    Leininger
Transcutaneous Electrical Nerve Stimulation (TENS), 279–280,
    304
Transdisciplinary model, 54–55, 54f
Transfemoral amputation, 303
Transferrin, 89, 89b
Transfers
  assessment of in patient, 138
  in joint replacement, 289, 290f
  safety during, 141, 142–145
  types of, 142
Transformational model of change, 184–185, 184t
Transhumeral amputation, 308
Transient incontinence, 122–123, 123–124t. *See also* Bladder
    management
Transient ischemic attacks, 219
Transition in chronic illness model, 43
Transition theory, 36, 41
Transparent film dressings, 111, 112t
Transradial amputations, 308
Transtibial amputation, 301
Transurethral sphincterotomy, 127
Trauma. *See also* Polytrauma; *specific kinds of traumatic injury*
  amputation and, 297, 299, 308
  bowel dysfunction and, 131t, 132
  nutrition and, 91
Traumatic brain injury (TBI), 255–268. *See also* Head injury
  aging with, 444
  anatomy, 256, 256f, 257t
  assessment/classification, 259–262, 259–264t, 260b, 262b,
    323, 323t
  bladder dysfunction and, 124
  bowel dysfunction and, 131, 131t
  cognitive impairments and, 149, 156–157, 156t. *See also*
    Cognition and behavior
  common effects of, 258–259
  education of patients/families, 265–266
  epidemiology, 255–256
  flat affect and, 157
  medical interventions, 262–263
  nursing strategies, 263–265, 263–265t, 264b
  nutrition and, 91

pathophysiology, 256–258
polytrauma and, 317–319, 322–323, 322b
Treatment. *See specific disabilities/diseases*
Tremors, 347, 349, 352, 353, 355–356t. *See also* Spasticity
Triglycerides, 85–86
Triphasic sexual response, 165–166, 165–166t
Tube feeding. *See* Feeding tubes
Tumors. *See also* Cancer
  bladder dysfunction and, 124, 125
  bowel dysfunction and, 131, 131t, 132

U
Ulcers. *See* Pressure ulcers; Skin integrity
UMNs. *See* Upper motor neurons (UMNs)
Unconscious state, 149, 150b. *See also* Cognition and behavior
Undernutrition, 87
Uninhibited bladder, 124–125
Uninhibited bowel, 131, 131t
Union of Physically Impaired Against Segregation, 17
University of Iowa Gerontological Nursing Intervention
    Research Center, 69
Upper motor neurons (UMNs), 271–273, 274, 348
Urecholine (bethanechol), 128
Urethra, 122, 122f
Urge incontinence, 123, 232
Urinary tract. *See* Bladder management
Urinary tract infection (UTI), 126–127, 128, 129, 171
U.S. Army Wounded Warrior Program (AW2), 328
U.S. Census Bureau, 14–15
U.S. Department of Agriculture Food Guide Pyramid, 98
U.S. Department of Health and Human Services, 14, 16, 20b,
    59, 178
UTI. *See* Urinary tract infection

V
VA. *See* Veterans Administration (VA) and Veterans Health
    Administration (VHA)
Vaccination and neurological disorders, 346, 350
Vaginal dryness, 162, 166–168, 168t, 281, 443
Valium (diazepam), 128, 353, 353t
Valproic acid (Depakene/Depakote), 240, 240t
Valsalva maneuver, 125, 127, 128, 132
Values. *See* Beliefs
Vardenafil (Levitra), 167
Venous thromboembolism, 236
Veracity principle, 387
Verbal impairments. *See* Speech and language impairments
Vesicoureteral reflux, 125, 125f
Veterans Administration (VA) and Veterans Health
    Administration (VHA), 3, 4–5t, 143, 317–321, 327, 410, 475
Veterans and war
  amputation and, 299, 308
  history of rehabilitation and, 3–4, 4–5t, 6, 17, 52
  Paralyzed Veterans of America, 130, 130b
  polytrauma and. *See* Polytrauma
  TBI statistics, 323
Veterinarians and animal therapy, 465. *See also* Animal-
    assisted therapy

VHA. *See* Veterans Administration (VA) and Veterans Health Administration (VHA)
Viagra (sildenafil), 166, 167
Videofluoroscopic swallow study, 233, 237
Videofluoroscopy, 93
Virchow's triad, 292
Visceral pain, 116–117
Visual impairment
    aging and, 442
    in neurological disorders, 346, 352, 355*t*
    in polytrauma, 319, 319*t*, 325
    in stroke, 218, 224–225, 226–227, 227*t*
Vitamins, 85–86, 86*t*, 90, 91, 95, 101
Vocational rehabilitation
    poststroke, 246
    services for, 55, 57*t*
    TBI and, 263, 264*t*
Vocational Rehabilitation Act (1943), 3, 4, 4*t*

W
Walking transfer, 142
Wallenberg syndrome, 218, 220*t*
War. *See* Veterans and war
Warfarin. *See* Coumadin
Warning signs. *See* Risk factors
Wars of disabilities, 318. *See also* Veterans and war
Water. *See* Fluids
Water-soluble vitamins, 86, 86*t*
Watson's Caring Theory, 202, 211
Ways of Coping Questionnaire, 37
WBAT (weight bearing as tolerated), 289
Weber syndrome, 218, 220*t*
WeeFIM scale, 137
Weight bearing as tolerated (WBAT), 289
Weight management. *See* Obesity and weight management
Well-being
    AAT and. *See* Animal-assisted therapy
    adaptation and, 38–39, 41–42, 44
    coping strategies and, 38, 38*b*
    as goal of rehabilitation, 2, 2*t*
    illness and concept of, 29
    promotion of, 16–17, 69, 445, 445–447*t*, 473. *See also* Education of clients and families
Wernicke's aphasia, 229, 230*t*, 243
Western societies
    adaptation and, 40
    chronic illness in, 29
    coping strategies in, 37
    medical model of, 30

Wheelchair sports teams, 382
White populations
    amputation in, 297
    cardiac disease in, 332
    coping strategies, 203
    SCI in, 270
    stroke in, 216
WHO. *See* World Health Organization
Whole person. *See* Holistic care
Women. *See* Gender and gender issues
Women to women conceptual model, 18
Work and disability. *See* Vocational rehabilitation
Workers' compensation, 405
Working memory, 154, 179, 181, 196
Work settings. *See also* Settings for care
    advanced practice nurses, 78
    case managers, 71
    direct care providers, 64
    geriatric nurses, 69
    liaison nurses, 66
    managers/administrators, 73
    nurse educators, 74–75
    pediatric nurses, 68
    researchers, 76–77
World Health Organization (WHO)
    on aging, 18
    ICF, 34–35, 35*f*, 40, 42
    on terminal illness, 367
Worldview. *See* Beliefs; Spirituality
Wound Care Education Institute, 117
Wound gel dressings, 111, 114*t*
Wound, Ostomy and Continence Nurses Society, 105, 117
Wounds. *See also* Pressure ulcers
    amputation, 302
    care and treatment of, 108–116, 111*b*, 112–116*t*
    healing stages of, 101, 103–104, 105, 106–107*t*
    pain management, 116–117
    polytrauma, 325, 326

Y
Youth with special healthcare needs, 432–433. *See also* Pediatric rehabilitation

Z
Zanaflex. *See* Tizanidine
Zoonotic diseases, 465–469, 466–467*t*

—